Diseases of the Gallbladder and Bile Ducts

Diseases of the Gallbladder and Bile Ducts

Diagnosis and Treatment

Edited by

Pierre-Alain Clavien, MD, PhD, FACS
Professor and Chairman
Department of Visceral and Transplant Surgery
University of Zurich
Zurich, Switzerland

John Baillie, MD, ChB, FRCP
Associate Professor
Division of Gastroenterology
Department of Medicine
Duke University
Durham, North Carolina

Consulting Editor: *Paul V. Suhocki, MD, Duke University Medical Center*
Assistant to the Editors: *Jaye M. Danko, Duke University Medical Center*

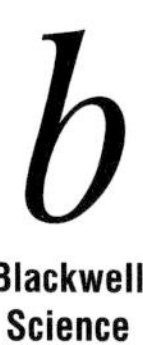

Blackwell
Science

Editorial Offices:

Commerce Place, 350 Main Street, Malden, Massachusetts 02148, USA
Osney Mead, Oxford OX2 0EL, England
25 John Street, London WC1N 2BL, England
23 Ainslie Place, Edinburgh EH3 6AJ, Scotland
54 University Street, Carlton, Victoria 3053, Australia

Other Editorial Offices:

Blackwell Wissenschafts-Verlag GmbH, Kurfürstendamm 57, 10707 Berlin, Germany
Blackwell Science KK, MG Kodenmacho Building, 7-10 Kodenmacho Nihombashi, Chuo-ku, Tokyo 104, Japan
Iowa State University Press, A Blackwell Science Company, 2121 S. State Avenue, Ames, Iowa 50014-8300, USA

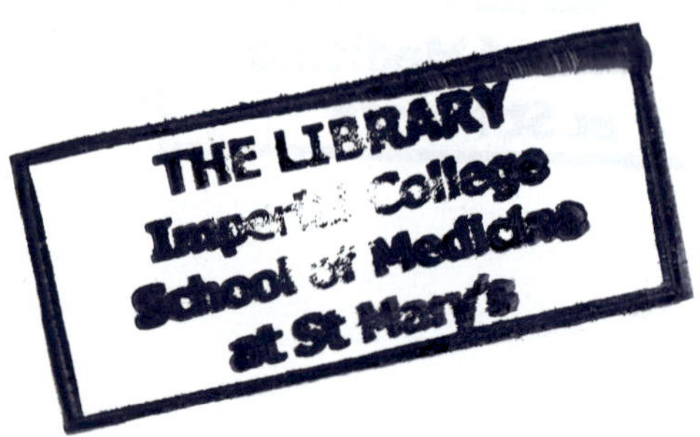

Distributors:
USA
Blackwell Science, Inc.
Commerce Place
350 Main Street
Malden, Massachusetts 02148
(Telephone orders: 800-215-1000 or 781-388-8250; fax orders: 781-388-8270)

Canada
Login Brothers Book Company
324 Saulteaux Crescent
Winnipeg, Manitoba R3J 3T2
(Telephone orders: 204-837-2987)

Australia
Blackwell Science Pty, Ltd.
54 University Street
Carlton, Victoria 3053
(Telephone orders: 03-9347-0300; fax orders: 03-9349-3016)

Outside North America and Australia
Blackwell Science, Ltd.
c/o Marston Book Services, Ltd.
P.O. Box 269
Abingdon
Oxon OX14 4YN
England
(Telephone orders: 44-01235-465500; fax orders: 44-01235-465555)

Acquisitions: Laura DeYoung
Development: Laura Woollett
Production: Irene Herlihy
Manufacturing: Lisa Flanagan
Marketing Manager: Toni Fournier
Cover design by Meral Dabcovich, VisPer

Typeset by Best-set Typesetter Ltd., Hong Kong
Printed and bound by Sheridan Books/Ann Arbor

Printed in the United States of America
01 02 03 04 5 4 3 2 1

To our mentors, to whom we are profoundly indebted for their inspired teaching, long-standing support, and advice during our careers

(PAC): Felix Harder, Adrien Rohner, Bernie Langer, and Steve Strasberg

(JB): Jack Vennes

Contents

Contributors

Bilal O. Al-Jiffry, MD
Department of General & Digestive Surgery
Flinders Medical Center
Bedford Park, Adelaide, SA
Australia

Mitchell S. Anscher, MD
Department of Radiation Oncology
Duke University Medical Center
Durham, North Carolina

John Baillie, MB, ChB, FRCP
Division of Gastroenterology, Department of Medicine
Duke University Medical Center
Durham, North Carolina

Malcolm M. Bilimoria, MD
Department of Surgical Oncology
The University of Texas
MD–Anderson Cancer Center
Houston, Texas

Rachel H. Chou, MD
Department of Radiation Oncology
Duke University Medical Center
Durham, North Carolina

Lisa A. Clark, MD
Division of General Surgery
Duke University Medical Center
Durham, North Carolina

Pierre-Alain Clavien, MD, PhD, FACS
Department of Visceral and Transplant Surgery
University Hospital Zurich
Zurich, Switzerland;
Division of Hepatobiliary Surgery and Transplantation
Department of Surgery
Duke University Medical Center
Durham, North Carolina

Christopher H. Crane, MD
Department of Radiation Oncology
The University of Texas
MD–Anderson Cancer Center
Houston, Texas

Robert Enns, MD, FRCP
Division of Gastroenterology
Department of Medicine
St. Paul's Hospital
University of British Columbia
Vancouver, British Columbia
Canada

Steve Eubanks, MD
Division of General and Thoracic Surgery
Duke University Medical Center
Durham, North Carolina

Alex Gandsas, MD
Division of General and Thoracic Surgery
Duke University Medical Center
Durham, North Carolina

Henning Gerke, MD
Division of Gastroenterology
Johannes-Gutenberg University
Mainz, Germany

E. Jenny Heathcote, MBBS, MD
University of Toronto
Toronto Western Hospital
Toronto, Ontario
Canada

Neil Kaplowitz, MD
USC Research Center for Liver Diseases
Division of Gastrointestinal and Liver Diseases
Keck School of Medicine
University of Southern California
Los Angeles, California

Catherine G. Lee, MD
Department of Radiation Oncology
Duke University Medical Center
Durham, North Carolina

Joseph W. Leung, MD, FRCP, FACP, FACG
Chief, Gastroenterology
University of California UC Davis Medical Center
Sacramento, California

Kevin McGrath, MD
Division of Gastroenterology, Department of Medicine
Duke University Medical Center
Durham, North Carolina

Klaus Mergener, MD
Division of Gastroenterology
Johannes-Gutenberg University
Mainz, Germany

Michael A. Morse, MD
Department of Medicine
Duke University Medical Center
Durham, North Carolina

Rendon C. Nelson, MD
Director, Abdominal Imaging
Department of Radiology
Duke University Medical Center
Durham, North Carolina

Theodore N. Pappas, MD
Division of General Surgery
Duke University Medical Center
Durham, North Carolina

C. Wright Pinson, MD, MBA
Division of Hepatobiliary Surgery and Liver Transplantation
Department of Surgery
Vanderbilt University Medical Center
Nashville, Tennessee

Robert J. Porte, MD, PhD
Division of Hepatobiliary Surgery and Liver Transplantation
Department of Surgery
University Hospital, Groningen
Groningen, The Netherlands

Hannes A. Rüdiger, MD
Department of Visceral and Transplant Surgery
University Hospital Zurich
Zurich, Switzerland;
Division of Hepatobiliary Surgery and Transplantation
Department of Surgery
Duke University Medical Center
Durham, North Carolina

Markus Selzner, MD
Department of Visceral and Transplant Surgery
University Hospital Zurich
Zurich, Switzerland;
Division of Hepatobiliary Surgery and Transplantation
Department of Surgery
Duke University Medical Center
Durham, North Carolina

Michael A. Skinner, MD
Chief, Division of Pediatric Surgery
Associate Professor of Surgery
Duke Children's Hospital
Durham, North Carolina

Andrew Stolz, MD
USC Research Center for Liver Diseases
Division of Gastrointestinal and Liver Diseases
Keck School of Medicine
University of Southern California
Los Angeles, California

Steven M. Strasberg, MD
Head of Section of Hepatobiliary-Pancreatic Surgery
Washington University School of Medicine
St. Louis, Missouri

Paul V. Suhocki, MD
Division of Interventional Radiology
Department of Radiology
Duke University Medical Center
Durham, North Carolina

James Toouli, MBBS, PhD, FRACS
Flinders Medical Center
Department of General & Digestive Surgery
Bedford Park, Adelaide, SA
Australia

William R. Treem, MD
Chief, Division of Pediatric Gastroenterology, Nutrition, and Hepatology
Duke Children's Hospital
Durham, North Carolina

Jean-Nicolas Vauthey, MD, FACS
Liver Service
Department of Surgical Oncology
The University of Texas
MD–Anderson Cancer Center
Houston, Texas

Kay Washington, MD, PhD
Department of Pathology
Vanderbilt University Medical Center
Nashville, Tennessee

Paul E. Wise, MD
Division of Hepatobiliary Surgery and Liver Transplantation
Department of Surgery
Vanderbilt University Medical Center
Nashville, Tennessee

Kenneth A. Wong, MD
Department of Radiology
Duke University Medical Center
Durham, North Carolina

Andy S. Yu, MD
Division of Gastroenterology and Hepatology
Stanford University Medical Center
Stanford, California

Preface

Diseases of the gallbladder and bile ducts are common and major focuses in gastroenterology, oncology, radiology, nuclear medicine, and surgery. This past decade has brought numerous new diagnostic and therapeutic modalities ranging from mini-invasive procedures such as endoscopic or laparoscopic procedures to new techniques of liver transplantation. Major advances have also been made in the understanding of the pathogenesis of a variety of conditions and the natural history of previously unclear entities. While this has led to better "evidence-based" treatments of patients, the proliferation of new diagnostic and therapeutic tools has also lead to confusion about which therapy to select for particular situations. The modern treatment of biliary diseases should be approached through a multidisciplinary team having special interest in this field. In addition, a number of innovative approaches are still experimental and often technically demanding, so that complex biliary problems should be managed in centers with experience in treating these patients and a strong commitment to research.

To this end, *Diseases of the Gallbladder and Bile Ducts: Diagnosis and Treatment* is intended to provide a comprehensive and critical approach to established and new diagnostic and therapeutic modalities. The book was written by a multidisciplinary panel of international experts with extensive experience in this population of patients. Each chapter was reviewed by the Editors and at least one external reviewer to achieve the comprehensive and balanced coverage of each topic, to avoid redundancy among chapters, and to provide appropriate cross-references. While each chapter can be read separately, the book was written with the intent that chapters can be read sequentially.

The book is designed to serve the need of all those involved in the management of patients with biliary diseases from medical students to specialists in various areas. The first series of chapters comprehensively covers anatomy, physiology and pathology, and imaging modalities of the biliary tree. The next six chapters present various therapeutic approaches involving medical, endoscopic, and percutaneous treatments, as well as open and laparoscopic surgery. Then, common and less common intra- and extrahepatic biliary diseases including the gallbladder are covered in separate chapters. Specific chapters are dedicated to complex problems such as laparoscopic injuries to the bile duct, cholangiocarcinoma, primary biliary cirrhosis, and diseases of the small bile ducts, and the differential diagnosis and treatment of intrahepatic cholestasis. Finally, a detailed chapter is provided regarding specific biliary disorders in the pediatric population.

We hope that *Diseases of the Gallbladder and Bile Ducts: Diagnosis and Treatment* will provide timely information and guidelines for the management of this population of patients.

P.-A.C.
J.B.

Notice: The indications and dosages of all drugs in this book have been recommended in the medical literature and conform to the practices of the general community. The medications described and treatment prescriptions suggested do not necessarily have specific approval by the Food and Drug Administration for use in the diseases and dosages for which they are recommended. The package insert for each drug should be consulted for use and dosage as approved by the FDA. Because standards for usage change, it is advisable to keep abreast of revised recommendations, particularly those concerning new drugs.

Section

1

Anatomy, Pathophysiology, and Imaging of the Biliary System

Chapter 1

Anatomy and Physiology of the Biliary Tree and Gallbladder

James Toouli Bilal O. Al-Jiffry

The biliary tract is the conduit between the liver and the duodenum and is designed to store and transport bile, under control of neuronal and hormonal regulation. Bile is formed in the hepatocytes and steadily secreted into canaliculi, which transport it to the larger extrahepatic ducts. The sphincter of Oddi regulates the flow of bile into the duodenum or to the cystic duct and the gallbladder. When stimulated, the gallbladder contracts steadily, the sphincter relaxes, and bile flow into the duodenum increases.

LIVER ANATOMY

To understand the anatomy and physiology of the biliary tract and the production of bile, it is necessary to briefly outline the anatomy of the liver. The liver is divided macroscopically into the right and left lobe by the falciform ligament anteriorly (Fig. 1.1). Inferiorly, this corresponds to the round ligament and umbilical fissure. The right lobe is further divided by the gallbladder fossa into the right hemiliver to the right of the gallbladder and the quadrate lobe to the left. The fourth lobe (caudate) is posterior and surrounds the inferior vena cava. Hence, anatomically the liver is divided into two main lobes and two accessory lobes.

With improved understanding of liver function, the concept of functional anatomy has developed. This was initiated by Cantlie in 1898 and was enhanced by McIndoe in 1929, Ton That Tung in 1939, and Couinaud in 1957. These concepts have been combined, resulting in the Brisbane 2000 terminology for liver anatomy. The liver was divided into three functional livers (1): the right, the left, and the caudate. The separation between the right and left hemiliver is at Cantlie's line, which is an oblique plane extending from the center of the gallbladder bed to the left border of the inferior vena cava. In this plane runs the middle hepatic vein, which is an important radiological landmark.

The right hemiliver is divided further into two sectors by the right portal scissura (anterior and posterior sectors), within which runs the right hepatic vein. Each sector then is divided on the basis of its blood supply and bile drainage into two segments. The anterior sector is divided into segment 5 (inferior) and segment 8 (superior) and the posterior sector into segment 6 (inferior) and segment 7 (superior) (Fig. 1.2).

The left hemiliver is divided into three segments. Segment 4 (quadrate lobe) is known as the left medial hemiliver, which lies to the right of the falciform ligament, and its right margin forms the right margin of the left hemiliver. Segment 3 lies in the anterior part, and segment 2 lies in the posterior part of the left lateral hemiliver on the left of the falciform ligament. Between segments 2 and 3 runs the left hepatic vein. The left portal scissura divides the left hemiliver into two sectors; the anteromedial sector is composed of segment 3 and segment 4, and the posterior sector is composed of segment 2. This latter classification in the left hemiliver is not surgically useful, thus the segment notation is more commonly applied (2).

The caudate hemiliver (segment 1) is considered separately because of its separate blood supply, and venous and bile drainage (1). The importance of this will be illustrated later in the chapter.

Blood Supply and Venous Drainage

The arterial supply to the liver in early gestation life is from three main sources: the left hepatic artery from the left gastric artery, the middle hepatic artery (common hepatic artery) from the celiac trunk, and the right hepatic artery

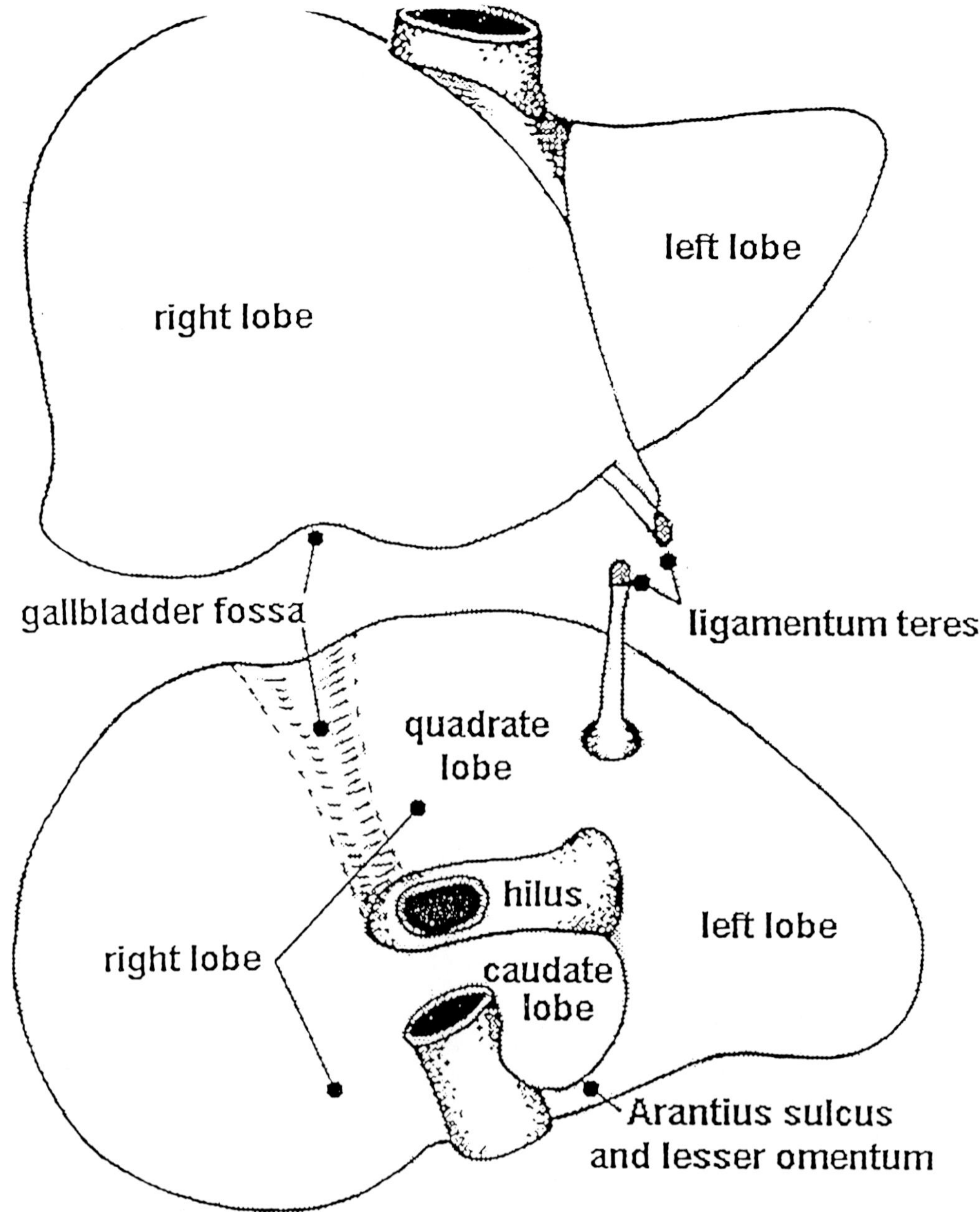

FIGURE 1.1. *The classic anatomical division of the liver into two main lobes (right and left lobes) and two accessory lobes (quadrate and caudate lobes). (Reproduced by permission from Nyhus LM, Baker RJ, Fischer JE, eds. Mastery of surgery. 3rd ed. Boston: Little, Brown, 1997.)*

from the superior mesenteric artery. With further development, the blood supply assumes the adult pattern, with atrophy of both the right and left hepatic arteries and the common hepatic artery (middle hepatic) supplying the whole liver (3). This adult pattern occurs in around 67% of individuals (4). The common hepatic artery gives the right and left hepatic arteries, which supply the right and left hemilivers, respectively. In 90% of cases, segment 4 is supplied by a named branch (middle hepatic) from either the right or left hepatic artery (45% each) (4). The other variations that occur are (5):

The common hepatic supplying the right liver and the left hepatic arising from the left gastric in 8%.

The common hepatic supplying the left liver and the right hepatic arising from the superior mesenteric artery in 11%.

Persistence of all three arteries in 3%.

Atrophy of the common hepatic artery in 12%, with the liver supplied by the

- right hepatic in 9%
- left hepatic in 1%
- both right and left in 2%

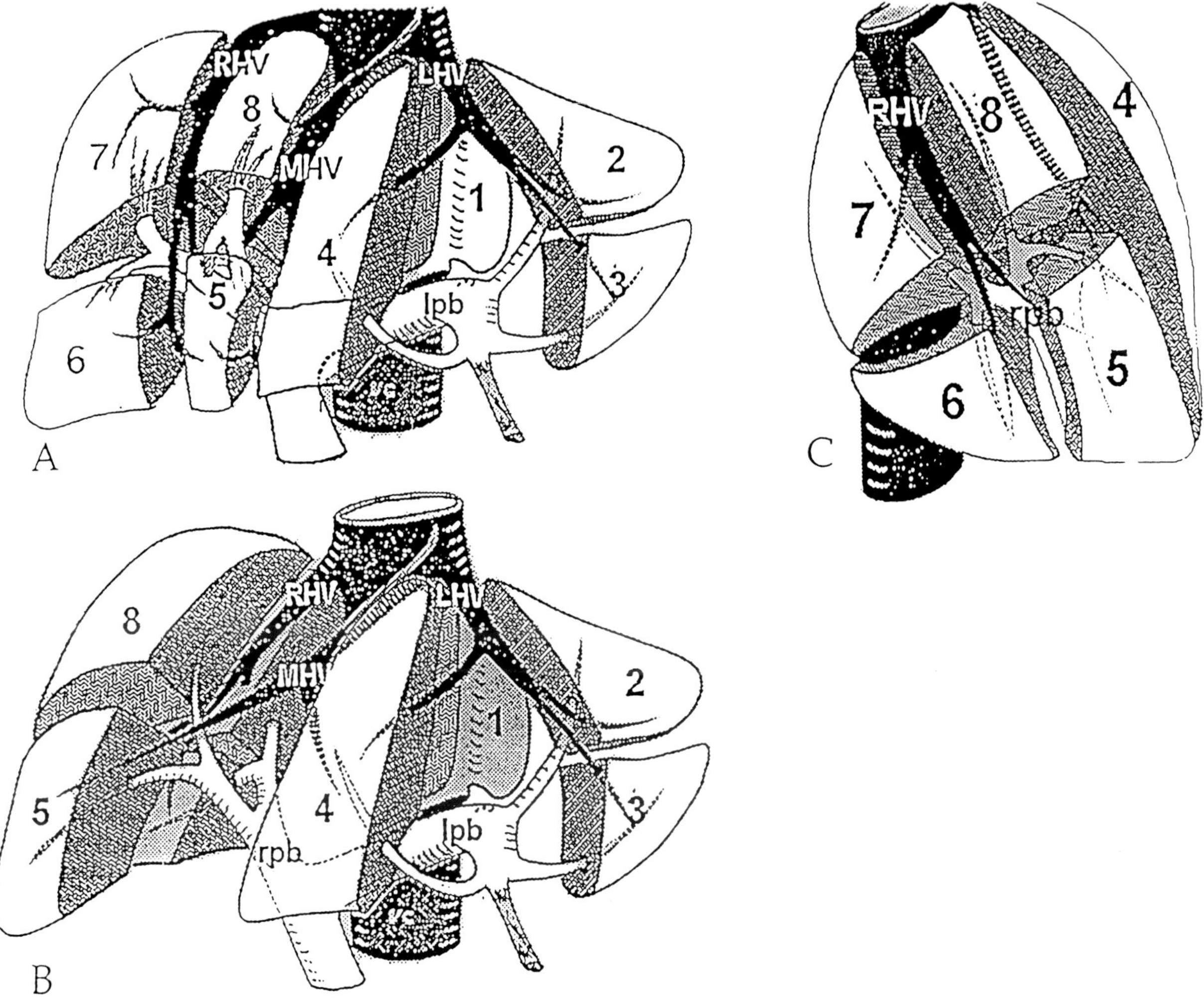

FIGURE 1.2. *The functional division of the liver using Couinaud's original drawings.* ***(A)*** *In the bench position.* ***(B)*** *The actual orientation in-patient.* ***(C)*** *The right hepatic vein dividing the right liver into the anterior sector (segments 5 and 8) and the posterior sector (segments 6 and 7). RHV, right hepatic vein; MHV, middle hepatic vein; LHV, left hepatic vein; lpb, left portal branch; rpb, right portal branch; IVC, inferior vena cava. (Reproduced by permission from Nyhus LM, Baker RJ, Fischer JE, eds. Mastery of surgery. 3rd ed. Boston: Little, Brown, 1997.)*

The left hepatic arising from the left gastric is usually easy to identify in the gastrohepatic ligament. When this artery is present, care should be taken not to damage it when performing a gastrectomy.

The right hepatic artery arising from the superior mesenteric artery, on the other hand, is more variable. It ascends behind the pancreas in relation to the portal vein, and in the portal pedicle it assumes a posterior location, usually slightly to the left of the portal vein.

The venous drainage of the liver is into the inferior vena cava through the right, middle, and left hepatic veins. The union of superior, middle, and inferior branches usually forms the right vein, where the superior is the largest branch. The right hepatic vein trunk joins at the right margin of the vena cava at a point separate and slightly above the trunk that is formed by the middle and left vein. The middle hepatic vein forms from two veins arising from segment 4 and segment 5. The middle hepatic vein joins the left hepatic vein to form a common trunk before draining into the vena cava in 90% of people. The left hepatic vein is more variable and is usually formed by the union of the branches from segment 2, segment 3, and segment 4.

Intrahepatic Bile Ducts

There are more than 2 km of bile ductules and ducts in the adult human liver. These structures are far from being inert channels, and are capable of significantly modifying biliary flow and composition in response to hormonal secretion. Bile secretion starts at the level of the bile canaliculus, the smallest branch of the biliary tree (6). They form a meshwork between hepatocytes with many anastomotic interconnections. Bile then enters the small terminal bile ductules (canals of Hering), which provide a conduit through which bile may traverse to enter the larger perilobular or interlobular bile ducts.

The interlobular bile ducts form a richly anastomosing network that closely surrounds the branches of the portal vein (7). These ducts increase in caliber and possess smooth muscle fibers within their wall as they reach the hilus of the liver. Furthermore, as they become larger, the epithelium becomes increasingly thicker, and the surrounding layers of connective tissue grow thicker and contain many elastic fibers. These ducts anastomose to form the segmental branches (from segment 1 to segment 8) (8).

In 80% to 85% of individuals, these segmental branches anastomose to form the anterior (segment 5 and segment 8) and posterior sectorial bile ducts (segment 6 and segment 7) (as described in the previous section) in the right hemiliver. With the union of these two sectorial ducts in 57% (1) of individuals, the right hepatic duct is formed. The right hepatic duct is usually short—approximately 9 mm in length (7). In the left hemiliver the segmental branches 2 and 3 anastomose to form the left hepatic duct in the region of the umbilical fissure. The anastomosis of segment 4 to the left hepatic duct usually occurs as a single trunk to the right of the umbilical fissure in 67% (7). The left hepatic duct is generally longer and more surgically accessible than the right hepatic duct. Variations of the sectorial and hepatic ducts will be discussed separately.

The caudate lobe (segment 1) is drained by both right and left hepatic ducts. Its arterial supply is also from both right and left portal vein and hepatic artery, with small venous branches draining directly to the inferior vena cava (7).

The anatomy of this third hemiliver is revealed in certain pathologic conditions, such as Budd-Chiari syndrome where the outflow of the three hepatic veins is obstructed, leading to diversion of blood to the caudate lobe resulting in its hypertrophy (9).

Variation of the Intrahepatic Bile Ducts

As illustrated previously, the incidence of the right anterior and posterior sectorial ducts joining to form the right hepatic duct occurs in only 57% of people (Fig. 1.3). In 12%, the right anterior and right posterior ducts join at the junction with the left hepatic duct without the existence of the right hepatic duct. In 20% of cases, drainage occurs directly into the common hepatic duct (1).

There has also been reported variation in the segmental anastomosis in the right liver. The main right segmental drainage was variable in 9% of segment 5, 14% in segment 6, and 29% in segment 8. Variation in segment 7 was not reported (7).

With regard to the left liver, 67% of individuals have the previously described anatomy. The main variation lies in the ectopic drainage of segment 4. It has been reported that 2% drain directly into the common hepatic duct, and 27% drain directly into segment 2 or segment 3 only. This should be taken into consideration when performing a left lobectomy to avoid compromising the drainage of segment 4 (7).

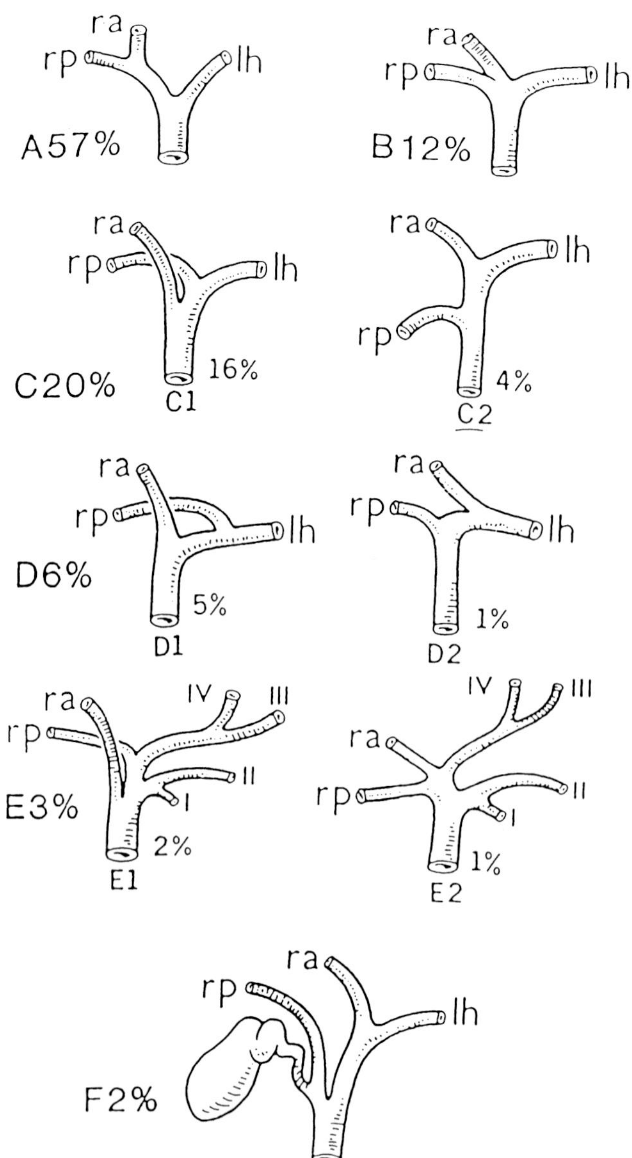

FIGURE 1.3. *Variations in the confluence of sectorial and hepatic ducts. (Reproduced by permission from Blumgart LH, ed. Surgery of the liver and biliary tract. New York: Churchill Livingstone: 1988.)*

Another form of ectopic drainage of the intrahepatic ducts is the involvement of the cystic duct and the gallbladder (Fig. 1.4). As illustrated, these variations are important to note during cholecystectomy (10).

Extrahepatic Bile Ducts

The joining of the right and left hepatic ducts forms the common hepatic duct. The accessory biliary apparatus, composed of the gallbladder and cystic duct, joins the common hepatic duct to form the common bile duct that drains bile into the duodenum. This comprises the extrahepatic biliary system.

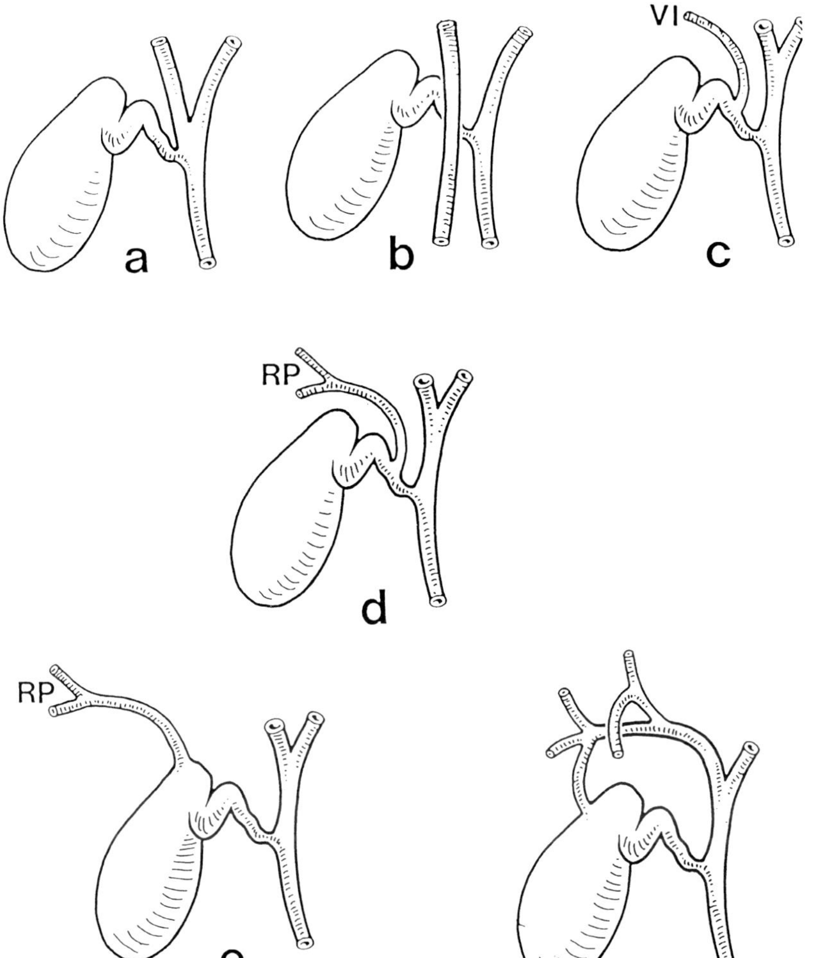

FIGURE 1.4. *Variations in the drainage of the intrahepatic ducts into the cystic duct. (Reproduced by permission from Blumgart LH, ed. Surgery of the liver and biliary tract. New York: Churchill Livingstone: 1988.)*

The confluence takes place at the right of the hilus of the liver, anterior to the portal venous bifurcation and overlying the origin of the right branch of the portal vein (Fig. 1.5). The biliary confluence is separated from the posterior aspect of segment 4 of the left liver by the hilar plate, which is the fusion of connective tissue enclosing the biliary and vascular structures with Glisson's capsule (11).

Gallbladder and Cystic Duct

The gallbladder is a reservoir of bile in the shape of a piriform sac partly contained in a fossa on the inferior surface of the right hepatic lobe. It extends from the right extremity of the porta hepatis to the inferior border of the liver. It is 7 to 10 cm long and 3 to 4 cm broad at its widest part, and can hold from 30 to 50 mL. The gallbladder is divided into a fundus, body, infundibulum, and neck.

The fundus extends about 1 cm beyond the free edge of the liver. The body is the largest segment. The infundibulum is the transitional area between the body and the neck. Hartmann's pouch is a bulge on the inferior surface of the infundibulum. Gallstones may become impacted here and can cause obstruction of the cystic duct. The neck is the tapered segment of the infundibulum that is narrow and joins the cystic duct.

The cystic duct is 3 to 4 cm long and passes posteriorly inferior and to the left from the neck of the gallbladder to join the common hepatic duct to form the common bile duct (CBD). The mucosa of the cystic duct is arranged with spiral folds known as the valves of Heister (12).

A number of anomalies occur in the gallbladder (Table 1.1). Furthermore, the cystic duct inserts into the bile duct at a variety of sites (see Fig. 1.4) (13,14).

The arterial supply to the gallbladder is from the cystic artery. Because the cystic artery is an end artery, the gallbladder is more susceptible to ischemic injury and necrosis as a result from inflammation or interruption of the artery. The cystic artery can originate from the right hepatic, left hepatic, or the common hepatic artery, and it can be anterior or posterior to the common hepatic duct. Figure 1.6 illustrates some of these variations.

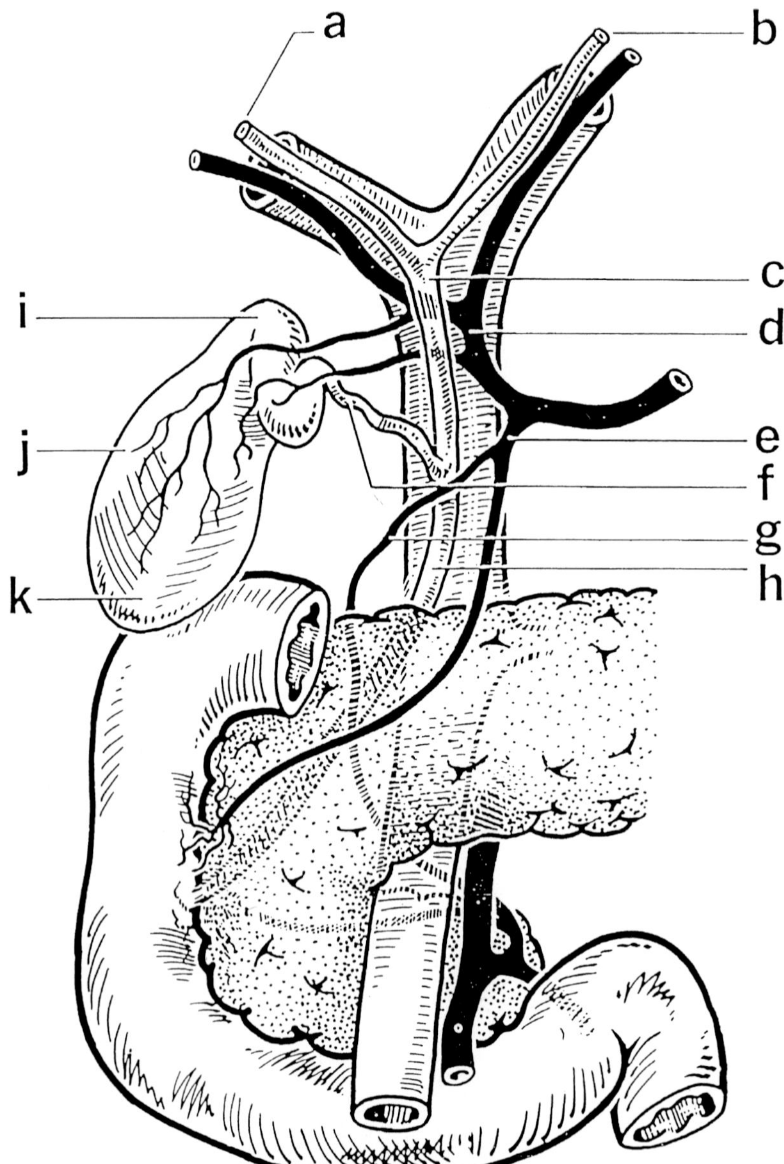

FIGURE 1.5. *The anatomy of the extrahepatic biliary system. (a) right hepatic duct, (b) left hepatic duct, (c) common hepatic duct, (d) hepatic artery, (e) gastroduodenal artery, (f) cystic duct, (g) retroduodenal artery, (h) common bile duct, (i) neck of the gallbladder, (j) body of the gallbladder, (k) fundus of the gallbladder. (Reproduced by permission from Blumgart LH, ed. Surgery of the liver and biliary tract. New York: Churchill Livingstone: 1988.)*

Table 1.1. Anomalies of the gallbladder

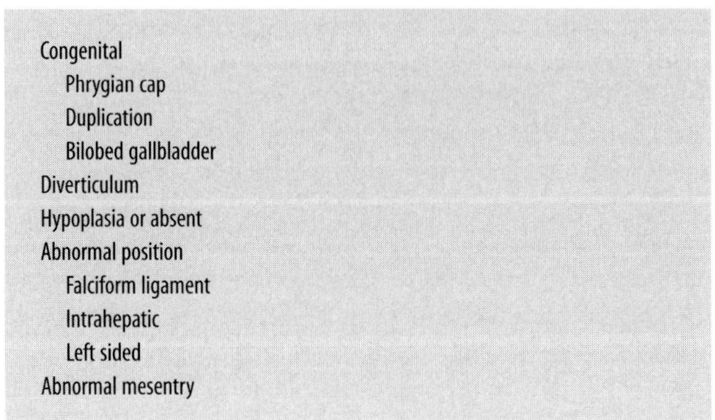

Anomalies of the gallbladder
Congenital
Phrygian cap
Duplication
Bilobed gallbladder
Diverticulum
Hypoplasia or absent
Abnormal position
Falciform ligament
Intrahepatic
Left sided
Abnormal mesentry

The venous drainage is through the cystic vein, which drains into the portal vein. There are also some small veins that drain directly into the liver to the hepatic veins.

The lymphatic drainage of the gallbladder proceeds mainly by four routes, which form two pathways that drain in the thoracic duct (these will be discussed later with the common bile duct) (15).

1. Superior and external, drains the fundus (around 6% of cases).
2. Superior and medial, drains the medial aspect of the gallbladder (around 10% of cases).
3. Inferior and external, drains the body of the gallbladder (present in 82% of cases).
4. Inferior and medial, from the body of the gallbladder (constant).

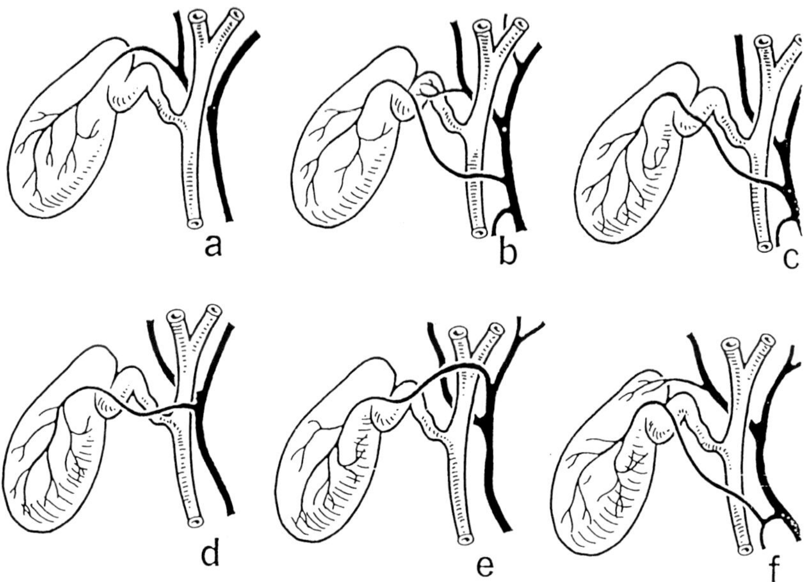

FIGURE 1.6. *Variations of the blood supply (cystic artery) to the gallbladder. (Reproduced by permission from Blumgart LH, ed. Surgery of the liver and biliary tract. New York: Churchill Livingstone: 1988.)*

All four routes drain to both pathways, except the inferior and external which drain only to the inferior pathway. This is important in cases of gallbladder cancer, which can spread to the liver; because of its extensive lymph drainage to both pathways, cure by radical surgery is difficult.

The gallbladder is innervated by the vagus nerve through its hepatic branch from the anterior vagal trunk. The gallbladder is also innervated by the sympathetic nervous system through the celiac plexus. Fibers in the right phrenic nerve may also be distributed to the gallbladder through the hepatic plexus.

The Duct of Luschka

The duct of Luschka is a small bile duct, running in the bed of the gallbladder, outside the wall. It is present in 50% of individuals (16). This duct is surgically significant because it may be injured during cholecystectomy and may result in bile fistula unless ligated. Recent reports demonstrated a 1.5% to 2.0% incidence of bile leak from the duct of Luschka after laparoscopic cholecystectomy. Ligation has no consequences, as it is an end duct that drains an isolated segment.

Common Bile Duct

The common hepatic duct forms by the junction of the cystic duct with the common hepatic duct. Its course is divided into supraduodenal, retroduodenal, pancreatic, and intraduodenal (joins the main pancreatic duct to form the sphincter of Oddi, which will be discussed separately).

The supraduodenal segment usually lies in the free border of the hepatoduodenal ligament. It runs to the right of the hepatic artery and anterior to the portal vein. The retroduodenal segment descends posterior to the first part of the duodenum and slightly obliquely from right to left. The pancreatic segment is related to the head of the pancreas; it can run entirely retropancreatic or travel through its parenchyma.

The diameter of the common bile duct is often used as an indication of biliary pathology. Its "normal" size varies depending on the modality used to measure it, and a range of 4 to 13 mm has been reported (16,17). The most common modality to examine the common bile duct diameter is ultrasound, and a diameter up to 6 mm is considered normal. Some consider the equivalent in contrast radiology to be 10 mm; this depends on the magnification (18).

Sphincter of Oddi

The common bile duct enters the duodenum approximately 8 cm from the pylorus in the second part of the duodenum. The site of entry is marked by a papilla (major papilla). Its position can be variable; in approximately 13% it can be located at the junction of the second and third part of the duodenum, or even more distally (19). A transverse fold of mucosa usually covers the papilla. The papilla is identified as a small nipple or pea-like structure in the lumen of the duodenum (20).

The main pancreatic duct of Wirsung joins the common bile duct and forms a common channel in approximately 85% of individuals. In 15% they open either separately or as a V junction with the duodenal mucosa. In 4% of individuals the body and tail of the pancreas drain via the duct of Santorini (pancreas divisum) to the minor papilla. In this instance only the ventral aspect of the pancreas drains through the duct of Wirsung. The minor papilla is located proximal and slightly anterior to the major papilla.

The human sphincter of Oddi is generally a continuous smooth muscle structure that is subdivided into several parts

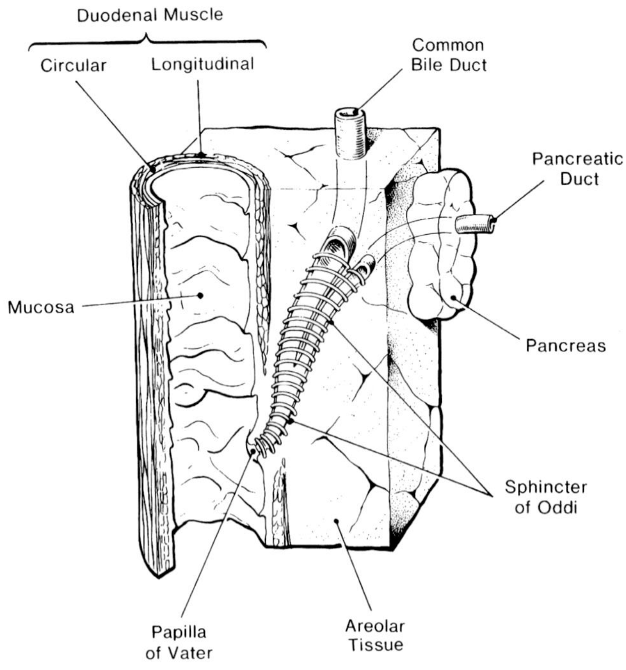

FIGURE 1.7. *The choledochoduodenal junction. The sphincteric muscle is predominantly circular in orientation, and extends beyond the wall of the duodenum. There is a small extension along the pancreatic duct.*

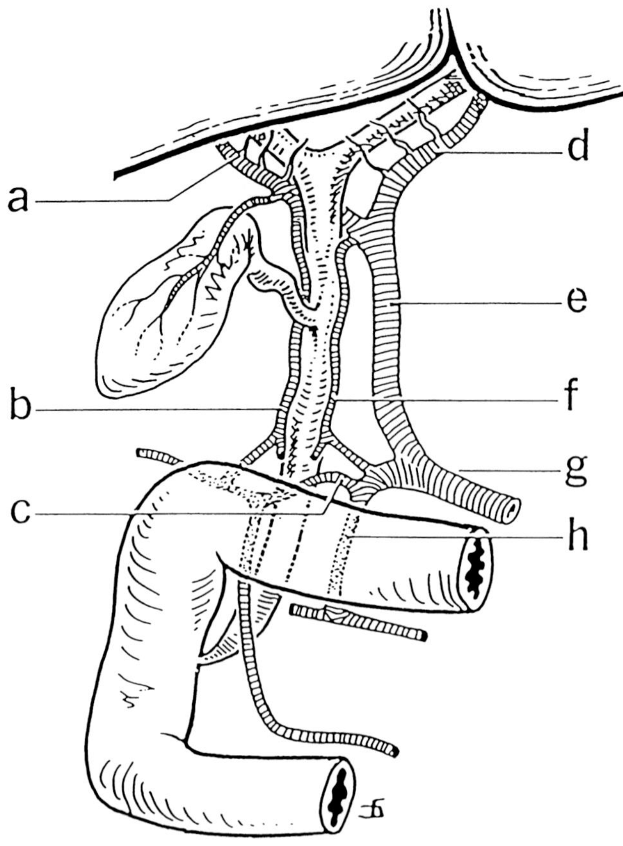

FIGURE 1.8. *Blood supply to the extrahepatic bile ducts: (a) right hepatic artery, (b) 9 o'clock artery, (c) retroduodenal artery, (d) left hepatic artery, (e) hepatic artery, (f) 3 o'clock artery, (g) common hepatic artery, (h) gastroduodenal artery. (Reproduced by permission from Blumgart LH, ed. Surgery of the liver and biliary tract. New York: Churchill Livingstone: 1988.)*

that largely reflect the arrangements found in other animal species (8) (Fig. 1.7).

1. Sphincter choledochus consists of circular muscle that surrounds the common bile duct.
2. Pancreatic sphincter surrounds the intraduodenal portion of the pancreatic duct before its juncture with the ampulla.
3. Fasciculi longitudinales are composed of longitudinal muscle fibers between the pancreatic and bile duct.
4. Sphincter ampullae are composed of longitudinal muscle fibers that surround the papilla.

Blood Supply

The blood supply to the common bile duct is also divided into three segments (Fig. 1.8) (5). The supraduodenal segment of the duct essentially has an axial blood supply. The blood supply originates from the retroduodenal artery, right hepatic artery, cystic artery, gastroduodenal artery, and the retroportal artery. On average there are eight small arteries, with the main two running along the side of the common bile duct at 3 and 9 o'clock. Sixty percent of the arterial blood supply occurs from the duodenal end of the duct, and 38% is from the hepatic end. Only 2% of the arterial supply is nonaxial, arising directly from the main hepatic trunk. The second segment is the retropancreatic part of the duct, which is supplied by the retroduodenal artery. It provides blood to the multiple small vessels running around the duct to form a mural plexus. The third segment is the hilar duct, which receives its blood supply from the surrounding blood vessels, forming a rich network.

The veins draining the bile duct correspond to the described arteries. They drain into veins at 3 and 9 o'clock on the side of the common bile duct.

Lymphatic Drainage

The lymph drainage of the extrahepatic biliary system is through two pathways (15):

1. The superior pathway of nodes along the cystic duct, the hepatic duct, the anterior and medial aspect of the portal vein, and the celiac axis.
2. The inferior pathway of nodes along the cystic duct, anterior and lateral aspect of the portal vein, the posterior aspect of the pancreas, between the aorta and the inferior vena cava, and the left aspect of the aorta under the left renal vein.

Lymph drainage of the common bile duct is by lymph nodes along the duct to both the inferior and superior pathway.

Nerves of the Common Bile Duct and Sphincter of Oddi

The nerve supply to the extrahepatic bile duct is from extrinsic and intrinsic nerves. The extrinsic nerves are mainly from the hepatic plexus. The posterior hepatic plexus contains preganglionic parasympathetic fibers from branches of the vagus nerve and postganglionic sympathetic fibers that arise from the right celiac plexus. The anterior hepatic plexus contains postganglionic fibers from the left celiac and preganglionic fibers from the left vagus. The intrinsic nerve supply is mainly from neural connection from surrounding organs such as the duodenum, stomach, and gallbladder. This complex neural supply is important in controlling sphincter motility.

PHYSIOLOGY OF THE BILIARY TRACT

Bile Production

Bile fulfills two major functions. It participates in the absorption of fat, and forms the vehicle for excretion of cholesterol, bilirubin, iron, and copper. Bile acids are the main active component of biliary secretion. They are secreted into the duodenum and efficiently reabsorbed from the terminal ileum by the portal venous system (21).

Bile Secretion

Bile is secreted by the hepatocytes through the canalicular membrane into the canalicular space. The secretory process is both active and passive and the active process generates bile flow. The products of active secretion are known as the primary solutes and these are made up of conjugated bile acids, conjugated bilirubin, glutathione, conjugates of steroid hormones, and leukotrienes. Filtrable solutes are generated by passive secretion induced by osmotic pressure and are called secondary solutes. These are mainly plasma, glucose, electrolytes, low-molecular-weight organic acids, and calcium.

The maximum secretory pressure developed by the liver is 30 cm. In the fasting state, the sphincter of Oddi has an average resting pressure of 12 to 15 cm H_2O. Because the opening pressure of the cystic duct is 8 cm H_2O, and the gallbladder is 10 cm H_2O, the pressure gradient favors the entry of bile into the gallbladder (22). Therefore, during fasting most of the bile is diverted into the gallbladder, where it is concentrated.

Bile is produced by hepatocytes and cells of the intrahepatic ducts at a rate of 600 mL/day. The hepatic bile entering the gallbladder during fasting consists of approximately 97% water and 1% to 2% bile acids. Phospholipids, cholesterol, bile pigment, and electrolytes make up the remainder (23,24). Hepatic bile is iso-osmolar with plasma. Sodium, chloride, and bicarbonate ions, with nearly an isotonic amount of water, are absorbed from the bile. The gallbladder is able to remove 90% of the water from hepatic bile (25). In monkeys the volume of water absorption is 30% of the gallbladder bile volume per hour (26). The gallbladder concentration of bile salts, bilirubin, and cholesterol may rise 10-fold or more, relative to hepatic bile levels.

The gallbladder partially empties during fasting in conjunction with the phases of the interdigestive cycle. After a meal, the gallbladder contracts and the sphincter of Oddi relaxes, leading to the delivery of bile to the duodenum. The gallbladder empties around 75% of its content. At the same time, hepatic bile bypasses the gallbladder and empties into the duodenum. At the end of the meal, the gallbladder relaxes and the sphincter of Oddi contracts, leading to the diversion of hepatic bile into the gallbladder once again for storage until the next meal.

In individuals who have undergone a cholecystectomy, bile acids are stored in the proximal small intestine (27). After meal ingestion, the acids get transported to the distal ileum for absorption and maintenance of the enterohepatic circulation.

Bile Reabsorption

The reabsorption of bile acids is through the enterohepatic circulation. Bile acids are also absorbed from the terminal ileum by the portal system back to the liver. This is achieved by passive and active transcellular absorption. The most important mechanism is a sodium-coupled transport system that is present in the apical membrane of the enterocytes; it is known as the ileal bile acid transporter (IBAT) (28).

In the distal ileum and large intestine, intestinal bacteria deconjugate bile acids, which are absorbed passively in solution (29). A small amount of the bile acid is lost from the body in feces. This fecal loss is compensated by synthesis of new bile acids. In healthy adults, less than 3% of bile acids present in hepatic bile are newly synthesized.

In the portal system bile acids are bound to albumin. The ability of the albumin binding depends on the nuclear substitutes. For trihydroxy bile acids, this is around 75%, whereas it is 98% for dihydroxy bile acids. On first pass, the hepatic circulation extraction is between 50% and 90%; the level of bile acids in the systemic circulation is directly proportional to the load presented to the liver, and it increases after meals (27). The plasma level of total bile acids is 3 to 4 μmol/L in the fasting state, and increases twofold to threefold after digestion.

Abnormality in Secretion and Gallstone Formation

Cholesterol is insoluble in water, but is made soluble in bile with the aid of bile salts and phospholipids. Thus, in simple terms, gallstones form when the cholesterol concentration in the bile exceeds the ability of the bile to hold it in soluble form. This occurs either by an increase in cholesterol secretion by the liver or a decrease in bile salts or phospholipids through a decrease in synthesis or interruption of the enterohepatic circulation. The result is crystals that grow into gallstones.

Bile cholesterol is normally derived from three main sources: synthesis in the hepatocytes from acetate, low-density lipoproteins that carry cholesterol from extrahepatic tissue to the liver, and chylomicrons that transport dietary cholesterol to the liver (30).

The main source of cholesterol is the synthesis by the liver. This process is through a sequence of enzymatic steps with 3-hydroxy-3-methyl-glutarylcoenzyme (HMG-CoA) reductase being the rate-limiting reaction (31). It is thought that obese people have an increase in the activity of this enzyme. When cholesterol is secreted into the bile, it forms mixed micelles and vesicles via the aid of bile salts and phospholipids (32,33). The micelles are lipid aggregates that have the polar group directed out toward the aqueous side, and the nonpolar group directed inward. As cholesterol saturation increases in bile, more cholesterol is carried in the vesicle form (34). The cholesterol saturation index is determined by the ratio of the measured concentration of bile salts and phospholipids compared to the concentration of cholesterol (Fig. 1.9; see also Fig. 11.1). If this ratio is greater than 1, bile is saturated with respect to cholesterol, thus producing the environment for the precipitation of cholesterol to form vesicles. Vesicles are 10 times bigger than micelles and have phospholipid bilayers, but contain no bile salts. With the increase in the cholesterol saturation index, more complex and unstable vesicles form (35). Compared with normal individuals, patients with gallstones secrete vesicles that are 33% more enriched with cholesterol (36), which are more prone to aggregate as well as crystallize (37). So a decrease in bile salts can increase the cholesterol saturation index without an increase in cholesterol concentration. However, bile salt hyposecretion is not usually present (28). Once the unstable vesicles are present, they aggregate together in the supersaturated bile (39). Crystallization occurs, resulting in cholesterol monohydrate crystals that can agglomerate to form macroscopic gallstones (40).

During the normal interdigestive period the gallbladder partially contracts, thus potentially evacuating any small crystals that might have formed. This cleansing function of the gallbladder should in theory prevent bile stasis and prevent crystals from growing into stones.

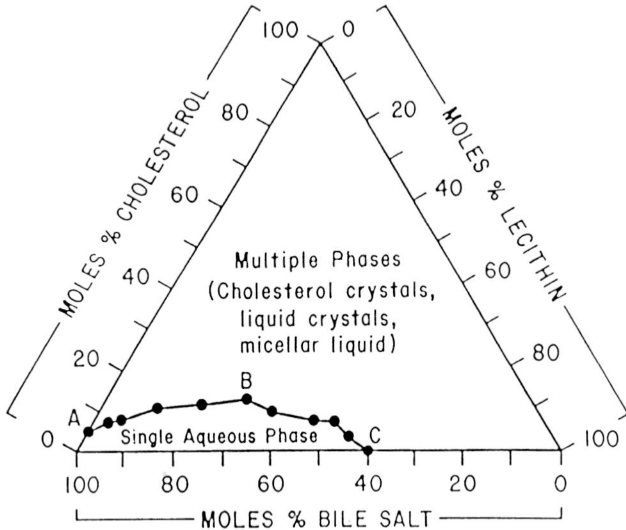

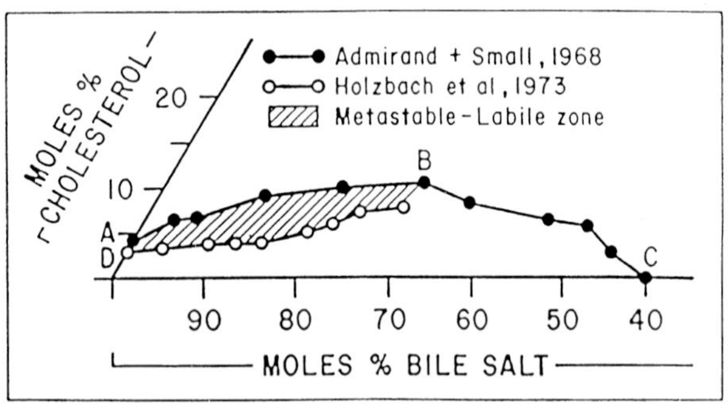

FIGURE 1.9. *Triangular diagram demonstrating the molar coordination of cholesterol, bile salt, and lecithin. If the point of bile analysis is above line ABC, cholesterol is supersaturated; if it lies below line DBC, cholesterol is completely soluble; in between the two lines is a metastable-labile zone in which stones may form if specific nucleating factors are present. (Reproduced by permission from Sabiston DC Jr, ed. Textbook of surgery: the biological basis of modern surgical practice. 14th ed. Philadelphia: Saunders, 1991.)*

Motility of the Biliary Tract

Normal flow of bile occurs following contraction of the gallbladder and relaxation of the sphincter of Oddi. Control of these motor events is complex and involves both nerves and hormones. Disturbance of any of these controlling factors may lead to dysmotility and result in clinical disorders.

Gallbladder Motility

The normal motility of the gallbladder regulates the flow of bile during fasting and after meals. Gallbladder filling is determined by the rate of bile secretion from the liver, the active relaxation of the gallbladder, and the resistance to flow through the lower end of the bile duct produced by the sphincter of Oddi. In the fasting state the gallbladder progressively fills with bile. This is accomplished without large pressure gradients in the biliary system. As the gallbladder accommodates filling, significant changes in volume occur with little change in its intraluminal pressure (41).

The gallbladder does not remain dormant during the fasting periods (interdigestive phase); it has its own motility cycle that is correlated with the migratory motor complex (MMC) of the gut. It was first observed in dogs (42) and then in humans (43) during cholecystographic studies. The gallbladder volume changes during the interdigestive phase (44), decreasing by 30% to 35% of maximal contractile capacity at the end of phase two and continuing to empty during phase three of the MMC. During phase one and early in phase two, the gallbladder refills and the cycle repeats (45–47). This process of partial emptying and refilling during fasting may promote bile mixing and prevent sludge and microcalculi formation (48).

When an individual feeds, a cephalic response occurs. Gallbladder contraction in humans in response to the smell of fried meats has been observed (43) and similar findings have also been reported in dogs (49). The release of cholecystokinin (CCK), the main gallbladder-contracting hormone, by the duodenum after the ingestion of food (mainly fat, intraluminal acid, and amino acid) (50) causes an increase in hepatic bile flow and gallbladder contraction, and a reduction in the resting pressure of the sphincter of Oddi. These events promote the flow of gallbladder bile into the duodenum (51), with more than 75% of the resting gallbladder volume ejected during endogenous CCK stimulation (52). During this process the gallbladder tone remains constant over short periods of time (53). This allows rapid passive refilling of the gallbladder (active refilling) in the postprandial period, thus helping to maintain a pool of bile salts continuously in the gallbladder to preserve the enterohepatic circulation of bile salts (54).

Control of Gallbladder Motility Motility of the gallbladder is controlled by a number of mechanisms involving gut hormones (mainly CCK), bioactive peptides, nerves (sympathetic, parasympathetic, and intrinsic), and other hormones (progesterone).

Gut Hormones and Peptides CCK is the major hormone controlling gallbladder motility, as first described by Ivy and Oldberg in 1928 (55). This hormone is composed of 33 amino acids and is produced by the I cell in the duodenum. The action of CCK on the gallbladder is mediated by direct binding to a specific receptor in the gallbladder smooth muscle (56). Blockade of the receptor by a specific antagonist, loxiglumide, completely prevents CCK-mediated gallbladder contraction (57). CCK-induced contraction is not significantly altered by cholinergic (58) or adrenergic (59) blockade. CCK may act as a parasympathetic neurotransmitter within vagal neurons in the gallbladder intramural plexus, where it has been identified (60). Parasympathetic postsynaptic transmission enhancement has also been demonstrated by CCK, which promotes gallbladder contraction (61).

Other gut hormones and peptides such as secretin, gastrin, and motilin also have been identified that affect the gallbladder motility (Table 1.2).

Neuronal Control The neuronal control of gallbladder motility is not yet clearly understood. As discussed in the anatomy section, the gallbladder is innervated by the vagus, the celiac plexus, and the phrenic nerve and intrinsic nerves.

The cholinergic input from the vagus nerve plays a major role in the interdigestive, cephalic, and gastric phases of gallbladder motility. Gallbladder interdigestive motility in humans and dogs is lost following atropine treatment (62,63). It has also been noted that patients develop a larger fasting gallbladder volume after truncal vagotomy (64,65).

Table 1.2. The action of hormones and peptides on the human biliary tract

Hormones/Peptides	Gallbladder	Sphincter of Oddi
CCK	E	R
Gastrin/pentagastrin	E	E
Glucagon		NE
Motilin	E	E
Secretin		E followed by R
Octreotide	R	E
Enkephalin	R	R
Gastrin-releasing peptide	E	
Vasoactive intestinal peptide		R

E = excitatory, R = relaxation, NE = no effect.

In the cephalic and gastric phases, sham feeding causes gallbladder contraction without an increase in CCK blood levels (66,67). This action is blocked by atropine and truncal vagotomy (68), indicating a cholinergic vagal innervation involving muscarinic receptors.

In the intestinal phase, multiple studies have shown that atropine causes relaxation of the CCK-stimulated gallbladder in humans (69,70), dogs (71), and opossums (72). This response is mainly through M1 receptors. The M1 receptor antagonist (telenzepine) causes an inhibitory effect (73). The cholinergic fibers mediating this action are thought to run in the vagus nerve, because the gallbladder response to intraduodenal nutrients is inhibited in humans (74), dogs (70), and opossums (75) following truncal vagotomy. However, direct electrical stimulation of the vagus nerve does not increase gallbladder contraction or enhance subthreshold levels of CCK (76). This indicates that the vagus nerve plays only a minor role in gallbladder motility.

The effect of sympathetic nerve input on gallbladder motility has been inconsistent. It is generally accepted that sympathetic stimulation causes gallbladder relaxation. Norepinephrine and isoprenaline relaxed the stimulated gallbladder in the guinea pig (77,78), whereas direct stimulation of the sympathetic nerves did not affect gallbladder pressure in cat (79) and norepinephrine and isoprenaline did not produce any effect at physiologic doses (53). It was demonstrated that the gallbladder has both α-adrenergic and β-adrenergic receptors (80). Subsequent studies demonstrated that the gallbladder has mainly β-adrenergic receptors that mediate gallbladder relaxation, and that the α-adrenergic receptors (mainly excitatory) do not act except after blocking the β-adrenergic receptors (81,82).

There is accumulating evidence for the involvement of nonadrenergic noncholinergic nerves in the regulation of gallbladder motility and inhibition of nitric oxide (NO) synthase–enhanced gallbladder responses to CCK (83). In the prairie dog, the gallbladder was found to contain NO synthase in nerves, causing relaxation of the gallbladder that was precontracted by CCK (84). Recently, Cullen et al. concluded that superoxide increases gallbladder motility by affecting NO synthase, and the presence of superoxide scavenging enzyme in the gallbladder may regulate gallbladder motility by clearing endogenous superoxide (85).

Other Factors in the Control of Gallbladder Motility

Although both estrogen and progesterone receptors have been identified in the gallbladder's smooth muscle (86), multiple studies have shown that estrogen has no effect on gallbladder motility. However, clinical observation has suggested that these hormones have considerable effect on gallbladder motility, probably via progesterone. Multiple studies testing progesterone's effect on the gallbladder motility have shown inhibition (41,87), and the contractile effect of a cholecystokinin-octapeptide (CCK-8) was reduced when the tissue was pretreated with progesterone (87). Recently two studies in the guinea pig demonstrated progesterone-impaired gallbladder emptying in response to CCK; also, progesterone might cause a downregulation of the contractile G-protein and an upregulation of the G-alphas that mediate relaxation (88,89). Although the action of the female sex hormone on gallbladder motility is evident, there is no clear documentation on its role in the normal physiology of gallbladder motility.

Prostaglandins have also been suggested to play a role in gallbladder motility. Arachidonic acid (AA) produces contraction of the guinea pig gallbladder in vitro that was blocked by indomethacin, a potent inhibitor of prostaglandins (90,91). In humans, a dose-dependent gallbladder contraction was demonstrated in vitro with the use of several different prostaglandins (92). Another study suggested that the inhibitory effect of indomethacin is related to the inhibition of prostaglandin synthesis (93), and it was effective in relieving pain in patients with biliary colic (94). Although one study demonstrated that CCK may increase the release of AA (95), aspirin had no effect on stone formation nor did it prevent the decrease in contractility despite a profound decrease in endogenous gallbladder prostaglandin synthesis (96).

Sphincter of Oddi Motility

The sphincter of Oddi has three main functions: the regulation of flow into the duodenum, prevention of reflux from the duodenum to the bile and pancreatic duct, and the filling of the gallbladder. Manometric studies in humans have shown that the sphincter of Oddi has a basal pressure of 10 mm Hg over which are superimposed contractions with a frequency of 2 to 6 per minute and an amplitude of 50 to 140 mm Hg above duodenal pressure. These contractions are mainly in an antegrade direction (Fig. 1.10). Bile flow occurs mainly in between contractions (97) when the pressure in the bile duct overcomes the low basal pressure. The phasic contractions expel small volumes of bile and thus keep the opening of the bile duct free of crystals or debris. Furthermore, this prevents any reflux of duodenal content into the bile or pancreatic ducts. Modulation of the sphincter of Oddi basal pressure causes filling of the gallbladder and decrease in pressure causes flow of bile and pancreatic juice into the duodenum.

During fasting, the sphincter of Oddi exhibits a cyclical activity pattern that is distinct from, but coincident with, duodenal interdigestive activity. The sphincter of Oddi contracts throughout all phases of the interdigestive cycle. The frequency increases just prior to phase three of the duodenal activity, thus increasing the resistance of reflux of duodenal contents into the ducts. Feeding enhances the flow of bile through the sphincter with an overall decrease in sphincteric pressure. In humans, this is characterized by a decrease in basal pressure and a fall in contraction ampli-

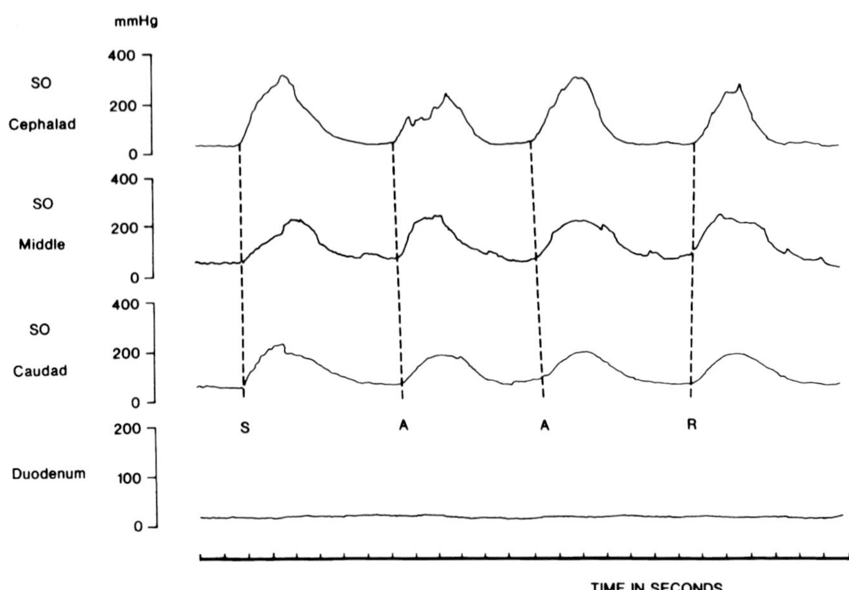

FIGURE 1.10. *Manometric recording from the human sphincter of Oddi using a triple-lumen catheter. Prominent phasic contractions are superimposed on a modest basal pressure. The contractions may be antegrade (A), simultaneous (S), or retrograde (R). They are independent of duodenal pressure changes.*

tude (97). These changes produce a decrease in resistance and facilitate flow from the ducts into the duodenum.

Control of Sphincter of Oddi Motility Like the gallbladder, control of the sphincter of Oddi's motility is complex and involves neural and hormonal pathways.

Gut Hormones and Peptides Cholecystokinin produces inhibition of the phasic contraction and a decrease in basal pressure. The mechanism of its action appears to be via a stimulation of nonadrenergic, noncholinergic inhibitory neurons. Secretin decreases the activity of the sphincter in most species, such as rabbits and cats, with no effect. In humans it causes an initial excitation followed by relaxation. Other hormones and peptides such as gastrin, motilin, and octreotide have been reported to alter the contraction of the sphincter of Oddi (see Table 1.2).

Neuronal Control Parasympathetic innervation is the main extrinsic innervation of the sphincter. Vagotomy experiments in animals have shown mixed results, with both excitatory and inhibitory effects (98). Vagal stimulation induces sphincter contraction. After administration of sympathetic blockers and atropine, vagal stimulation relaxes the sphincter, which suggests a noncholinergic nonadrenergic effect. These results indicate that vagal innervation to the sphincter is mainly excitatory; however, there exists an underlying inhibitory action via noncholinergic nonadrenergic nerves. Sympathetic blockade on its own does not influence sphincter of Oddi activity, suggesting that the sympathetic system does not have a major regulatory role under normal circumstances. Intrinsic nerves have a prominent role in controlling sphincter of Oddi activity.

Recent studies have identified a role for NO as the major noncholinergic nonadrenergic inhibitory transmitter acting on the sphincter of Oddi. NO donors such as sodium nitroprusside induce relaxation of the opossum sphincter, whereas inhibition of NO synthase with L-arginine analogues reduces the relaxation induced by transmural electrical stimulation.

Electrical stimulation of the gallbladder produces a fall in sphincter of Oddi pressure of dogs (99). Subsequent studies in humans demonstrated that distention of the gallbladder decreased resistance to flow by reducing the amplitude and decreasing the basal pressure, thus promoting the flow of bile (100). This response of the sphincter of Oddi to gallbladder distention, a cholecystic-sphincter of Oddi reflex, is mediated via neural connections between the gallbladder and the sphincter. This connection was abolished by application of local anesthetic to the common bile duct.

Distention of the stomach causes sphincter of Oddi contraction, thus producing a resistance to reflux of duodenal contents through the sphincter of Oddi. It has been identified as the pyloro-sphincter reflex. This response is abolished by atropine, which suggests it is mediated by cholinergic nerves.

Distention or the instillation of dilute hydrochloric acid into the duodenum of humans results in sphincter spasm. This enterosphincter reflex is abolished by atropine.

Other Factors in the Control of Sphincter of Oddi

- **Prostaglandin.** Prostaglandin E_1 inhibits sphincter of Oddi activity by suppressing its membrane activity. In addition, prostaglandin E_2 has an inhibitory action.
- **Sex Hormones.** Recent reports suggest that sex hormones and pregnancy affect the motility of the sphincter of Oddi. This action is demonstrated by differences in the response to cholecystokinin stimulation of male and female prairie dogs. In a separate study, sphincter motility was significantly reduced during high-dose estrogen infusion (primarily due to decreased phasic wave frequency), and it remained low for at least 20 minutes following the infusion.
- **Hymecromone Glucuronides.** These antispastic drugs, given intravenously as well as lignocaine given via T-tube in the bile duct, were effective in reducing sphincter of Oddi activity in patients.

Dysmotility of the Biliary Tract

Dysmotility of the gallbladder has been documented in several studies, and is thought to play a role in gallstone formation. Impaired gallbladder-emptying in response to exogenous CCK or meal stimulus has been well documented in gallstone patients. Increased fasting and residual gallbladder volumes mainly characterize the motility defect. In a study of patients on total parenteral nutrition, their gallbladder motility was shown to be defective, promoting sludge and microcrystal formation. Infusion of CCK improved gallbladder motility and decreased the incidence of gallstone and sludge formation. It may be that crystals are continually formed, but the ability to eject them is what prevents gallstone formation. Consequently, formation of gallstones may require dysmotility of the gallbladder.

Sphincter of Oddi dysmotility results in either biliary sphincter of Oddi dysfunction or episodes of recurrent pancreatitis (101). Both of these clinical entities are associated with abnormally elevated sphincter of Oddi basal pressure and are treatable by division of the sphincter of Oddi (101,102).

SUGGESTED READINGS

Corazziari E, Shaffer EA, Hogan WJ, Sherman S, Toouli J. Functional disorders of the biliary tract and pancreas. Gut 1999;45(suppl 2):48–54. This is a review article, derived from a consensus working party report, as part of the Rome criteria for the diagnosis and management of gastrointestinal motility disorders. It is an excellent overview by the world experts in the field.

Strasberg S, on behalf of the IHPBA. Brisbane 2000 Terminology on liver anatomy, HPB 2000 (volume number and page to be determined.) This review of liver terminology is the product of a working party of the International Hepato-pancreato Biliary Association, and incorporates the consensus view on terminology that has been accepted by the community of liver, biliary, and pancreatic specialists. It is a landmark manuscript on liver terminology.

Tierney S, Pitt H, Lillemoe K. Physiology and pathophysiology of gallbladder motility. Surg Clin North Am 1993;73:1267–90. This is an up-to-date review of the physiology and pathophysiology of gallbladder motility written by active researchers in the field. It is well referenced.

REFERENCES

1. Couinaud C. Le foie—studies anatomique et chirurgirales. Paris: Masson et Cie, 1957.
2. Strasberg SM. Terminology of liver anatomy and liver resections: coming to grips with hepatic Babel. J Am Coll Surg 1997;184:413–34.
3. Couinaud C. Surgical anatomy of the liver revisited. Paris: C. Couinaud, 1989.
4. Michels NA. The hepatic, cystic and retroduodenal arteries and their relations to the biliary ducts. With samples of the entire celiacal blood supply. Ann Surg 1951;133:503.
5. Northover JM, Terblanche J. Bile duct blood supply. Its importance in human liver transplantation. Transplantation 1978;26:67–9.
6. Jones AL, Schmucker DL, Renston RH, Murakami T. The architecture of bile secretion. A morphological perspective of physiology. Dig Dis Sci 1980;25:609–29.
7. Healey Jr JE, Schroy PC. Anatomy of the biliary ducts within the human liver. Analysis of the prevailing patterns of branching and the major variation of the biliary ducts. Arch Surg 1953;66:599.
8. Suchy FJ. Anatomy, anomalies and pediatric disorders of the biliary tract. In: Feldman M, Sleisenger MH, Scharschmidt BF, eds. Sleisenger and Fordtran's gastrointestinal and liver disease: pathophysiology, diagnosis, management. 6th ed. Philadelphia: Saunders, 1998:905–29.
9. Bismuth H. Surgical anatomy and anatomical surgery of the liver. World J Surg 1982;6:3–9.
10. Albaret P, Chevalier JM, Cronier P, et al. A proper des canaux hepatiques directement abouches dans la voie biliaire accessoire. Ann Chir 1981;35:88–92.
11. Hepp J, Couinaud C. L'abord et l'utilisation du canal hepatique gauche dans les reparations de la voie biliaire principale. Presse Med 1956;64:947.
12. Wood D. Presidential address: eponyms in biliary tract surgery. Am J Surg 1979;138:746–54.
13. Gross RE. Congenital anomalies of the gallbladder. A review of a hundred and forty-eight cases with report of a double gallbladder. Arch Surg 1936;32:131.
14. Kune GA. The influence of structure and function in the surgery of the biliary tract. Ann R Coll Surg Engl 1970;47:78–91.
15. Caplan I. Drainage lymphatique intra et extra-hepatique de la vessicule biliaire. Bulletin Mem Acad Med Belg 1982;137:324–34.
16. Kune GA. The anatomical basis of liver surgery. Aust N Z J Surg 1969;39:117–26.
17. Dowdy GS, Waldron GW, Brown WG, et al. Surgical anatomy of the pancreato-biliary ductal system. Arch Surg 1962;84:229.
18. Padbury RTA. Anatomy. In: Toouli J, ed. Surgery of the biliary tract. New York: Churchill Livingstone, 1993:1–20.
19. Lindner HH, Penz VA, Ruggeri RA, et al. A clinical and anatomical study of anomalous termination of the common bile duct into the duodenum. Ann Surg 1976;198:626.
20. Boyden EA. The anatomy of the choledochoduodenal junction. Surg Gynecol Obstet 1957;104:641.
21. Hofmann AF, Hofmann N. Measurement of bile acid kinetics by isotope dilution in man. Gastroenterology 1974;67:314–23.
22. Everson GT. Gallbladder function in gallstone disease. Gastroenterol Clin North Am 1991;20:85–110.
23. Shaffer EA. The effect of vagotomy on gallbladder function and bile composition in man. Ann Surg 1982;195:413–18.
24. Jansson R. Effects of gastrointestinal hormones on concentrating function and motility in the gallbladder. An experimental study in the cat. Acta Physiol Scand Suppl 1978;456:1–38.
25. Banfield WJ. Physiology of the gallbladder. Gastroenterology 1975;69:770–7.
26. Svanvik J, Allen B, Pellegrini C, et al. Variation in concentrating function of the gallbladder in the conscious monkey. Gastroenterology 1984;86:919–25.
27. Hofmann AF. Bile secretion and the enterohepatic circulation of bile acid. In: Feldman M, Sleisenger MH, Scharschmidt BF, eds. Sleisenger and Fordtran's gastrointestinal and liver disease: pathophysiology, diagnosis, management. 6th ed. Philadelphia: Saunders, 1998:937–48.
28. Wong MH, Oelkers P, Craddock AL, Dawson PA. Expression cloning and characterization of the hamster ileal sodium-dependent bile acid transporter. J Biol Chem 1994;269:1340–7.
29. Hofmann AF. Intestinal absorption of bile acids and biliary constituents: the intestinal component of the enterohepatic circulation and the integrated system. In: Johnson LR, Alpers DH, Christensen J, eds. Physiology of the gastrointestinal tract. New York: Raven Press, 1994:648–56.
30. Hay DW, Carey MC. Pathophysiology and pathogenesis of cholesterol gallstone formation. Semin Liver Dis 1990;10:159–70.
31. Brown MS, Goldstein JL. Receptor mediated control of cholesterol metabolism. Science 1976;191:150–4.
32. Admirand WH, Small DM. The physicochemical basis of cholesterol gallstone formation in man. J Clin Invest 1968;47:1043–52.
33. Cabral DJ, Small DM. Physical chemistry of bile. In: Johnston DE, Kaplan MM. Pathogenesis and treatment of gallstones. N Engl J Med 1993;328:412–21.
34. Donovan JM, Carey MC. Separation and quantitation of cholesterol "carriers" in bile. Hepatology 1990;12:94S–104S.
35. Cohen DE, Kaler EW, Carey MC. Cholesterol carriers in human bile: are "lamellae" involved? Hepatology 1993;18:1522–31.
36. Lamont JT, Carey MC. Cholesterol gallstone formation: 2. Pathobiology and pathomechanics. Prog Liver Dis 1992;10:165–91.
37. Harvey PR, Somjen G, Lichtenberg MS, et al. Nucleation of cholesterol from vesicles isolated from bile of patients with and without cholesterol gallstones. Biochim Biophys Acta 1987;921:198–204.
38. Carey MC, Cahalane MJ. Enterohepatic circulation. In: Carey MC. Pathogenesis of gallstones. Am J Surg 1993;165:410–19.
39. Sedaghat A, Grundy SM. Cholesterol crystals and the formation of cholesterol gallstones. N Engl J Med 1980;302:1274–7.
40. Small DM. Cholesterol nucleation and growth in gallstone formation. N Engl J Med 1980;302:1305–7.
41. Ryan J, Cohen S. Gallbladder pressure-volume response to gastrointestinal hormones. Am J Physiol 1976;230:1461–5.
42. Bainbridge FA, Dale HH. The contractile mechanism of the gallbladder and its extrinsic nervous control. J Physiol 1906;33:138–55.
43. Boyden EA. An analysis of the reaction of the human gallbladder to food. Anat Rec 1928;40:147–92.
44. Szurszewski JH. A migrating electric complex of canine small intestine. Am J Physiol 1969;217:1757–63.
45. Takahashi I, Kern MK, Dodds WJ, et al. Contraction pattern of opossum gallbladder during fasting and after feeding. Am J Physiol 1986;250:G227-35.
46. Toouli J, Bushell M, Stevenson G, et al. Gallbladder emptying in man related to fasting duodenal migrating motor contractions. Aust N Z J Surg 1986;56:147–51.
47. Traynor OJ, Byrne PJ, Keegan B, et al. Effect of vagal denervation on canine gallbladder motility. Brit J Surg 1987;74:850–4.
48. Takahashi I, Nakaya M, Suzuki T, et al. Postprandial changes in contractile activity and bile concentration in gallbladder of the dog. Am J Physiol 1982;243:G365–71.
49. McMaster PD, Elman R. On the expulsion of bile by the gallbladder: and a reciprocal relationship with the sphincter activity. J Exp Med 1926;44:173–98.
50. Thompson JC, Fender HR, Ramus NI, et al. Cholecystokinin metabolism in man and dogs. Ann Surg 1975;182:496–504.
51. Ryan JP. Motility of the gallbladder and biliary tree. In: Johnson LP, Christensen J, Grossman MI, eds. Physiology of the gastrointestinal tract. New York: Raven Press, 1986:473–95.
52. Fisher RS, Rock E, Levin G, Malmud L. Effects of somatostatin on the gallbladder emptying. Gastroenterology 1987;92:885–90.
53. Schoetz DJ Jr, Birkett DH, Williams LF, et al. Gallbladder motor function in the intact primate: autonomic pharmacology. J Surg Res 1978;24:513–19.
54. LaMorte WW, Schoetz DJ Jr, Birkett DH, Williams LF Jr. The roll of the gallbladder in the pathogenesis of cholesterol gallstones. Gastroenterology 1979;77:580–92.
55. Ivy AC, Oldberg E. A hormone mechanism for gallbladder contraction and evacuation. Am J Physiol 1928;86:599.
56. Steigerwalt RW, Goldfine ID, Williams JA. Characterization of cholecystokinin receptor on bovine gallbladder membranes. Am J Physiol 1984;247:G709–14.
57. Schmidt WE, Creutzfeldt W, Schleser A. Role of CCK in regulation of pancreaticobiliary function and GI motility in human: effect of loxiglumide. Am J Physiol 1991;260:G197–206.
58. Hedner P. Effect of the C-terminal octapeptide of cholecystokinin on guinea pig ileum and gallbladder in vitro. Acta Physiol Scand 1970;78:232–5.

59. Amer MS. Studies with cholecystokinin in vitro. 3. Mechanism of the effect on the isolated rabbit gallbladder strip. J Phamacol Exp Ther 1972;183:527–34.
60. Strah KM, Melendez RL, Pappas TN, Debas HT. Interaction of vasoactive intestinal polypeptide and cholecystokinin octapeptide on the control of gallbladder contraction. Surgery 1986;99:469–73.
61. Bauer AJ, Hanani M, Muir TC, Szurszewski JH. Intracellular recording from gallbladder ganglia of opossums. Am J Physiol 1991;260:G299–306.
62. Svenberg T, Christofides ND, Fitzpatrick ML, Areola-Ortiz F, Bloom SR, Welbourn RB, Christofides ND, Fitzpatrick ML, et al. Interdigestive biliary output in man: relationship to fluctuations in plasma motilin and effect of atropine. Gut 1982;23:1024–8.
63. Magee DF, Naruse S, Pap A. Vagal control of the gallbladder. J Physiol 1984;355:65–70.
64. Johnson FE, Boyden EA. The effect of double vagotomy on the motor activity on the human gallbladder. Surgery 1952;32:591–601.
65. Parkin GJ, Smith RB, Johnston D, et al. Gallbladder volume and contractility after truncal, selective and highly selective (parietal-cell) vagotomy in man. Ann Surg 1973;178:581–6.
66. Hopman WP, Jansen JB, Rosenbusch G, et al. Cephalic stimulation of gallbladder contraction in humans: role of cholecystokinin and the cholinergic system. Digestion 1987;38:197–203.
67. Yamamura T, Takahashi T, Kusunoki M, et al. Gallbladder dynamics and plasma cholecystokinin responses after meals, oral water, or sham feeding in healthy subjects. Am J Med Sci 1988;295:102–7.
68. Fisher RS, Rock E, Malmud LS, et al. Gallbladder emptying response to sham feeding in humans. Gastroenterology 1986;90:1854–7.
69. Hopman WP, Jansen JB, Rosenbusch G, et al. Role of cholecystokinin and the cholinergic system in intestinal stimulation of gallbladder contraction in man. Hepatology 1990;11:261–5.
70. Fisher RS, Rock E, Malmud LS, et al. Cholinergic effects on gallbladder emptying in humans. Gastroenterology 1985;89:716–22.
71. Lamers CBHW, Poitras WP, Jansen JBMJ, et al. Relative potencies of cholecystokinin-33 and cholecystokinin-8 measured by radioimmunoassay and bioassay. Scand J Gastrenterol 1983;18(suppl):191–2.
72. Nanyu N, Dodds WJ, Layman RD, et al. Mechanism of cholecystokinin-induced contraction of the opossum gallbladder. Gastroenterology 1990;98:1299–306.
73. Tankurt E, Yegen BC, Biren T, et al. Influence of pirenzepine on gallbladder contraction in man induced by sham feeding or an intraduodenal meal. Digestion 1992;51:103–9.
74. Fried GM, Ogden WD, Greeley GH Jr, et al. Correlation of release and action of cholecystokinin in dogs before and after vagotomy. Surgery 1983;93:786–91.
75. Takhashi I, Dodds WJ, Hogan WJ, et al. Effect of vagotomy on biliary-tract motor activity in the opossum. Dig Dis Sci 1988;33:481–9.
76. Pallin B, Skoglund S. Neural and hormonal control of the gallbladder emptying mechanism in the cat. Acta Physiol Scand 1964;60:348.
77. Bartaccini G, DeCaro G, Endean R, et al. The action of caerulin on the smooth muscle of the gastrointestinal tract and the gallbladder. Br J Pharmacol 1986;34:291–310.
78. Andersson KE, Andersson R, Hender P, et al. Cholecystokinetic effect and concentration of cyclic AMP in the gallbladder muscle in vitro. Acta Physiol Scand 1972;85:511–16.
79. Winkelstein A, Achsner PW. The pressure factors in the biliary system of the dog. Am J Med Sci 1924;168:812.
80. Amer MS. Studies with cholecystokinin in vitro. 3. Mechanism of the effect on the isolated gallbladder strips. J Pharmacol Exp Ther 1972;183: 527–34.
81. Persson CG, Ekman M. Effect of morphine, cholecystokinin, and sympathomimetics on the sphincter of Oddi and intestinal pressure in cat duodenum. Scand J Gastrenterol 1972;7:345–51.
82. Persson CG. Adrenergic, cholecystokinetic and morphine-induced effect on extra-hepatic biliary motility. Acta Physiol Scand Suppl 1972;383:1–32.
83. Mourelle M, Guarner F, Molero X, et al. Regulation of gallbladder motility by the arginine-nitric oxide pathway in guinea pig. Gut 1993;34:911–15.
84. Salomons H, Keaveny AP, Henihan R, et al. Nitric oxide and gallbladder motility in prairie dogs. Am J Physiol 1997;272:G770–8.
85. Cullen JJ, Conklin JL, Ephgrave KS, et al. The role of antioxidant enzymes in the control of opossum gallbladder motility. J Surg Res 1999;86: 155–61.
86. Daignault P, Fazekas A, Rosenthall L, et al. Relationship between gallbladder contraction and progesterone receptors in patients with gallstones. Am J Surg 1988;155:147–51.
87. Davis M, Ryan J. Influence of progesterone on guinea pig gallbladder motility in vitro. Dig Dis Sci 1986;31:513–18.
88. Tierney S, Nakeeb A, Wong O, et al. Progesterone alters biliary flow dynamics. Ann Surg 1999;229:205–9.
89. Xiao ZL, Chen Q, Biancani P, Behar J. Mechanism of gallbladder hypomotility in pregnant guinea pigs. Gastroenterology 1999;116:411–19.
90. Wood JR, Stamford IF. Prostaglandins in chronic cholecystitis. Prostaglandins 1977;13:97–106.
91. Yoshida M, Koeda T. Studies on the electrical stimulation-induced contractile responses of hamster and mouse gallbladders. J Smooth Muscle Res 1992;28:111–20.
92. Kotwall CA, Clanachan AS, Baer HP, Scott GW. Effects of prostaglandins on motility of gallbladders removed from patients with gallstones. Arch Surg 1984;119:709–12.
93. Nakata K, Ashida K, Nakazawa K, et al. Effects of indomethacin on prostaglandin synthesis and on contractile response of the guinea pig gallbladder. Pharmacology 1981;23:95–101.
94. Thornell E, Jansson R, Svanvik J. Indomethacin intravenously–a new way for effective relief of biliary pain: a double-blind study in man. Surgery 1981;90:468–72.
95. Hidaka T, Nakano M, Shingu M, et al. Stimulation of prostaglandin synthesis by cholecystokinin in primary culture cells of bovine gallbladder muscle. Prostaglandins Leukot Essent Fatty Acids 1989;38:113–17.
96. Li YF, Russell DH, Myers SI, et al. Gallbladder contractility in aspirin- and cholesterol-fed prairie dogs. Gastroenterology 1994;106:1662–7.
97. Worthley CS, Baker RA, Iannos J, et al. Human fasting and postprandial sphincter of Oddi motility. Br J Surg 1989;76:709–14.
98. Dahlstrand C, Edin R, Dahlstrom A, Ahlman H. An in vivo model for the simultaneous study of motility of the gallbladder, sphincter of Oddi and duodenal wall in the cat. Acta Physiol Scand 1985;123:355–62.
99. Wyatt AP. The relationship of the sphincter of Oddi to the stomach, duodenum and gall-bladder. J Physiol 1967;193:225–43.
100. Thune A, Saccone GTP, Toouli J. Distention of the gallbladder inhibits sphincter of Oddi motility in man. Gut 1991;32:690–3.
101. Toouli J, Di Francesco V, Saccone G, et al. Division of the sphincter of Oddi for treatment of dysfunction associated with recurrent pancreatitis. Br J Surg 1996;83:1205–10.
102. Toouli J, Roberts-Thomson IC, Kellow J, et al. Manometry based randomised trial of endoscopic sphincterotomy for sphincter of Oddi dysfunction. Gut 2000;46:98–102.

Chapter 2

Pathology of the Intrahepatic and Extrahepatic Bile Ducts and Gallbladder

KAY WASHINGTON

Disorders of the biliary system may be divided into small duct diseases and large duct diseases, with little overlap in the level of the biliary tree affected. The large duct diseases include extrahepatic obstruction, most infectious cholangiopathies (Chapter 15), and primary sclerosing cholangitis (Chapter 19). Most immune-mediated diseases of the biliary tract affect small bile ducts; examples include primary biliary cirrhosis (Chapter 21), acute rejection of the hepatic allograft, graft-versus-host disease, and drug-induced bile duct injury (Chapter 22). The modalities that are most useful for diagnosis also differ for these two broad categories of biliary disorders, based on anatomic distribution: liver biopsy is generally necessary for diagnosis of small duct disorders, whereas imaging studies are usually required for diagnosis of large duct diseases (Chapters 3 to 5). Disorders of the bile ducts often present considerable diagnostic difficulty for the practicing pathologist, and interpretation of biopsies and resection specimens with these lesions is best undertaken with thorough consideration of possible differential diagnoses and full knowledge of the clinical setting.

Core needle biopsies of liver continue to have a major role in the evaluation of small duct disorders such as primary biliary cirrhosis, and surgical wedge biopsies are rarely indicated. Fine-needle aspiration biopsies may be used for diagnosis of hepatic mass lesions, including peripheral cholangiocarcinoma, but are of limited use for the diagnosis of inflammatory disorders. Because seeding of neoplastic cells along the needle track, although rare, has been documented for hepatocellular carcinoma and for metastatic tumors, some investigators advocate limiting the use of needle aspiration biopsy (1) and reserving it for nonresectable hepatic mass lesions (2). Cytologic examination of bile duct brushing specimens is the most useful technique for nonsurgical evaluation of biliary strictures, and has a high specificity but relatively low sensitivity for the diagnosis of malignancy (3). Forceps biopsies taken during percutaneous transhepatic cholangioscopy from the margin of stenotic areas in bile duct malignancies may also be useful for diagnosis, especially when two biopsy specimens are obtained (4). Cytologic examination of bile has a lower sensitivity than evaluation of bile duct brushings or biopsies, due to the rapid degeneration of cells shed into bile (5).

PATHOLOGY OF CHOLESTASIS

It is not surprising that cholestasis is a feature of many disorders involving the liver and bile ducts, given that the process of bilirubin formation and bile secretion is complex and involves multiple cell types. For instance, cholestatic disorders may be due primarily to hepatocyte dysfunction, as in some examples of drug-induced hepatic injury; impaired transport of bile into the canaliculus; disorders such as primary biliary cirrhosis that affect primarily the small intrahepatic bile ducts; diseases affecting the larger intrahepatic and extrahepatic bile ducts, such as primary sclerosing cholangitis, or conditions affecting the common bile duct or ampulla of Vater. The accumulation of bile products within the liver results in morphologic patterns of injury that are not difficult to recognize but are unfortunately not specific.

Morphologic patterns of bile accumulation in the liver may be broadly divided into *acute cholestasis* and *chronic cholestasis.* The defining morphologic feature of acute cholestasis is the accumulation of bile pigment in zone 3, most characteristically in canaliculi but also involving hepatocytes and Kupffer cells as the cholestasis becomes progressively severe. Bile pigment may on occasion be confused with other brown pigments that accumulate within the liver; however, in comparison to lipofuscin and iron, bile pigment is less granular and refractile, and has a brown-green hue. Iron is more commonly found in periportal hepatocytes. Lipofuscin is preferentially located in zone 3 hepatocytes and may be quite prominent in livers of elderly persons, but the lack of associated canalicular bile plugs and the granularity of the pigment are diagnostic clues.

Bile ductular proliferation is often but not invariably present in acute cholestasis, but is not specific for cholestatic injury. Proliferating bile ductules may be found at the perimeter of portal tracts in any condition causing periportal fibrosis, but when ductular proliferation is especially prominent and accompanied by canalicular cholestasis, biliary obstruction should be considered. In contrast to the interlobular bile duct, these serpiginous ductular structures are found at the periphery of the portal tract and are not sectioned in the same profile as the branch of the hepatic artery. Proliferating bile ductules invariably attract neutrophils, and the presence of acute inflammatory cells should not lead to a diagnosis of acute cholangitis, which is defined as acute inflammation involving *interlobular* bile duct epithelium.

The histologic hallmark of *chronic cholestasis* is feathery degeneration of hepatocytes (cholate stasis) due to accumulation of bile salts within the cytoplasm, imparting a pale appearance to periportal or periseptal hepatocytes. Canalicular bile plugs are scarce to nonexistent. Periportal and periseptal hepatocytes also accumulate copper in chronic cholestasis, and this copper storage can be demonstrated with a variety of special stains. Orcein or aldehyde fuchsin stains, which are generally used to demonstrate accumulation of hepatitis B surface antigen, will also highlight increased copper binding protein, which, like hepatitis B surface antigen, contains a large number of sulfhydryl groups. Positive staining is seen as granular deposition in periportal hepatocytes (Table 2.1). Any of the special stains for copper itself, such as rhodanine or rubeanic acid stain, may also be used. This copper accumulation is not specific, but when found in a precirrhotic liver biopsy is highly suggestive of chronic cholestasis, if rare entities such as Wilson's disease and Indian childhood cirrhosis have been excluded. Mallory's hyaline may also be found in periportal hepatocytes in chronic cholestasis, and is morphologically indistinguishable from that found in alcoholic liver disease.

DISEASES AFFECTING SMALL BILE DUCTS

Primary Biliary Cirrhosis

Clinical Features

In primary biliary cirrhosis (PBC), the intrahepatic bile ducts are progressively destroyed by a nonsuppurative inflammatory process (Chapter 21). The disease has distinctive clinical features, being found primarily in women (90% of patients) who are mostly in their fifth to seventh decades. PBC is probably autoimmune in etiology, judging by its association with other autoimmune disorders such as Sjögren's disease and keratoconjuctivitis sicca; in some patients, PBC may represent a generalized disorder of lacrimal, salivary, and pancreaticobiliary small duct epithelia. Large intrahepatic and extrahepatic bile ducts are not affected. The most specific feature of PBC is the presence of antimitochondrial antibodies in the serum of 90% of patients affected. Antibodies (M-2) directed to the pyruvate dehydrogenase enzyme complex E2 subunit present on the inner mitochondrial membrane are highly specific (96%) for PBC. Immunoperoxidase staining methods have demonstrated PDC-E2 or a cross-reacting antigen in apical cytoplasm of biliary epithelial cells from patients with PBC (6), suggesting a key role for this antigen in the pathogenesis of the bile duct injury. Circulating autoantibodies such as anti-smooth muscle and anti-nuclear antibodies and rheumatoid factor are often present. Hypergammaglobulinemia with a selective elevation of IgM is often seen.

Table 2.1. Useful stains in evaluation of bile duct lesions

Stain	Shows	Disease
PAS with diastase	Basement membrane	Bile duct injury; PBC
Trichrome	Type I collagen	Useful for identification of bile ducts
Shikata stain (orcein, aldehyde fuchsin, Victoria blue)	Increased copper binding protein in chronic cholestasis	PBC, PSC
Cytokeratin (AE1/AE3)	Biliary epithelium (bile ducts express CK 7, 8, 18, 19)	Ductopenia
Epithelial membrane antigen	Biliary epithelium	Ductopenia
Cross-reactive CEA	Cytoplasmic staining in cholangiocarcinoma; canalicular staining in hepatocellular carcinoma	Useful in distinguishing hepatocellular carcinoma from cholangiocarcinoma or metastatic adenocarcinoma
Monoclonal CEA	Cytoplasmic staining in cholangiocarcinoma	Negative in hepatocellular carcinoma

Most patients with PBC present with fatigue and pruritus, the latter due to the accumulation of bile salts. Many asymptomatic patients are now identified after screening tests show an elevation of their serum alkaline phosphatase levels. Patients are rarely jaundiced early in the course of the disease; indeed, the presence of bile pigment in a liver biopsy suspected of harboring low-stage PBC should prompt a reconsideration of the diagnosis. PBC follows a progressive clinical course in most patients, and most but not all asymptomatic patients will develop significant liver disease.

Pathology

The characteristic lesion of primary biliary cirrhosis is the so-called *florid duct lesion,* sometimes also called chronic nonsuppurative destructive cholangitis (7). Interlobular bile ducts, 40 to 80 microns in diameter, are typically involved. In early stage PBC, the diagnostic lesions may be focal and may not be sampled on needle biopsy. The three components of the florid duct lesion are inflammation, injury to bile duct epithelial cells, and disruption of the bile duct basement membrane. The inflammatory infiltrate is composed of lymphocytes, scattered eosinophils, macrophages, and a variable number of plasma cells, and is intimately associated with the bile duct (Fig. 2.1). The macrophages may be dispersed throughout the portal inflammatory infiltrate or may be aggregated into loose clusters or occasionally into well-formed granulomas. In early stages, the inflammatory infiltrate is largely confined to the portal tract, although granulomas and Kupffer cell aggregates may be present in the lobule. The biliary epithelial cells of injured bile ducts are swollen and focally stratified, may be vacuolated, and are commonly infiltrated by lymphocytes. The basement membrane becomes disrupted and fragmented, which is best visualized by PAS stain. In small portal tracts, bile ducts are often absent and seem to have vanished without a trace, although aggregates of lymphocytes or PAS-positive basement membrane material may mark their former location. Canalicular cholestasis is not a feature of early stage PBC.

As the duct destruction progresses, bile ductular proliferation accompanied by fibrosis develops at the periphery of portal triads, and portal tracts enlarge by this process of biliary piecemeal necrosis. In some cases the inflammatory infiltrate spills over into the adjacent parenchyma, and lymphocytic piecemeal necrosis may mimic chronic hepatitis. At this stage the changes of chronic cholestasis begin to appear, with swollen and rarefied periportal hepatocytes and accumulation of copper. As periportal fibrosis progresses, portal–portal fibrous bridges are formed. Bile ductular proliferation often subsides in late stage PBC, and in the cirrhotic stage little ductular or ductal epithelium can be identified. The cirrhosis has a typical biliary pattern in which the nodules have an irregularly shaped "jigsaw puzzle piece" profile.

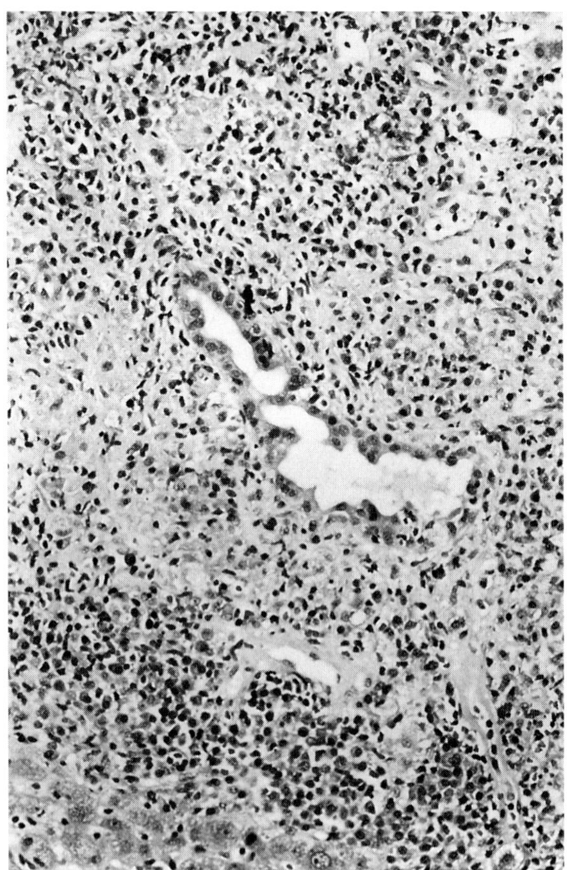

FIGURE 2.1. *Primary biliary cirrhosis. A damaged medium-sized interlobular bile duct is surrounded by a granulomatous inflammatory infiltrate in this florid duct lesion. The bile duct epithelium is infiltrated by lymphocytes.*

Histologic Differential Diagnosis

The term "AMA-negative PBC" or *autoimmune cholangitis* has been applied to cases that are clinically, histologically, and biochemically compatible with PBC except for the lack of identifiable antimitochondrial antibodies. To date, no significant differences between patients with PBC and these AMA-negative patients have been described (8–12). AMA-negative patients were slightly younger in one group (50 vs. 55 years) but were otherwise indistinguishable (8). Although data are largely lacking, it is thought that the response to ursodeoxycholic acid (UDCA) therapy in these patients is the same as for those who are AMA-positive, and there are accordingly no differences in the treatments prescribed for these two groups at the present time.

The differential diagnosis for PBC depends on the stage of the disease. In stage 1 and 2 disease, portal inflammation, piecemeal necrosis, and bile ductular proliferation may mimic *chronic hepatitis,* particularly hepatitis C. Bile duct damage is less prominent in chronic hepatitis and bile duct loss is rarely seen, but lymphocytic infiltration of bile duct epithelium is often a feature of hepatitis C. Clinical information such as antimitochondrial antibody status and serologic markers for viral hepatitis is helpful in most cases.

It may be more difficult to distinguish *autoimmune hepatitis* from PBC, however, and indeed this distinction may prove impossible on histologic grounds. Because treatment for autoimmune hepatitis differs markedly from that for primary biliary cirrhosis, accurate diagnosis is important. Difficulties arise because the portal inflammatory infiltrate of PBC often contains numerous plasma cells, and infiltration of bile duct epithelium by lymphocytes is not uncommon in autoimmune hepatitis, if looked for, and some degree of bile duct injury is often present. However, although nondestructive bile duct lesions are quite common in autoimmune hepatitis, duct loss is generally not a feature, and granulomatous bile duct destruction is not seen. Serum alkaline phosphatase, cholesterol, and IgM levels are elevated to higher levels in PBC. To add to the problem, some patients with clinical and histologic features of autoimmune hepatitis will have serum antimitochondrial antibodies. In some cases this is caused by misreading of immunofluorescence-type tests (confusing anti-LKM antibodies with antimitochondrial antibodies). In other patients, however, the AMA is truly positive, but usually in low titer. Serologic markers may not be definitive in such cases, as patients with PBC may have a positive AMA result, and patients with autoimmune hepatitis may have a low titer AMA. The term "overlap syndrome" is used for cases of autoimmune liver disease with both cholestatic and hepatitic features that do not fit readily into the usual diagnostic categories (13,14).

The existence of this *overlap syndrome* between PBC and autoimmune hepatitis is generally recognized, although investigators disagree over exact classification. Some researchers (13) consider these patients to have PBC, based on duct destruction and presence of AMA, and have proposed that these cases be classified as "PBC, hepatitic form." Others have concluded that overlap of PBC and autoimmune hepatitis is not rare, and that combination therapy with UDCA and steroids is indicated in most of these patients to obtain a biochemical response (14). In a recent study of 12 such patients, the authors found that "overlap" cases constituted 9% of 130 consecutive patients who had a diagnosis of PBC. Because of the observation that some patients diagnosed with PBC have a flare of hepatitic activity when treated with UDCA, it has been proposed that response to UDCA may unmask the hepatitis component in overlap patients (14).

Distinction of PBC from those cases of sarcoidosis with destruction of bile ducts by granulomas may be difficult (15,16). In a study of 100 cases of hepatic sarcoidosis, 58% of the biopsies showed evidence of cholestasis, generally feathery degeneration and increased copper storage (15). Nineteen of these biopsies had bile duct lesions similar to those seen in PBC. The granulomas of sarcoidosis tended to be better formed and more numerous than those of PBC. The lack of AMA positivity and the presence of pulmonary involvement also favor a diagnosis of hepatic sarcoidosis. Of note, sarcoidosis may also cause intrahepatic biliary strictures that have cholangiographic features resembling primary sclerosing cholangitis (17).

Histologic Staging of Primary Biliary Cirrhosis

The value of histologic staging in assessing prognosis in PBC is debatable, given the lack of uniformity of duct loss and fibrosis in the liver in this disease. However, the presence of portal–portal bridging fibrosis on biopsy has been shown to be a poor prognostic sign. Several staging schemes have been described, and there is little practical difference between the two that are most commonly employed, those described by Scheuer (18) and Ludwig (19) (Table 2.2). In stage 1 disease, damage to interlobular bile ducts is seen in the form of the florid duct lesion. In stage 2, the effects of duct injury result in extension of the process to the periportal areas; ductular proliferation, probably representing a compensatory reaction to bile duct loss, is prominent. Stage 3 is characterized as a scarring or precirrhotic stage, with bridging fibrosis. Stage 4 is cirrhosis.

Immune-Mediated Transplant-Associated Cholangiopathies

Acute rejection of the hepatic allograft and acute graft-versus-host disease (GVHD) after bone marrow transplantation share morphologic features, as might be predicted because both are the product of interaction between an immune system and a liver that differ at the major histocompatibility complex (MHC). In a sense, both are iatrogenic cholangiopathies. The bile ducts are the major target of injury in both processes, and small bile ducts are more severely affected than larger ducts. The pathogenesis of bile duct injury is not completely understood, but direct immunologic injury from invading lymphocytes and indirect damage due to cytokine release are plausible mechanisms. In acute rejection, damage to the peribiliary vascular plexus may result in ischemic injury to bile ducts, although this is less likely in GVHD. The presence of immunologically active molecules on the cell surface of biliary epithelium is also a factor in these post-transplant cholangiopathies. For instance, the major blood group antigens and Class I MHC antigens are normally expressed on biliary epithelial cells.

Table 2.2. Staging of primary biliary cirrhosis

Stage	Ludwig	Scheuer	Features
1	Portal	Florid duct lesion	Bile duct injury
2	Periportal	Ductular proliferation	Bile duct loss and portal expansion
3	Septal	Fibrosis	Bridging fibrosis
4	Cirrhosis	Cirrhosis	Nodular architecture

Sources: Ludwig J, Dickson ER, McDonald GS. Staging of chronic nonsuppurative cholangitis (syndrome of primary biliary cirrhosis). Virchows Arch A 1978;379:103–12; Scheuer: Scheuer PJ. Primary biliary cirrhosis. Proc Roy Soc Med 1967;60:1257–60.

Class II MHC antigens, ICAM-1, CD51, and LFA-3 are upregulated and expressed in the setting of inflammation and contribute to the immune-mediated injury (20).

Clinical Features

Acute rejection in the liver is more common in younger patients and patients mismatched at the HLA-DR locus. It generally develops 5 to 21 days after transplantation. Very late presentations are often due to inadequate immunosuppression, either from an attempt to decrease immunosuppression or due to poor patient compliance. Clinical presentation is highly varied, ranging from no symptoms and normal liver tests in patients undergoing protocol biopsies, to malaise and fever with elevated bilirubin, aminotransferases, and alkaline phosphatase (21).

Acute graft-versus-host disease in bone marrow transplantation is more likely to occur in patients receiving HLA-mismatched grafts. Acute GVHD usually occurs 3 to 6 weeks after transplantation and often presents first with skin involvement, followed by gastrointestinal manifestations. Liver involvement is manifested by increased serum alkaline phosphatase, hyperbilirubinemia with jaundice, and mild hepatomegaly. Approximately one-half of the 80% of bone marrow transplantation patients with abnormal liver function tests will have acute hepatic GVHD. Because most patients with hepatic involvement will also have skin and gastrointestinal GVHD, a liver biopsy often is not obtained to diagnose GVHD but rather to rule out other causes of hepatic dysfunction (22).

Histopathologic Features

The most helpful diagnostic features in acute hepatic allograft rejection are the presence of a mixed *portal inflammatory infiltrate* with eosinophils, largely sparing the hepatic parenchyma; *infiltration and injury of bile ducts* by lymphocytes; and *endotheliitis.* The inflammatory infiltrate expands the portal areas and may focally spill over into the adjacent parenchyma. Marked involvement of the hepatic parenchyma is not generally a feature of acute rejection, although this may be seen in very severe cases. The infiltrate is composed of small lymphocytes, large activated lymphocytes, macrophages, eosinophils, and varying numbers of neutrophils. Plasma cells are rare, and immunophenotyping shows that most of the portal lymphocytes are T cells, with both $CD4^+$ and $CD8^+$ cells represented. $CD4^+$ cells mediate graft injury by releasing cytokines which activate other effector cells; the $CD8^+$ cells probably cause injury by direct cytopathic attack on graft cells (21).

Bile duct injury may be focal in mild acute rejection, or bile ducts may be obscured by the inflammatory infiltrate and difficult to identify (Fig. 2.2). The bile duct epithelium is infiltrated by lymphocytes, and the biliary epithelial cells show cell swelling, cytoplasmic vacuolization, nuclear crowding and reactive change such as prominent nucleoli and slight increase in the nuclear/cytoplasmic ratio, and irregular spacing of nuclei. In very mild cases, only cuffing of bile ducts by inflammatory cells and slight reactive changes may be seen. In rejection treated with corticosteroids prior to biopsy, infiltration of bile ducts by neutrophils may be prominent and may mimic biliary obstruction.

Endotheliitis, infiltration of venular endothelium by mononuclear inflammatory cells, is probably overdiagnosed. In addition to the presence of lymphocytes in close proximity to vascular endothelium, there should be evidence of endothelial cell injury such as endothelial cell enlargement and detachment. Both portal veins and central veins may be affected. Occasionally central vein involvement is particularly striking and may be associated with centrilobular hepatocyte necrosis and perivenular hemorrhage. Portal changes typical of acute rejection are sometimes but not always present in such cases. Isolated central venulitis typically responds to usual antirejection therapy (23).

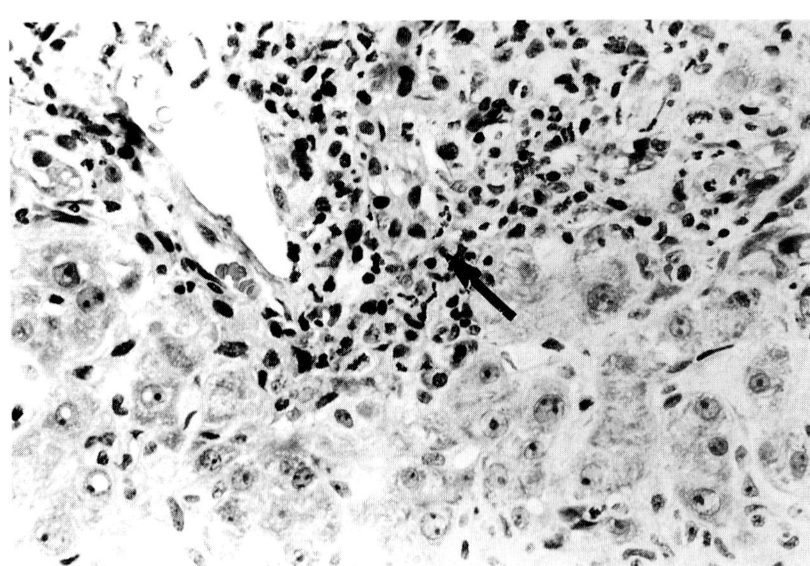

FIGURE 2.2. *Acute allograft rejection. A mixed portal inflammatory infiltrate composed of mononuclear cells and scattered eosinophils and neutrophils is present. The interlobular bile duct (arrow) is difficult to recognize in the midst of the inflammatory infiltrate. The bile duct epithelial cells are swollen and vacuolated.*

Portal inflammation is also a hallmark of acute GVHD, although it is less intense than in acute rejection. As in rejection, the inflammatory infiltrate is predominantly mononuclear; eosinophils and neutrophils are rare. The inflammatory infiltrate centers about bile ducts, which show the diagnostic alterations in hepatic GVHD. Interlobular bile ducts are distorted and angular and focally infiltrated by lymphocytes; the epithelial cell nuclei are irregularly spaced and pleomorphic (Fig. 2.3). As in acute rejection, the lymphocytes infiltrating the bile ducts in acute GVHD are T cells. The bile duct lumen may contain necrotic debris or sloughed epithelial cells. Biopsies taken early in the course of hepatic GVHD (before day 35 after transplant) may not show characteristic bile duct abnormalities, and may show only nonspecific lobular changes such as spotty hepatocyte necrosis (24). In my experience, endotheliitis is rarely if ever seen in acute hepatic GVHD, although a rate of 40% has been reported (25). Cholestasis is a common finding in acute GVHD. Parenchymal necrosis may be seen, but is not specific.

Chronic Allograft Rejection

Chronic rejection in the hepatic allograft generally develops after multiple episodes of acute rejection, or evolves from an episode of unresolved acute rejection. It may rarely occur de novo in the patient who has never had clinical acute rejection. It is usually diagnosed months to years following transplantation. Two major sites of attack are recognized in the liver: interlobular bile ducts and hepatic arteries (21). The bile duct damage generally takes the form of "vanishing bile duct syndrome," in which the bile duct loss is accompanied by only a mild lymphoplasmacytic inflammatory infiltrate. Bile ductular proliferation is not seen, and the portal inflammatory infiltrate subsides with loss of bile ducts, leaving empty-appearing portal tracts (Fig. 2.4). The arterial changes in chronic rejection are rarely seen on liver biopsy, as they preferentially involve the large arteries near the hepatic hilum. This obliterative arteriopathy is characterized by the accumulation of foamy histiocytes in the thickened intimal layer. The resulting ischemia may contribute to bile duct loss. Centrilobular areas in both forms of chronic rejection show spotty hepatocyte necrosis, cholestasis, and perivenular inflammation or fibrosis. Diagnosis of chronic rejection may be difficult to establish with certainty on needle biopsy. For definitive diagnosis, bile duct loss should be seen in at least 50% of portal tracts, although the diagnosis may be suggested in biopsies with a lesser degree of duct loss. Differential diagnosis of chronic ductopenic rejection includes bile duct stricture, drug reaction, and cytomegalovirus infection.

Chronic Graft-versus-Host Disease

Chronic GVHD usually occurs after bouts of acute GVHD but may be seen de novo in a minority of patients (26). The histopathology of chronic GVHD is not well delineated. Like chronic rejection, it is characterized by bile duct distortion and loss and cholestasis. Hepatic involvement occurs in about 90% of patients with chronic GVHD and the skin and oral mucosa are usually involved as well, resulting in scleroderma-like changes and Sjögren's syndrome. Liver biopsy shows a sparse portal mononuclear inflammatory infiltrate with severely distorted interlobular bile ducts and canalicular cholestasis in the lobule. With loss of bile ducts and continued disease progression, changes of chronic cholestasis may be seen and portal fibrosis followed by cirrhosis may develop. Unlike in chronic rejection, arterial changes are not seen. The differential diagnosis includes chronic viral hepatitis; the degree of portal inflammation, piecemeal necrosis, and bile ductular proliferation is generally greater in viral hepatitis, whereas bile duct injury and loss predominate in chronic GVHD.

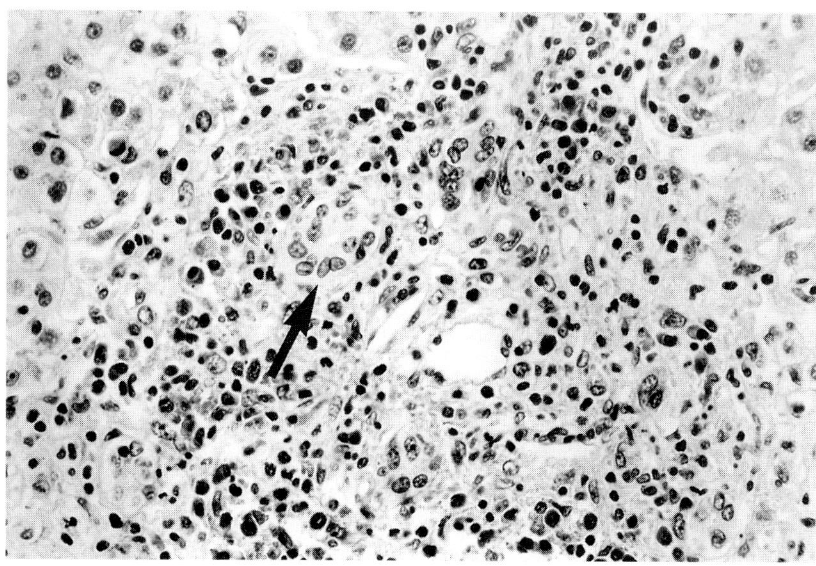

FIGURE 2.3. *Acute graft-versus-host disease. Interlobular bile ducts are the primary target in the liver in acute GVHD. A mononuclear inflammatory infiltrate is often seen around affected bile ducts and infiltrating bile duct epithelium. The bile duct epithelial cells in this example show reactive nuclear enlargement and irregular spacing of nuclei (arrow).*

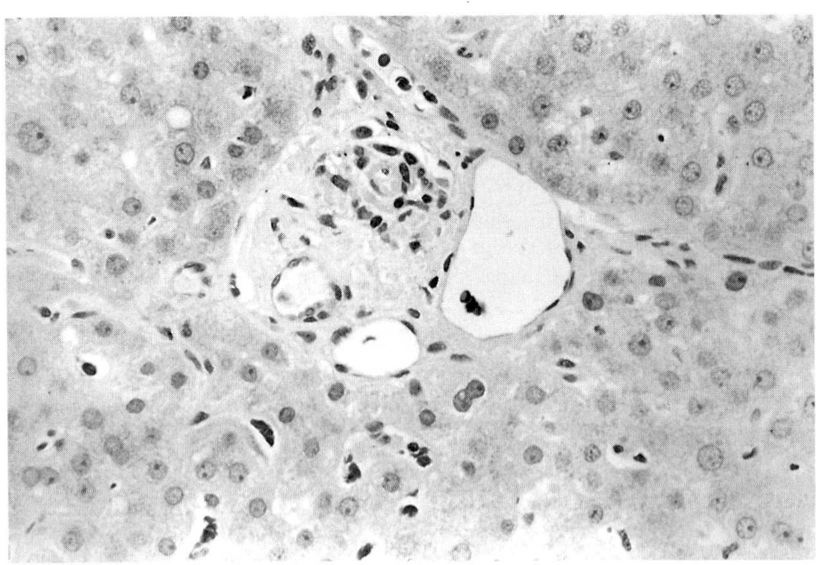

FIGURE 2.4. *Chronic rejection (vanishing bile duct syndrome). The bile duct in this portal tract has vanished, leaving an empty-appearing portal tract with only scattered mononuclear inflammatory cells.*

Table 2.3. Banff scheme: grading of acute hepatic allograft rejection

Global Assessment	Criteria
Indeterminate	Portal inflammatory infiltrate that fails to meet criteria for diagnosis of acute rejection
Mild	Rejection infiltrate in a minority of triads that is generally mild and confined to the portal area
Moderate	Rejection infiltrate that expands most or all of the triads
Severe	As above for moderate, with spillover into periportal areas and moderate to severe perivenular inflammation that extends into the hepatic parenchyma and is associated with perivenular hepatocyte necrosis

Source: Demetris AJ, Batts KP, Dhillon AP, et al. Banff schema for grading liver allograft rejection: an international consensus document. Hepatology 1997;25:658–63.

Grading

Several grading schemes for acute rejection have been developed. Most rely on the density of the portal inflammatory infiltrate, the number of portal tracts involved, the extent of bile duct injury, and the extent of endotheliitis. One of the more recent schemes is the Banff Consensus Schema, which relies upon a global assessment and generation of a rejection activity index by grading individual features (27). At least two of the following three features are required for a histologic diagnosis of acute rejection: mixed portal inflammatory infiltrate, predominantly mononuclear but also containing neutrophils and eosinophils; bile duct damage or inflammation; and endotheliitis involving portal vein branches or terminal hepatic venules. Once the diagnosis of acute rejection has been established by the Banff schema, the grade is assigned based on the global assessment (Table 2.3), which is largely based on the portal inflammatory infiltrate. In addition, a rejection activity index may be generated and a total numerical score based on the sum of the individual component scores assigned (Table 2.4). In comparison to other grading schemes, the Banff schema often results in upgrading of rejection (28).

Acute GVHD is graded clinically by assessing skin, liver, gastrointestinal involvement, and clinical performance status (22). Histopathologic grading of acute hepatic GVHD provides little prognostic information and is often not done, although various schemes have been proposed. Chronic GVHD is graded as limited or extensive based on organ involvement or the presence of severe liver disease. The hepatic involvement is regarded as limited if there is duct injury without piecemeal necrosis, fibrosis, or loss of bile ducts. The designation of extensive chronic hepatic GVHD is reserved for liver biopsies with these features (29).

Adult Idiopathic Ductopenia

The term *idiopathic adulthood ductopenia* has been used to describe a small group of patients with chronic cholestasis of unknown etiology associated with loss of intrahepatic bile ducts. This disorder affects young to middle-aged adults and is more common in males (30). Reported cases probably represent a heterogeneous group of related disorders, with some representing late onset of paucity of intrahepatic bile ducts, primary sclerosing cholangitis involving

Table 2.4. Rejection activity index: Banff scheme

Category	Criteria	Score
Portal inflammation	Mostly lymphocytic infiltrate involving but not expanding a minority of portal tracts	1
	Expansion of most or all of triads by mixed inflammatory infiltrate containing activated lymphocytes, neutrophils, and eosinophils	2
	Marked expansion of most or all triads by mixed infiltrate with numerous lymphoblasts and eosinophils with spillover into periportal parenchyma	3
Bile duct inflammation/damage	A minority of bile ducts are cuffed and infiltrated by inflammatory cells; mild reactive changes such as increased N : C ratio	1
	Most or all ducts infiltrated by inflammatory cells. More than an occasional duct shows degenerative changes such as nuclear pleomorphism, altered polarity, and cytoplasmic vacuolization	2
	As above for 2, with most or all of the ducts showing degenerative changes or focal lumenal disruption	3
Venous endothelial inflammation	Subendothelial lymphocytic infiltration involving some but not a majority of portal and/or hepatic venules	1
	Subendothelial infiltration involving most or all or portal and/or hepatic venules	2
	As above for 2, with moderate or severe perivenular inflammation that extends into the perivenular parenchyma and is associated with perivenular hepatocyte necrosis	3

Source: Demetris AJ, Batts KP, Dhillon AP, et al. Banff schema for grading liver allograft rejection: an international consensus document. Hepatology 1997;25:658–63.

small ducts without large duct involvement, and autoimmune-mediated cholangitis. The criteria generally used for idiopathic adulthood ductopenia are onset of cholestasis in late adolescence or adulthood, ductopenia defined as lack of bile ducts in more than 50% of portal tracts (Fig. 2.5), a normal cholangiogram, and no known etiology. The frequency of this disorder is low and it probably represents less than 5% of cases of chronic cholestasis in adulthood (31).

A mild form of idiopathic loss of intrahepatic bile ducts has also been reported in asymptomatic adults with elevated serum liver tests, mainly γ-glutamyltransferase and alanine aminotransferase concentrations. On biopsy, most portal triads still contained interlobular bile ducts (55% to 78%). Normalization of liver tests was seen in some of the patients treated with ursodeoxycholic acid. It is not clear if some of these patients represented AMA-negative primary biliary cirrhosis, as most were women and mean age at diagnosis was 41 years (32).

Drug-Associated Bile Duct Paucity

Drugs may induce cholestasis by one of three mechanisms: interference with hepatic transport processes and canalicular secretion, resulting in pure hepatocellular cholestasis or cholestatic hepatitis; a small duct cholangiopathy from injury to intrahepatic bile ducts at the level of bile ductules or interlobular bile ducts; and extrahepatic obstruction from sclerosing ischemic lesions of the large bile ducts related to intrahepatic artery chemotherapy (33). As might be predicted given these multiple possible mechanisms, a variety of histologic patterns are seen in drug-related cholestasis, and there are no specific features on liver biopsy that are pathognomonic for drug injury. Therefore, correlation with clinical findings is essential and a high index of suspicion must often be maintained on the part of the pathologist and the gastroenterologist to arrive at a correct diagnosis.

Several different histologic patterns may be seen in drug-induced cholestatic liver disease. One of the more common patterns is that of pure cholestasis, in which bile is seen in canaliculi, hepatocytes, and Kupffer cells, predominantly in zone 3, without portal inflammation or significant hepatocyte necrosis. This "bland" cholestasis without associated inflammatory changes is seen most commonly in patients receiving estrogens and androgenic steroids. The differential diagnosis includes large bile duct obstruction, but the lack of portal edema, inflammation, and bile ductular proliferation generally eliminates this from consideration.

Another common histologic pattern in drug-induced hepatic injury is cholestatic hepatitis, in which canalicular

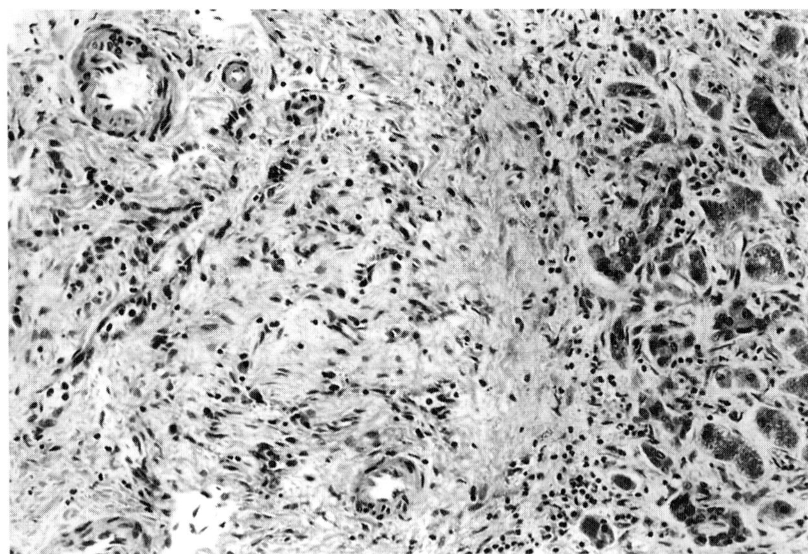

FIGURE 2.5. *Idiopathic adulthood ductopenia is an uncommon cause of biliary cirrhosis. In this example, very few residual interlobular bile ducts were present, and minimal bile ductular proliferation is seen in fibrous septa.*

cholestasis and hepatocyte injury are seen in varying severity. Many different drugs have been associated with this pattern of injury. In many cases, injury to interlobular bile ducts is also present. The bile duct injury may be relatively subtle, consisting of reactive change and focal degenerative changes and cell loss in bile duct epithelium, or there may be overt loss of bile ducts, resulting in ductopenia. Infiltration of bile ducts by inflammatory cells, generally lymphocytes, may be seen in some cases but is often minimal. A second pattern of drug-related bile duct injury results in acute cholangitis, with bile ductular proliferation and infiltration of bile ducts by neutrophils. Drug-induced prolonged cholestasis is diagnosed when jaundice persists for more than 6 months or liver tests indicate continued cholestasis for more than 1 year after withdrawal of the offending agent (34). In some patients, liver biopsies show changes similar to primary biliary cirrhosis. In time, most patients recover, although it may take several years for liver tests to return to normal, and in some patients the disease is irreversible and results in biliary cirrhosis.

Acute cholestatic liver disease with loss of intrahepatic bile ducts on liver biopsy has been linked to a number of drugs, most commonly neuroleptics, anticonvulsants, and antibiotics; specific examples include ibuprofen, carbamazepine, chlorpromazine, trimethoprim-sulfamethoxazole, and tetracycline (35–37). The pathogenesis of drug-induced bile duct injury is unclear. Most of the drugs associated with drug-related bile duct paucity undergo biotransformation to toxic intermediates, which may result in direct cellular injury. More likely, immune response targeting bile duct epithelial cells may be responsible, as prolonged cholestasis has been most often seen with drugs considered to induce acute hepatitis or cholestatic hepatitis through a hypersensitivity mechanism.

In early stages of drug-induced bile duct injury, bile duct epithelial cells are swollen and vacuolated. Pyknotic nuclei and mitotic figures may be seen; some bile ducts may appear atrophic and ductopenia has been reported as early as 10 days following onset of jaundice (36). Occasionally severe injury of bile ducts by inflammatory cells may be seen (Fig. 2.6). Marked canalicular cholestasis is generally present in zone 3, and a mild lobular hepatitis with occasional eosinophils may be seen. The portal inflammatory infiltrate is variable in density but often contains eosinophils. In a report of eight patients with prolonged drug-induced cholestasis, most biopsies taken 9 to 14 months after the onset of jaundice did not show lobular hepatitis. Some biopsies showed mild portal fibrosis and in all cases were ductopenic. All cases in this series showed some degree of portal inflammation and bile ductular proliferation in the chronic phase. Biopsies taken after 24 months did not demonstrate canalicular bile plugs, lobular inflammation, or hepatocyte necrosis. Extensive portal fibrosis occurred in some patients, and ductopenia persisted in some. Three of the eight patients reported had complete clinical recovery and normalization of liver tests, by 22, 23, and 27 months after the onset of jaundice (37).

On a practical note for the surgical pathologist, it is important to remember that prolonged cholestasis with ductopenia on liver biopsy may be seen in hepatic injury from many different types of drugs. The liver biopsy may be obtained late after the initial insult and withdrawal of the offending agent, and is often primarily done to rule out other causes of liver dysfunction. The differential diagnosis includes other small duct cholangiopathies and causes of chronic cholestasis such as primary biliary cirrhosis, primary sclerosing cholangitis, and idiopathic adulthood ductopenia. Acute onset of disease, an appropriate drug history, and a period of jaundice suggest a drug-induced lesion. Thoughtful correlation with appropriate clinical information is essential for proper interpretation.

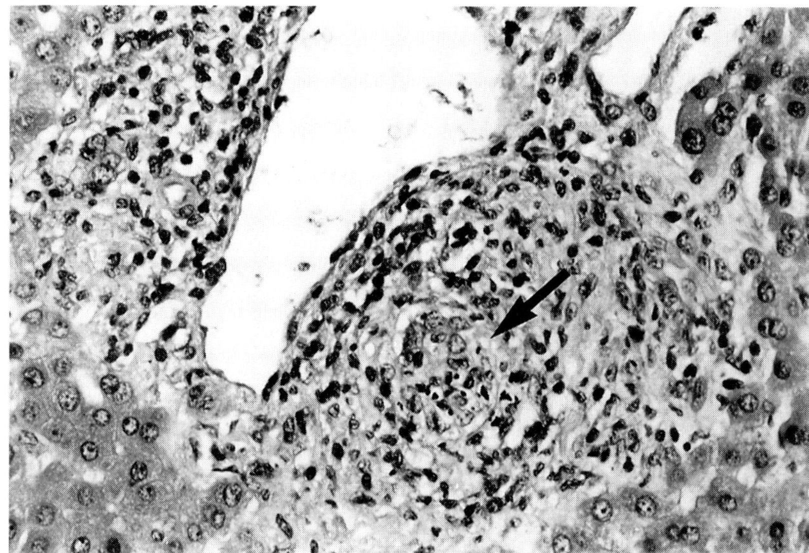

FIGURE 2.6. *Bile duct injury associated with antibiotic therapy. The portal triad contains a mixed inflammatory infiltrate. The interlobular bile duct (arrow) is almost unrecognizable because of heavy infiltration of duct epithelium in this example of drug-induced cholestasis associated with amoxicillin/clavulanate (Augmentin) therapy.*

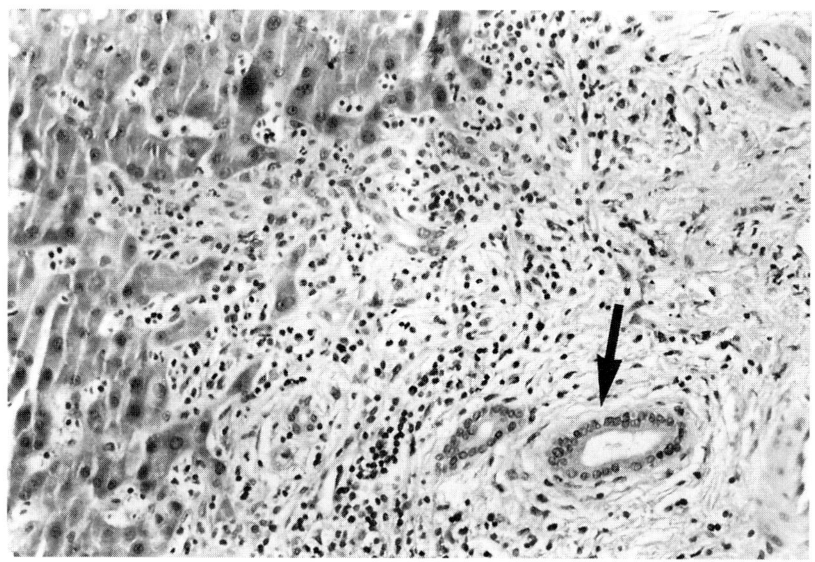

FIGURE 2.7. *In large duct obstruction, periductal edema (arrow), though a characteristic finding, is not always present. Bile ductular proliferation may be seen at the perimeter of portal tracts.*

DISEASES AFFECTING LARGE BILE DUCTS

Large Duct Obstruction

The earliest change in the liver in obstruction of extrahepatic or large intrahepatic bile ducts is accumulation of bile in zone 3 canaliculi. Liver biopsy is rarely performed at this early stage, however. Portal changes are diffuse throughout the portion of liver affected and include edema, often accentuated around bile ducts; inflammation; and bile ductular proliferation. Early in the course of obstruction, the portal inflammatory infiltrate consists primarily of neutrophils, although increasing numbers of mononuclear cells are seen if obstruction persists. Scattered eosinophils may also be seen. Neutrophils are associated with proliferating bile ductules, which are seen at the periphery of the portal tract as serpiginous structures often lacking a well-defined lumen. Proliferating ductules, unlike the interlobular bile duct, are not cut in the same cross-sectional profile as the branch of the hepatic artery. Periductal edema (Fig. 2.7) is more specific for biliary obstruction than proliferating bile ductules but is often not present. Ductal cholestasis, if present, is considered a near-pathognomonic feature of large bile duct obstruction. If bacterial infection of the biliary tract is superimposed, neutrophils may be seen in interlobular bile duct epithelium and lumina. This pattern of inflammation is often considered suggestive of ascending cholangitis, but is not pathognomonic.

If obstruction continues, bile accumulation continues, involving zone 1, bile duct, and bile ductules. In longstanding severe obstruction, bile infarcts and bile lakes, due to rupture of bile ducts with resulting extravasation of bile, may be seen in the lobule, although these are rarely sampled on liver biopsy. In severe cholestasis, hepatocyte necrosis may be seen in the lobule, primarily involving zone 3. In chronic large duct obstruction, portal fibrosis is seen, and the portal inflammatory infiltrate contains more lymphocytes, although neutrophils are still present. Periductal fibrosis around large ducts may be seen and should not be considered diagnostic of primary sclerosing cholangitis. Cholate stasis and Mallory's hyaline are seen in periportal hepatocytes. With long-standing obstruction, portal–portal bridging may develop and lead to the development of biliary cirrhosis.

Recurrent Pyogenic Cholangitis

Recurrent pyogenic cholangitis is a bacterial form of cholangitis that occurs almost exclusively in patients of Asian origin (Chapter 15). Many of the histologic features in this disorder are a result of bile stasis. Biliary parasites are present in some but not all cases. Repetitive bacterial infection and pigment stone formation occur, resulting in biliary strictures, which in turn predispose to infection and more stone formation. Large intrahepatic ducts are affected (Fig. 2.8A) and are scarred, are thickened, and contain biliary sludge and stones. Microscopically, fibrosis and inflammation are present in the walls of large ducts. Small portal tracts show acute cholangitis, portal edema, and varying degrees of fibrosis (38) (see Fig. 2.8B). Cholangiocarcinoma arising in large stone-bearing ducts may complicate the disease. Inflammatory pseudotumors have also been reported in recurrent pyogenic cholangitis (39).

Primary Sclerosing Cholangitis

Clinical Features

In contrast to primary biliary cirrhosis, which more commonly affects women, primary sclerosing cholangitis (PSC) is a disease of men, with a male predominance of 2:1 (Chapter 19). The median age of onset is low (30 years) but there is an extraordinarily wide age range of 1 to 90 years.

(A)
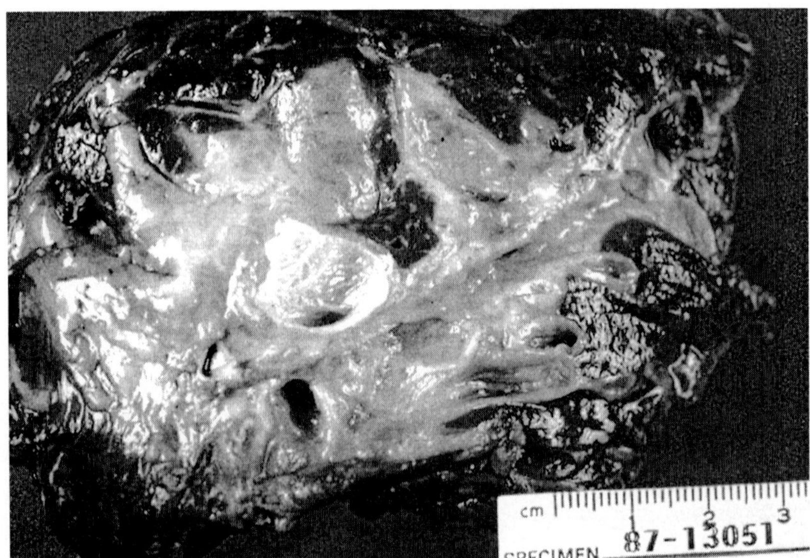

(B)
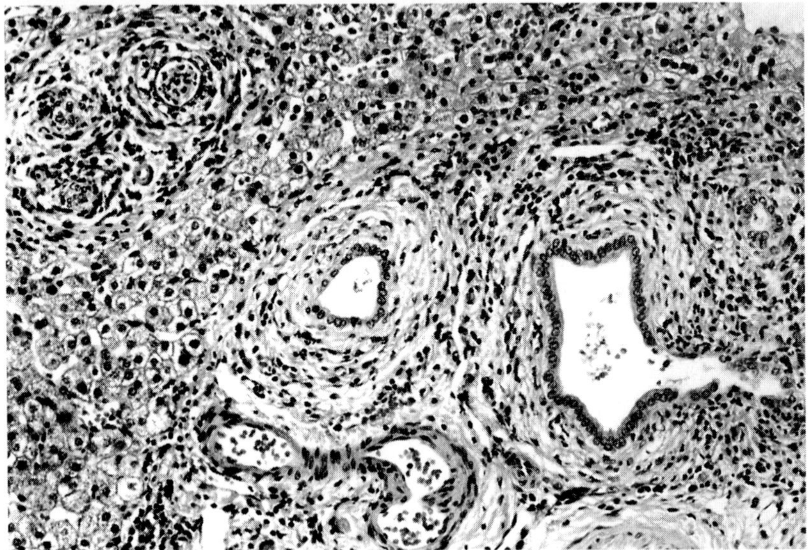

FIGURE 2.8. *Recurrent pyogenic cholangitis. **(A)** The large bile ducts are dilated and scarred by fibrous tissue. Biliary sludge and stones have been removed in this example. **(B)** The small portal tracts in recurrent pyogenic cholangitis show changes of large duct obstruction, and contain a mixed inflammatory infiltrate with numerous neutrophils. Portal edema and fibrosis may also be seen.*

PSC was previously thought to be rarer than PBC, but is probably about equal in prevalence. The prevalence of PSC in the United States is estimated at 2 to 7 cases/100,000 population (40), but this is likely to be an underestimate.

The association of PSC with ulcerative colitis remains an enigma. Approximately 70% of patients with PSC have ulcerative colitis. Conversely, 3% to 7.5% of patients with ulcerative colitis have PSC. The ulcerative colitis typically involves a majority of the colon, but often has a relatively mild clinical course. Patients with PSC and ulcerative colitis may be at even higher risk for adenocarcinoma of the colon than the usual patient with ulcerative colitis. Like PBC, PSC is considered to be a disease of autoimmunity, and a marked increase in prevalence of HLA antigens B8 and DR3 has been found in patients with PSC (41). The HLA B8, DR3 haplotype has been associated with a number of autoimmune diseases such as autoimmune hepatitis, thyroiditis, celiac disease, and myasthenia gravis.

The natural history of PSC is more variable than that of PBC. For the most part PSC is a progressive disease. Because of the presence of bile duct strictures and the formation of biliary stones and sludge, PSC is commonly complicated by bacterial cholangitis. The development of cholangiocarcinoma is a major complication, seen in up to 16% of PSC patients. Accurate diagnosis of cholangiocarcinoma remains a problem in many cases, as tumors may be indistinguishable from strictures on the cholangiogram and accurate cytologic diagnosis from bile duct brushings may be exceedingly difficult. Elevated CA19–9 levels, if greatly elevated, may be of utility, although considerable overlap with PSC without cancer is seen (42).

Diagnosis and Role of Liver Biopsy

Diagnosis of PSC is established on radiographic grounds, by the cholangiographic appearance of beading and irregularity of the biliary system; indeed, cholangiography is the diagnostic gold standard for PSC. Although serum antineutrophilic antibodies (ANCA) are present in 80% of PSC patients, this test is considered of limited use in diagnosis because of overlap with autoimmune hepatitis. Liver biopsy is undertaken to rule out other causes of liver disease and for staging purposes. Most hepatologists understand that liver biopsy is rarely diagnostic in this disease, as the disease process may be patchy in the liver and small intrahepatic bile ducts may not show diagnostic changes.

Pathologic Features

A wide variety of morphologic changes that reflect the varying levels of duct involvement are seen in PSC. Most of the histologic changes early in the course of the disease occur in the portal tract. Unfortunately, the classic lesion of periductal concentric "onion-skinning" fibrosis is rarely seen in needle biopsy specimens. This pattern of fibrosis often has only a sparse inflammatory infiltrate. The bile duct epithelium is atrophic and epithelial cells are shrunken, with pyknotic nuclei (Fig. 2.9). A rounded scar often marks the site of a destroyed bile duct. Alternatively the smaller interlobular bile ducts may vanish without a trace (43), especially in pediatric cases, and residual scars are not identified. Interlobular bile ducts may be distorted in a subtle fashion, with only angulated profiles and irregular spacing of duct cell nuclei to indicate epithelial injury. The bile duct epithelium may be vacuolated and focally infiltrated by lymphocytes. The portal inflammatory infiltrate is usually sparse and primarily made up of mononuclear inflammatory cells, with scattered eosinophils. Early in the disease portal eosinophils may be unusually prominent. Portal granulomas are distinctly unusual, although a granulomatous response to leakage of bile products does occur in 3% to 4% of biopsies (44). Lobular changes early in the disease are generally minor; late in the disease, changes of chronic cholestasis are common. The pattern of fibrosis is similar to that seen in primary biliary cirrhosis.

Changes of large duct obstruction are often superimposed on small duct changes of PSC. Bile ductular proliferation is common, and periductal edema and acute cholangitis may also be seen, especially in the setting of bacterial cholangitis. Canalicular bile plugs may be present.

The large bile ducts most commonly involved by PSC are of course not present in needle biopsy specimens. In the liver explant, larger intrahepatic bile ducts are often dilated and contain inspissated bile plugs and sludge. The walls of large bile ducts are fibrotic and contain chronic inflammatory cells. Reactive changes in entrapped peribiliary glands can pose a diagnostic dilemma in evaluation of surgical biopsies of these large ducts to rule out cholangiocarcinoma. Clues to malignancy are unequivocal perineural invasion, cribriform glandular structures, and pronounced nuclear pleomorphism and atypia (45). The peribiliary glands are grouped in lobular clusters, although this may be difficult to discern in the fibrotically distorted specimen.

Staging

The histologic staging schemes used for primary sclerosing cholangitis (40) are similar to those used for primary biliary cirrhosis (Table 2.5).

Differential Diagnosis

As for primary biliary cirrhosis, the differential diagnosis for PSC changes with disease stage. Histologic overlap with *primary biliary cirrhosis* is occasionally a problem, although knowledge of the clinical setting, serologic tests, and radiographic appearance generally results in resolution. The portal inflammatory infiltrate in PSC is usually sparser than that seen in PBC, and florid duct lesions are not seen.

Chronic large duct obstruction may be difficult to distinguish from PSC, as extrahepatic obstruction from bile duct strictures is part of the pathologic process in this disease. Periductal fibrosis, bile ductular proliferation, and cholestasis are seen in both obstruction and PSC. However, in large duct obstruction from other causes, loss of interlobular bile ducts and atrophic changes in ductal epithelium do not

(A)

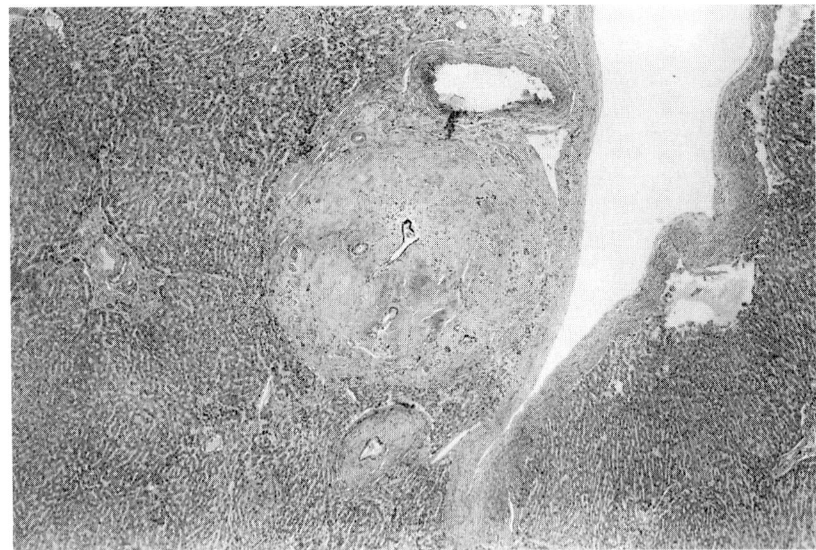

(B)

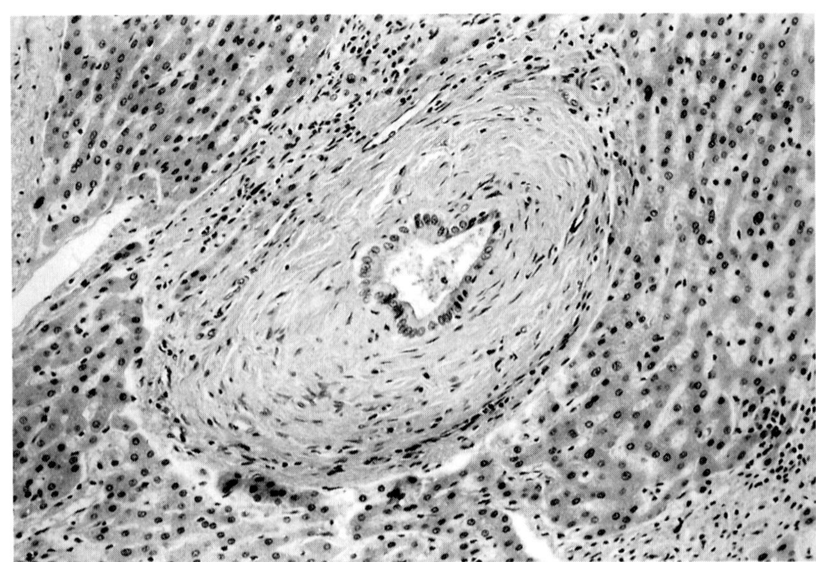

FIGURE 2.9. ***(A)*** *In primary sclerosing cholangitis, affected bile ducts are obliterated by dense fibrous tissue.* ***(B)*** *Concentric periductal "onion-skinning" fibrosis with atrophy and injury to bile duct epithelium is the classic lesion seen in PSC, but this pattern of ductal injury is not seen in all cases and may be absent in needle biopsy specimens.*

Table 2.5. Staging of primary sclerosing cholangitis

Stage	Designation	Features
1	Portal	Duct abnormalities
2	Periportal	Ductular proliferation
3	Septal	Bridging fibrous septa
4	Cirrhosis	Nodular architecture

Source: Weisner RH, Porayko MK, LaRusso NF, Ludwig J. Primary sclerosing cholangitis. In: Schiff L, Schiff ER, eds. Diseases of the liver. 7th ed. Philadelphia: J.B. Lippincott, 1993:411–26.

occur. The presence of numerous eosinophils in the portal inflammatory infiltrate also favors PSC.

In pediatric patients with PSC, overlap of clinical and histopathologic features with *autoimmune hepatitis* may occur (46). Although alkaline phosphatase is usually elevated in adults with PSC, normal alkaline phosphatase levels may be seen in children with the disease; in one study of 32 children with PSC, 15 had normal alkaline phosphatase levels at presentation (46). Most pediatric patients with PSC will also have ulcerative colitis (55%), although this figure is less than the commonly quoted 70% in adults. The cholangiogram may show very subtle irregularity of bile ducts, without overt stricture formation; predominance of intrahepatic disease is common in childhood PSC. Concentric periductal fibrosis is rarely seen in biopsies from children; instead, the most notable feature is the loss of interlobular bile ducts, which often seem to vanish without a trace. The portal tracts may contain a dense mononuclear inflammatory infiltrate, with piecemeal necrosis and scattered plasma cells, further resembling autoimmune hepatitis. A high index of suspicion on the part of the gastroenterologist and the pathologist is often necessary to make the diagnosis of PSC in the pediatric patient.

Secondary Sclerosing Cholangiopathies

Other causes of biliary strictures are *intrahepatic artery chemotherapy, immunodeficiency syndromes,* and *Langerhans' cell histiocytosis.* Hepatic artery infusion of floxuridine for treatment of hepatic metastases from colorectal carcinoma has been associated with a sclerosing cholangitis-like lesion resulting in hepatic failure. The etiology of these changes may be ischemic rather than toxic, as the bile ducts are supplied by the hepatic artery (47). Although treatment regimens now attempt to minimize the risk of this complication, one study reported a 1-year rate of sclerosing cholangitis of 25% (48).

Langerhans' cell histiocytosis may present with isolated hepatic involvement or with involvement of other organ systems, most commonly lymph node and skin. In one recent study, 7 of 9 cases demonstrated injury to small and medium intrahepatic bile ducts by infiltrating Langerhans' cells (49). Concentric periductal fibrosis similar to that of primary sclerosing cholangitis was a feature of most cases, and bile ductular proliferation was often prominent. Of note, two cases with a PSC-like pattern of injury had no detectable Langerhans' cells in the liver, and the diagnosis was established by biopsy of extrahepatic sites.

Infectious cholangiopathies may also mimic PSC. The most common infectious agents associated with this pattern of hepatic injury are cytomegalovirus and cryptosporidium, seen primarily in the AIDS population. Microsporidial species, Cyclospora, and mycobacterial avium complex are also biliary pathogens in this setting (50) and may be identified in biopsy or cytologic samples. Periampullary small bowel biopsies, bile duct brushings, or biopsies of the common bile duct are commonly used for diagnosis. Clinical presentation of AIDS-related cholangiopathies is variable, ranging from asymptomatic to severe right upper quadrant pain. Many patients will also have diarrhea as the infectious agents are also enteric pathogens.

The mechanism of bile duct injury in cryptosporidial infection has recently been elucidated by studies using cultured biliary epithelial cells (51) and an animal model (52). In immunodeficient SCID mice, T cell cytokines appear to be required for inflammatory and sclerosing response to cryptosporidial infection (52). Studies on cultured biliary epithelial cells have shown that the sporozoite form of the organism invades the luminal but not the basolateral surface of biliary epithelium; it resides in a tight-fitting vacuole formed by invagination of the plasma membrane, where it is able to undergo a complete reproductive cycle. Widespread apoptosis of epithelial cells occurred within hours after infection (51).

Some children with primary immunodeficiency develop sclerosing cholangitis. Although many of these cases are undoubtedly related to persistent biliary tract infections, in others no infectious agent has been demonstrated. In one report of 56 children with PSC, 8 (14%) had a primary immunodeficiency syndrome that was associated with cryptosporidial infection in 3, cytomegalovirus in 3, and no demonstrable organisms in 2 (53). In our practice, we have seen PSC-like lesions in two children with immunodeficiency: one with severe combined immunodeficiency treated with bone marrow transplantation, and one with common variable immunodeficiency.

FIBROPOLYCYSTIC DISEASES

Cystic diseases of the liver may be broadly divided into the categories of infectious cystic lesions (which are of course not cysts, as they lack an epithelial lining) and true epithelial cysts. Epithelial cysts may be further subdivided into mucinous cystic neoplasms, and non-neoplastic cysts. The non-neoplastic cysts include sporadic *simple cysts,* which are generally clinically silent and discovered incidentally. These are typically solitary and are lined by a single layer of columnar or flattened biliary-type epithelium. Also included in lists of sporadic hepatic cysts is the *ciliated hepatic foregut cyst,* considered developmental in origin. These rare lesions are lined by pseudostratified columnar epithelium with mucus cells; the underlying fibrous wall contains smooth muscle fibers (54). *Perihilar cysts* arise from periductal glands in the hepatic hilum and may be found in a variety of conditions. They probably represent retention cysts from blockage of drainage of these periductal glands. Generally asymptomatic, large perihilar cysts occasionally cause large duct obstruction.

The disorders known collectively as *fibropolycystic diseases of the liver* (Chapter 16) are characterized by dilatation and varying degrees of fibrosis of different levels of the intrahepatic biliary tree. These disorders include congenital hepatic fibrosis, Caroli's disease, Caroli's syndrome, multiple von Meyenburg complexes, and polycystic liver disease; these may occur singly or in various combinations. The essential precursor of the hepatic lesions is the failure of bile ductal plate remodeling during embryogenesis. This ductal plate malformation may occur at different levels in the biliary tree, from small interlobular bile ducts to large segmental ducts, thus leading to a spectrum of clinicopathologic entities (55–57). Features in common include association with various cystic diseases of the kidney, mendelian inheritance patterns, and increased risk of cholangiocarcinoma.

Congenital Hepatic Fibrosis

Congenital hepatic fibrosis is a disorder that is usually inherited in an autosomal recessive fashion, in most cases associated with autosomal recessive polycystic kidney disease (ARPKD), but in some cases paradoxically associated with autosomal dominant polycystic kidney disease (ADPKD). It is characterized by persistence of the embryologic ductal plate, with dilatation of the residual duct-like structures around the periphery of the portal tract (Fig. 2.10). Normal interlobular bile ducts may or may not be present. Exten-

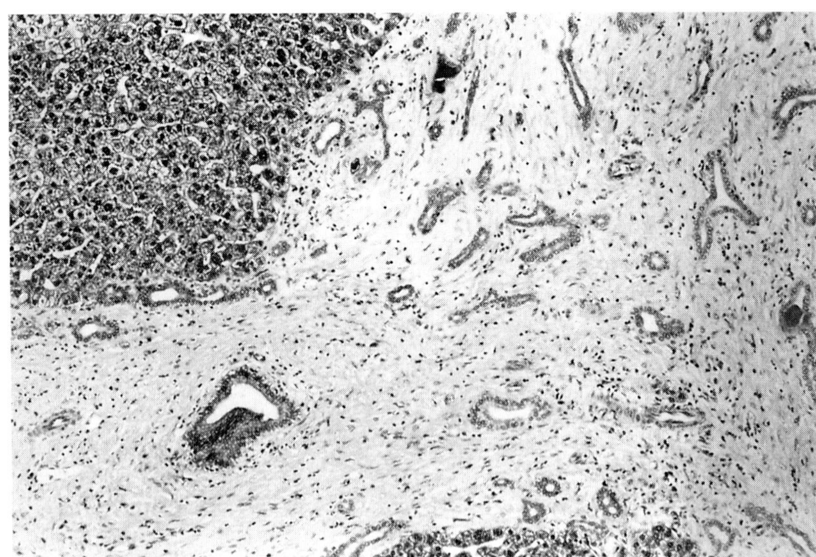

FIGURE 2.10. *Congenital hepatic fibrosis. The hepatic parenchyma is distorted by fibrous expansion of portal tracts containing numerous abnormal biliary channels. These dysmorphic anastomosing biliary channels are arranged around the perimeter of the enlarged portal tracts. The adjacent liver is noncirrhotic.*

sive portal–portal bridging fibrosis is usually present and may lead to an erroneous diagnosis of cirrhosis. However, in contrast to cirrhosis, the hepatic parenchymal architecture is normal, without evidence of regeneration.

Four forms of congenital hepatic fibrosis are described, based on clinical presentation: *portal hypertensive, cholangitic, mixed,* and *latent.* In young children with ARPKD, the renal symptoms may predominant and the hepatic lesion may be discovered only upon investigation. The most common mode of presentation of the liver disease is portal hypertension, with patients presenting as teenagers with splenomegaly or bleeding from esophageal varices. The isolated cholangitic form of congenital hepatic fibrosis is uncommon. Many patients, as in this case, have the latent form of congenital hepatic fibrosis that is found incidentally in later life. The natural history of the disorder is often dominated by the renal disease (58). Patients with portal hypertension may have normal growth and hepatic function. Those with the cholangitic form are at greater risk for hepatic dysfunction.

Caroli's Disease and Caroli's Syndrome

Caroli's disease and syndrome are both disorders characterized by the presence of multiple saccular dilatations of the larger segmental intrahepatic bile ducts. Caroli's syndrome combines this cyst formation in large ducts with congenital hepatic fibrosis, and is thus thought to represent a sustained insult to development of the intrahepatic biliary system. In contrast, Caroli's disease affects only segmental bile ducts, and may be a result of a hereditary factor acting at a particular point in the development of the biliary tree (55–57). The dilated ducts (Fig. 2.11) are subject to bile sludging and predispose the individual to multiple bouts of cholangitis. Continued obstruction may lead to secondary biliary cirrhosis. Approximately 15% of cases involve only a portion of the liver, most commonly the left lobe; such cases are amenable to surgical resection. An increased risk of cholangiocarcinoma is reported, and amyloidosis may occur as a result of chronic infection.

Von Meyenburg Complexes

Von Meyenburg complexes are small lesions, also called bile duct hamartomas, that are generally asymptomatic and are often diagnosed during intraoperative frozen section consultation or at autopsy. When multiple, they may represent the forme fruste of polycystic liver disease. The von Meyenburg complex consists of dilated biliary channels, sometimes containing inspissated bile, embedded in fibrous stroma at the periphery of a portal tract (Fig. 2.12). Although it was previously thought that von Meyenburg complexes did not communicate directly with the biliary tree, recent studies have shown their continuity with the intrahepatic bile ducts, thus supporting origin from the ductal plate. The lesion probably represents a slowly involuting remnant of the ductal plate of a small peripheral interlobular bile duct (55,56). Multiple von Meyenburg complexes are found in polycystic liver disease, and give rise to the macroscopic cysts of that disorder.

Polycystic Liver Disease

Patients with polycystic liver disease usually have ADPKD. The liver cysts are not present at birth, but develop over time as fluid accumulates in the dilated biliary spaces of von Meyenburg complexes. Up to 30% of young adults will have liver cysts; this prevalence increases to 90% in older patients. Multiple unilocular cysts resembling simple biliary cysts and ranging in size from a few millimeters to over 10 cm in diameter are scattered diffusely throughout the liver (Fig. 2.13). The cysts usually do not compromise hepatic

(A)

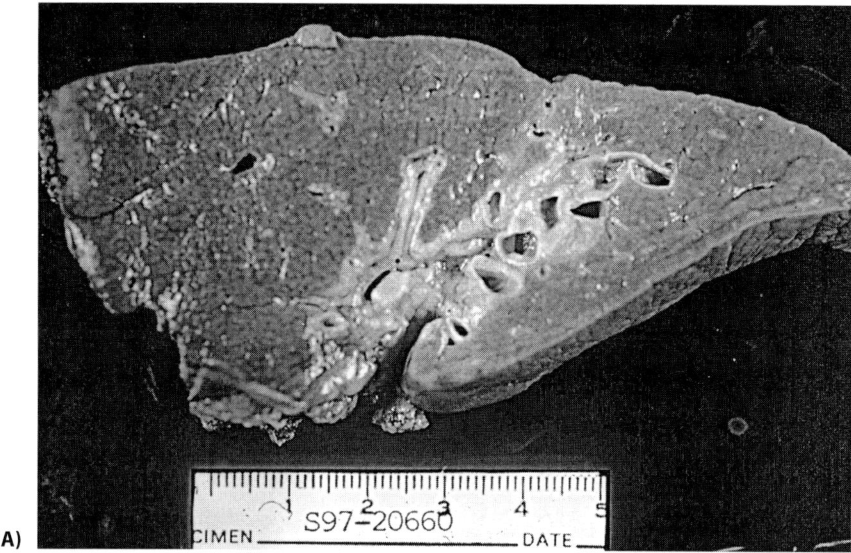

(B)

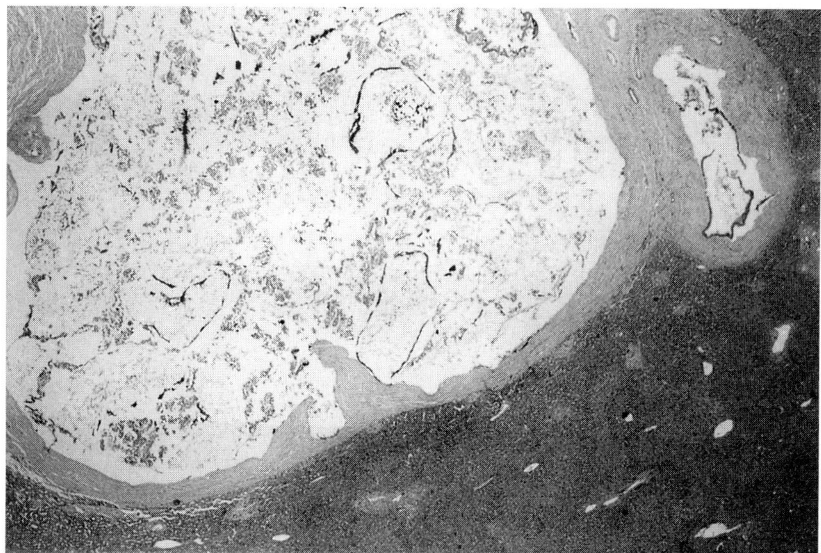

FIGURE 2.11. *Caroli's disease.* ***(A)*** *Involvement of large intrahepatic bile ducts by the ductal plate malformation process gives rise to congenital dilatation of bile ducts in Caroli's disease. The lesion may be confined to one lobe of the liver, generally the left lobe, and may thus be amenable to resection.* ***(B)*** *The dilated cuts are predisposed to bile stasis, stone formation, and infection.*

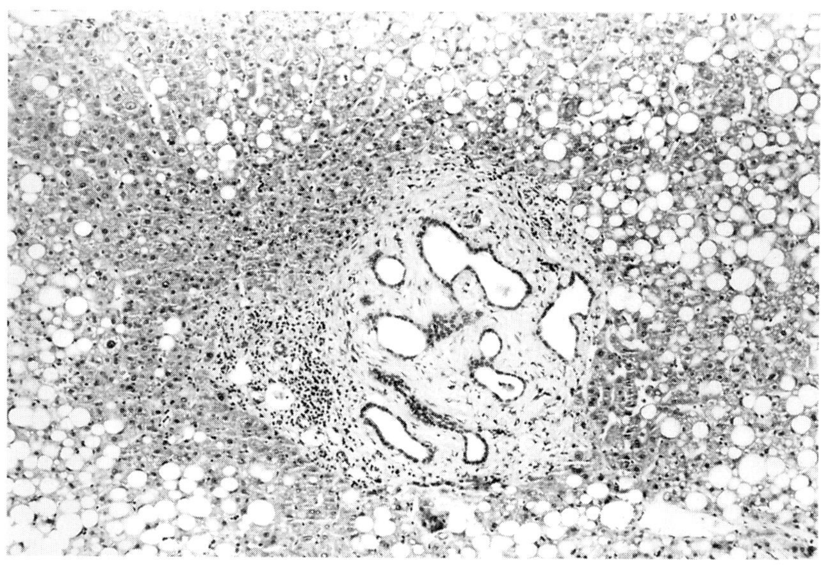

FIGURE 2.12. *The von Meyenburg complex, or biliary microhamartoma, consists of dilated biliary channels associated with a portal tract. These, when single or few in number, are generally incidental findings, but when multiple are considered part of the spectrum of ductal plate malformation disorders. The adjacent liver in this example is steatotic.*

(A)

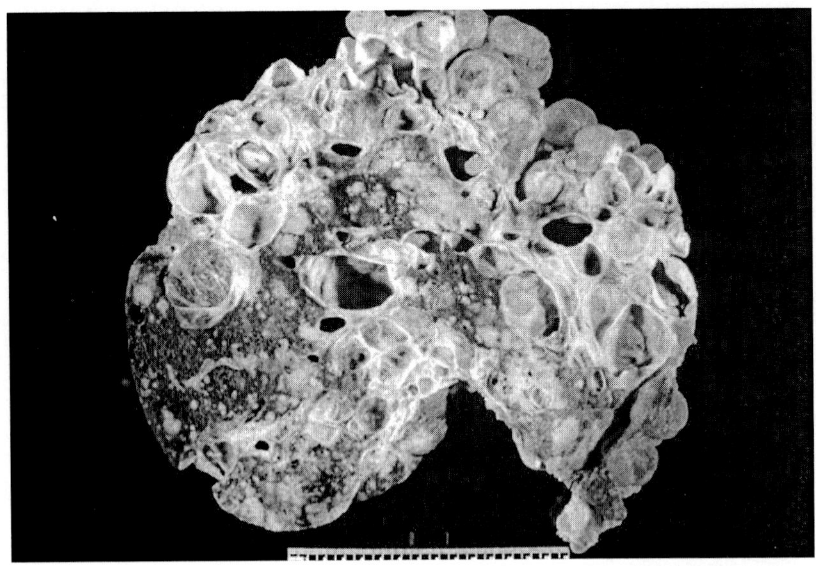

(B)

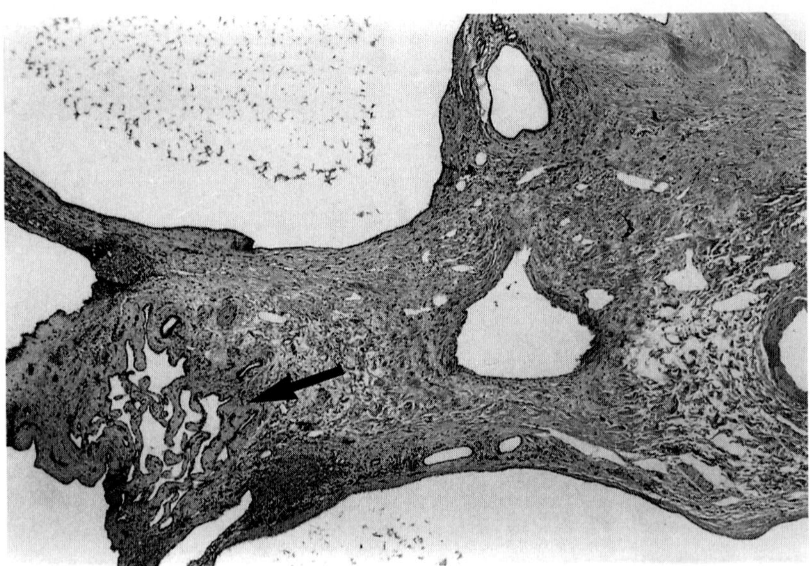

FIGURE 2.13. *Polycystic liver disease.* ***(A)*** *Multiple unilocular cysts of varying sizes are found in the liver in polycystic liver disease. In this example, the noncystic portion of the liver is also involved by metastatic pancreatic carcinoma.* ***(B)*** *The cysts are lined by a simple cuboidal to low columnar biliary type epithelium. Von Meyenburg complexes (arrow) are frequently found in the vicinity of the cysts and probably give rise to them by progressive accumulation of fluid.*

function but may produce hepatomegaly and abdominal discomfort. Women are more likely to be symptomatic from the cysts, and morbidity is related to number of pregnancies, use of oral contraceptives, and severity of renal involvement (59).

Pathogenesis

The currently favored theory for the pathogenesis of the fibropolycystic disorders is that a single gene defect causes maturational arrest of biliary and renal tubular epithelial cells. Approximately 95% of autosomal dominant polycystic kidney disease has been linked to mutations in one of two genes. PKD1, located on chromosome 16 and mutated in 85% of patients with ADPKD, encodes an integral membrane glycoprotein, polycystin-1. The second gene implicated in ADPKD, PKD2, is responsible for 5% to 10% of cases and is located on chromosome 4. PKD2 also encodes an integral membrane protein, known as polycystin-2. Patients with PKD2 mutations are similar clinically to patients with PKD1 mutations, but present later in life with renal disease (60). Germline mutations in these genes are inactivating. Although ADPKD is inherited in a dominant fashion, it is believed that the disease is recessive on a cellular level, in that loss of the wild-type allele in renal or hepatic epithelial cells (the second hit hypothesis) is necessary for cyst formation (61,62). Mice with targeted mutations of either gene die in embryogenesis, suggesting that these genes are required for normal fetal development. Polycystin-1 is involved in cell–cell or cell–matrix interactions with other proteins. Polycystin-2 is thought to function as a subunit of an ion channel whose activity is regulated by polycystin-1. It is postulated that polycystin-2 forms complexes with itself, polycystin-1, or some unknown protein to function as an ion channel (60). In view of this hypothesis, it is interesting that the coexistence of cystic fibrosis and ADPKD appears to reduce or delay formation of renal and hepatic cysts (63). The interaction of polycystin-1 and polycystin-2 may serve to explain the nearly identical shared phenotype associated with mutations in these genes.

Abnormally elevated expression of the proto-oncogenes c-*myc*, c-*fos*, and c-Ki-*ras* has been demonstrated in cyst epithelium in polycystic kidneys. This altered expression may reflect a maturational arrest in renal tubulo-epithelial cells, with loss of polarization and increased proliferative capacity. It is postulated that dysregulated proliferation of the epithelial cells leads to cyst formation (57). Defective remodeling of the ductal plate probably results in the distinctive hepatic lesions, although the dominant role of the portal vein branches in development of the biliary tree must also be considered, and it is likely that mesenchyme–epithelial cell interaction also plays a role in the pathogenesis of these lesions. Further clarification of these disorders will depend on genetic studies.

Choledochal Cyst

Cystic dilatation of the common bile duct, or choledochal cyst (Fig. 2.14), is generally considered a congenital disorder, although reflux of pancreatic juices into the bile duct because of an anomalous pancreaticobiliary junction has also been implicated (Chapter 16). Classification is based on anatomic location and extent (64) (Table 2.6). Microscopically, the cyst wall is fibrotic and variably inflamed. The biliary epithelial lining is often denuded; goblet cell metaplasia and squamous metaplasia have been described. Complications include biliary obstruction, cholangitis, cirrhosis, and cholangiocarcinoma. Complete surgical excision is the treatment of choice.

BILIARY DISORDERS OF CHILDHOOD

Cholestasis is a common finding in pediatric liver disease, and the list of diagnostic possibilities is extensive (Chapter

(A)
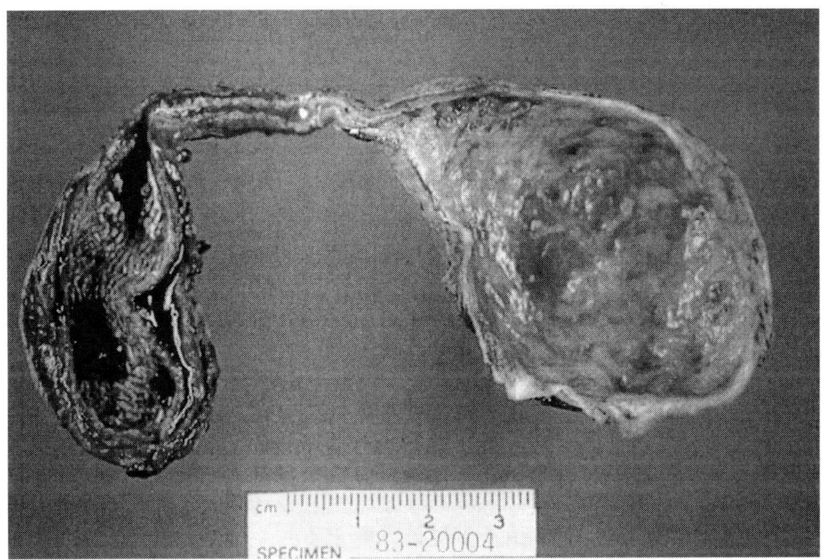

(B)
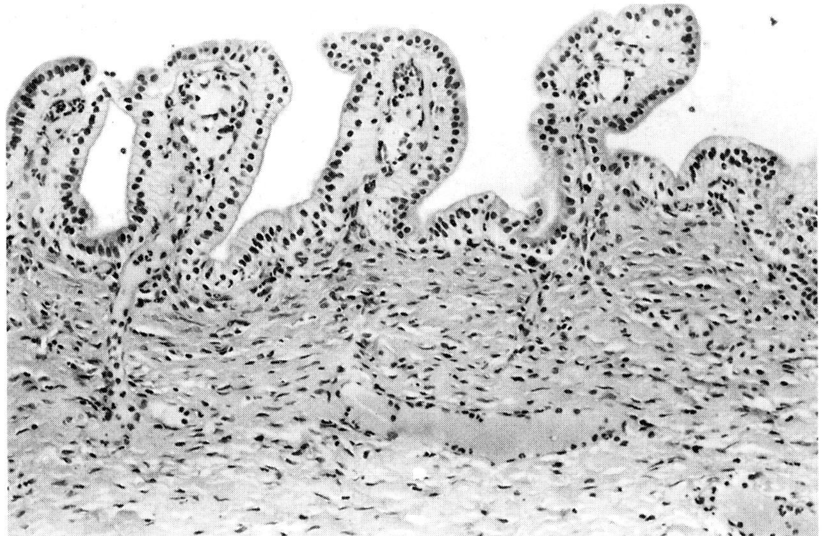

FIGURE 2.14. *Choledochal cyst.* ***(A)*** *This fusiform dilatation of the common bile duct is classified as a type I large choledochal cyst (left). The gallbladder is on the right.* ***(B)*** *The choledochal cyst is usually lined by biliary-type epithelium, although squamous metaplasia may be seen in the setting of inflammation.*

Table 2.6. Classification of choledochal cysts

Type	Features	Comments
I	Segmental or diffuse dilatation of common bile duct	Most common form
II	Diverticulum, usually of lateral wall	
III	Choledochocele, usually in duodenal wall	Usually lined by duodenal mucosa
IV-A	Multiple extrahepatic duct cysts	In association with intrahepatic cysts (Caroli's disease)
IV-B	Multiple extrahepatic duct cysts	Without associated intrahepatic cysts

Source: Matsumoto Y, Uchida K, Nakase A, Houjo I. Clinicopathologic classification of congenital cystic dilatation of the common bile duct. Am J Surg 1977;134:569–74.

23). Extrahepatic biliary atresia is the most common cause of large bile duct disease in children. Small duct disorders in the pediatric age group are represented by the group of disorders known as paucity of intrahepatic bile ducts, characterized by a decrease in the number of interlobular bile ducts. Neonatal hepatitis, not further considered here, is a heterogeneous group of disorders characterized by hepatocellular injury, cholestasis, and giant cell transformation of hepatocytes, without biliary obstruction or injury to small bile ducts, although bile ductular proliferation is sometimes seen in expanded portal tracts.

Extrahepatic Biliary Atresia

Extrahepatic biliary atresia is a progressive fibroinflammatory obliteration of all or part of the extrahepatic bile ducts, with eventual involvement of small intrahepatic biliary radicals. It is thought to be acquired, for the condition is rare in neonates and stillborns, but the etiology remains unknown. An infectious agent has long been suspected, based on the progressive inflammatory changes in the biliary system and the rarity of the condition in newborns and premature infants (65). Recent efforts have focused on the possible role of such viruses as cytomegalovirus (66), human papilloma virus, rotavirus, and reovirus 3 (65) as etiologic agents in extrahepatic biliary atresia, but the results remain inconclusive. Other proposed etiopathologic mechanisms include a defect in morphogenesis of the extrahepatic biliary tree, disorders of immune response, exposure to environmental toxins, and interruption of the vascular supply to the biliary tree (65). In approximately 20% of cases, other congenital anomalies such as polysplenia and intestinal malrotation are found; these cases are considered by some investigators to be an embryonic or fetal type of biliary atresia. These infants have an earlier onset of cholestasis than those with the more common perinatal type of biliary atresia (67).

Morphologic Features

At exploratory surgery, the extrahepatic bile ducts are partially or totally replaced by a fibrous atretic cord, and the gallbladder is often shrunken and fibrotic. On microscopic examination, at least a portion of the extrahepatic bile duct is often completely obliterated by fibrous tissue. In less severely affected areas, the bile duct lumen is narrowed by edematous fibrous tissue containing mononuclear inflammatory cells, neutrophils, and an occasional eosinophils (Fig. 2.15A). The ductal epithelium is sloughed or degenerative. The liver shows changes of extrahepatic obstruction including portal enlargement and edema, canalicular cholestasis, bile ductular proliferation, and portal inflammation (see Fig. 2.15B). Occasional hepatocyte giant cells are found in some cases, but these are generally not as numerous as in neonatal cholestasis, and lobular changes are not as prominent in biliary atresia. Even early in the course of the disease the interlobular bile ducts show subtle signs of injury such as angulated outlines, irregular spacing of epithelial cell nuclei, and pyknosis and degenerative changes in epithelium. In some cases, abnormal ductal structures suggestive of ductal plate malformation are present. As the disease progresses, destruction of intrahepatic bile ducts continues, resulting in loss of interlobular bile ducts. The time course is variable, but bridging portal fibrosis eventually progresses to cirrhosis. Residual intrahepatic bile ducts may become cystically dilated.

The size of ductal remnants in the porta hepatis at the time of hepatoportoenterostomy is considered by some investigators to be an indicator of the likelihood of restoration of bile flow. A diameter of 150 to 200 microns for residual biliary structures (preferably bile ducts lined by columnar epithelium, not representing peribiliary glands) is considered desirable, although correlation of size of draining radicals with good outcome is not perfect (68). Poor outcome has been associated with severe injury to intrahepatic ducts, lack of ducts in the hepatic hilum, coexistence of associated congenital anomalies, and the presence of cirrhosis on the initial biopsy. Recurrent bouts of bacterial cholangitis following hepatoportoenterostomy are also associated with poor outcome (69).

Syndromic and Nonsyndromic Paucity of Intrahepatic Bile Ducts

Pediatric conditions characterized by decreased numbers of intrahepatic bile ducts are generally subdivided into syn-

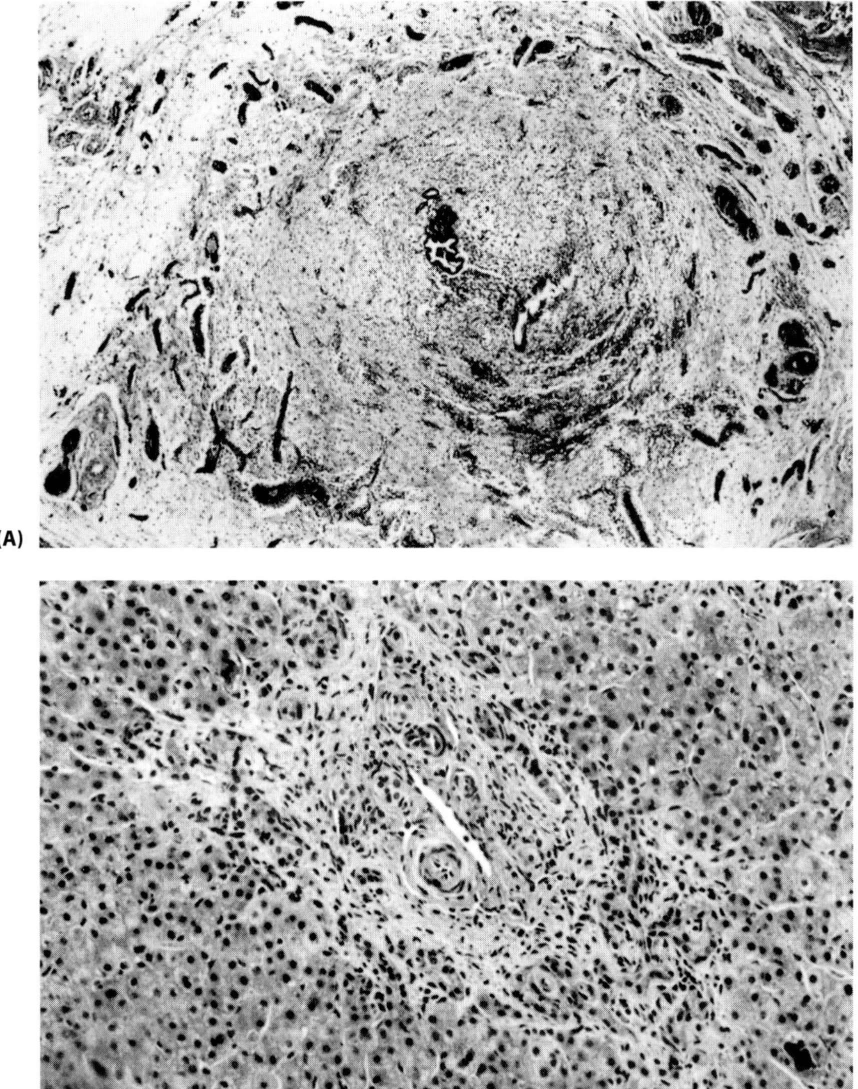

FIGURE 2.15. *Extrahepatic biliary atresia.* ***(A)*** *The extrahepatic bile duct is virtually obliterated by edematous fibrous tissue in this example. Only a small residual lumen is identified.* ***(B)*** *The portal tracts are enlarged by fibrous tissue, with early bile ductular proliferation around the perimeter.*

dromic and nonsyndromic categories. Syndromic paucity of intrahepatic bile ducts is synonymous with Alagille syndrome, characterized by chronic cholestasis, distinctive facies, cardiac murmur, vertebral abnormalities, and ocular abnormalities (70). Nonsyndromic reduction in the number of intrahepatic bile ducts is a heterogeneous group of disorders with varying etiologies such as congenital infection, metabolic disorders, and chromosomal abnormalities. The term "nonsyndromic paucity of intrahepatic bile ducts" is generally reserved for those cases in which no specific etiology can be found.

In Alagille syndrome, the characteristic lesion is the loss of interlobular bile ducts, recognized by finding hepatic artery branches that are not accompanied by a bile duct (Fig. 2.16). Evaluation of a liver biopsy should include a count of the numbers of bile ducts and the numbers of portal triads available for evaluation. Because the normal ratio of bile ducts to portal triads is approximately 1.0 to 1.8, a ratio of less than 0.5 or 0.4 is considered indicative of ductopenia. The portal triads are often small and inconspicuous and lack a significant inflammatory infiltrate. The degree of portal fibrosis is variable, however, and late changes include portal–portal bridging fibrosis; cirrhosis develops in a minority of patients, estimated at 15% (70). Chronic cholestasis generally occurs, but the lobular changes are often mild. Biopsy specimens taken early, before 3 months of age, may not show the characteristic reduction in the number of bile ducts. Such biopsies usually show degenerative changes in bile ducts, and bile ductular proliferation may lead to confusion with extrahepatic biliary atresia.

The gene responsible for many cases of Alagille syndrome, *JAG1* (Jagged1), has been identified (71,72). This gene is located on chromosome 20p12 and encodes a ligand for the Notch transmembrane receptor. Described mutations in this gene result in translational frameshifts and gross

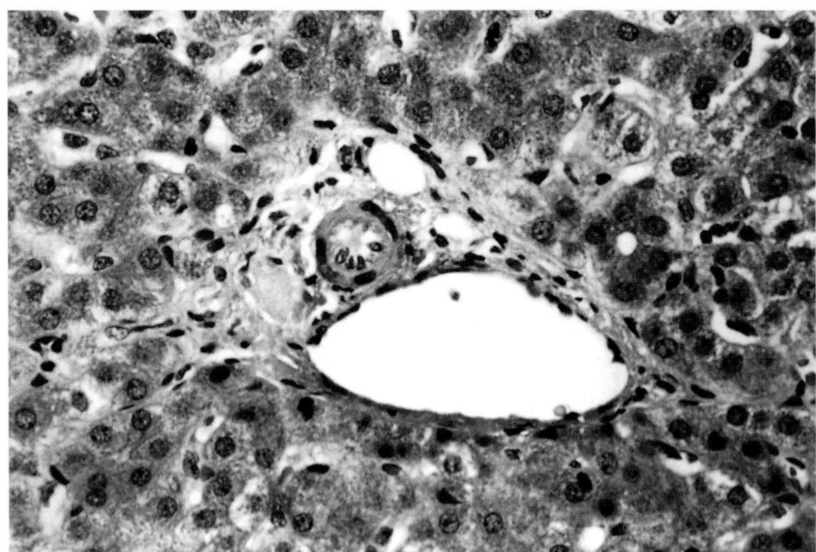

FIGURE 2.16. *Paucity of intrahepatic bile ducts. Most portal triads are devoid of interlobular bile ducts in this example of Alagille syndrome. The portal tract is not enlarged by fibrous tissue, and there is no inflammatory infiltrate.*

alteration of the protein; haploinsufficiency of *JAG1* appears to be sufficient to produce clinical manifestations of Alagille syndrome. The Jagged/Notch signaling pathway mediates cell fate decisions in early development, and abnormalities in this pathway may explain the multisystem developmental abnormalities found in Alagille syndrome.

Cytomegalovirus infection is probably the most common congenital infection associated with a reduction in the number of interlobular bile ducts; characteristic viral inclusions may be found in bile duct epithelial cell nuclei in residual bile ducts (73), but inclusions may also be scarce. Chromosomal abnormalities associated with paucity of bile ducts include trisomy 18 and trisomy 21. A number of metabolic disorders may also be associated with decreased numbers of interlobular bile ducts; these include α_1-antitrypsin deficiency, with increased α_1-antitrypsin accumulation in periportal hepatocytes on periodic acid-Schiff (PAS) or immunoperoxidase stain, and Zellweger syndrome, which shows reduction in hepatocyte peroxisomes by electron microscopy. Rarely cystic fibrosis may present as paucity of intrahepatic bile ducts. Duct paucity may also be seen in Byler syndrome (progressive familial intrahepatic cholestasis); in some cases, the biopsy shows features of both neonatal hepatitis and paucity of intrahepatic bile ducts.

The relationship between idiopathic adulthood ductopenia (IAD) and nonsyndromic paucity of intrahepatic bile ducts in children remains unclear. Liver changes in IAD are those of chronic cholestasis with loss of interlobular bile ducts, essentially the same changes seen in pediatric patients with the nonsyndromic form of paucity of intrahepatic bile ducts. In Alagille syndrome, the liver typically shows less cholestatic changes, and less portal fibrosis and bile ductular proliferation. Availability of genetic testing for the human Jagged1 gene implicated in Alagille syndrome may expand our knowledge of the spectrum of abnormalities in this disorder.

NEOPLASMS OF THE BILIARY SYSTEM

Benign Neoplasms

Bile Duct Adenoma

The bile duct adenoma is an innocuous lesion, usually an incidental finding at autopsy or in the resected liver. It is not clear that the bile duct adenoma is a true neoplasm, and it is regarded by some investigators as hamartoma of peribiliary glands (74). These lesions are usually solitary and if subcapsular may be discovered at surgery, where they may be mistaken for metastatic adenocarcinoma. Bile duct adenomas generally measure 1 cm or less, although larger ones, up to 4 cm, have been reported. Microscopically they consist of a dense proliferation of bland ductular structures in a variably dense stroma (75). Cytologic atypia is lacking and mitotic figures are rare (Fig. 2.17). The bile duct adenoma may be confused with the biliary microhamartoma, or von Meyenburg complex. The biliary microhamartoma represents failure of the ductal plate to involute and is made up of dilated bile duct-like structures, occasionally containing bile, located adjacent to a portal tract (see Fig. 2.12). The biliary structures are usually more angulated than the densely packed ducts of the bile duct adenoma.

Biliary Cystadenoma

The biliary cystadenoma (Chapter 16) is an uncommon hepatic neoplasm occurring predominantly in women. Extrahepatic tumors involving the common hepatic duct have also been reported (76). Biliary cystadenomas are large multiloculated cysts histologically similar to mucinous cystic tumors arising in the pancreas (77). The cysts are lined by mucin-secreting cells similar to bile duct epithelium, ranging from flattened cuboidal to tall columnar; occasional goblet cells are seen and scattered endocrine cells can be identified in some cases by immunostaining for chromogranin (78). The epithelial lining is usually simple, although areas of nuclear pseu-

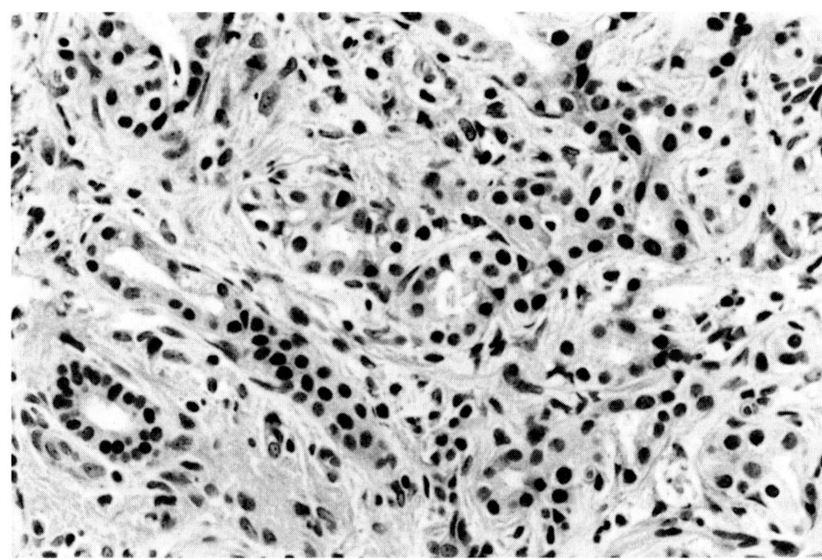

FIGURE 2.17. *The bile duct adenoma is composed of tightly packed small bile duct-like structures. These lesions are small, noninfiltrative, and lack significant nuclear atypia.*

dostratification and crowding may be seen. In tumors from men, the supporting stroma is composed of dense fibrous tissue; in women, the stroma may be densely cellular and resemble ovarian stroma (Fig. 2.18). The biliary cystadenoma should be distinguished from the simple biliary cyst, which is unilocular and lacks a distinctive supporting stroma.

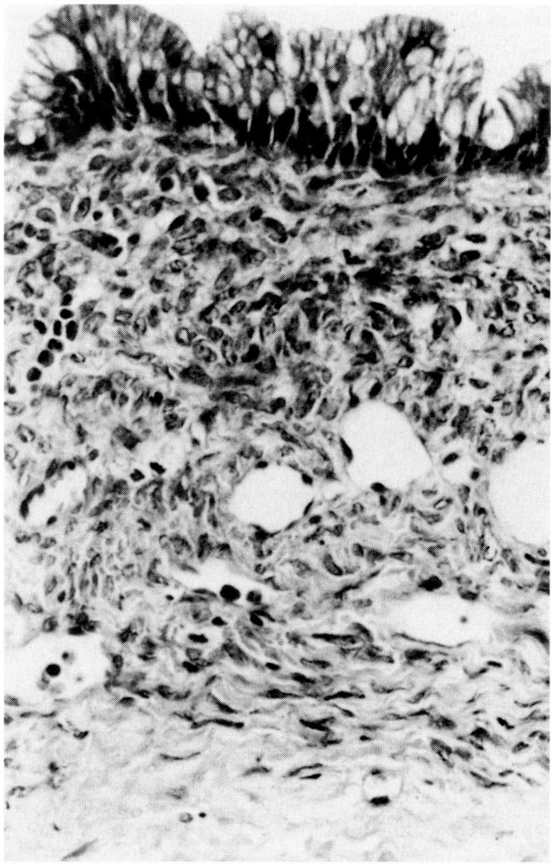

FIGURE 2.18. *The multilocular cysts of the biliary cystadenoma are lined by columnar to cuboidal cells resembling biliary epithelium. In women, a distinctive mesenchymal ovarian-type stroma is often present in the cyst wall just beneath the epithelium.*

Malignant Neoplasms

Cholangiocarcinoma

Cholangiocarcinoma, the second most frequent primary hepatic malignancy, after hepatocellular carcinoma, makes up from 5% to 30% of malignant hepatic tumors (Chapter 20). Although several classification schemes for these malignant bile duct tumors have been proposed, the most widely accepted divides these lesions into two broad categories: intrahepatic (peripheral), the most common type worldwide (79); and hilar (central). This division is supported by the different clinical presentations and surgical strategies associated with these locations. The term "cholangiocarcinoma" is reserved by some investigators for intrahepatic tumors confined to the liver and not involving the extrahepatic biliary tree. Hilar tumors, the majority of surgically treated cholangiocarcinomas in most series from the United States (80), are further subdivided based on the duct involved, or the position of the neoplasm along the common bile duct.

An alternative proposed classification based on anatomy and preferred surgical treatment divides cholangiocarcinomas into intrahepatic, perihilar, and distal tumors (80). In this classification, perihilar tumors involve the hepatic duct bifurcation. Distal tumors involve the distal extrahepatic or intrapancreatic portion of the common bile duct.

Central/Hilar (Perihilar) Cholangiocarcinoma

Central/hilar (perihilar) cholangiocarcinoma shares many etiologic associations, such as primary sclerosing cholangitis, fibropolycystic liver diseases, and parasite infestation, with intrahepatic cholangiocarcinoma. The incidence of cholangiocarcinoma in patients with primary sclerosing cholangitis is estimated at 8% to 10%. In contrast to most patients with intrahepatic cholangiocarcinoma, patients with perihilar tumors usually present with jaundice and other evidence of large bile duct obstruction.

Gross and Microscopic Features The typical gross appearance of perihilar cholangiocarcinoma is dense white scar infiltrating the hepatic hilum and extending into the adjacent parenchyma (Fig. 2.19A). In cases of primary sclerosing cholangitis, the presence of a tumor on gross examination may be obscured by dense fibrosis. The bile duct may be encircled and thickened by dense desmoplastic tumor. In some cases, the tumor is papillary and protrudes into the lumen of the bile duct. In general the microscopic appearance is similar to that of intrahepatic cholangiocarcinoma, with most of the tumors composed of small well-formed ducts (see Fig. 2.19B). Desmoplasia is a prominent feature in many perihilar cholangiocarcinomas, and perineural invasion is commonly found. The differential diagnosis includes benign reactive changes and bile ductular proliferation; in patients with biliary stents, diagnosis may be particularly difficult because of the significant degree of cellular atypia associated with reactive change in bile duct epithelium.

Prognostic Factors Incomplete resection and positive regional lymph nodes appear to be the two most important factors predictive of shortened survival (81–83). Although univariant analysis has shown various factors such as tumor grade and size to be significant prognostic factors in hilar cholangiocarcinoma, multivariant analysis in several studies showed only residual tumor stage after surgery and the presence of lymph node metastases to be of independent

(A)

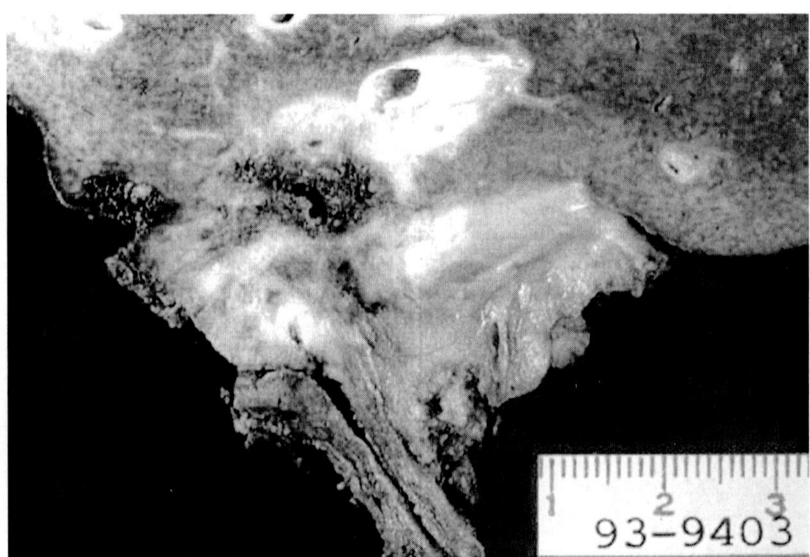

(B)

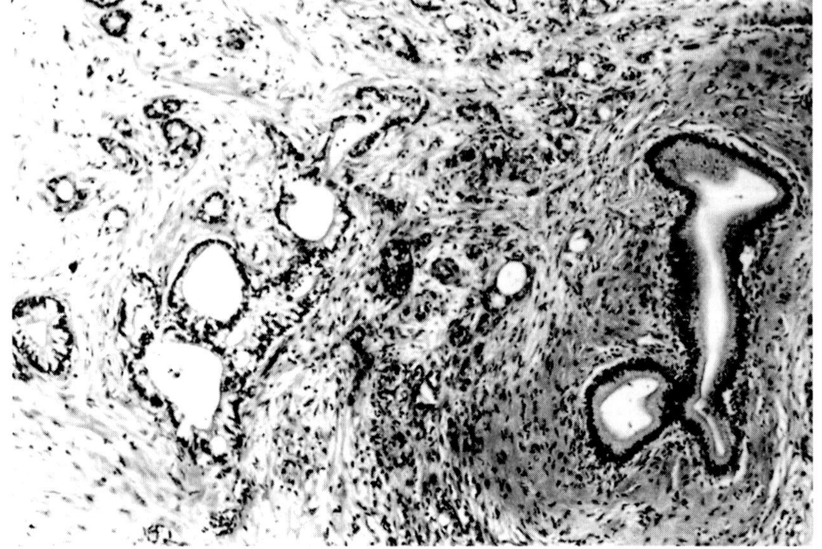

FIGURE 2.19. *Perihilar cholangiocarcinoma.* ***(A)*** *The gross appearance of perihilar cholangiocarcinoma is that of an ill-defined, densely fibrotic infiltrating mass lesion. It may be indistinguishable grossly from hilar fibrosis in primary sclerosing cholangitis.* ***(B)*** *The typical cholangiocarcinoma forms small tubular to cribriform glands, and the tumor cells closely resemble biliary epithelium. A dense desmoplastic stroma usually accompanies the tumor.*

statistical significance (82,83). Other investigators report that histologic grade influences survival (83,84), with patients with well-differentiated carcinomas having a median survival of 58 months, compared to 9 months for patients with poorly differentiated tumors (81). Perineural invasion, present in 36 of 43 cases, was not shown to be an independent prognostic factor (81), probably because of its high prevalence in these tumors. Two studies have shown that high total bilirubin concentration preoperatively is a poor prognostic indicator (81,84).

Stage Perihilar cholangiocarcinoma is staged using a tumor/node/metastasis (TNM) classification scheme (Table 2.7) devised by the American Joint Commission on Cancer for staging extrahepatic bile duct carcinomas (85). Stage I tumors are confined to the bile duct, whereas stage II tumors have spread to periductal tissues. Stage III tumors have regional lymph node metastases. Stage IV tumors have evidence of distant metastases or invasion of adjacent structures.

Carcinoma of the Extrahepatic Bile Duct

Malignancies involving the extrahepatic bile duct are relatively uncommon, occurring less frequently than carcinoma of the gallbladder. This type of tumor appears preponderantly in men, and is more common in the elderly. Although a palpable mass may be evident at surgery, in many cases only diffuse thickening of the bile duct wall is appreciated. Lesions of the confluence of the hepatic bile duct and upper common hepatic duct account for over half of cases of extrahepatic biliary cancer (86). Lesions involving the middle third of the common bile duct account for approximately 20%, as do cases involving the lower third of the common bile duct. Over 95% of these tumors are adenocarcinomas, and most have an associated desmoplastic stroma; when these tumors are well differentiated, frozen section diagnosis may be particularly difficult, especially in the setting of stent placement and inflammation.

Diagnosis of Hilar Cholangiocarcinoma and Bile Duct Carcinoma by Endobiliary Brush Cytology

As endoscopic cholangiogram techniques become ever more sophisticated and widely used, cytologic examination is used more and more in the evaluation of biliary strictures. Such specimens often pose diagnostic challenges for even the experienced pathologist, much less those of us who rarely see these difficult specimens. The key cytologic criteria for malignancy that have been identified by multiple investigators include a background of tissue damage, nuclear overlap and crowding, irregular nuclear membranes, nuclear molding, coarse chromatin pattern, and increased nuclear to cytoplasmic ratio (87,88). In general, sensitivity (37% to 85%) is lower than specificity (93% to 100%) (3,5). There are essentially no false-positive diagnoses, but a negative result does not reliably exclude malignancy.

Peripheral or Intrahepatic Cholangiocarcinomas

The Liver Cancer Study Group of Japan has defined peripheral cholangiocarcinoma as cholangiocarcinoma arising in a segmental duct or a more peripheral duct (89).

Table 2.7. Staging of perihilar cholangiocarcinoma

TNM Definitions	
Primary Tumor	
T1a	Tumor invades mucosa
T1b	Tumor invades muscular layer
T2	Tumor invades perimuscular connective tissue
T3	Tumor invades adjacent structures
Regional Lymph Nodes	
N0	No regional lymph node metastasis
N1	Metastasis in cystic duct, pericholedochal, and/or perihilar lymph nodes
N2	Metastasis in regional lymph nodes near duodenum or head of pancreas
Metastasis	
M0	No distant metastasis
M1	Distant metastasis
Stage Grouping	
Stage I	T1, N0, M0
Stage II	T2, N0, M0
Stage III	T1 or T2, N1 or N2, M0
Stage IVA	T3, any N, M0
Stage IVB	Any T, any N, M1

Source: Beahrs OH, Henson DE, Hutter RVP, et al. Manual for staging of cancer. Philadelphia: Lippincott, 1992.

Etiology The etiology of intrahepatic cholangiocarcinoma is usually unknown. However, these tumors are associated with all forms of fibropolycystic liver disease, including the presence of multiple biliary microhamartomas (79). Chronic inflammatory lesions of the bile ducts and conditions associated with bile stasis also predispose the individual to the development of intrahepatic cholangiocarcinoma; these conditions include primary sclerosing cholangitis, parasitic infections with liver flukes such as Clonorchis and Opisthorchis, and recurrent bacterial cholangitis with hepatolithiasis. Intrahepatic cholangiocarcinomas have also been reported in association with exposure to Thorotrast (90) and have been associated with anabolic steroid use. In contrast to hepatocellular carcinoma, most cases of intrahepatic cholangiocarcinoma arise in a noncirrhotic liver and are not associated with hepatitis B infection. In one series of 85 intrahepatic cholangiocarcinomas, less than 5% were associated with nonbiliary cirrhosis. The cholangiocarcinomas in this series did not differ in morphologic features from cholangiocarcinomas arising in noncirrhotic livers, and displayed similar immunohistochemical staining patterns with respect to carcinoembryonic antigen, CA19-9, DU-PAN-2, and biliary-type cytokeratins (91).

Clinical Associations Intrahepatic cholangiocarcinoma generally occurs in older adults, with most patients between 50 and 70 years of age. The tumor is often clinically silent until late in the course; patients typically complain of fever, weight loss, anorexia, and vague abdominal pain. In contrast to hilar cholangiocarcinoma, patients with intrahepatic cholangiocarcinoma rarely present with jaundice.

Prognostic Factors and Staging Intrahepatic cholangiocarcinoma is staging using the same TNM classification and stage grouping as hepatocellular carcinoma (85) (Table 2.8). Complete resection of the tumor appears to be an important factor in prognosis in intrahepatic cholangiocarcinoma. Median survival for resectable intrahepatic cholangiocarcinoma is as high as 30 months in some series, and the 5-year survival ranges between 35% and 45% (80,92). Median survival for unresectable intrahepatic tumors is only 6 to 7 months, even with adjuvant therapy.

Tumor grade is probably not a major determinant of prognosis in intrahepatic cholangiocarcinomas, although some investigators have proposed that a prominent desmoplastic stroma may be associated with poor outcome (93). In one series of 19 patients with intrahepatic cholangiocarcinoma who underwent surgical resection, positive hilar lymph nodes were a poor prognostic sign; most of these patients died within 9 months of surgery, in contrast to node-negative patients, who had a median survival of over 36 months. Tumor grade and size in this small series had no effect

Table 2.8. Staging of intrahepatic cholangiocarcinoma

TNM Definitions	
Primary Tumor	
T1	Solitary tumor 2 cm or less, without vascular invasion
T2	Solitary tumor 2 cm or less with vascular invasion or multiple tumors limited to one lobe, none >2 cm, no vascular invasion or solitary tumor >2 cm, without vascular invasion
T3	Solitary tumor >2 cm with vascular invasion or multiple tumors limited to one lobe, none >2 cm, with vascular invasion or multiple tumors limited to one lobe, any >2 cm, with or without vascular invasion
T4	Multiple tumors in more than one lobe or tumor involving a major branch of the portal or hepatic vein
Regional Lymph Nodes	
N0	No regional lymph node metastases
N1	Regional lymph node metastases
Distant Metastases	
M0	No distant metastases
M1	Distant metastases
Stage Grouping	
Stage I	T1, N0, M0
Stage II	T2, N0, M0
Stage III	T1 or T2, N1, M0
	T3, N0 or N1, M0
Stage IVA	T4, any N, M0
Stage IVB	any T, any N, M1

Source: Beahrs OH, Henson DE, Hutter RVP, et al. Manual for staging of cancer. Philadelphia: Lippincott, 1992.

on survival (92). Another series of 34 patients with intrahepatic cholangiocarcinoma reports that tumor size greater than 5 cm was associated with recurrence and that multiple tumors and incomplete resection were associated with poor outcome (94).

Gross and Microscopic Features On gross examination, intrahepatic cholangiocarcinomas are generally gray-white to tan masses; larger lesions may contain areas of central necrosis or, less commonly, hemorrhage. Most tumors are firm because of the prominent desmoplastic stroma, which may be gritty because of dystrophic calcifications. In general the intrahepatic cholangiocarcinoma consists of a single nonencapsulated mass in a noncirrhotic liver (Fig. 2.20), although satellite lesions may be present. The margins may be deceptively well circumscribed on gross examination, but microscopic examination shows infiltrative borders. Rarely, involvement of portal or hepatic veins may be seen. An intraductal growth occurs in up to 15% of cases and may be associated with a more favorable outcome (95). Some investigators have subdivided intrahepatic cholangiocarcinomas based on the pattern of growth, and report that tumors without biliary strictures behave more like hepatocellular carcinomas, in that they are more likely to occur in a diseased liver and have frequent intrahepatic spread without lymph node metastases (89).

Most cholangiocarcinomas are adenocarcinomas; rarely, areas of squamous differentiation may be seen, and sarcomatoid variants have been reported (96). Other variants include papillary adenocarcinoma, found generally within larger ducts, and signet ring cell carcinoma. The most common microscopic pattern is a well to moderately differentiated adenocarcinoma forming small tubular glands and duct-like structures. The tumor cells are low cuboidal to columnar, with clear to eosinophilic cytoplasm and round to oval nuclei. Intracellular mucin production may be scant, but is usually demonstrable with special stains for mucin; typically a mixture of neutral and acidic mucins is found. A desmoplastic stroma is generally prominent, but is not always present. Perineural and lymphovascular invasion is common, and cholangiocarcinomas often involve portal tracts, either by spread within portal vein radicals or by spread within the intrahepatic biliary tree. Bile ducts in adjacent portal tracts may demonstrate varying degrees of epithelial dysplasia; however, it is usually not possible to identify a specific bile duct of origin.

Differential Diagnosis The primary challenge for the pathologist in diagnosing most intrahepatic cholangiocarcinomas is distinction from metastatic adenocarcinoma (Table 2.9). Primary sites producing tumors with similar histology include the pancreas, extrahepatic biliary tree, breast, and occasionally lung. Immunohistochemical stains are of limited use in distinguishing cholangiocarcinoma from other primaries, and mucin stains are helpful only in distinguishing cholangiocarcinoma from hepatocellular carcinoma. The distinction between cholangiocarcinoma and metastatic adenocarcinoma therefore depends heavily on the exclusion of a primary site elsewhere.

The distinction between hepatocellular carcinoma and cholangiocarcinoma is usually more straightforward, although there is some overlap in morphology and combined tumors do exist. Hepatocellular carcinomas display a trabecular architecture with scant fibrous stroma, a distinctly different morphology from the usual cholangiocarcinoma. In problematic cases, a panel of immunohistochemical stains can be employed to distinguish between the two. Polyclonal or cross-reactive CEA positivity in cholangiocarcinoma will usually show a cytoplasmic staining pattern, without the "chicken wire" pattern of cross-reactivity to biliary glycoprotein seen in hepatocellular carcinoma. Immunostain for alpha-fetoprotein is negative in cholangiocarcinoma.

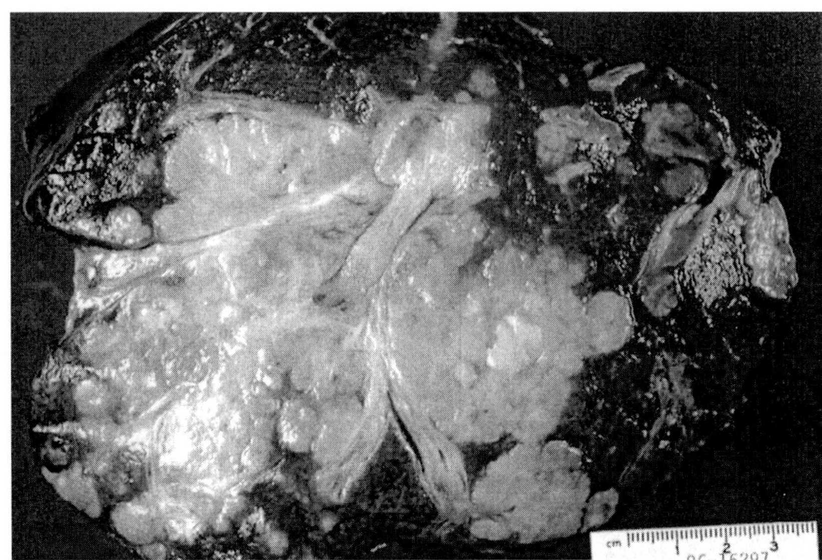

FIGURE 2.20. *The peripheral cholangiocarcinoma usually arises in a noncirrhotic liver and forms a dense, gray-white mass. The tumor is often deceptively well circumscribed; satellite lesions may be seen.*

Table 2.9. Differential diagnosis of cholangiocarcinoma

Diagnosis	Distinguishing Features
Non-neoplastic reactive change in periductal glands	Cribriform glands, mitoses, isolated tumor cells in stroma, perineural invasion, nuclear atypia in cholangiocarcinoma
Bile duct adenoma	Small lesions, no mitoses, no nuclear atypia
Bile duct hamartoma	
Metastatic adenocarcinoma	CK7/CK20 useful in some circumstances
Hepatocellular carcinoma	HCC has trabecular architecture, minimal fibrous stroma; cross-reactive CEA; alpha-fetoprotein

Source: Ferrell L. Malignant liver tumors that mimic benign lesions: analysis of five distinct lesions. Semin Diag Pathol 1995;12:64–76.

Ultrastructural examination is seldom indicated, but electron microscopy of cholangiocarcinoma cells shows typical features of adenocarcinoma, such as microvilli and true lumen formation.

Intrabiliary growth of tumors metastatic to liver or large bile ducts may mimic cholangiocarcinoma. In particular, metastasis from colorectal carcinoma may involve the large bile ducts, leading to obstructive changes in the liver (97,98). Colorectal carcinoma has a propensity for growth along mucosal surface, leading to the erroneous interpretation of origin of the tumor in dysplasia of primary biliary neoplasia. Hepatocellular carcinoma may also present as an intraluminal mass involving a large bile duct, at times posing diagnostic difficulties (99,100).

Mixed Hepatocellular/Cholangiocarcinoma

Occasional primary epithelial malignancies in the liver will show divergent differentiation, with features of both cholangiocarcinoma and hepatocellular carcinoma. These tumors assume one of two patterns, termed "collision tumors" and "transition tumors" by Goodman in one of the earlier studies of this relatively rare entity (101). In the collision tumor, different areas of the neoplasm or separate tumor masses in the liver show different patterns of differentiation, with separate areas of hepatocellular carcinoma and cholangiocarcinoma. The transition tumors show more intermixed patterns. In general, combined hepatocellular/cholangiocarcinomas have the same associations with cirrhosis, hepatitis B, hepatitis C, and elevated alpha-fetoprotein levels as hepatocellular carcinomas. These tumors have a poor prognosis and disseminate widely, spreading to regional lymph nodes and distant organs. Metastases maintain the mixed pattern or exhibit hepatocellular differentiation (102).

Biliary Cystadenocarcinoma

Biliary cystadenocarcinoma is a rare tumor, generally arising in a preexisting biliary cystadenoma (Chapter 16). These tumors arise in adults; benign biliary cystadenomas are more common in women, but for cystadenocarcinomas the sex ratio is approximately 1 : 1 (77). The most common presenting symptoms are abdominal pain or an abdominal mass. The etiology remains unknown, although there are reports of cystadenocarcinomas arising in the setting of polycystic liver disease, such as Caroli's disease (103).

Gross Morphology Most biliary cystadenocarcinomas are multilocular, although rare unilocular cases have been reported (77). Cystadenocarcinomas in one series ranged in size from 3 to 30 cm, essentially no different in size from benign biliary cystadenomas (77). The cyst fluid may be clear mucinous, bile stained, or blood tinged. The cyst lining may contain papillary projections into the cyst lumen. Areas of solid thickening and large papillary projections are clues to malignancy (Fig. 2.21A).

Microscopic Features The epithelial lining of the cysts generally consists of tall columnar cells and should display cytologic features of malignancy. The tumor infiltrates the underlying cyst wall. Most biliary cystadenocarcinomas are well differentiated; the most common patterns are a tubulopapillary or tubular adenocarcinoma (see Fig. 2.21B, C). Rarely, the tumor shows adenosquamous differentiation. The stroma is variable in biliary cystadenocarcinomas. Ovarian-type stroma is often present in tumors in women; in men, the stroma consists of dense fibrosis.

Determination of Malignancy The prediction of behavior from morphologic features is difficult in cystic mucinous neoplasms. Many otherwise benign biliary cystadenomas have areas of nuclear enlargement, crowding, and stratification, considered areas of dysplastic change. Many pathologists reserve the term "cystadenocarcinoma" for cases with frankly invasive adenocarcinoma involving the stroma or adjacent parenchyma. Surgical resection offers the greatest opportunity for cure; long-term survival is relatively high for women with biliary cystadenocarcinomas arising in preexisting cystadenomas with ovarian-type stroma. Cystadenocarcinomas in men may have a more aggressive course (77).

(A)

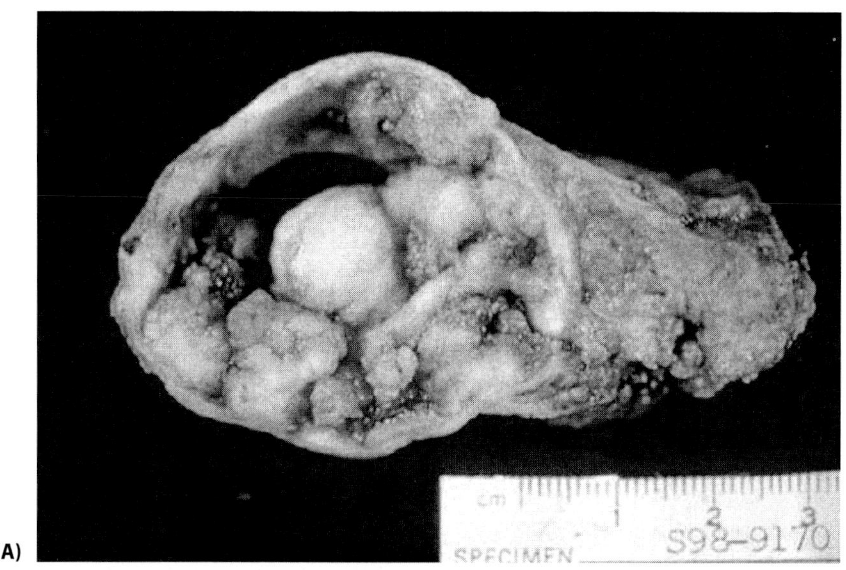

(B)

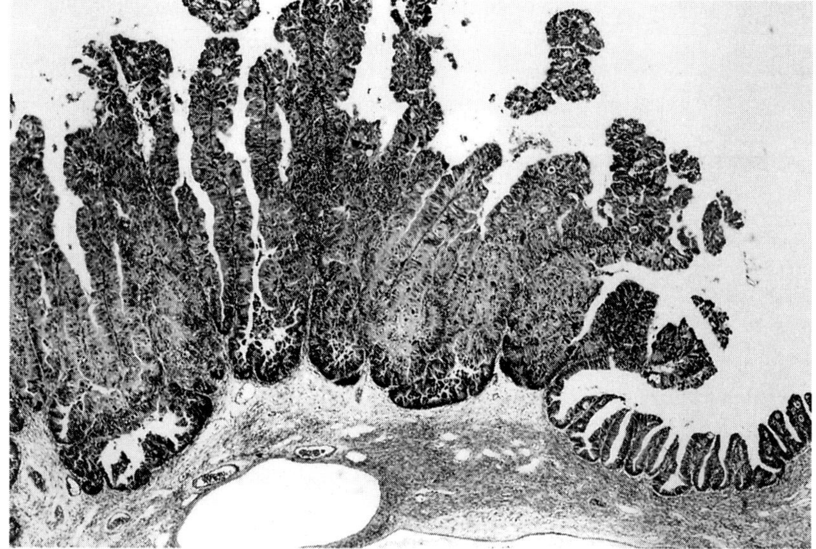

(C)

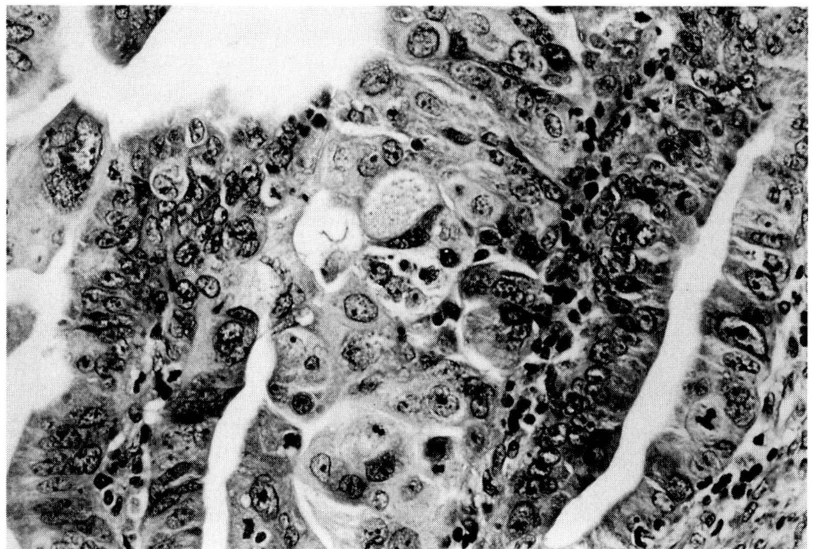

FIGURE 2.21. *Biliary cystadenocarcinoma.* ***(A)*** *The solid fleshy areas in this cystic tumor represent areas of carcinoma arising in a biliary cystadenoma.* ***(B)*** *Microscopically, biliary cystadenocarcinomas often have a papillary configuration on low power. The epithelium on the right shows features of borderline malignancy.* ***(C)*** *Marked cytologic atypia and invasion of adjacent stroma are clues to malignancy.*

PATHOLOGY OF THE GALLBLADDER

Cholelithiasis

The two major types of gallstones (Chapter 11) are cholesterol and pigment stones. Cholesterol stones composed of at least 50% cholesterol monohydrate are more common (80% in Western countries). These stones are rarely pure and generally contain bile pigments, calcium, and a mucoprotein matrix component. They are generally multiple and faceted and measure less than 2 cm in diameter. Pure cholesterol stones (approximately 10% of stones) are often larger. Pigment stones are more common in Asian populations and in patients with hemolytic disorders. These stones are small, irregular, and soft. Two subtypes are recognized: black stones, composed of polymerized calcium bilirubinate, and brown stones, associated with infection and composed of calcium palmitate and precipitated calcium bilirubinate. Morphologic changes in the gallbladder in the setting of gallstones are variable, ranging from nearly normal histopathologic findings to severe acute and chronic cholecystitis.

Inflammatory Conditions

The most common inflammatory conditions involving the gallbladder, acute and chronic cholecystitis, account for the vast majority of pathologic changes in surgically removed gallbladders (Chapter 11). Rarer conditions include *eosinophilic cholecystitis*, in which the gallbladder is heavily infiltrated by eosinophils, without neutrophils or other inflammatory cells. The etiology of this condition is usually unknown; although rare cases have been associated with parasites or hypersensitivity response. Although specific infectious agents such as cytomegalovirus, Cryptosporidium, various fungi, tuberculosis, and helminths may involve the gallbladder, such cases are rarely encountered.

Acute Cholecystitis

Acute cholecystitis is associated with cholelithiasis in 90% of cases, and obstruction of the cystic duct is an important factor in its pathogenesis. Bacterial infection is usually a secondary event and not the inciting factor. The gallbladder is edematous and congested. The mucosa is often but not invariably ulcerated, and there may be areas of granulation tissue and fibroblast proliferation in the gallbladder wall. The neutrophilic infiltrate is variable and may depend on timing of surgery; in subacute cases, eosinophils may be particularly prominent.

Chronic Cholecystitis

Chronic cholecystitis (Fig. 2.22) is associated with gallstones in approximately 95% of cases. Its histopathologic incidence is highly dependent upon the criteria used for diagnosis, which are not well established. For instance, Rokitansky-Aschoff sinuses, in the absence of chronic inflammation or significant fibrosis, are regarded by some as sufficient grounds for diagnosis. Well-developed examples show stromal and mural infiltration by mononuclear inflammatory cells, predominantly lymphocytes and plasma cells. Macrophages may also be present, and a granulomatous response to extravasated bile may be seen. When the granulomatous response is exuberant and associated with foamy macrophages, the term *xanthogranulomatous cholecystitis* is often used. The gallbladder wall in chronic cholecystitis is usually thickened by fibrous tissue. Epithelial changes include goblet cell metaplasia and mucinous metaplasia, and dysplastic changes may rarely be seen, occurring more commonly in older patients.

Acute Acalculous Cholecystitis

Acalculous cholecystitis (Chapter 12) is associated with many clinical conditions, but is often seen in patients with severe trauma or burns or after major surgery, and may follow episodes of hypotension. Marked edema of the gallbladder wall, epithelial necrosis, and infiltration by neutrophils are common features. The inflammatory process is often severe, and perforation, hemorrhage, and frank necrosis of the gallbladder wall are not uncommon.

Cholesterolosis

The term *cholesterolosis* refers to the accumulation of foamy macrophages in the lamina propria of the gallbladder. Grossly this accumulation is seen as yellow mucosal flecks or linear streaks. Gallbladders with cholesterolosis may be otherwise normal or may contain gallstones. The accumulation of cholesterol is thought to be related to faulty transport of cholesterol into the gallbladder lumen.

Polyps and Benign Neoplasms

Cholesterol Polyp

Cholesterol polyps, which are not true neoplasms, are the most common polyp occurring in the gallbladder, accounting for some 80% of gallbladder polyps. These lesions are frequently associated with cholesterolosis but also occur in its absence. Usually measuring less than 1.0 cm, the cholesterol polyp is a yellow multinodular pedunculated lesion on a stalk, with numerous foamy macrophages in the stroma (Fig. 2.23). Multiple cholesterol polyps are not uncommon (104).

Inflammatory Polyp

The inflammatory polyp is an uncommon lesion in the gallbladder. Like inflammatory polyps in other sites, it is considered non-neoplastic and is composed of granulation tissue infiltrated by lymphocytes. The inflammatory polyp most likely represents a response to ulceration and mucosal injury, typically following cholecystitis.

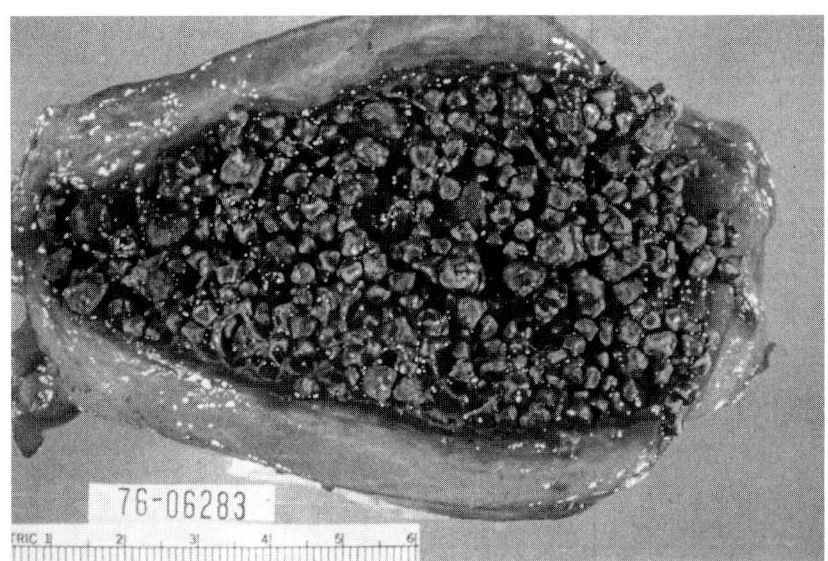

(A)

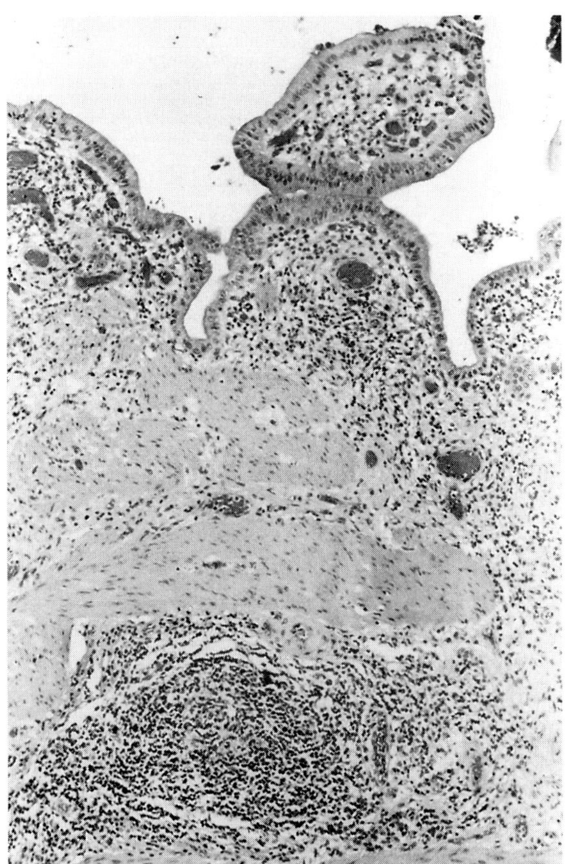

(B)

FIGURE 2.22. *Chronic cholecystitis.* ***(A)*** *The gallbladder wall is markedly thickened by fibrous tissue in this case of chronic cholecystitis. Numerous gallstones are present in the gallbladder lumen.* ***(B)*** *The gallbladder wall contains a chronic inflammatory infiltrate.*

Adenomyoma

The adenomyoma (Chapter 14) is a non-neoplastic nodule, generally located in the fundus of the gallbladder (Fig. 2.24). It is composed of glandular elements interspersed among thick bundles of smooth muscle. When generalized, this process of diverticula formation with associated smooth muscle thickening is referred to as adenomyomatosis, and results in thickening of the gallbladder wall. Adenomyomatosis is considered an acquired lesion similar to diverticulosis coli, and may be related to increased intraluminal pressure.

Adenoma

True adenomas of the gallbladder are rare (Chapter 14). These neoplastic polyps may be pedunculated or sessile, measuring up to 2 cm or more. Three histologic subtypes

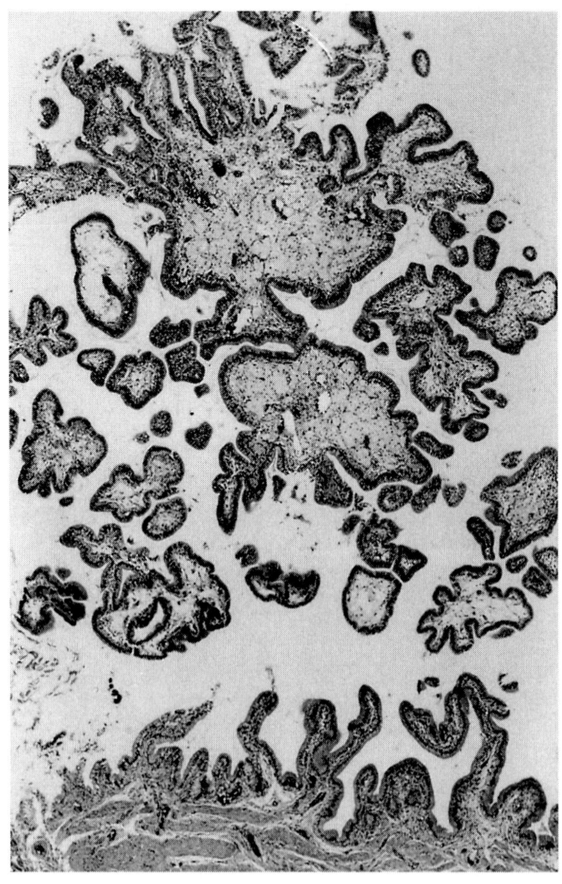

FIGURE 2.23. *The cholesterol polyp is non-neoplastic polyp. The stroma contains numerous foamy macrophages, similar to cholesterolosis. The connecting stalk is not visualized in this example.*

are recognized: papillary, tubulopapillary, and tubular. In some cases of adenocarcinoma of the gallbladder, areas of residual adenoma are found, suggesting that in some instances adenomas serve as precursor lesions for invasive adenocarcinoma.

Other Mass Lesions

A number of benign tumors occur in the gallbladder and extrahepatic ducts. Granular cell tumors may occur anywhere in the biliary system. Paragangliomas also occur in the gallbladder. Traumatic neuromas may occur in the region of the cystic duct following cholecystectomy. Malignant tumors include rhabdomyosarcoma in children, carcinoid, malignant melanoma, and a variety of sarcomas such as leiomyosarcoma, angiosarcoma, and malignant fibrous histiocytoma.

Malignant Neoplasms

Primary cancers of the gallbladder (Chapter 14), although relatively infrequent in the United States, constitute the fifth most common digestive tract cancer, with an annual incidence of 2.5/100,000 population. Most patients are elderly, with a mean age of approximately 65 years. Women are affected more frequently than men, with a sex ratio of 3:1. Gallbladder cancer is much more common in some ethnic and racial groups, such as the Pima Indians of the American Southwest, who have a sixfold greater rate than non-Indians in the same area, and it is very common in Chile. Most gallbladder cancers are discovered at cholecystectomy; a preoperative diagnosis is rare (105).

Etiology

Although the pathogenesis remains largely unknown, gallbladder carcinoma has been associated with the presence of gallstones. However, one-fourth of patients with carcinoma of the gallbladder do not have cholelithiasis, arguing against direct causality. Calcification in the gallbladder wall is also associated with gallbladder carcinoma (105).

Several investigators have shown that overexpression of the p53 gene product is found in many gallbladder carcinomas and intramucosal lesions, suggesting a role for this tumor suppressor gene in carcinogenesis and tumor progression in this organ (106,107).

Precursor Lesions in Gallbladder Mucosa

Metaplastic changes in the gallbladder mucosa are very common in the setting of cholelithiasis. Antral-type metaplasia, in which the gallbladder mucosa resembles deep gastric antral glands, is extremely common in well-sampled specimens; this change was found in 95% of gallbladders with cholelithiasis in a study from Chile (108). Intestinal metaplasia, with goblet cells, a less common change, was found in 58% of cases in this study (108). Dysplasia and carcinoma in situ were found in 16% and 2.5% of cases, respectively. Evidence that dysplastic mucosa changes are a precursor lesion for gallbladder carcinoma is indirect and based on relative ages of patients with these lesions and the presence of dysplasia and intramucosal carcinoma in gallbladders with invasive carcinoma. Another study from Chile estimated the period required for progression of dysplasia to advanced gallbladder carcinoma to be around 15 years, based on the mean ages of patients with dysplasia and various stages of carcinoma (109).

Gross Morphology

Carcinoma of the gallbladder may be visible as a polypoid mucosal growth (Fig. 2.25A), a mucosal plaque, or may cause diffuse thickening of the gallbladder wall. As many as one-third of cases have no recognizable macroscopic lesion (110). Extension into the liver is a common pattern of spread, and these cases may show a concentric ring of tumor growth encasing the gallbladder.

Microscopic Appearance

Most gallbladder cancers are readily recognizable as adenocarcinomas (see Fig. 2.25B). Many are well differentiated,

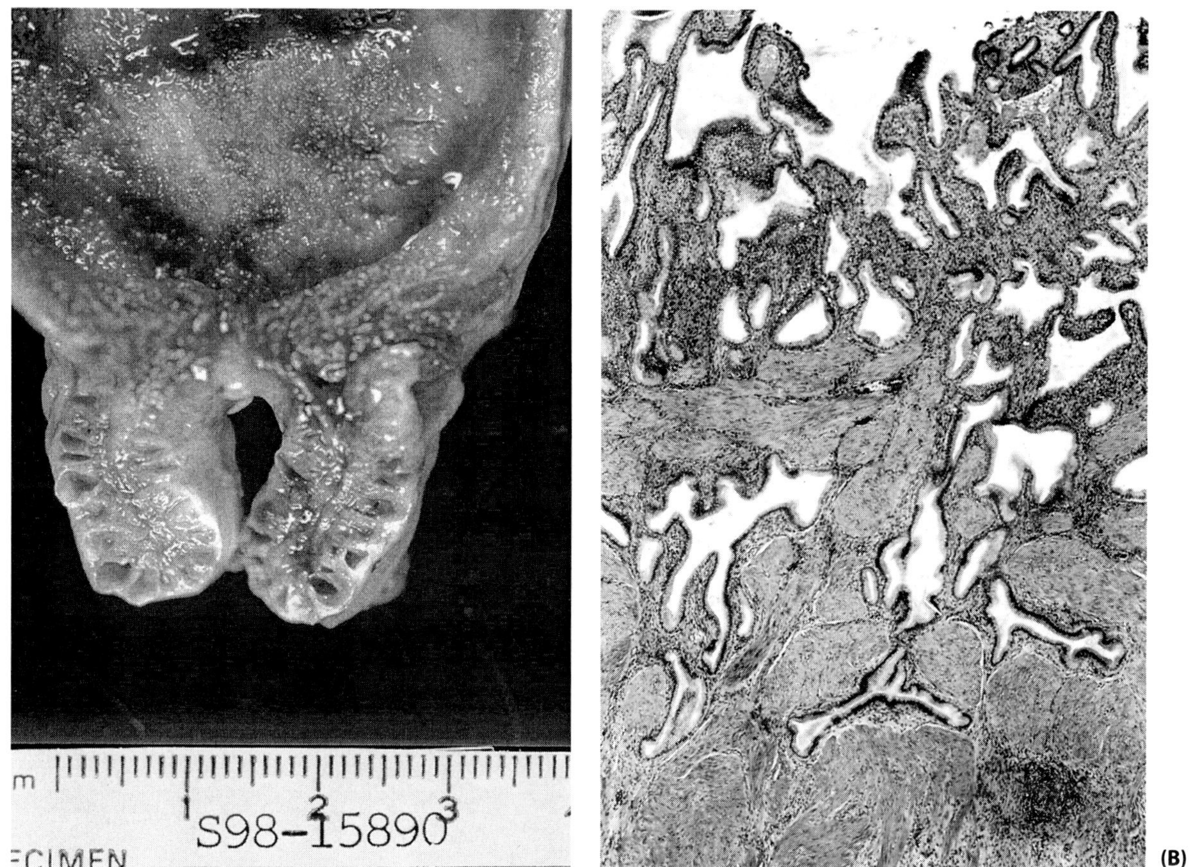

FIGURE 2.24. *Adenomyoma. **(A)** Solitary adenomyomas of the gallbladder are usually located in the fundus and have a distinctive cut surface with dilated spaces. **(B)** Microscopically, these spaces are seen to represent diverticular extensions of the surface mucosa into the muscular wall of the adenomyoma.*

Table 2.10. Staging of gallbladder cancer

TNM Definitions	
Primary Tumor	
Tx	Primary tumor cannot be assessed
Tis	Tumor in situ
T1a	Tumor invades lamina propria
T1b	Tumor invades muscular layer
T2	Tumor invades perimuscular connective tissue
T3	Tumor perforates the serosa or directly invades into one adjacent organ, or both (extension 2 cm or less into liver)
T4	Tumor extends more than 2 cm into liver and/or into two or more adjacent organs
Regional Lymph Nodes	
N0	No regional lymph node metastasis
N1	Metastasis in cystic duct, pericholedochal, and/or hilar lymph nodes
N2	Metastasis in regional lymph nodes near duodenum or head of pancreas
Metastasis	
M0	No distant metastasis
M1	Distant metastasis
Stage Grouping	
Stage I	T1, N0, M0
Stage II	T2, N0, M0
Stage III	T1 or T2, N1, M0
	T3, N0 or N1, M0
Stage IVA	T4, N0 or N1, M0
Stage IVB	Any T, N2, M0; Any T, any N, M1

Source: Beahrs OH, Henson DE, Hutter RVP, et al. Manual for staging of cancer. Philadelphia: Lippincott, 1992.

(A)

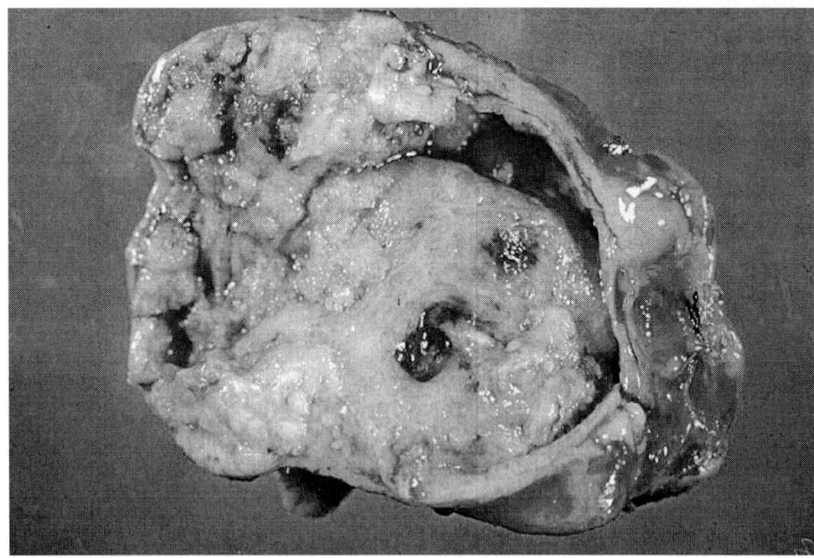

(B)

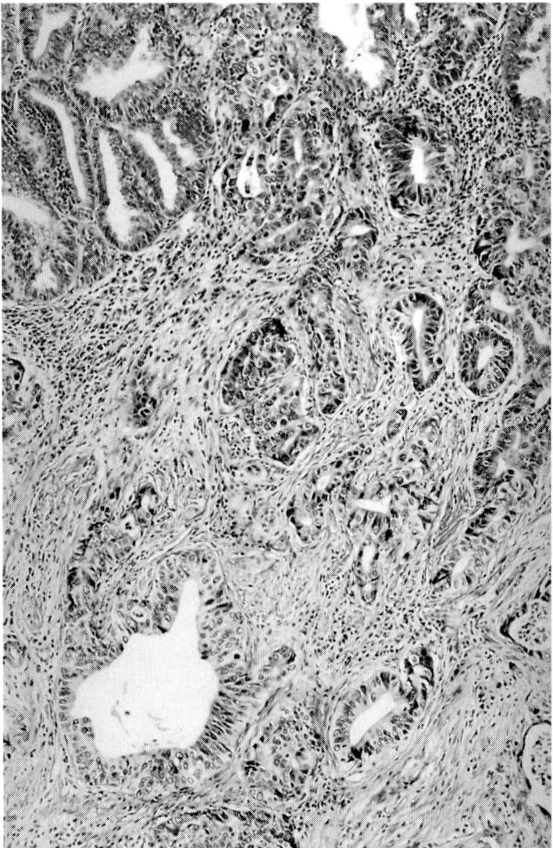

FIGURE 2.25. *Adenocarcinoma of gallbladder is widely variable in gross appearance.* ***(A)*** *The tumor may form a fleshy mass protruding into the gallbladder lumen, as seen in this example, or may be grossly indistinguishable from wall thickening in chronic cholecystitis.* ***(B)*** *The majority of gallbladder carcinomas are adenocarcinomas.*

with variable sized glands lined by columnar or cuboidal cells. The tumor cells have clear to eosinophilic cytoplasm and occasional tumor cells show goblet cell differentiation. Gallbladder carcinomas are associated with a desmoplastic response in most cases. Extension into Rokitasky-Aschoff sinuses should not be confused with tumor invasion. Other histologic patterns include papillary adenocarcinoma, adenosquamous or squamous differentiation, poorly differentiated signet ring cell carcinoma, primary carcinoid tumors, and giant cell carcinoma with osteoclast-like giant cells (111). Clear cell adenocarcinomas with abundant glycogen accumulation may be confused with metastatic renal cell carcinoma. Small cell undifferentiated carcinoma is usually associated with recognizable adenocarcinoma. Malignant mesenchymal tumors of the gallbladder are quite rare; rhabdomyosarcoma, angiosarcoma, and malignant histiocytoma are among those reported (112).

Staging

In the United States, gallbladder cancer is staged using a tumor/lymph node/metastasis system (Table 2.10) (see also Table 14.1) (85). The predominant pattern of tumor spread is by direct extension, primarily involving the gallbladder fossa and the liver, followed by involvement of the extrahepatic bile ducts. The duodenum, pancreas, transverse colon, and hepatic artery and portal vein may also be involved by direct extension. Regional lymph nodes are positive in up to 70% of cases. Frequent sites of hematogenous spread include the liver, lungs, and bone.

Prognosis

The most important prognostic feature identified so far is the tumor stage at presentation. Patients who present with stage III or stage IV disease have a median survival of 4 months or less (113). Patients with involvement of regional lymph nodes fare only slightly better, with a median survival of 7 months. A relationship between histologic grade and survival was suggested in this same study, although multivariant analysis was not performed and improvement in survival with well-differentiated tumors was very slight, with only 4 months difference in median survival between patients with well-differentiated tumors and poorly differentiated tumors. Papillary adenocarcinoma has been associated with the best survival, probably because of its propensity to present at an earlier stage than other gallbladder carcinomas. Small cell carcinoma is associated with a very poor prognosis. This study also suggested that vascular invasion was a poor prognostic sign (113).

DNA content as measured by flow cytometry (114), overexpression of the p53 gene product (106), and expression of c-erbB-2 gene product (115) have not emerged as prognostically relevant markers.

SUGGESTED READINGS

Weisner RH, LaRusso NF, Ludwig J, Dickson ER. Comparison of the clinicopathologic features of primary sclerosing cholangitis and primary biliary cirrhosis. Gastroenterology 1985;88:108–14. This is an important paper delineating the clinical features and describing histologic findings in PBC and PSC. The descriptions of the pathologic features of these disorders are brief but the observations remain sound more than 15 years later.

Demetris AJ, Batts KP, Dhillon AP, et al. Banff schema for grading liver allograft rejection: an international consensus document. Hepatology 1997;25:658–63. This paper details the standardized nomenclature and grading of acute allograft rejection currently in use in most major liver transplantation centers.

Desmet VJ. Congenital disease of the intrahepatic bile ducts: variations on the theme "ductal plate malformation." Hepatology 1994;16:1069–83. This paper is a review of bile duct embryogenesis and the role of ductal plate malformation in the pathogenesis of fibropolycystic liver diseases. The descriptions of the relationship between the various forms of congenital biliary tract diseases are particularly informative.

REFERENCES

1. Torzilli G, Minigawa M, Takaya T, et al. Accurate preoperative evaluation of liver mass lesions without fine-needle biopsy. Hepatology 1999;30:889–93.
2. John TG, Garden OJ. Needle track seeding of primary and secondary liver carcinoma after percutaneous needle biopsy. HPB Surg 1993;6:199–203.
3. Trent V, Khurana KK, Pisharodi LR. Diagnostic accuracy and clinical utility of endoscopic bile duct brushings in the evaluation of biliary strictures. Arch Pathol Lab Med 1999;123:712–5.
4. Tamada K, Kurihara K, Tomiyama T, et al. How many biopsies should be performed during percutaneous transhepatic cholangioscopy to diagnose biliary tract cancer? Gastrointest Endosc 1999;50:653–8.
5. Kurzawinski TR, Deery A, Dooley JS, et al. A prospective study of biliary cytology in 100 patients with bile duct strictures. Hepatology 1993;18:1399–1403.
6. Joplin R, Gershwin ME. Ductular expression of autoantigens in primary biliary cirrhosis. Semin Liver Dis 1997;17:97–103.
7. Wiesner RH, LaRusso NF, Ludwig J, Dickson ER. Comparison of the clinicopathologic features of primary sclerosing cholangitis and primary biliary cirrhosis. Gastroenterology 1985;88:108–14.
8. Goodman ZD, McNally PR, Davis DR, Ishak KG. Autoimmune cholangitis: a variant of primary biliary cirrhosis. Clinicopathologic and serologic correlations in 200 cases. Dig Dis Sci 1995;40:1232–42.
9. Lacerda MA, Ludwig J, Dickson ER, et al. Antimitochondrial antibody-negative primary biliary cirrhosis. Am J Gastroenterol 1995;90:247–9.
10. Michieletti P, Wanless IR, Katz A, et al. Antimitochondrial antibody negative primary biliary cirrhosis: a distinct syndrome of autoimmune cholangitis. Gut 1994;35:260–5.
11. Taylor SL, Dean PJ, Riely CA. Primary autoimmune cholangitis. An alternative to antimitochondrial antibody-negative primary biliary cirrhosis. Am J Surg Pathol 1994;18:91–9.
12. Invernizzi P, Crosignani A, Battezzati PM, et al. Comparison of the clinical features and clinical course of antimitochondrial antibody-positive and -negative primary biliary cirrhosis. Hepatology 1997;25:1090–5.
13. Lohse AW, zum Buschenfeld KH, Franz B, et al. Characterization of the overlap syndrome of primary biliary cirrhosis (PBC) and autoimmune hepatitis: evidence for it being a hepatitic form of PBC in genetically susceptible individuals. Hepatology 1999;29:1078–84.
14. Chazouilleres O, Wendum D, Serfaty L, et al. Primary biliary cirrhosis-autoimmune hepatitis overlap syndrome: clinical features and response to therapy. Hepatology 1998;28:296–301.
15. Devaney K, Goodman ZD, Epstein MS, et al. Hepatic sarcoidosis: clinicopathologic features in 100 patients. Am J Surg Pathol 1993;17:1272–80.
16. Ishak KG. Sarcoidosis of the liver and bile ducts. Mayo Clin Proc 1998;73:467–72.
17. Alam I, Levenson SD, Ferrell LD, Bass NM. Diffuse intrahepatic biliary strictures in sarcoidosis resembling sclerosing cholangitis. Case report and review of the literature. Dig Dis Sci 1997;42:1295–301.
18. Scheuer PJ. Primary biliary cirrhosis. Proc Roy Soc Med 1967;60:1257–60.
19. Ludwig J, Dickson ER, McDonald GS. Staging of chronic non-suppurative cholangitis (syndrome of primary biliary cirrhosis). Virchows Arch A 1978;379:103–12.
20. Demetris AJ. Immune cholangitis: liver allograft rejection and graft-versus-host disease. Mayo Clin Proc 1998;73:367–79.
21. Washington MK, Howell DN. The role of histopathology in the evaluation of the liver transplant recipient. In: Killenberg PC, Clavien PA, eds. Medical care of the liver transplant patient. Malden, MA: Blackwell Science, 1997.
22. McDonald GB, Shulman HM, Wolford JL, Spencer GD. Liver disease after human marrow transplantation. Semin Liver Dis 1987;7:210–29.
23. Tasamandas AC, Jain AB, Felekouras ES, et al. Central venulitis in the allograft liver: a clinicopathologic study. Transplantation 1997;64:252–7.
24. Shulman HM, Sharma P, Amos D, et al. A coded histologic study of hepatic graft-versus-host disease after human bone marrow transplantation. Hepatology 1988;8:463–70.
25. Snover DC, Weisdorf SA, Ramsay NK, et al. Hepatic graft versus host disease: a study of the predictive value of liver biopsy in diagnosis. Hepatology 1984;4:123–30.
26. Sullivan KM, Agura E, Anasetti C, et al. Chronic graft-versus-host disease and other late complications of bone marrow transplantation. Semin Hematol 1991;28:250–9.
27. Demetris AJ, Batts KP, Dhillon AP, et al. Banff schema for grading liver allograft rejection: an international consensus document. Hepatology 1997;25:658–63.
28. Ormonde DG, de Boer WB, Kierath A, et al. Banff schema for grading liver allograft rejection: utility in clinical practice. Liver Transpl Surg 1999;5:261–8.
29. Snover DC. Biopsy diagnosis of liver disease. Baltimore: Williams & Wilkins, 1992:228–9.
30. Ludwig J. Idiopathic adulthood ductopenia: an update. Mayo Clin Proc 1998;3:285–91.

31. Bruguera M, Llach J, Rodes J. Nonsyndromic paucity of intrahepatic bile ducts in infancy and idiopathic ductopenia in adulthood: the same syndrome? Hepatology 1992;15:830–4.
32. Moreno A, Carreno V, Cano A, Gonzalez C. Idiopathic biliary ductopenia in adults without symptoms of liver disease. N Engl J Med 1997;336:835–8.
33. Erlinger S. Drug-induced cholestasis. J Hepatol 1997;26(suppl 1):1–4.
34. Desmet VJ. Vanishing bile duct syndrome in drug-induced liver disease. J Hepatol 1997;26(suppl 1):31–5.
35. Hunt CM, Washington K. Tetracycline-induced bile duct paucity and prolonged cholestasis. Gastroenterology 1994;107:1844–7.
36. Altraif I, Lilly L, Wanless IR, Heathcote J. Cholestatic liver disease with ductopenia (vanishing bile duct syndrome) after administration of clindamycin and trimethoprim-sulfamethoxazole. Am J Gastroenterol 1994;89:1230–4.
37. Degott C, Feldmann G, Larrey D, et al. Drug-induced prolonged cholestasis in adults: a histological semiquantitiative study demonstrating progressive ductopenia. Hepatology 1992;15:244–51.
38. Carpenter HA. Bacterial and parasitic cholangitis. Mayo Clin Proc 1998;73:473–8.
39. Yoon KH, Ha HK, Lee JS, et al. Inflammatory pseudotumor of the liver in patients with recurrent pyogenic cholangitis: CT-histopathologic correlation. Radiology 1999;211:373–9.
40. Weisner RH, Porayko MK, LaRusso NF, Ludwig J. Primary sclerosing cholangitis. In: Schiff L, Schiff ER, eds. Diseases of the liver. 7th ed. Philadelphia: J.B. Lippincott, 1993:411–26.
41. Donaldson PT, Farrant JM, Wilkinson ML, et al. Dual association of HLA DR2 and DR3 with primary sclerosing cholangitis. Hepatology 1991;13:129–33.
42. Nichols JC, Gores GJ, LaRusso NF, et al. Diagnostic role of serum CA 19-9 for cholangiocarcinoma in patients with primary sclerosing cholangitis. Mayo Clin Proc 1993;68:874–9.
43. Casali AM, Carbone G, Cavalli G. Intrahepatic bile duct loss in primary sclerosing cholangitis: a quantitative study. Histopathology 1998;32:449–53.
44. Ludwig J, Colina F, Poterucha JJ. Granulomas in primary sclerosing cholangitis. Liver 1995;15:307–12.
45. Ferrell L. Malignant liver tumors that mimic benign lesions: analysis of five distinct lesions. Semin Diag Pathol 1995;12:64–76.
46. Wilchanski M, Chait P, Wade JA, et al. Primary sclerosing cholangitis in 32 children: clinical, laboratory, and radiographic feature, with survival analysis. Hepatology 1995;22:1415–22.
47. Ludwig J, Kim CH, Wiesner RH, Krom RA. Floxuridine-induced sclerosing cholangitis: an ischemic cholangiopathy? Hepatology 1989;9:215–8.
48. Rougier P, Laplanche A, Hugier M, et al. Hepatic arterial infusion of floxuridine in patients with liver metastases from colorectal carcinoma: long-term results of a prospective randomized trial. J Clin Oncol 1992;10:1112–8.
49. Kaplan KJ, Goodman ZD, Ishak KG. Liver involvement in Langerhans' cell histiocytosis: a study of nine cases. Mod Pathol 1999;12:370–8.
50. Lefkowitch JH. Pathology of AIDS-related liver disease. Dig Dis 1994;12:321–30.
51. Chen X-M, Levine SA, Tietz P, et al. Cryptosporidium parvum is cytopathic for cultured human biliary epithelia via an apoptotic mechanism. Hepatology 1998;28:906–13.
52. Stephens J, Cosyns M, Jones M, Hayward A. Liver and bile duct pathology following *Cryptosporidium parvum* infection of immunodeficient mice. Hepatology 1999;30:27–35.
53. Debray D, Pariente D, Urvoas E, et al. Sclerosing cholangitis in children. J Pediatr 1994;124:49–56.
54. Vick DJ, Goodman ZD, Deavers MT, et al. Ciliated hepatic foregut cyst: a study of six cases and review of the literature. Am J Surg Pathol 1999;23:671–7.
55. Desmet VJ. Ludwig symposium on biliary disorders- part I. Pathogenesis of ductal plate abnormalities. Mayo Clin Proc 1998;73:90–9.
56. Desmet VJ. Congenital diseases of intrahepatic bile ducts: variations on the theme "ductal plate malformation." Hepatology 1992;16:1069–83.
57. D'Agata IAD, Jonas MM, Perez-Atayde AR, Guay-Woodford LM. Combined cystic disease of the liver and kidney. Semin Liver Dis 1994;14:215–28.
58. Perisic VN. Long-term studies on congenital hepatic fibrosis in children. Acta Paediatr 1995;84:695–6.
59. Gabow PA, Johnson AM, Kaehny WD, et al. Risk factors for the development of hepatic cysts in autosomal dominant polycystic kidney disease. Hepatology 1990;11:1033–7.
60. Bacallao RL, Carone FA. Recent advances in the understanding of polycystic kidney disease. Curr Opin Nephrol Hypertens 1997;6:377–83.
61. Wu G, d'Agati V, Cai Y, et al. Somatic inactivation of Pkd2 results in polycystic kidney disease. Cell 1998;93:177–88.
62. Watnick TJ, Torres VE, Gandolph MA, et al. Somatic mutation in individual liver cysts supports a two-hit model of cytogenesis in autosomal dominant polycystic kidney disease. Mol Cell 1998;2:247–51.
63. O'Sullivan DA, Torres VE, Gabow PA, et al. Cystic fibrosis and the phenotypic expression of autosomal dominant polycystic kidney disease. Am J Kidney Dis 1998;32:976–83.
64. Matsumoto Y, Uchida K, Nakase A, Houjo I. Clinicopathologic classification of congenital cystic dilatation of the common bile duct. Am J Surg 1977;134:569–74.
65. Bates MD, Bucuvalas JC, Alonso MH, Ryckman FC. Biliary atresia: pathogenesis and treatment. Semin Liver Dis 1998;18:281–93.
66. Jevon GP, Dimmick JE. Biliary atresia and cytomegalovirus infection: a DNA study. Pedatr Dev Pathol 1999;2:11–4.
67. Carmi R, Magee CA, Neill CA, Karrer FM. Extrahepatic biliary atresia and associated anomalies: Etiologic heterogeneity suggested by distinctive patterns of association. Am J Medi Genetics 1993;45:683–93.
68. Tan CE, Davenport M, Driver M, Howard ER. Does the morphology of the extrahepatic biliary remnants in biliary atresia influence survival? A review of 205 cases. J Pediatr Surg 1994;29:1459–64.
69. Lunzmann K, Schweizer P. The influence of cholangitis on the prognosis of extrahepatic biliary atresia. Eur J Pediatr Surg 1999;9:19–23.
70. Krantz ID, Piccoli DA, Spinner NB. Alagille syndrome. J Med Genet 1997;34:152–7.
71. Li L, Krantz ID, Genin A, et al. Alagille syndrome is caused by mutations in human Jagged1, which encodes a ligand for Notch1. Nat Genet 1997;16:243–51.
72. Oda T, Elkahloun AG, Pike BL, et al. Mutations in the human Jagged1 gene are responsible for Alagille syndrome. Nat Genet 1997;16:235–42.
73. Dimmick JE. Intrahepatic bile duct paucity and cytomegalovirus infection. Pediatr Pathol 1993;13:847–52.
74. Bhathal PS, Hughes NR, Goodman ZD. The so-called bile duct adenoma is a peribiliary gland hamartoma. Am J Surg Pathol 1996;20:858–64.
75. Allaire GS, Rabin L, Ishak KG, Sesterhenn IA. Bile duct adenoma. A study of 152 cases. Am J Surg Pathol 1988;12:708–15.
76. Davies W, Chow M, Nagorney D. Extrahepatic biliary cystadenomas and cystadenocarcinoma. Report of seven cases and review of the literature. Ann Surg 1995;222:619–25.
77. Devaney K, Goodman ZD, Ishak KG. Hepatobiliary cystadenoma and cystadenocarcinoma. A light microscopic and immunohistochemical study of 70 patients. Am J Surg Pathol 1994;18:1078–91.
78. Terada T, Kitamura Y, Ohta T, Nakanuma Y. Endocrine cells in hepatobiliary cystadenomas and cystadenocarcinomas. Virchows Arch 1997;430:37–40.
79. Colombari R, Tsui WM. Biliary tumors of the liver. Semin Liver Dis 1995;15:402–13.
80. Nakeeb A, Pitt HA, Sohn TA, et al. Cholangiocarcinoma. A spectrum of intrahepatic, perihilar, and distal tumors. Ann Surg 1996;224:463–73.
81. Su CH, Tsay SH, Wu CC, et al. Factors influencing postoperative morbidity, mortality, and survival after resection for hilar cholangiocarcinoma. Ann Surg 1996;223:384–94.
82. Klempnauer J, Ridder GJ, von Wasielewski R, et al. Resectional surgery of hilar cholangiocarcinoma: a multivariate analysis of prognostic factors. J Clin Oncol 1997;15:947–54.
83. Klempnauer J, Ridder GJ, Werner M, et al. What constitutes long term survival after surgery for hilar cholangiocarcinoma? Cancer 1997;79:26–34.
84. Nagorney DM, Donohue JH, Farnell MB, et al. Outcomes after curative resections of cholangiocarcinoma. Arch Surg 1993;128:871–9.
85. Beahrs OH, Henson DE, Hutter RVP, et al. Manual for staging of cancer. Philadelphia: Lippincott, 1992.
86. Jarnagin WR, Fong Y, Blumgart LH. The current management of hilar cholangiocarcinoma. Adv Surg 1999;33:345–73.
87. Layfield LJ, Wax TD, Lee JG, Cotton PB. Accuracy and morphologic aspects of pancreatic and biliary duct brushings. Acta Cytol 1995;39:11–18.
88. Bardales RH, Stanley MW, Simpson DD, et al. Diagnostic value of brush cytology in diagnosis of duodenal, biliary, and ampullary neoplasms. Am J Clin Pathol 1998;109:540–8.
89. Yamanaka N, Okamoto E, Ando T, et al. Clinicopathologic spectrum of resected extraductal mass-forming intrahepatic cholangiocarcinoma. Cancer 1995;76:2449–56.
90. Rubel LR, Ishak KG. Thorotrast-associated cholangiocarcinoma. An epidemiologic and clinicopathologic study. Cancer 1982;50:1408–15.
91. Terada T, Kida T, Nakanuma Y, et al. Intrahepatic cholangiocarcinomas associated with nonbiliary cirrhosis. A clinicopathologic study. J Clin Gastroenterol 1994;18:335–42.

92. Chou FF, Sheen-Chen SM, Chen CL, et al. Prognostic factors of resectable intrahepatic cholangiocarcinoma. J Surg Oncol 1995;59:40–4.
93. Kajiyama K, Maeda T, Takenaka K, et al. The significance of stromal desmoplasia in intrahepatic cholangiocarcinoma: a special reference of "scirrhous-type" and "non-scirrhous-type" growth. Am J Surg Pathol 1999;23:892–902.
94. Madariaga JR, Iwatsuki S, Todo S, et al. Liver resection for hilar and peripheral cholangiocarcinomas: a study of 62 cases. Ann Surg 1998;227:70–9.
95. Suh KS, Roh HR, Lee KU, et al. Clinicopathologic features of the intraductal growth type of peripheral cholangiocarcinoma. Hepatology 2000;31:12–17.
96. Nakajima T, Tajima Y, Sugano I, et al. Intrahepatic cholangiocarcinoma with sarcomatous change. Cancer 1993;72:1872–7.
97. Riopel MA, Klimstra DS, Godellas CV, et al. Intrabiliary growth of metastatic colonic adenocarcinoma: a pattern of intrahepatic spread easily confused with primary neoplasia of the biliary tract. Am J Surg Pathol 1997;21:1030–6.
98. Okano K, Yamamoto J, Moriya Y, et al. Macroscopic intrabiliary growth of liver metastases from colorectal cancer. Surgery 1999;126:829–34.
99. Ikeda Y, Matsuma T, Adachi E, et al. Hepatocellular carcinoma of the intrabiliary growth type. Int Surg 1997;82:76–8.
100. Lai ST, Lam KT, Lee KC. Biliary tract invasion and obstruction by hepatocellular carcinoma: report of five cases. Postgrad Med J 1992;68:961–3.
101. Goodman ZD, Ishak KG, Langloss JM. Combined hepatocellular-cholangiocarcinoma: a histologic and immunohistochemical study. Cancer 1984;55:124–35.
102. Maeda T, Adachi E, Kajiyama K, et al. Combined hepatocellular and cholangiocarcinoma: proposed criteria according to cytokeratin expression and analysis of clinicopathologic features. Hum Pathol 1995;26:956–64.
103. Theise ND, Miller F, Worman HJ, et al. Biliary cystadenoma arising in a liver with fibropolycystic disease. Arch Pathol Lab Med 1993;117:163–5.
104. Albores-Saavedra J, Vardaman CJ, Vuitch F. Non-neoplastic polypoid lesions and adenomas of the gallbladder. Pathol Ann 1993;28:145–78.
105. Jones RS. Carcinoma of the gallbladder. Surgical Clinics of North America 1990;70:1419–28.
106. Washington K, Gottfried MR. Expression of p53 in adenocarcinoma of the gallbladder and bile ducts. Liver 1996;16:99–104.
107. Wistuba II, Gazdar AF, Roa I, et al. p53 protein overexpression in gallbladder carcinoma and its precursor lesions: an immunohistochemical study. Human Pathology 1996;27:360–5.
108. Duarte I, Llanos O, Domke H, et al. Metaplasia and precursor lesions of gallbladder carcinoma: frequency, distribution, and probability of detection in routine histologic samples. Cancer 1993;72:1878–84.
109. Roa I, Araya JC, Villaseca M, et al. Preneoplastic lesions and gallbladder cancer: an estimate of the time period required for progression. Gastroenterology 1996;111:232–36.
110. Roa I, Araya JC, Villaseca M, et al. Gallbladder cancer in a high risk area: morphological features and spread patterns. Hepatogastroenterology 1999;46:1540–6.
111. Albores-Saavedra J, Molberg K, Henson DE. Unusual malignant epithelial tumors of the gallbladder. Semin Diag Pathol 1996;13:326–38.
112. Albores-Saavedra J, Henson DE, Sobin LH. The WHO histologic classification of tumors of the gallbladder and extrahepatic bile ducts: a commentary on the second edition. Cancer 1992;70:410–14.
113. Henson DE, Albores-Saavedra J, Corle D. Carcinoma of the gallbladder: histologic types, stage of disease, grade, and survival. Cancer 1992;70: 1493–7.
114. Roa I, Araya JC, Shiraishi T, et al. DNA content in gallbladder carcinoma: a flow cytometric study of 96 cases. Histopathology 1993;23: 459–64.
115. Suzuki T, Takano Y, Kakita A, et al. An immunohistochemical and molecular biological study of c-erbB-2 amplification and prognostic relevance in gallbladder cancer. Pathol Res Prac 1993;189:283–92.

Chapter 3

Noninvasive Imaging of the Gallbladder and Bile Ducts

KENNETH A. WONG RENDON C. NELSON

Noninvasive imaging of the gallbladder and bile ducts is a challenging task because these are thin-walled tubular structures that often course either perpendicular or tangential to the axial plane, which is the typical plane of section. As a result, techniques that are capable of generating images in more anatomically suitable planes, such as the coronal or oblique planes, often add more diagnostic information. Normal caliber ducts, particularly the intrahepatic bile ducts, are usually not visualized with the various cross-sectional imaging techniques, although they may be depicted on occasion using higher resolution modalities. In addition to differences in risk and cost, the major advantage of noninvasive over invasive procedures is the ability to evaluate the periductal or pericholecystic soft tissue such as the liver, porta hepatis, and pancreas. Furthermore, distant metastatic foci, either lymphatic or hematogenous, can be determined.

This chapter discusses the various imaging techniques that can be applied to evaluating the gallbladder and bile ducts, including ultrasound, computed tomography, magnetic resonance imaging, and nuclear medicine. Technical considerations as well as the advantages and disadvantages of each modality are emphasized in the first part of this chapter. Then the imaging features with examples of various disease entities affecting these structures will be discussed. The chapter finishes with a review of cholescintigraphy and its role in imaging the gallbladder and bile ducts.

MODALITIES

Ultrasound

Ultrasound uses high-frequency sound waves that are imperceptible to the human ear but able to penetrate human soft tissue. A small hand-held transducer is used to both transmit the sound waves and receive the echoes reflected by internal tissue interfaces. Sound waves at these frequencies are not well-propagated by gas-containing structures, such as the lungs or the gastrointestinal tract. This is particularly a problem in patients with an adynamic ileus or bowel obstruction. Bony structures also inhibit the transmission of the sound waves. Therefore, ultrasound is best suited to evaluating solid organs such as the liver, spleen, and kidneys, as well as fluid-filled structures such as the gallbladder, bile ducts, and pancreatic duct. The ability to evaluate the pancreas with ultrasound is variable, depending upon the nature of surrounding structures such as the gastric antrum, transverse colon, or proximal jejunum. An oral contrast agent has recently been introduced that both displaces and absorbs gas in the lumen of the stomach, duodenum, and proximal jejunum, thereby providing a window for visualizing the pancreas and surrounding structures (1). Although large patients with extensive subcutaneous and/or visceral fat are often difficult to image with ultrasound due to absorption of the sound beam by the echogenic fat, recent software upgrades that use harmonics have resulted in improved image quality in these patients as well (2,3). The addition of color and power Doppler has further expanded the diagnostic capability of ultrasound so that it can evaluate blood flow in both a qualitative and semi-quantitative fashion. Intravascular contrast agents are currently being developed that, when administered intravenously, will cause both blood vessels and parenchymal tissue to enhance (4). These agents promise to not only improve the depiction of blood vessels but also increase the ability of ultrasound to detect focal masses in solid organs.

The advantages of ultrasound include the lack of ionizing radiation, the multiplanar capability, portability, the lack of motion sensitivity and the relative low cost. Furthermore, ultrasound is an excellent method for guiding percutaneous biopsies and drainages. Disadvantages include the limitations in sound transmission, and the fact that it is highly operator dependent and somewhat time consuming.

Computed Tomography

A computed tomography (CT) scanner basically consists of an x-ray tube, which rotates around the patient, and a moving tabletop, which exposes different parts of the body. There are two main types of CT scanners, axial and spiral. With older axial scanners, large power cables connected to the x-ray tube prohibited more than one rotation in the same direction (e.g., clockwise). During the time the x-ray tube is changing directions, the tabletop moves a distance equal to the thickness of one or more axial slices. Therefore, axial scanning has intermittent x-ray exposure and incremental table motion. By comparison, the newer spiral scanners have a slip-ring connection between the x-ray tube and the power supply allowing it to rotate in the same direction indefinitely. While the tube is spinning, the tabletop smoothly moves the patient through the gantry. Therefore, spiral scanning has both continuous x-ray tube exposure and continuous table motion (5). As a result, spiral scanning yields a volumetric data set in a much shorter period of time (seconds rather than minutes). If the data set is acquired using thin slices and slower table speeds, high quality multiplanar and three-dimensional images can be reconstructed. On the other hand, if a certain clinical situation demands that speed is more important than quality, the data set can be acquired with thick slices and faster table speeds. This data set, however, would not yield high quality multiplanar or three-dimensional images.

When imaging the abdomen, spiral scanning is preferable to axial scanning in almost every clinical situation. Exceptions include the spine and use in very large patients. In 1998, multislice spiral scanners were introduced, which can obtain up to four slices per x-ray tube rotation (6). These scanners not only are faster, allowing the operator to scan the entire abdomen and pelvis during a single breath-hold of about 20 seconds, but also extend the three-dimensional capability of CT.

The advantages of CT include very high spatial resolution, rapid acquisition and turnover times, somewhat lower operator dependence, three-dimensional capability, and the lack of patient claustrophobia. Disadvantages include the presence of ionizing radiation, which is mainly a concern in children and young adults, the need for gastrointestinal and intravascular contrast agents, the limitation to the axial plane, which is somewhat offset by three-dimensional imaging, and the relative high cost. Although CT of the abdomen can be performed without contrast agents, the diagnostic capability can be considerably extended. This is particularly true for detecting tumors in solid organs, such as the liver, spleen, and pancreas. Furthermore, as intravascular contrast agents are limited to the extracellular space and rapidly undergo both equilibrium and excretion, the optimal effect is very transient (7). Consequently, spiral scanners do a much better job at capitalizing on these enhancement effects than axial scanners.

Magnetic Resonance Imaging (MRI)

Magnetic resonance imaging (MRI) has a number of advantages over other imaging techniques. MRI, like ultrasound, requires no ionizing radiation. Instead, it uses strong magnetic fields and radiofrequency pulses to excite protons in hydrogen atoms. Relaxation of these excited hydrogen protons causes them to emit an echo, which yields information about the location and nature of various tissues. Tissue characterization includes the ability to differentiate fat, fluid, and blood as well as other tissues depending on the radiofrequency signal intensity encountered when different sequences are used. Gadolinium-chelates can be used as enhancing contrast agents in MRI (similar to iodinated contrast agents in CT), allowing better detection and characterization of solid and cystic masses. Gadolinium-chelates, however, have fewer side effects or adverse reactions compared to iodinated contrast agents. Furthermore, because the sensitivity and specificity are superior to that of noncontrast CT, MRI with gadolinium enhancement is an excellent alternative to CT in patients who have one or more contraindication to a bolus of iodinated contrast material.

The main disadvantages of MRI include limited availability, longer imaging time, lower spatial resolution, and higher cost. In major centers in the United States, MRI is widely available although it may not be as ubiquitous as CT or ultrasound in smaller centers or in some foreign countries. When MRI is available, many centers use this modality primarily for evaluating the central nervous or musculoskeletal systems where MRI has proven to provide important clinical information. As a result, less time remains for abdominal MRI; mainly due to the introduction of faster imaging techniques, MRI has recently been able to provide important clinical information. Time is also an important consideration, as some abdominal MRI protocols require up to an hour to complete. This means that a medically stable and cooperative patient is required to produce quality diagnostic images. Many patients who can tolerate a CT scan have difficulty with MRI due to claustrophobia. In addition, there are a number of conditions such as the presence of cardiac pacemakers, neurosurgical clips, or metallic foreign bodies in the eyes that disqualify patients from entering the magnet. The image resolution of MRI is similar to that of ultrasound and approximately half that of CT. CT has a resolution capability of 0.7 line pairs/mm whereas MRI has a resolution capability of only 0.3 line pairs/mm.

MRI Technique

In general, T1-weighted sequences allow good anatomical depiction with or without an MRI contrast agent. T2-weighted sequences demonstrate high signal intensity in water-containing structures as well as in areas of inflammation and neoplasia. Fat suppression techniques are often added to both T1- and T2-weighted sequences to reduce motion artifacts and improve tissue contrast. Images are typically acquired in the axial planes, although the coronal and sagittal planes can also be obtained electronically and are useful for further defining anatomy and pathology.

MRI of the gallbladder and bile ducts is somewhat limited at present and is usually reserved for clinical cases in which ultrasound and/or CT are equivocal or nondiagnostic. However, MRI has proven valuable as a problem solver when indeterminate cases occur. It is particularly valuable in the setting of cholangiocarcinoma for delineating the extent of disease and for evaluating the biliary tree when invasive methods such as endoscopic retrograde cholangiopancreatography (ERCP) are equivocal or contraindicated.

Magnetic resonance cholangiopancreatography (MRCP) is a relatively new technique that employs heavily T2-weighted sequences to impart a very high-signal intensity to water-containing structures such as the gallbladder and bile ducts, contrasted against a low-signal intensity background (8). The technique is a valuable noninvasive method of imaging the gallbladder, bile ducts, and pancreatic duct and can be displayed in a format similar to that of ERCP using a computer workstation.

Gadolinium-chelates are the most commonly used contrast agents in MRI. When these extracellular agents are administered intravenously and coupled with dynamic imaging, they have been shown to improve the detection and characterization of both inflammatory and neoplastic processes (9). Other contrast agents such as manganese-DPDP or gadolinium-EOB-DTPA can also be used to better demonstrate ductal anatomy and pathology. When these agents are injected intravenously they are partly excreted into the bile by the hepatocytes and then imaged using T1-weighted sequences.

GALLBLADDER

Ultrasound is the technique of choice for initial imaging of the gallbladder. This tubular structure is well visualized by ultrasound because it is both fluid-filled and relatively superficial. Ultrasound is not only capable of visualizing the lumen and its contents but also the gallbladder wall and adjacent liver. The gallbladder is also well visualized by CT, regardless of the location. It appears as a thin-walled water attenuation structure surrounded by low attenuation fat and bowel (especially the first and second portions of the duodenum and the hepatic flexure of the colon).

The attenuation of bile may be increased in patients with sludge, or several hours to days after the intravascular administration of iodinated contrast material. Although the kidneys excrete the vast majority of contrast material, approximately 2% to 3% is excreted by the liver into the bile and concentrated in the gallbladder (10). This percentage significantly increases in patients with renal dysfunction, as a result of so-called vicarious excretion of contrast material. Imaging of the gallbladder with MRI is reserved for problem solving in cases where ultrasound and/or CT have already been or could not be performed, and they do not answer the clinical question. MRI is very capable of assessing both the gallbladder and surrounding structures, including the pericholecystic fat.

Cholelithiasis

On ultrasound, gallstones are typically seen as mobile echogenic foci of various sizes layered along the dependent portion of the gallbladder lumen and associated with acoustical shadowing (Fig. 3.1). Ultrasound is by far the best and easiest technique for diagnosing cholelithiasis with an accuracy of greater than 95% (11,12). Stones that are undetected by ultrasound are typically those that are small and/or located in the neck of the gallbladder. MRI is superior to ultrasound in localizing stones in the cystic duct and gallbladder neck with a reported sensitivity near 100%, a specificity of 93%, and an accuracy of 97% (13). By comparison, ultrasound had a sensitivity of 62%, specificity of 100%, and accuracy of 94% in the same study. Because bile has a very bright signal intensity on T2-weighted MRI sequences, calculi are seen as low-intensity intraluminal filling defects. On ultrasound, a small percentage of calculi will not demonstrate acoustical shadowing and may be confused with a cholesterol polyp. These stones are usually small, composed of pure cholesterol, or found outside the focal

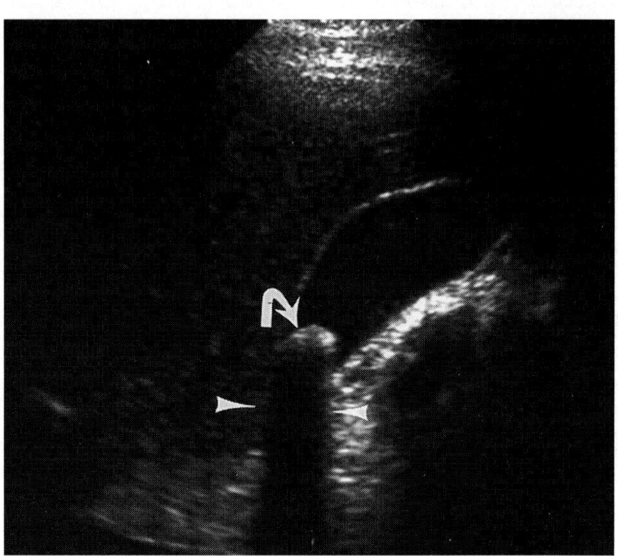

FIGURE 3.1. *Gray-scale ultrasound of the upper abdomen in the sagittal plane reveals a 1.5-cm gallstone (arrow) in the dependent portion of the gallbladder. The typical imaging features include a hyperechoic wall associated with posterior acoustic shadowing (arrowhead).*

zone of the ultrasound transducer. The mobile nature of gallstones is important in distinguishing them from cholesterol or adenomatous polyps. Therefore, it is critical to examine the patient in different positions such as supine, left lateral decubitus, or upright.

CT is not the method of choice for diagnosing gallstones, as an approximate sensitivity of 75% or less is considerably lower than that of ultrasound and MRI (14,15). This is primarily due to the fact that gallstones have a wide range of attenuation values, ranging from hypoattenuating to hyperattenuating. This includes some calculi that have the same attenuation as concentrated bile and therefore are invisible. Many stones have a high attenuation rim of calcium and a low attenuation center. At times, the stones may develop cracks or fissures centrally that cause nitrogen gas to coalesce, the so-called Mercedes-Benz sign (Fig. 3.2).

Cholecystitis

Ultrasound is the imaging modality of choice when assessing patients with possible acute cholecystitis. With this technique, acute cholecystitis is diagnosed when there is a combination of gallbladder distention, one or more calculi, gallbladder wall thickening, and/or focal tenderness over the gallbladder upon graded transducer compression (positive sonographic Murphy's sign) (Fig. 3.3) (16). The presence of pericholecystic fluid further supports the diagnosis. Perihepatic fluid, however, is less specific. CT and MRI are useful in equivocal cases, mainly for evaluating the inflammatory changes seen in the pericholecystic fat that ultrasound cannot reliably detect. Overall, the sensitivity and specificity of ultrasound for acute cholecystitis are approximately 85% to 95% and 64% to 100%, respectively (17,18). The absence of one or more of the above findings diminishes the accuracy. Blood flow in the gallbladder wall by color Doppler ultrasound has been postulated as evidence for hyperemia in acute cholecystitis but this finding remains controversial (19–21). In emphysematous cholecys-

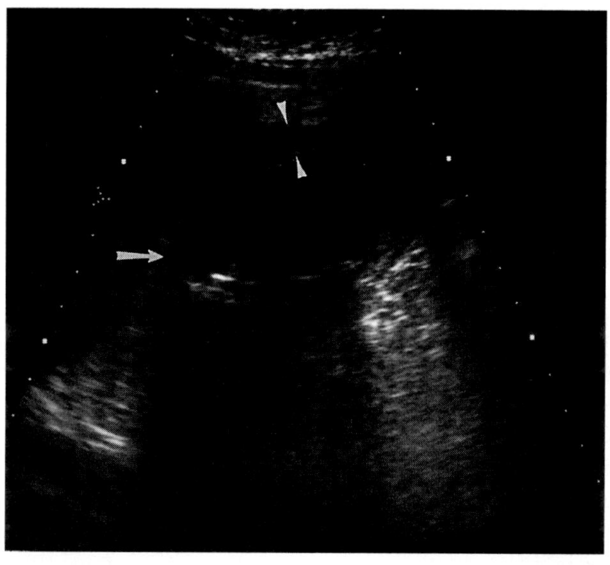

FIGURE 3.3. *Gray-scale ultrasound of the upper abdomen in the sagittal plane reveals a mildly distended gallbladder from a stone (arrow) with shadowing impacted in the neck. There is associated wall thickening (arrowheads) greater than 3 mm. The patient was acutely tender over the gallbladder during scanning indicating a positive sonographic Murphy's sign.*

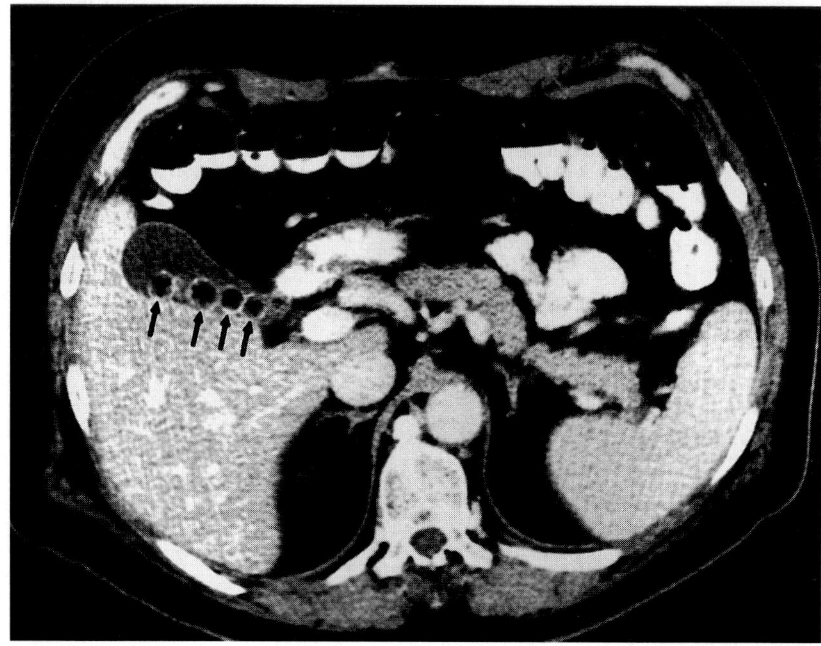

FIGURE 3.2. *Axial contrast-enhanced CT of the upper abdomen shows four calculi in the fundus of the gallbladder, each having a rim of calcium and a star-like collection of air centrally (arrows). This represents gallstone cracking with resultant nitrogen gas formation, the so-called Mercedes Benz sign.*

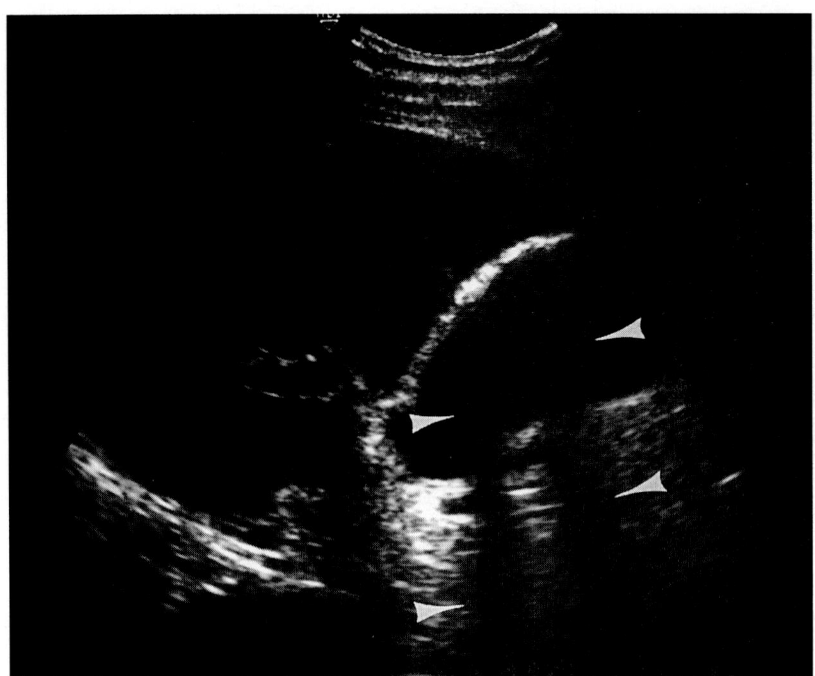

(A)

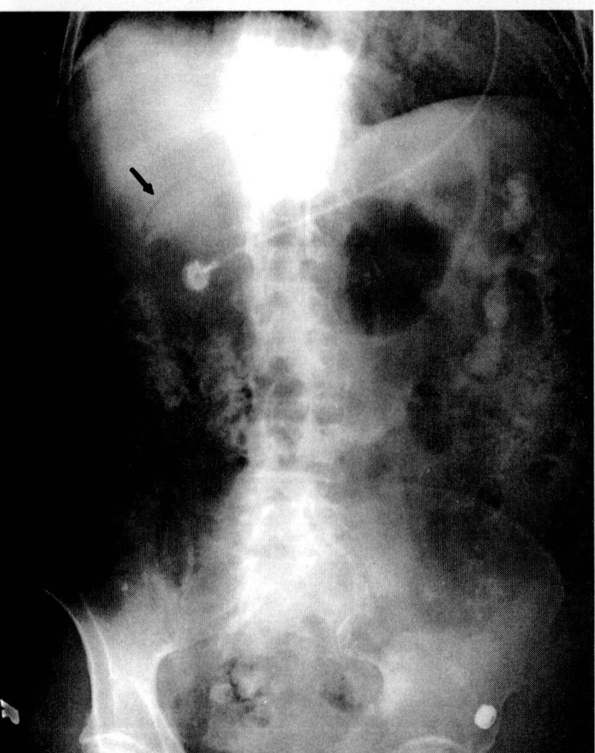

(B)

FIGURE 3.4. ***(A)*** *Gray-scale ultrasound of the gallbladder in the sagittal plane demonstrates a hyperechoic wall with "dirty" posterior acoustic shadowing (arrowheads). This represents gas in the gallbladder wall with resultant poor transmission of sound posteriorly in a patient with emphysematous cholecystitis.* ***(B)*** *This was confirmed with a plain film that shows a concentric rim of gas (arrow) overlying the expected location of the gallbladder wall.* ***(C)*** *It was also confirmed by a CT scan that demonstrated air in the wall of the gallbladder (arrow).*

titis, the intramural gas results in a characteristic indistinct or "dirty" acoustical shadowing from the gallbladder wall (Fig. 3.4).

On CT, acute cholecystitis is suggested when there is a distended gallbladder, with or without calculi, gallbladder wall thickening greater than 3 mm, pericholecystic or perihepatic fluid, and inflammatory stranding in the pericholecystic fat (Fig. 3.5). The latter finding is one of the most important because it is not readily apparent on ultrasound. Furthermore, dynamic contrast-enhanced CT may reveal hyperenhancement in the adjacent liver parenchyma, likely due to regional hyperemia (Fig. 3.6). If a stone is impacted in the neck of the gallbladder and associated with obstruction of the common hepatic or common bile duct, Mirizzi's syndrome is suggested (Fig. 3.7). If the gallbladder is decompressed, contains intraluminal gas, and is associated with an

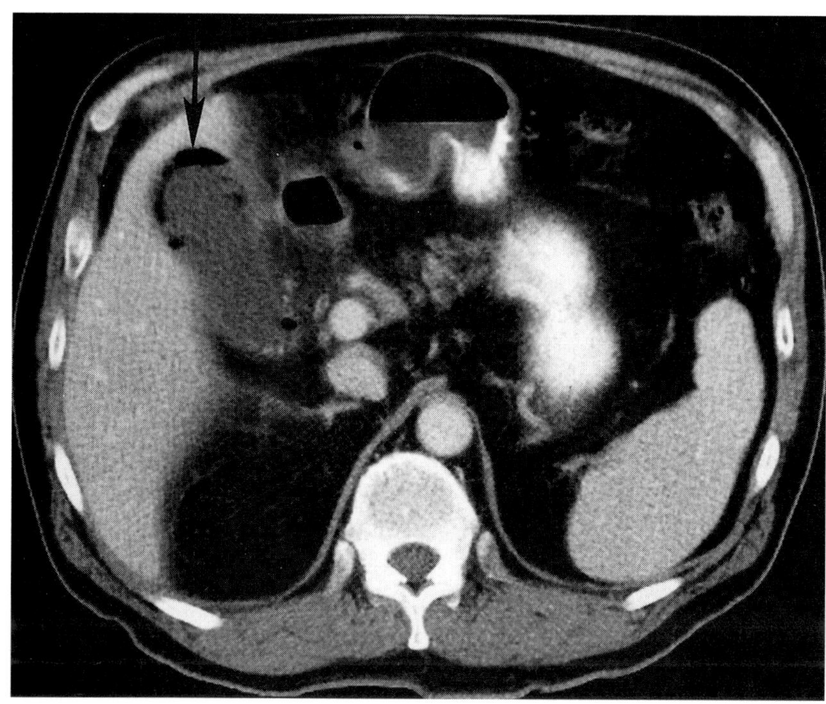

(C)

FIGURE 3.4. *Continued*

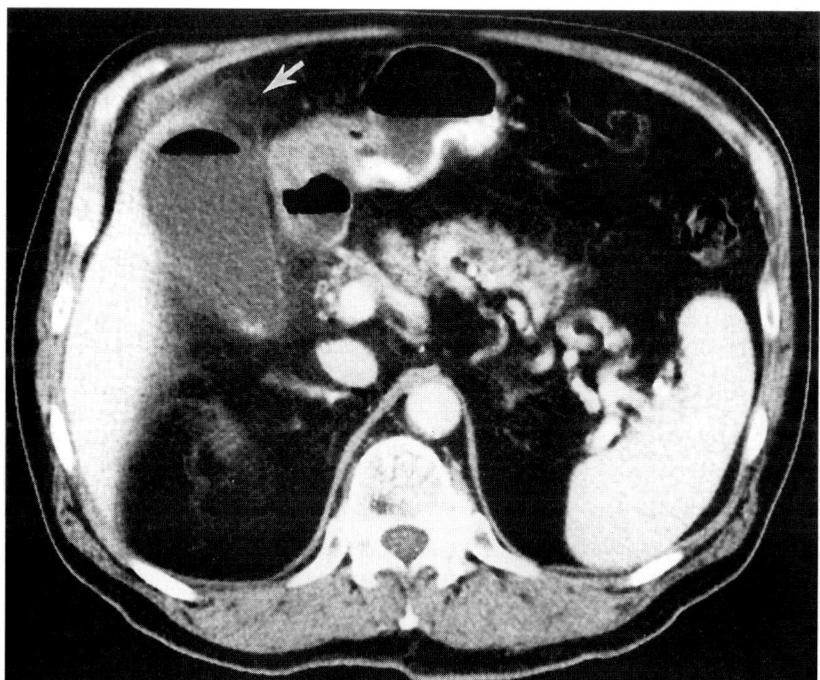

FIGURE 3.5. *Axial contrast-enhanced CT of the upper abdomen demonstrates a distended gallbladder with wall thickening as well as inflammatory stranding in the pericholecystic fat (arrow) in a patient with acute cholecystitis. Air is also noted in the gallbladder fundus.*

obstructing stone in the small bowel, gallstone ileus is suggested (Fig. 3.8). Furthermore, if linear collections of gas are noted in the wall of a distended gallbladder, emphysematous cholecystitis is suggested (see Fig. 3.4).

Findings on MRI include a high signal adjacent to the gallbladder on T2-weighted images likely representing inflammation or pericholecystic fluid. This finding has a sensitivity of 91% and specificity of 79% (22). Thickening and contrast enhancement of the gallbladder wall may also be seen in acute cholecystitis. In the same study, transient increased enhancement of hepatic parenchyma about the gallbladder fossa on post-gadolinium T1-weighted images was seen in 70% of the patients with acute cholecystitis (23).

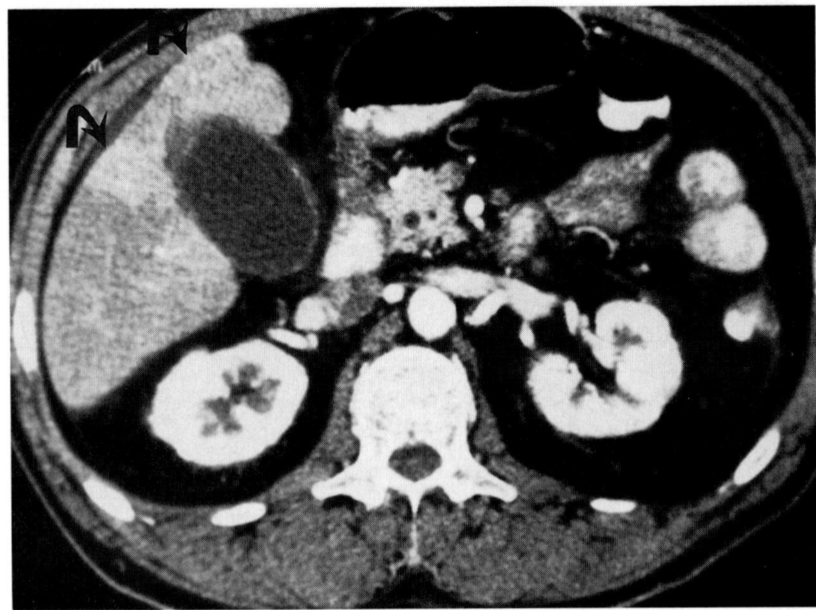

FIGURE 3.6. *Axial contrast-enhanced CT of the upper abdomen in a patient with acute cholecystitis demonstrating the hyperenhancement of the liver parenchyma adjacent to the gallbladder (arrows).*

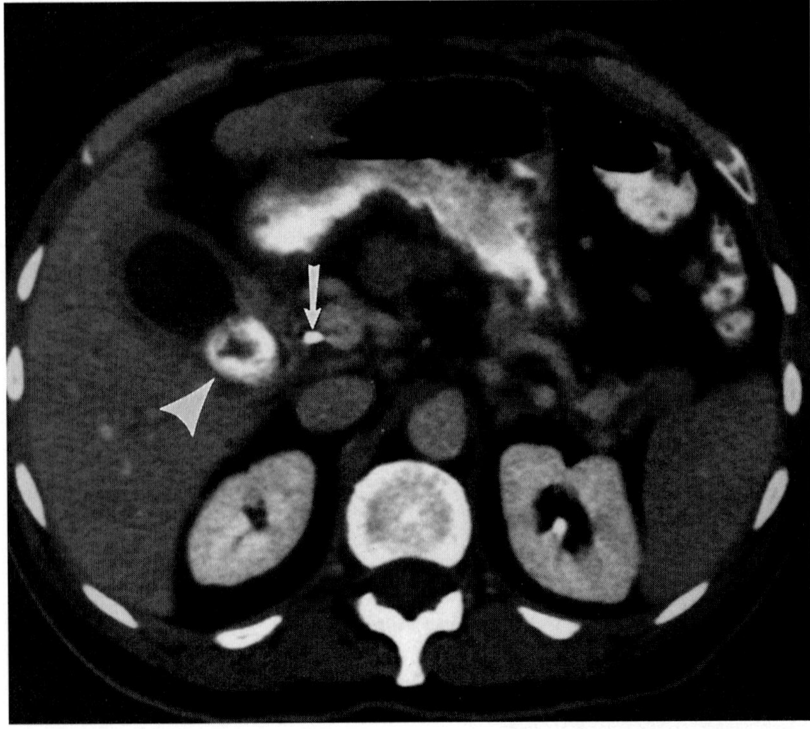

FIGURE 3.7. *Axial contrast-enhanced CT of the upper abdomen in a patient with Mirizzi's syndrome demonstrates a large calcified gallstone impacted in the neck of the gallbladder (arrowhead) associated with gallbladder wall thickening. A radiodense stent (arrow) has been placed in the common bile duct to relieve the biliary obstruction caused by the gallstone.*

In chronic cholecystitis, calculi are often identified in a nondistended gallbladder and there is mild-to-moderate thickening of the gallbladder wall. There is no significant pericholecystic inflammation or fluid. The degree of enhancement on T1-weighted post-gadolinium MRI can help differentiate acute from chronic cholecystitis. One study of patients with chronic cholecystitis demonstrated uniform enhancement of the mucosa and muscularis in the gallbladder wall on early post-gadolinium images and late enhancement of the subserosa on delayed images (24). The latter finding is likely due to fibrosis.

Gallbladder Carcinoma

In general, gallbladder carcinoma is an uncommon malignancy although it is the most common malignancy of the biliary tract. There is a female predominance and the majority of tumors are well-differentiated adenocarcinomas.

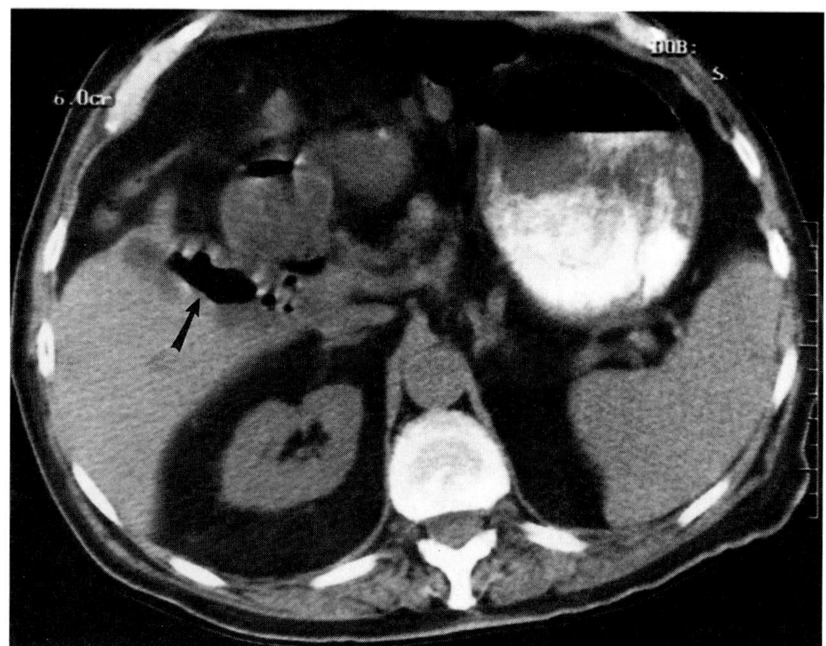

(A)

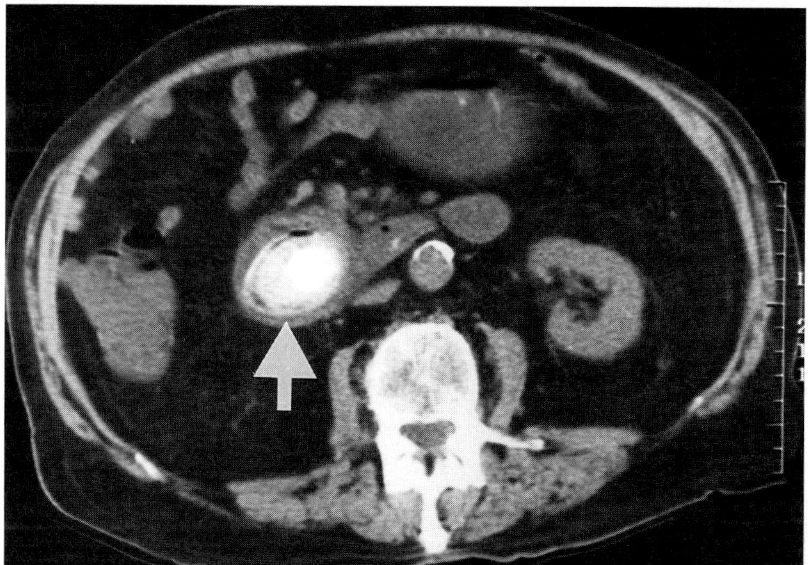

(B)

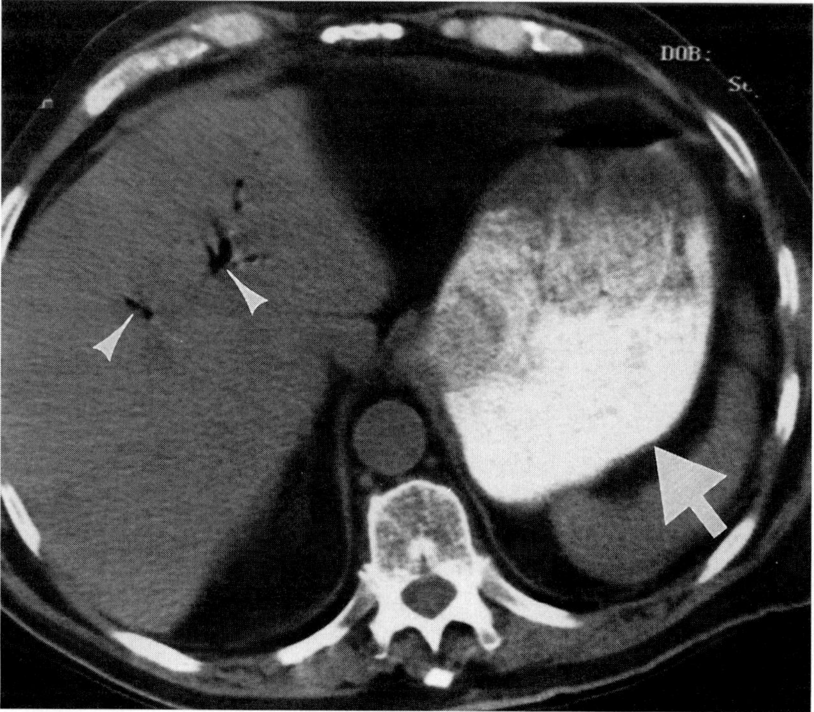

(C)

FIGURE 3.8. *Axial noncontrast CT of the upper abdomen in a patient with gallstone ileus.* ***(A)*** *The gallbladder is decompressed and gas-filled (arrow).* ***(B)*** *A large calcified gallstone is noted in the lumen of the second portion of the duodenum (arrow).* ***(C)*** *There is associated gastric dilation (arrow) and pneumobilia (arrowheads).*

Patients with a porcelain gallbladder or polyps greater than 2 cm in diameter are predisposed to this malignancy. Patients typically present with jaundice, right upper quadrant pain, or abnormal liver enzymes. Although gallbladder carcinomas are detected incidentally on occasion, most tumors are advanced at the time of presentation, either having directly invaded the adjacent liver parenchyma, metastasized hematogenously to the liver, or spread to porta hepatis lymph nodes (25). In fact, 75% of gallbladder carcinomas are unresectable at the time of presentation and the 1-year survival rate is only 5% (26).

On ultrasound, there is typically nodular or irregular thickening of the gallbladder wall in either an eccentric or circumferential fashion (27). The usually distinct echogenic margin between the gallbladder wall and the inferior surface of the liver is obliterated (Fig. 3.9). Hypoechoic or hyperechoic metastases are noted in the liver, often remote from the gallbladder fossa. Acoustical shadowing is often present due to concomitant gallstones or calcification in the wall (porcelain changes).

On CT, gallbladder carcinoma usually appears as a nodular and infiltrative hypoattenuating mass in the gallbladder fossa. This soft tissue mass may entirely replace the gallbladder although a small residual lumen is often apparent (see Fig. 3.9). Gallstones as well as wall calcifications are often present. The mass is relatively hypovascular and there is often direct invasion of the adjacent hepatic parenchyma. Furthermore, there are often hypoattenuating liver metastases scattered about the parenchyma (28). The bile ducts may or may not be dilated depending upon the location and extent of the tumor. Care should be taken to evaluate the porta hepatis for enlarged lymph nodes and the

(A)

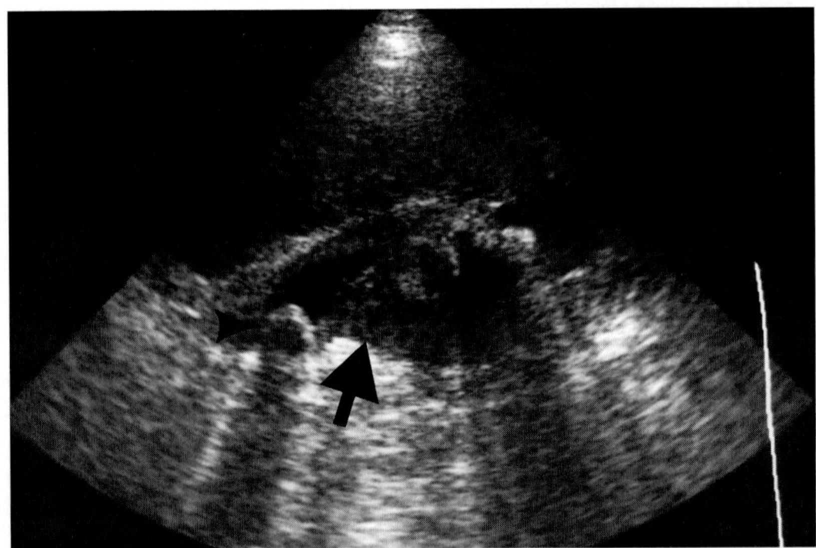

(B)

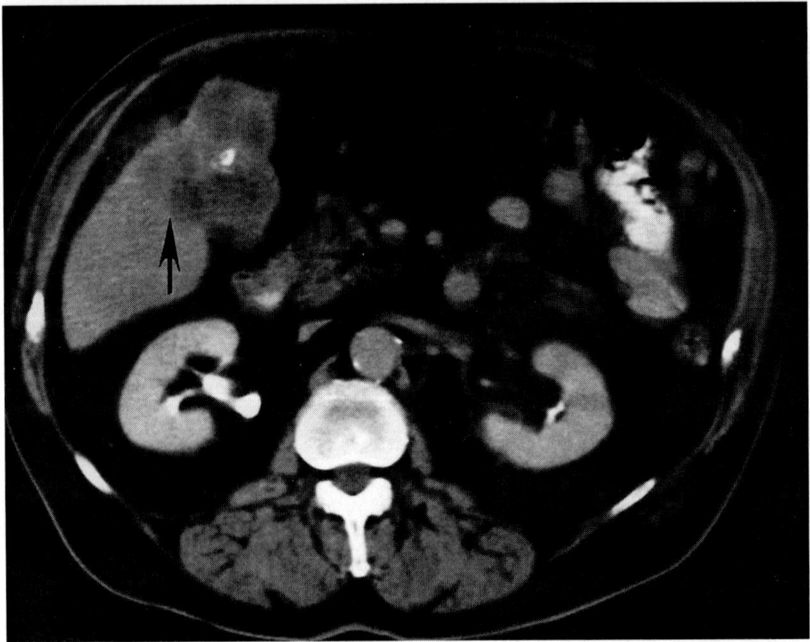

FIGURE 3.9. *Gallbladder carcinoma.* ***(A)*** *Gray-scale ultrasound in the sagittal plane demonstrates eccentric and nodular mass replacing the normally thin gallbladder wall (arrow). In addition, a hyperechoic lesion with posterior acoustic shadowing is noted adjacent to the carcinoma (arrowhead) representing a gallstone.* ***(B)*** *Axial contrast-enhanced CT also reveals a soft tissue mass replacing the gallbladder and associated with a calcified gallstone. Note that the mass has already invaded the adjacent liver parenchyma (arrow).*

peritoneal surfaces, especially the greater omentum, for carcinomatosis.

MRI should be reserved for equivocal cases when CT cannot define the extent of local invasion, thus affecting surgical treatment. Common findings include diffuse nodular thickening of the gallbladder wall, a mass in the gallbladder fossa, and invasion of the liver and adjacent structures (29). The tumor appears hypointense on T1-weighted images and hyperintense on T2-weighted images compared to a normal liver (30). Post-gadolinium-chelate axial T1-weighted gradient echo images with fat suppression are commonly used to define the extent of invasion into the liver, pancreas, or duodenum.

Positron emission tomography (PET) is a relatively new technique in nuclear medicine which indicates foci of increased metabolic activity, such as seen with malignant tumors. Although data is preliminary, it may be useful in patients with gallbladder carcinoma for detecting peritoneal metastases.

BILE DUCTS

The intrahepatic bile ducts may not be visualized by ultrasound when they are normal in caliber. When dilated, they often have a "tram track" appearance because the biliary radicals parallel the portal veins (Fig. 3.10). Color Doppler ultrasound is helpful in discerning which tubular structure is the bile duct. When they are markedly dilated, the ducts can be quite tortuous. The wall of the bile duct is normally very thin, measuring less than 1 mm.

CT has the advantage of high spatial resolution, which allows depiction of both the lumen and the wall of the bile ducts, but has the disadvantage of imaging only in the axial plane. This is somewhat offset by spiral CT with which a high quality volumetric data set can be acquired and then rendered or displayed in a multi-planar or three-dimensional (3D) fashion. CT is very sensitive to ductal dilation, and on occasion even nondilated bile and pancreatic ducts can be visualized. The depiction of ductal structures is markedly reduced, however, when intravenous iodinated contrast material is not used. Furthermore, CT cholangiography can also be performed noninvasively by acquiring a thin-section spiral CT the morning after ingesting several Telopaque tablets, the same agent used for oral cholecystography (OCG) (31). This data set can be reconstructed in 3D to evaluate the bile ducts in a fashion similar to direct cholangiography or MR cholangiography (MRC) (Fig. 3.11). Unfortunately, there must be reasonable liver function in order for the ducts to be adequately opacified.

Like MRI of the intrahepatic and extrahepatic bile ducts, MRC relies on heavily T2-weighted sequences on which stationary fluid within the ducts is of very high signal intensity relative to the adjacent liver (32–35) (Fig. 3.12). Gradient-echo sequences were originally used to produce these images but more recently fast spin echo sequences have been shown to yield better visualization of the ducts without long breath holds or magnetic susceptibility artifacts (36). The data obtained from these sequences can be manipulated on a computer workstation and displayed like the images obtained in an ERCP. In addition, it is also possible to obtain physiological information on pancreatic exocrine function after the intravenous injection of secretin.

Choledocholithiasis

Ultrasound is usually the initial imaging choice in patients with jaundice to determine the integrity of the bile ducts. Although ultrasound does not reliably visualize the bile

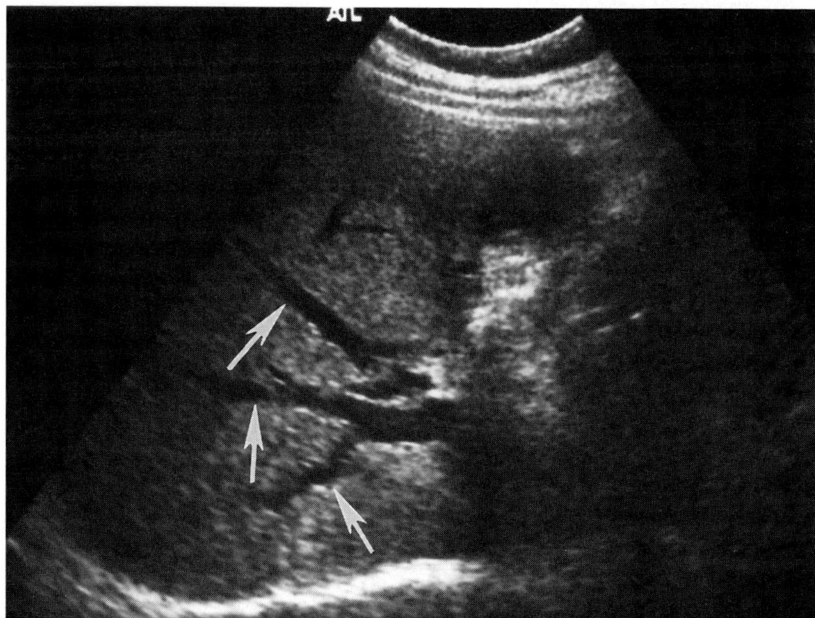

FIGURE 3.10. *Gray-scale ultrasound of the liver demonstrates the "tram track" appearance of intrahepatic bile duct dilatation (arrows).*

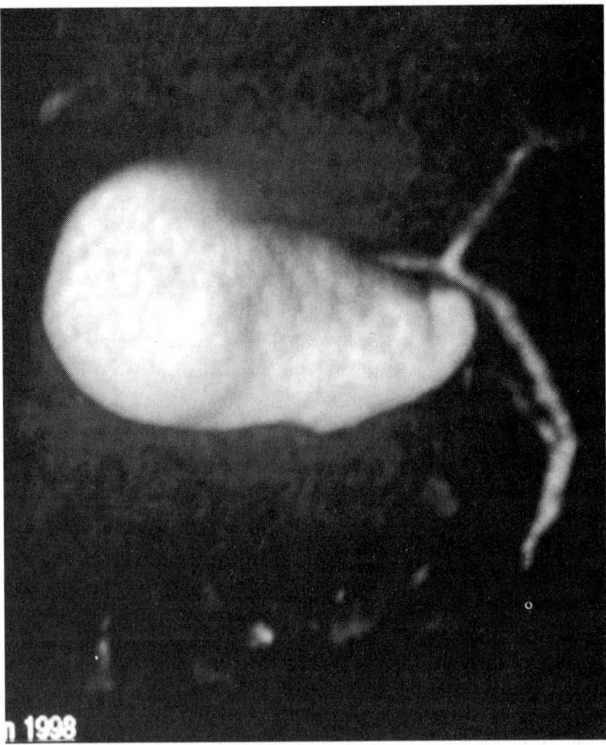

FIGURE 3.11. *Volume rendered three-dimensional image of the gallbladder and bile ducts in the frontal projection. The 3D image was reconstructed from an axial CT data set acquired after the oral ingestion of Telepaque tablets (CT cholangiogram). The gallbladder and extrahepatic bile ducts in this patient are normal.*

ducts at their extremes (i.e., the peripheral intrahepatic ducts at one end and the distal common bile duct at the other), the central intrahepatic ducts and especially the common hepatic duct are well visualized. Either CT or MRI better delineates these extreme portions of the ductal system. The normal common hepatic duct courses just anterior to the main portal vein and measures 5 to 6 mm in diameter. A duct measuring more than 6 mm yet not obstructed is a condition seen in elderly patients, in a minority of patients following cholecystectomy, and in patients with previous long-standing ductal obstruction. For elderly patients in particular, the upper limit of normal in duct caliber can increase by 1 mm for every decade after the age of 60 (i.e., 7 mm after age 70, 8 mm after 80, and so on) (37). Most patients with choledocholithiasis have dilated ducts, and on occasion the calculi themselves will be visualized as echogenic intraluminal foci, with or without acoustical shadowing (Fig. 3.13).

In general, CT is very sensitive to dilation of the biliary tree, including both intrahepatic and extrahepatic ducts. Although ultrasound is superior to CT for detecting stones in the gallbladder, CT is superior to ultrasound for detecting stones in the bile ducts (38,39). This is mainly because there is better visualization of the distal common bile duct by CT and the level of dilation or obstruction is better depicted. Even when a stone is not readily apparent, the diagnosis may be entertained when there is no evidence of a mass at the level of obstruction. However, this combination of findings is not specific for choledocholithiasis,

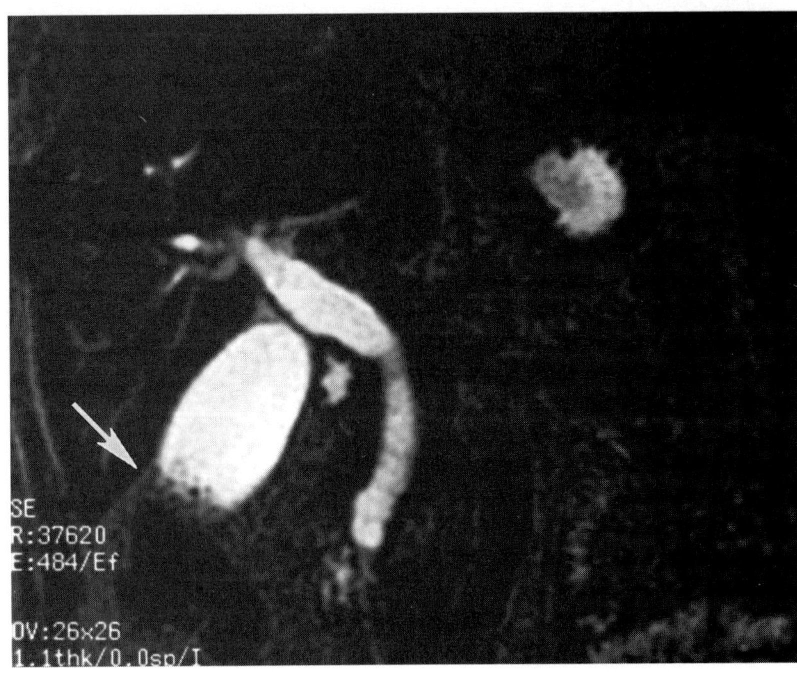

FIGURE 3.12. *MRC in the coronal projection demonstrating small calculi in the fundus of the gallbladder (arrow) and a dilated extrahepatic bile duct.*

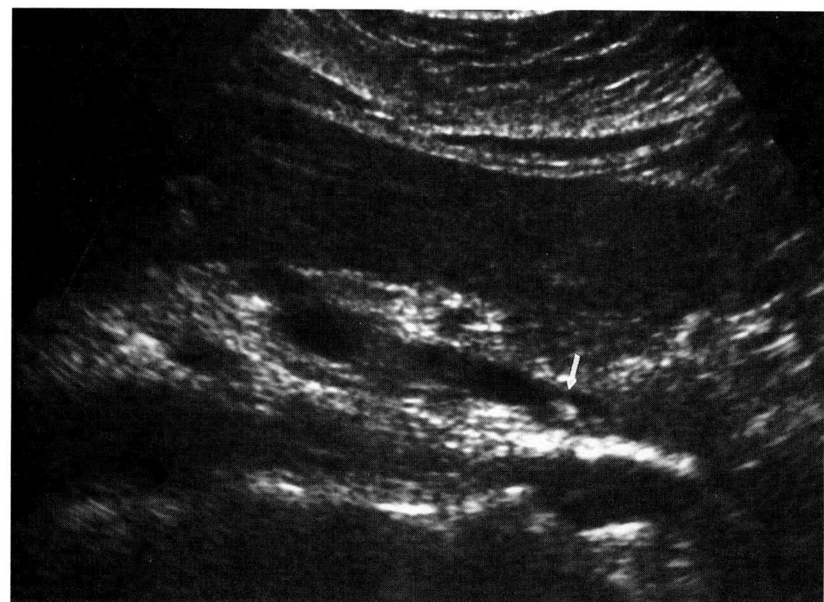

FIGURE 3.13. *Gray-scale ultrasound of the upper abdomen in the sagittal plane reveals a small gallstone (arrow) within the common bile duct associated with extrahepatic bile duct dilation.*

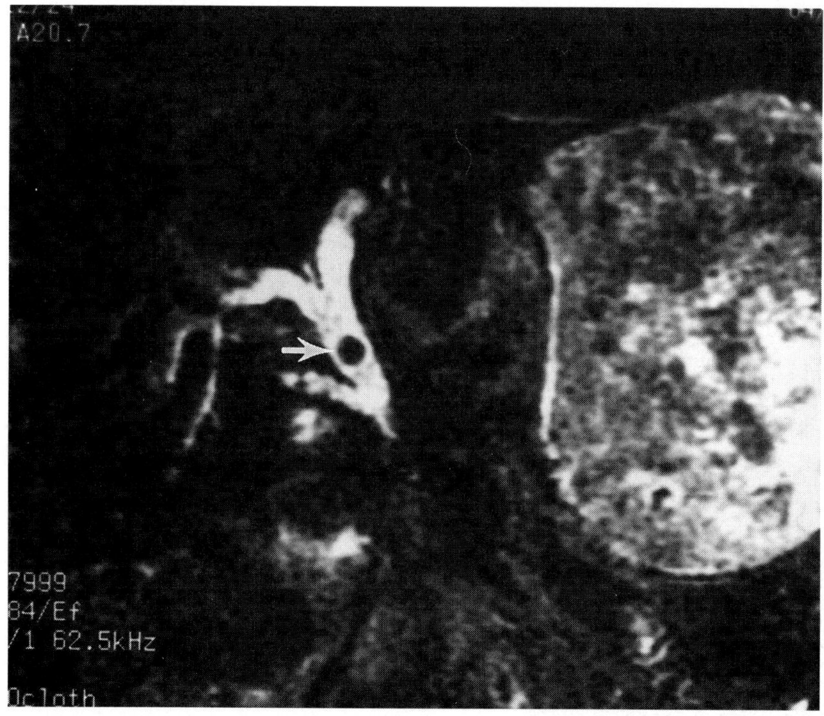

FIGURE 3.14. *MRC in the coronal projection demonstrating a filling defect within the common bile duct (arrow) representing choledocholithiasis.*

because both a benign stricture and ampullary stenosis may have a similar appearance. There is some evidence that a preliminary CT prior to the administration of either oral or intravenous contrast material may increase the sensitivity for detecting stones (40).

In general, ERCP remains the technique of choice when evaluating patients with suspected common bile duct stones, as the diagnosis can be made and then treatment applied in the same setting. However, in certain clinical settings where ERCP is contraindicated, MRC is the imaging modality of choice. MRC has greater than 90% sensitivity and specificity in the detection of choledocholithiasis (41–44). These percentages are superior to both ultrasound and CT. With MRC, calculi are seen as low-signal intensity defects within high-signal intensity bile (Fig. 3.14). It must be remembered, however, that both air bubbles and blood clots can have a similar low-signal intensity appearance.

Cholangitis

Inflammation of the bile ducts is caused by a number of conditions including infection, such as acute suppurative cholangitis, recurrent pyogenic cholangitis, or sclerosing cholangitis. In acute cholangitis, the bile ducts are often dilated and there may be thickening of the ductal wall. If biliary gas is present it will be seen as foci of indistinct or "dirty" acoustical shadowing on ultrasound. Occasionally, intrahepatic abscesses develop, which are usually multiple and relatively small (less than 2 cm), with their distribution depending on the site and level of ductal obstruction. Gas bubbles may also be noted within these abscesses. Abscesses tend to be hypoechoic on ultrasound, hypoattenuating on CT, and hyperintense on T2-weighted MRI. CT and MRI can also demonstrate marked enhancement of the ductal walls (45) (Fig. 3.15).

In sclerosing cholangitis, chronic obliterative fibrotic inflammation involves the wall of the intrahepatic and extra-hepatic bile ducts resulting in chronic obstructive jaundice.

(A)

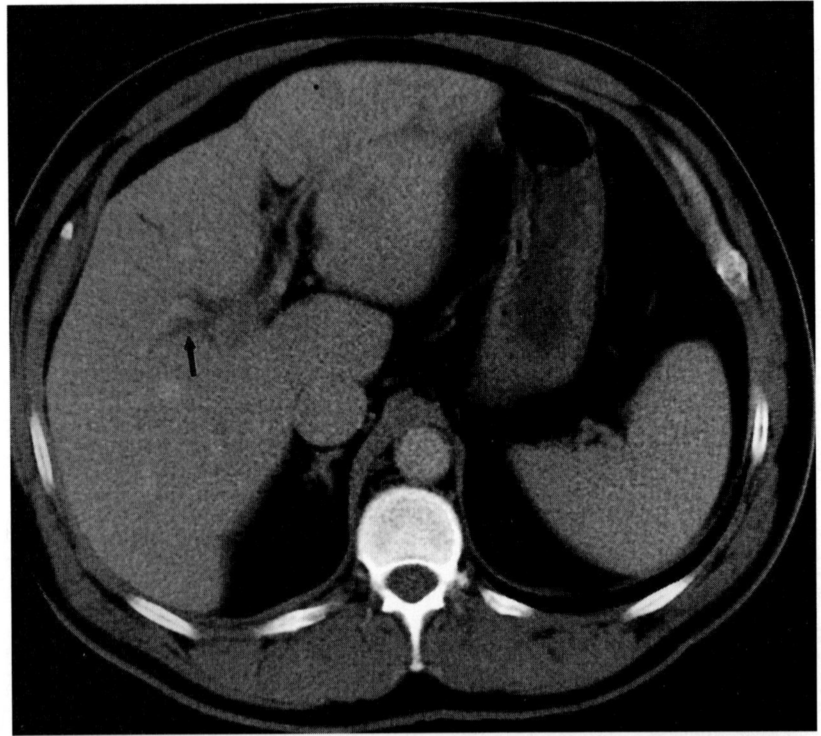

(B)

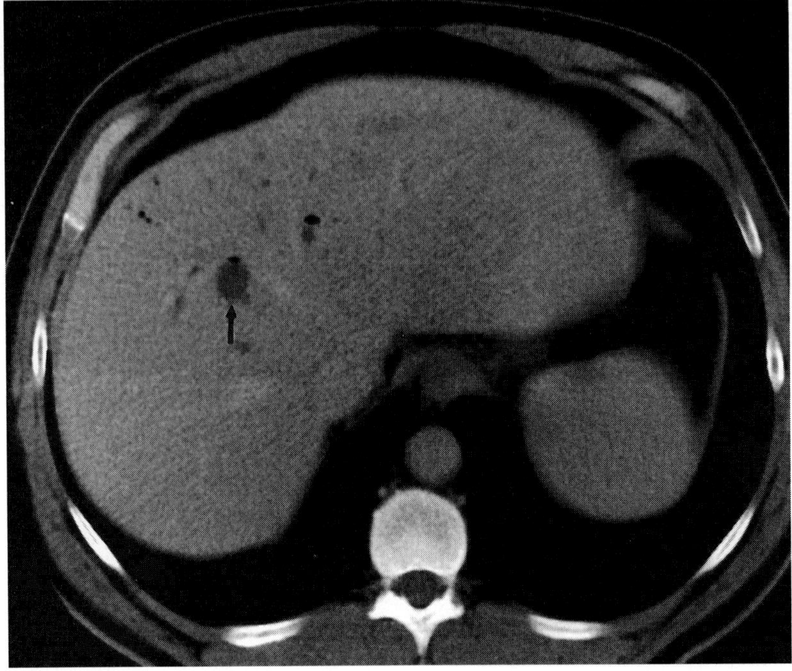

FIGURE 3.15. *(A) Axial contrast-enhanced CT of the upper abdomen demonstrates low attenuation (arrow) along the central intrahepatic bile ducts representing the inflammation associated with cholangitis. (B) A more cephalad image shows discrete low attenuation lesion with foci of gas (arrow) representing small abscesses.*

The patients are predominantly men under the age of 45. Secondary associations include ulcerative colitis, cirrhosis, pancreatitis, retroperitoneal fibrosis, Peyronie's disease, Riedel's thyroiditis, and retro-orbital pseudotumor (46). Cholangiocarcinoma develops in up to 12% of patients with sclerosing cholangitis (47). Other complications include biliary cirrhosis and portal hypertension.

Ultrasound can detect the segmental biliary dilatation and the morphologic changes of primary sclerosing cholangitis, although the irregularity of the ducts noted on either direct cholangiography or MRC is difficult to appreciate. When the inflammation is chronic such as in primary sclerosing cholangitis, the CT and MRI findings are much different than in acute cholangitis. Although segmental and scattered intrahepatic duct dilatation is apparent, the degree of dilatation is relatively mild. Intrahepatic calculi may be seen on ultrasound and CT (48). The segmental narrowing and irregularity of the bile ducts inherent to this disease, however, are difficult to appreciate with these two techniques.

The most striking changes relate to the morphology of the liver. First, the caudate lobe is enlarged and in some case may account for the vast majority of liver parenchyma. Second, there are deep lobulations in the capsular surface owing to profound segmental atrophy, particularly in the anterior segment of the right hepatic lobe and the medial segment of the left hepatic lobe. Furthermore, there are often enlarged lymph nodes in the porta hepatic and paraduodenal region.

ERCP is currently the initial diagnostic technique, although improvements in spatial resolution have increased the diagnostic capability of MRC so that intrahepatic ducts are readily displayed. The biliary tree can be depicted on MRI by using both MRC and multiphasic gadolinium-enhanced T1-weighted images. Common findings include intrahepatic bile duct dilatation (77%) and intervening bile duct stenoses (64%), giving the ducts a "beaded" appearance (49,50) (Fig. 3.16). Other findings include periportal edema, enhancement and thickening of the wall of the extrahepatic bile ducts, and increased enhancement of the periphery of the liver during the hepatic arterial phase.

Cystic Dilatation of the Bile Duct

Cystic dilatation of the bile ducts can be seen in patients with a choledochal cyst, a choledochocele, or Caroli's disease. These diseases are rare and the patients often present with colicky right upper quadrant pain and jaundice (51). The incidence of cholangiocarcinoma is increased in these patients (52). Because ultrasound tends to depict only a portion of the biliary tree, it is not the modality of choice for diagnosing or characterizing choledochal cysts or choledochoceles (53). The diagnosis should be considered, however, whenever focal dilatation of either an intrahepatic or extrahepatic bile duct is detected.

On CT, a choledochal cyst should be considered for any unilocular cystic mass that occurs in the region of the extrahepatic bile duct. At times there may be calculi within these cysts, which are typically thin-walled and can be quite large, on the order of several centimeters (54) (Fig. 3.17). In the normal patient, the common hepatic duct may dilate focally as it exits the liver parenchyma, so it is more difficult to make the diagnosis of a choledochal cyst in this region. If the cystic mass projects into the duodenal lumen, a choledochocele is suspected. A history of pancreatitis may confuse the picture because a pseudocyst in the head of the pancreas may have a similar appearance on ultrasound and CT.

Only a few studies have used MRC to evaluate choledochal cysts. These studies compared the findings of ERCP with MRC and concluded that both modalities provide similar information (55,56). MRC readily demonstrates fusiform dilatation (type I), the most common form, as well as saccular (type II) dilatation of the extrahepatic bile duct (Fig. 3.18). With a choledochocele (type III), there is

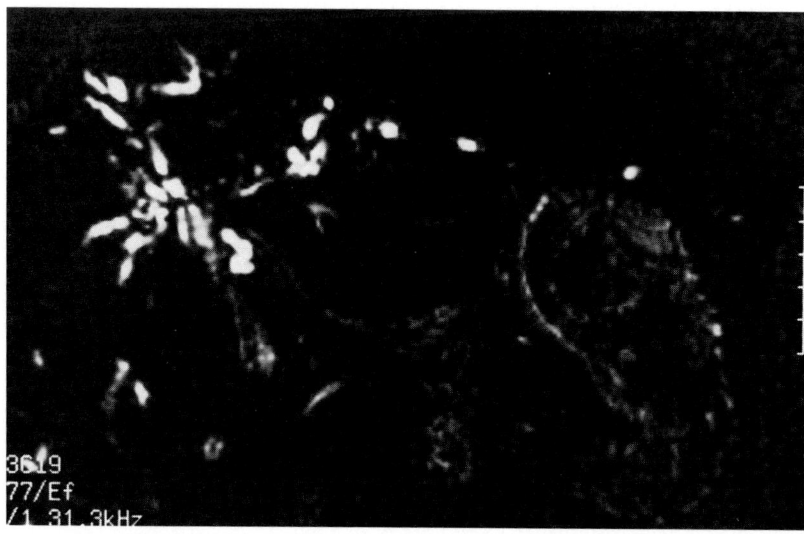

FIGURE 3.16. *MRC in the coronal projection in a patient with primary sclerosing cholangitis demonstrates the typical beaded appearance of the intrahepatic bile ducts with intervening segments of dilated and stenotic ducts.*

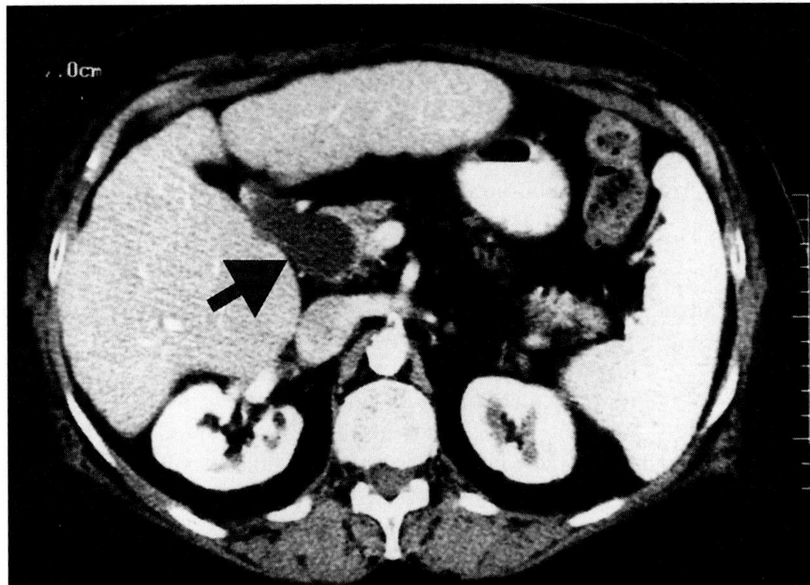
(A)

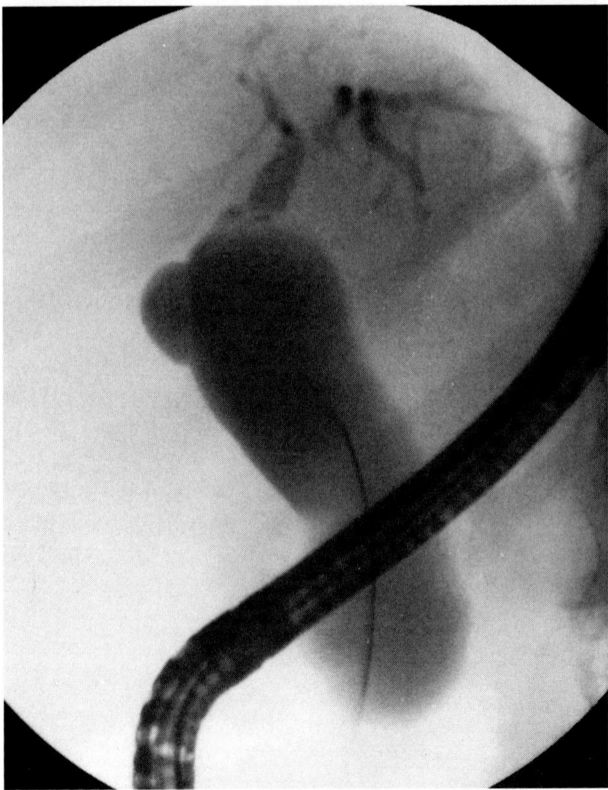
(B)

FIGURE 3.17. ***(A)*** *Axial contrast-enhanced CT of the upper abdomen demonstrated a well-defined low attenuation structure in the head of the pancreas (arrow) which appears to be a continuation extrahepatic bile duct.* ***(B)*** *An ERCP demonstrated marked fusiform dilatation of the common bile duct, consistent with a type I choledochal cyst.*

cystic dilatation of the distal common bile duct as it projects into the duodenal lumen. In Caroli's disease, there is cystic dilation of the intrahepatic ducts usually in a segmental manner and with no intervening stenotic regions (57).

Cholangiocarcinoma

Patients with cholangiocarcinomas commonly present with painless jaundice. The majority of cholangiocarcinomas originate from the extrahepatic bile ducts and are often unresectable at the time of diagnosis because the tumor has already spread to regional lymph nodes or infiltrated adjacent liver parenchyma (58). Tumors occurring at the confluence of the right and left intrahepatic ducts are termed Klatskin tumors. The survival rate for cholangiocarcinomas is approximately 5% at 5 years with a median survival of 5 months (59). ERCP is often required to obtain cytologic proof and for stent placement but has limited value for determining the extent of disease because the tumors

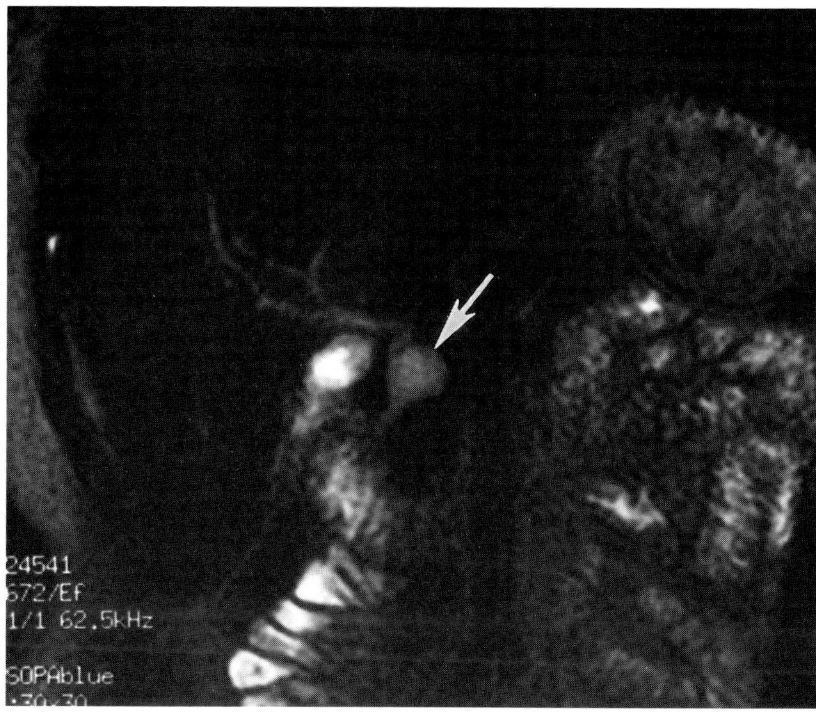

FIGURE 3.18. *MRC in the coronal projection demonstrates a saccular dilatation of the common bile duct (arrow) consistent with a type II choledochal cyst.*

tend to form strictures, thereby limiting opacification of more peripheral ducts. In this clinical scenario, CT or MRI can provide valuable information concerning both the size and extent of the tumor and resectability (60,61).

On ultrasound, cholangiocarcinoma may be suspected when there is thickening or nodularity of the duct wall (62). Although the cause of biliary obstruction is not always apparent by ultrasound, following the dilated biliary radicals from the periphery to the porta hepatis and down into the extrahepatic ducts may reveal a soft tissue mass. Intraluminal debris and even calculi may be seen within these proximally dilated ducts. The atrophic changes associated with long-standing biliary obstruction may be difficult to appreciate with ultrasound. Furthermore, some cholangiocarcinomas have a similar echo pattern to that of normal hepatic parenchyma and may not be apparent sonographically.

On CT, cholangiocarcinomas are seen as irregular or well-defined soft tissue masses found along the course of the intrahepatic ducts, the extrahepatic ducts, or both (63). Although many tumors are centrally located, others are peripheral and mimic a liver metastasis. They may be multifocal or seen as a subtle infiltrative mass extending along the course of the biliary tree. At times, the tumor is so obscure that the only evidence for a mass is proximal duct dilatation. If ductal obstruction is severe or long-standing there may be associated lobar atrophy (64). Cholangiocarcinomas are relatively vascular tumors, although they uncommonly demonstrate hyperenhancement during the hepatic arterial phase of a dynamic CT. Furthermore, about a third of the tumors will demonstrate a unique phenomenon whereby there is slow wash-in and delayed wash-out of contrast material (65). As a result, they will be isoattenuating to subtly hypoattenuating during the portal venous phase of enhancement and then hyperattenuating during a delayed phase, about 15 to 20 minutes later (Fig. 3.19).

Although CT remains the initial imaging modality for determining the extent of tumor, MRI is capable of providing similar information (66). Cholangiocarcinomas typically present as poorly defined, and at times subtle, masses that may be of low signal intensity on T1-weighted images and of high signal intensity on T2-weighted images. Common findings also include markedly dilated ducts with thickening of the wall measuring greater than 5 mm. T1-weighted multiphasic gadolinium-enhanced sequences with fat suppression typically show peripheral enhancement of the liver during the hepatic arterial phase and delayed or incomplete central fill-in on later phases (67,68). Delayed images are also useful in showing the extent of tumor infiltration along the biliary tree.

Although data is preliminary, PET scanning may be helpful in patients with intrahepatic ductal dilatation for differentiating benign from malignant causes of obstruction, such as cholangicarcinoma.

CHOLESCINTIGRAPHY

Cholescintigraphy is a nuclear medicine examination used in a number of clinical scenarios related to the hepatobiliary system. The exam uses a 99mTc-labeled iminodiacetic

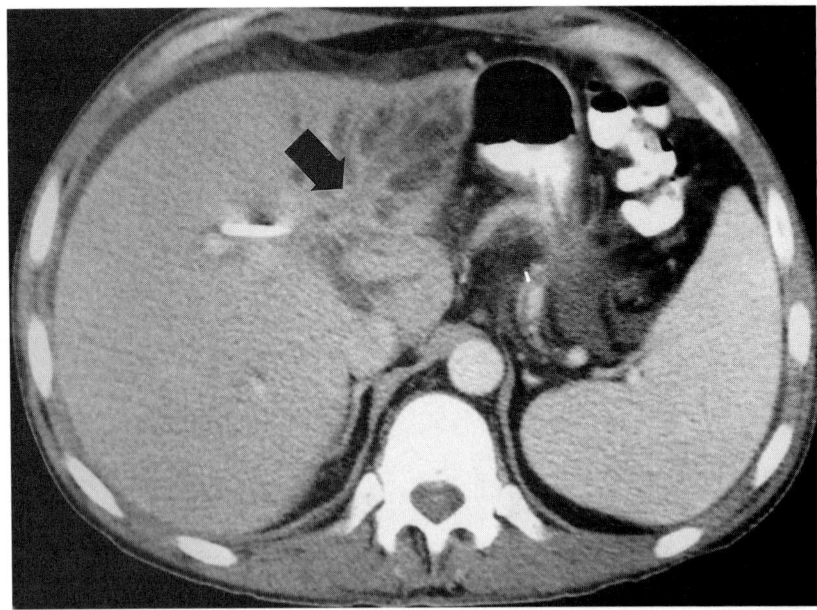

(A)

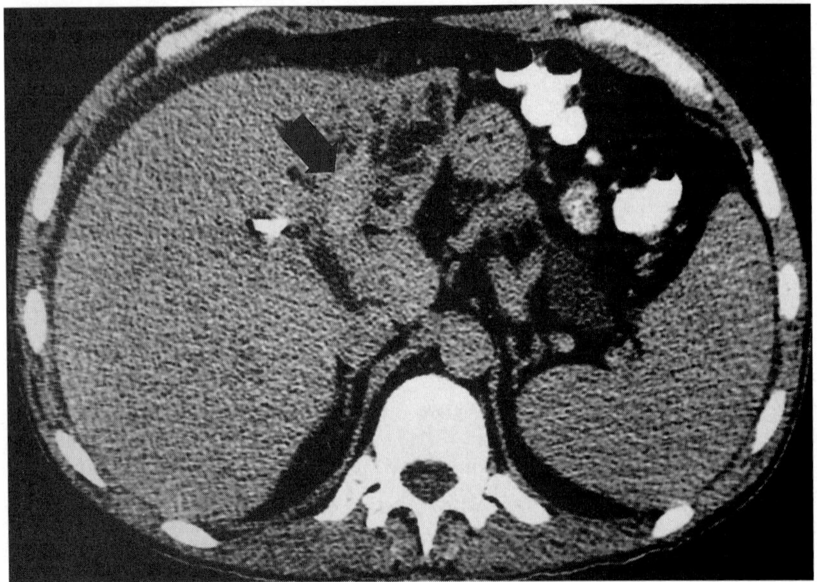

(B)

FIGURE 3.19. ***(A)*** *Axial contrast-enhanced CT of the liver during the portal venous phase demonstrates an ill-defined isoenhancing mass centrally (arrow) resulting in marked biliary dilatation.* ***(B)*** *On a CT obtained at the same level after a 15-minute delay following the administration of intravenous contrast material, there is a hyperenhancement of this mass (arrow) in comparison to the remaining hepatic parenchyma.*

acid analogue (IDA) radiopharmaceutical that shares the same hepatocyte uptake, transport, and excretion pathways as bilirubin. This technique not only provides images of the biliary tree but also yields functional information about the liver, gallbladder, and bile ducts, a major advantage of cholescintigraphy over other imaging modalities. For example, it can detect obstruction to bile flow without relying on secondary signs such as ductal dilatation (69,70). Function can even be quantitated in the form of gallbladder ejection fractions and biliary transit times (71,72).

The main disadvantage of cholescintigraphy is the low spatial resolution. Compared to CT, which has 0.7 line pairs/mm and MRI, which has 0.3 line pairs/mm, cholescintigraphy has less than 0.1 line pairs/mm. Other disadvantages include the presence of ionizing radiation (approximately a third less than CT), the limited availability of the radiopharmaceutical agent (which must be prepared just prior to the examination) at some sites, the cost of the examination (greater than ultrasound but less than CT or MRI), the need for adequate patient preparation (nothing by mouth for greater than 4 hours but less than 24 hours), and the fact that certain medications such as morphine sulfate can interfere with the test (73). Furthermore, functioning hepatocytes must be present to excrete the radiopharmaceutical agent into the biliary system. As a result, it is not possible to image the biliary system with this method in patients with liver failure. The exam can take an average of 30 to 60 minutes to complete, with delayed imaging at 2 to 4 hours required in some cases.

Cholescintigraphy is indicated in patients with suspected cholecystitis, biliary diversion procedures, postoperative leaks, common duct obstruction, or postcholecystectomy syndrome. In fact, it is considered to be the study of choice for diagnosing acute cholecystitis. It has a very high sensitivity and specificity for this diagnosis, exceeding 95% and 98%, respectively (74–76). By comparison, the ultrasound findings of gallbladder wall thickening, pericholecystic fluid, gallstones, and a sonographic Murphy's sign are less specific with individual specificities ranging from 70% to 90%. A normal 99mTc-IDA study will demonstrate gallbladder visualization within 60 minutes and have biliary-to-bowel transit times of also less than 60 minutes (Fig. 3.20). Non-filling of the gallbladder after 60 minutes is considered diagnostic of acute cholecystitis (Fig. 3.21). On occasion, images are obtained 2 to 4 hours later to ensure the diagnosis. Morphine sulfate can be used to shorten the examination time; by contracting the sphincter of Oddi, it results in preferential flow of bile through the cystic duct into the gallbladder (77,78). Ancillary findings such as increased blood flow to the gallbladder fossa and increased hepatic parenchymal uptake in the gallbladder fossa ("rim" sign) increase the specificity of this exam (Fig. 3.21) (79). However, false-positive results can occur in patients who have been fasting less than 4 or greater than 24 hours, in those with hepatic failure, in those receiving hyperalimentation, and those with chronic cholecystitis or who are severely debilitated (80).

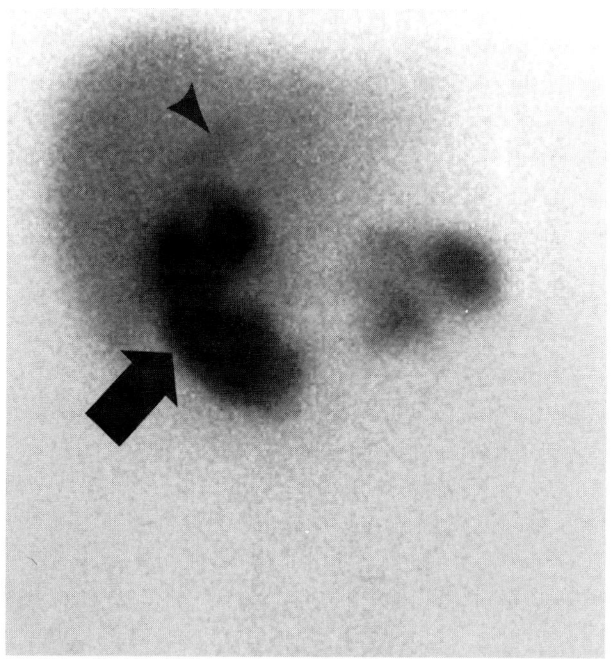

FIGURE 3.20. *Normal cholescintigram demonstrating radiopharmaceutical excretion into the biliary tree (arrowhead) and uptake in the gallbladder (arrow) in less than 1 hour. (Case courtesy of Rosalie J. Hagge, M.D., Durham, NC.)*

The diagnosis of common bile duct obstruction is usually made with ultrasound. Cholescintigraphy is rarely indicated unless ductal obstruction has occurred in less than 24 hours, not allowing the ducts to dilate sufficiently, or if recent or long-standing obstruction has occurred and ductal diameter has not returned to normal. The study is positive when there is an absence of normal biliary-to-bowel transit. However, cholescintigraphy is the examination of choice for children with suspected common bile duct obstruction due to biliary atresia, thereby differentiating it from other causes of neonatal jaundice (81,82). Pretreatment of the neonate with phenobarbital is required to ensure that the hepatocytes are fully functional. A positive exam will demonstrate a lack of biliary-to-bowel transit even after 24 hours.

Cholecystokinin (CCK) is a natural hormone that is released from the duodenal mucosa upon ingestion of a fatty meal, thereby causing the gallbladder to contract. Administration of CCK or Sincalide (Squibb Diagnostic) has proven useful with cholescintigraphy. It is indicated in patients who have fasted greater than 24 hours, for evaluation of sphincter of Oddi dysfunction (SOD), for differentiating functional from anatomic common bile duct obstruction, or the calculation of gallbladder ejection fraction (83). It is given to patients who have fasted greater than 24 hours to empty the gallbladder prior to the examination, allowing the radiopharmaceutical to enter the now empty gallbladder. In 20% of normal individuals, a hypertonic sphincter will cause delay in excretion of the labeled isotope agent, giving the appearance of SOD or biliary obstruction. This results in delayed biliary-to-bowel transit time, and gives the appearance of common bile duct obstruction. The administration of CCK will cause gallbladder contraction, which increases the pressure in the biliary system and overcomes the hypertonic sphincter, thus revealing common bile duct patency (84). Calculation of gallbladder ejection fraction is useful in the diagnosis of chronic acalculous cholecystitis. These patients have chronic pain but normal imaging examinations. If the gallbladder ejection fraction is less than 35% there is a high correlation with this disorder indicating that a cholecystectomy will likely result in symptomatic relief (85).

Perhaps one of the most useful indications for ordering a cholescintigram is to identify a biliary leak in post-operative/post-traumatic patients. These patients typically present with a fluid collection adjacent to the gallbladder which cannot be differentiated from blood or ascites using ultrasound, CT, or MRI. A cholescintigram will demonstrate leakage of the administered radiopharmaceutical agent outside the biliary system into the region of the fluid collection, confirming the presence of a bile leak (Fig. 3.22).

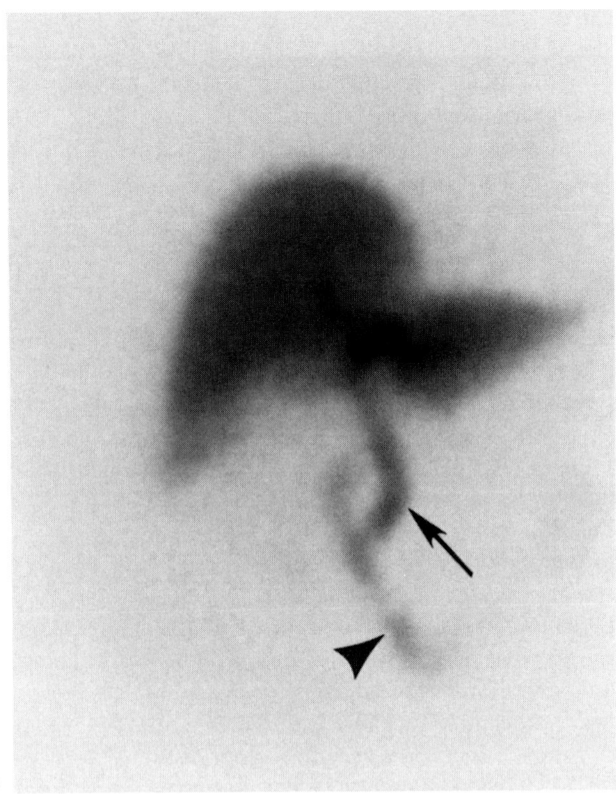

(A)

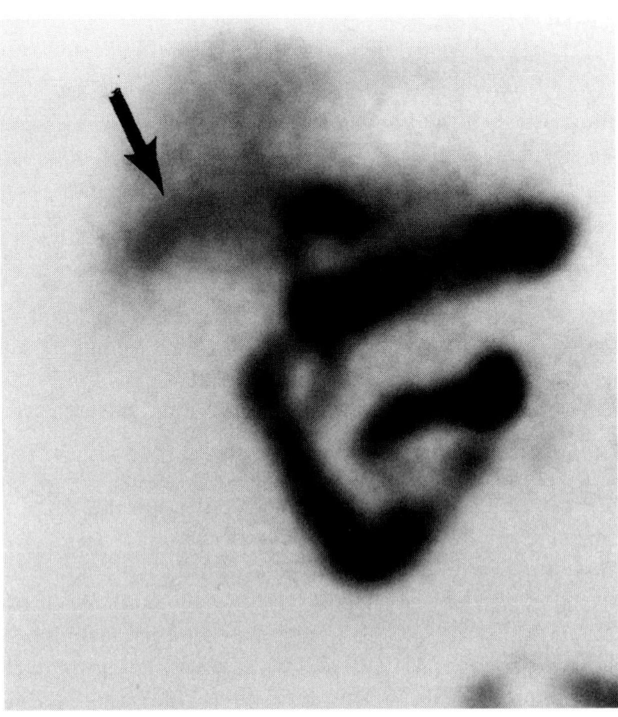

(B)

FIGURE 3.21. *(**A**) Cholescintigram in a patient with acute cholecystitis demonstrating the normal excretion of radiopharmaceutical into the biliary system (arrow) with normal excretion of the radiopharmaceutical into the duodenum (arrowhead) after 10 minutes. (**B**) However, at the 1-hour delayed images, no gallbladder uptake is seen and the adjacent hepatic parenchyma demonstrates the "rim" sign (arrow) associated with acute cholecystitis. (Case courtesy of Andrew J. Adamson, M.D., Durham, NC.)*

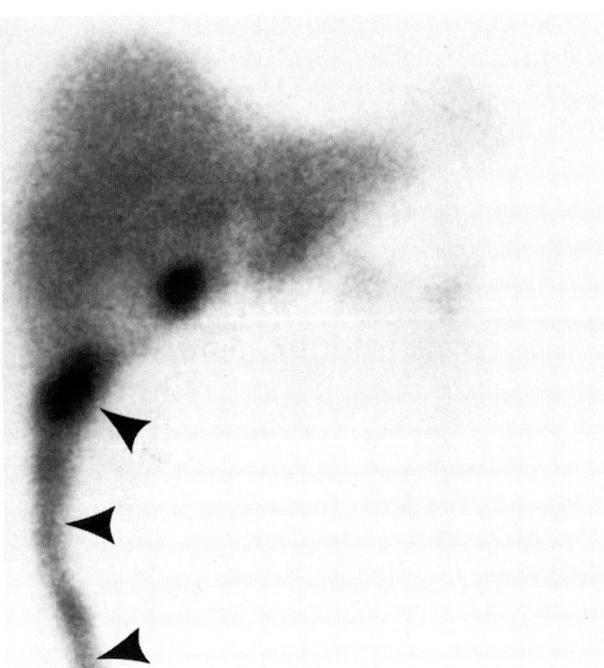

FIGURE 3.22. *Cholescintigram in a patient after laparoscopic cholecystectomy shows the radiopharmaceutical leaking into the right paracolic gutter confirming the existence of a bile duct leak (arrowheads). (Case courtesy of Rosalie J. Hagge, M.D., Durham, NC.)*

SUGGESTED READINGS

Higgins CB, Hricak H, Helms CA, eds. Magnetic resonance imaging of the body. 3rd ed. Philadelphia: Lippincott Williams & Wilkins, 1996:3–222,571–638.

Lee JKT, Sagel SS, Stanley RT, Heiken JP, eds. Computed body tomography with MRI correlation. 3rd ed. Philadelphia: Lippincott-Raven, 1998;2:779–844.

Mettler FA, Guiberteau MJ. Essentials of nuclear medicine imaging. 3rd ed. Philadelphia: WB Saunders, 1991:196–202.

Rumack CM, Wilson SR, Charboneau JW, eds. Diagnostic ultrasound. 2nd ed. St. Louis: Mosby, 1998;1:3–34,175–224.

REFERENCES

1. Harisinghani MG, Saini S, Schima W, et al. Simethicone coated cellulose as an oral contrast agent for ultrasound of the upper abdomen. Clin Radiol 1997;52:224–6.
2. Kono Y, Moriyasu F, Nada T, et al. Gray scale second harmonic imaging of the liver: a preliminary animal study. Ultrasound Med Biol 1997;23:719–26.
3. Burns PN, Powers JE, Hope Simpson D, et al. Harmonic imaging: principles and preliminary results. Angiology 1996;47:63–73.
4. Wilson SR, Burns PN, Muradali D, et al. Harmonic hepatic US with microbubble contrast agent: initial experience showing improved characterization of hemangioma, hepatocellular carcinoma and metastasis. Radiology 2000;215:153–61.
5. Kalender WA, Seissler W, Klotz E, Vock P. Spiral volumetric CT with single-breath-hold technique, continuous transport, and continuous scanner rotation. Radiology 1990;176:181–3.
6. Hu H, He HD, Foley WD, Fox SH. Four multidetector-row helical CT: image quality and volume coverage speed. Radiology 2000;215:55–62.
7. Foley WD. Dynamic hepatic CT. Radiology 1989;170:617–22.
8. Fulcher AS, Turner MA, Capps GW, et al. Half-Fourier RARE MRCP: experience in 300 subjects. Radiology 1998;207:21–32.
9. Van Beers BE, Gallez B, Pringot J. Contrast-enhanced MR imaging of the liver. Radiology 1997;203:297–306.
10. Perkerson RB Jr, Erwin BC, Baumgartner BR, et al. CT densities in delayed iodine hepatic scanning. Radiology 1985;155:445–6.
11. Birnholz JC. Population survey: ultrasonic cholecystography. Gastrointest Radiol 1982;7:789–90.
12. McIntosh DM, Penney HF. Gray-scale ultrasonography as a screening procedure in the detection of gallbladder disease. Radiology 1980;136:725–7.
13. Park MS, Yu JS, Kim YH, et al. Acute cholecystitis: comparison of MR cholangiography and US. Radiology 1998;209:781–5.
14. Havrilla TR, Reich NE, Haaga JR, et al. Computed tomography of the gallbladder. AJR 1978;130:1059–67.
15. Barakos JA, Ralls PW, Lapin SA, et al. Cholelithiasis: evaluation with CT. Radiology 1987;162:415–8.
16. Ralls PW, Coletti PM, Halls JM, Siemsen JK. Prospective evaluation of 99mTc-ISA cholescintigraphy and gray-scale ultrasound in the diagnosis of acute cholecystitis. Radiology 1982;144:369–71.
17. Laing FC, Federle MP, Jeffrey RB, Brown TW. Ultrasonic evaluation of patients with acute right upper quadrant pain. Radiology 1981;140:449–55.
18. Ralls PW, Coletti PM, Lapin SA, et al. Real-time sonography in suspected acute cholecystitis: prospective evaluation of primary and secondary signs. Radiology 1985;155:767–71.
19. Uggowitzer M, Kugler C, Schramayer G, et al. Sonography of acute cholecystitis: comparison of color and power Doppler sonography in detecting a hypervascularized gallbladder wall. AJR 1997;168:707–12.
20. Soyer P, Brouland JP, Boudiaf M, et al. Color velocity imaging and power Doppler sonography of the gallbladder wall: new look at sonographic diagnosis of acute cholecystitis. AJR 1998;171:183–8.
21. Paulson EK, Kliewer MA, Hertzberg BS, et al. Diagnosis of acute cholecystitis with color Doppler sonography: significance of arterial flow in thickened gallbladder wall. AJR 1994;162:1105–8.
22. Regan F, Schaefer DC, Smith DP, et al. The diagnostic utility of HASTE MRI in the evaluation of acute cholecystitis. Half-Fourier acquisition single-shot turbo SE. J Comput Assist Tomogr 1998;22:638–42.
23. Loud PA, Semelka RC, Kettritz U, et al. MRI of acute cholecystitis comparison with the normal gallbladder and other entities. Magn Reson Imaging 1996;14:349–55.
24. Demachi H, Matsui O, Hoshiba K, et al. Dynamic MRI using a surface coil in chronic cholecystitis and gallbladder carcinoma: radiologic and histopathologic correlation. J Comput Assist Tomogr 1997;21:643–51.
25. Vaittinen E. Carcinoma of the gallbladder. A study of 390 cases diagnosed in Finland from 1953–1967. Ann Chir Gynaecol Fenn Suppl 1970;168:1–81.
26. Hart J, Modan B. Factors affecting survival of patients with gallbladder neoplasm. Arch Intern Med 1972;129:931–4.
27. Bach AM, Loring LA, Hann LE, et al. Gallbladder cancer: can ultrasonography evaluate extent of disease? J Ultrasound Med 1998;17:303–9.
28. Ohtani T, Shirai Y, Tsukada K, et al. Spread of gallbladder carcinoma: CT evaluation with pathologic correlation. Abdom Imaging 1996;21:195–201.
29. Rooholamini SA, Tehrani NS, Razavi MK, et al. Imaging of gallbladder carcinoma. RadioGraphics 1994;14:291–306.
30. Sagoh T, Itoh K, Togashi K, et al. Gallbladder carcinoma: evaluation with MR imaging. Radiology 1990;174:131–6.
31. Caoili EM, Paulson EK, Heyneman LE, et al. Helical CT cholangiography with three-dimensional volume rendering using an oral biliary contrast agent: feasibility of a novel technique. AJR 2000;174:487–92.
32. Coakley FV, Schwartz LH. Magnetic resonance cholangiopancreatography. J Magn Reson Imaging 1999;9:157–62.
33. Takehara Y. Can MRCP replace ERCP? J Magn Reson Imaging 1998;8:517–34.
34. Takehara Y. MR pancreatography: technique and applications. Magn Reson Imaging 1996;8:290–301.
35. Barish MA, Soto JA, Yucel EK. Magnetic resonance cholangiopancreatography of the biliary ducts: techniques, clinical applications, and limitations. Magn Reson Imaging 1996;8:302–11.
36. Reinhold C, Guibaud L, Genin G, Bret PM. MR cholangiopancreatography: Comparison between two-dimensional fast spin-echo and three-dimensional gradient-echo pulse sequences. J Magn Reson Imaging 1995;4:379–84.
37. Bowie JD. What is the upper limit of normal for the common bile duct on ultrasound: how much do you want it to be? Am J Gastroenterol 2000;95:897–900.
38. Mitchell SE, Clark RA. A comparison of computed tomography and sonography in choledocholithiasis. AJR 1984;142:729–33.
39. Jeffrey RB, Federele MP, Laing FC, et al. Computed tomography of choledocholithiasis. AJR 1983;140:1179–83.
40. Neitlich JD, Topazian M, Smith RC, et al. Detection of choledocholithiasis: comparison of unenhanced helical CT and endoscopic retrograde cholangiopancreatography. Radiology 1997;203:753–7.
41. Varghese JC, Farrell MA, Courtney G, et al. A prospective comparison of magnetic resonance cholangiopancreatography with endoscopic retrograde cholangiopancreatography in the evaluation of patients with suspected biliary tract disease. Clin Radiol 1999;54:513–20.
42. Reinhold C, Taourel P, Bret PM, et al. Choledocholithiasis: evaluation of MR cholangiography for diagnosis. Radiology 1998;209:435–42.
43. Dwerryhouse SJ, Brown E, Vipond MN. Prospective evaluation of magnetic resonance cholangiography to detect common bile duct stones before laparoscopic cholecystectomy. Br J Surg 1998;85:1364–6.
44. Chan YL, Chan AC, Lam WW, et al. Choledocholithiasis: comparison of MR cholangiography and endoscopic retrograde cholangiography. Radiology 1996;200:85–9.
45. Higgins CB. The vascular system. In: Higgins CB, Hricak H, Helms CA, eds. Magnetic resonance imaging of the body. 2nd ed. New York: Raven Press, 1992:629–78.
46. Weisner RH, La Russo NF. Clinicopathologic features of the syndrome of primary sclerosing cholangitis. Semin Liver Dis 1985;5:241–53.
47. MacCarty RL, LaRusso NF, May GR, et al. Cholangiocarcinoma complicating primary sclerosing cholangitis: cholangiographic appearances. Radiology 1985;156:43–6.
48. Dodd GD III, Niedzwiecki GA, Campbell WL, Baron RL. Bile duct calculi in patients with primary sclerosing cholangitis. Radiology 1997;203:443–7.
49. Ito K, Mithcell DG, Outwater EK, Blasbalg R. Primary sclerosing cholangitis: MR imaging features. AJR 1999;172:1527–33.
50. Fulcher AS, Turner MA, Franklin KJ, et al. Primary sclerosing cholangitis: evaluation with MR cholangiography—a case control study. Radiology 2000;215:71–80.
51. Crittenden SL, McKinley MJ. Choledochal cyst—clinical features and classification. Am J Gastroenterol 1985;80:643–7.
52. Voyles CT, Smadja C, Shands WC, Blumgart LH. Carcinoma in choledochal cysts: age-related incidence. Arch Surg 1983;118:986–8.
53. Reuter K, Raptopoulous VD, Cantelmo N, et al. The diagnosis of a choledochal cyst by ultrasound. Radiology 1980;136:437–8.
54. Tsutomu A, Yugi L, Akira T. CT of choledochal cyst. AJR 1980;135:729–34.
55. Matos C, Nicaise N, Deviere J, et al. Choledochal cysts: comparison of findings at MR cholangiopancreatography and endoscopic retrograde cholangiopancreatography in eight patients. Radiology 1998;209:443–8.

56. Irie H, Honda H, Jimi M, et al. Value of MR cholangiopancreatography in evaluating choledochal cysts. AJR 1998;171:1381–5.
57. Pavone P, Laghi A, Catalano C, et al. Caroli's disease: evaluation with MR cholangiopancreatography (MRCP). Abdom Imaging 1996;21:117–9.
58. Lavine E, Maklad MF, Wright CH, Lee KR. Computed tomographic and ultrasonic appearances of primary carcinoma of the common bile duct. Gastrointest Radiol 1979;4:147–51.
59. Warren KW, Tan EGC. Disease of the gallbladder and bile ducts. In: Schiff L, ed. Diseases of the liver. Philadelphia: JB Lippincott, 1975.
60. Soyer P, Bluemke DA, Reichle RL, et al.. Imaging of intrahepatic cholangiocarcinoma. 1. Peripheral cholangiocarcinoma. AJR 1995;165:1427–31.
61. Soyer P, Bluemke DA, Reichle R, et al. Imaging of intrahepatic cholangiocarcinoma. 2. Hilar cholangiocarcinoma. AJR 1995;165:1433–6.
62. Subramanyam BR, Raghavendra BN, Balthazar EJ, et al. Ultrasonic features of cholangiocarcinoma. J Ultrasound Med 1984;3:405–8.
63. Choi BI, Lee JH, Han MC, et al. Hilar cholangiocarcinoma: comparative study with sonography and CT. Radiology 1989;172:689–92.
64. Vazquez JL, Thorsen MK, Dodds WJ, et al. Atrophy of the left hepatic lobe caused by cholangiocarcinoma. AJR 1985;144:547–8.
65. Keogan MT, Seabourn JT, Paulson EK, et al. Contrast-enhanced CT of intrahepatic and hilar cholangiocarcinoma: delay time for optimal imaging. AJR 1997;169:1493–9.
66. Choi BI, Han JK, Shin YM, et al. Peripheral cholangiocarcinoma: comparison of MR and CT. Abdom Imaging 1995;20:357–60.
67. Soyer P, Bluemke DA, Sibert A, Laissy JP. MR imaging of intrahepatic cholangiocarcinoma. Abdom Imaging 1995;20:126–30.
68. Adjei ON, Tamura S, Sugimura H, et al. Constrast-enhanced MR imaging of intrahepatic cholangiocarcinoma. Clin Radiol 1995;50:6–10.
69. Carr TG, Kazarian KK, Smego DR, Barone JE. Radionuclide cholescintigraphy in patients with suspected biliary tract obstruction. Am Surg 1991;57:673–5.
70. Lecklitner ML, Austin AR, Benedetto AR, Growcock GW. Positive predictive value of cholescintigraphy in common bile duct obstruction. J Nucl Med 1986;27:1403–6.
71. Toftdahl DB, Hojgaard L, Winkler K. Dynamic cholescintigraphy: induction and description of gallbladder emptying. J Nucl Med 1996;37:261–6.
72. Kim CK, Palestro CJ, Solomon RW, et al. Delayed biliary-to-bowel transit in cholescintigraphy after cholecystokinin treatment. Radiology 1990;176:553–6.
73. Kim CK, Lim JK, Machac J. Variable bile retention on cholescintigraphy after morphine administration. Eur J Nucl Med. 1996;23:1464–7.
74. Flancbaum L, Choban PS, Sinha R, Jonasson O. Morphine cholescintigraphy in the evaluation of hospitalized patients with suspected acute cholecystitis. Ann Surg 1994;220:25–31.
75. Adam A, Roddie ME. Acute cholecystitis: radiological management. Clin Gastroenterol 1991;5:787–816.
76. Lauritsen KB, Sommer W, Hahn L, Henriksen JH. Cholescintigraphy and ultrasonography in patients suspected of having acute cholecystitis. Scand J Gastroenterol 1988;23:42–6.
77. Krishnamurthy S, Krishnamurthy GT. Cholecystokinin and morphine pharmacological intervention during 99m TC-HIDA cholescintigraphy: a rational approach. Semin Nucl Med 1996;26:16–24.
78. Kim CK. Pharmacological intervention for the diagnosis of acute cholecystitis: cholecystokinin pretreatment or morphine, or both? J Nucl Med 1997;38:647–9.
79. Bohdiewica PJ. The diagnostic value of grading hyperperfusion and the rim sign in cholescintigraphy. Clin Nucl Med 1993;18:867–71.
80. Klingensmith WC 3rd, Turner WM. Cholescintigraphy for acute cholecystitis: false positive results caused by chronic cholecystitis. Gastrointest Radiol 1990;15:129–32.
81. Nadel HR. Hepatobiliary scintigraphy in children. Semin Nucl Med 1996;26:25–42.
82. Cox KL, Stadalnik RC, McGahan JP, et al. Hepatobiliary scintigraphy with technetium-99m disofenin in the evaluation of neonatal cholestasis. J Pediatr Gastroenterol Nutr 1987;6:885–91.
83. Toftdahl DB, Hojgaard L, Winkler K. Dynamic cholescintigraphy: induction and description of gallbladder emptying. J Nucl Med 1996;37:261–6.
84. Krishnamurthy S, Krishnamurthy GT. Biliary dyskinesia: role of the sphincter of Oddi, gallbladder and cholecystokinin. J Nucl Med 1997;38:1824–30.
85. Sorenson MK, Fancher S, Lang NP, et al. Abnormal gallbladder nuclear ejection fraction predicts success of cholecystectomy in patients with biliary dyskinesia. Am J Surg 1993;166:672–4.

Chapter

4

Percutaneous Imaging of the Biliary Tree and Gallbladder

Paul V. Suhocki

Physicians have been using cholangiography to evaluate the biliary tree for eight decades. In current practice, cholangiography is performed to 1) define the level of obstruction in patients with dilated bile ducts, 2) evaluate for the presence of suspected gallstones, 3) determine the etiology of cholangitis, 4) evaluate suspected bile duct inflammatory disorders, and 5) demonstrate the site of a bile leak (1). Contrast is injected into the bile ducts in an antegrade or retrograde fashion before radiography is performed. Antegrade contrast injection is done through a percutaneously placed needle (percutaneous transhepatic cholangiography, PTC) or a T-tube. The technical success rate of PTC is 95% in patients with dilated bile ducts and 65% in patients with nondilated ducts (1). Retrograde contrast injection is done through a cannula placed endoscopically into the common bile duct (endoscopic retrograde cholangiopancreatography, ERCP). The latter method is performed more frequently than PTC because it is associated with fewer complications. Magnetic resonance cholangiopancreatography (MRCP), computed tomography (CT), and sonography are noninvasive radiologic means of evaluating the biliary tree that have also contributed to the decline in number of PTC procedures performed over the last several years (see Chapter 3).

Burckhardt and Muller first described PTC in 1921. The researchers opacified the biliary tree by injecting a contrast agent into the gallbladder (2). This is a technique sometimes used today but it requires the cystic duct to be patent for its success. Huard et al. (3) were the first to describe direct percutaneous puncture of the bile ducts with a needle in 1937. They used lipid soluble contrast. Carter and Saypol (3a) described the use of this technique with water-soluble contrast in 1952. These authors performed their cholangiograms by advancing a needle into the liver without imaging guidance. They then slowly retracted the needle. Once bile emanated from the needle, they injected contrast and performed radiography.

Arner et al. (4) used fluoroscopy to guide the percutaneous puncture of the bile ducts in 1962. They first passed the needle into the liver under fluoroscopy. They then injected contrast while retracting the needle, looking for bile duct opacification. Once a duct was visible, they injected more contrast to fill the biliary tree. Radiologists still use this technique today, but with a smaller gauge needle. Okuda et al. (5) introduced this "skinny needle" technique in 1974; their flexible 22-gauge needle was less traumatic to the liver.

In spite of the lower complication rate with the skinny needle technique, PTC still carries risks of sepsis, cholangitis, bile leak, hemorrhage, and pneumothorax. Today, PTC is usually performed only after the safer method of ERCP has been unsuccessful in accessing the biliary tree (see Chapter 3). ERCP can fail from the endoscopist's inability to 1) cannulate the ampulla because of unfavorable anatomy or a tumor, 2) cross an obstruction or tear in the extrahepatic bile duct, or 3) pass the endoscope through the afferent limb of a biliary enteric bypass.

Once the biliary tree has been opacified by either PTC or ERCP, the bile ducts are evaluated for the presence of occlusions, stenoses, filling defects, contour abnormalities, and leaks. A treatment plan is chosen after a diagnosis has been made. Complicated cases may require the combined skills of the interventional radiologist, endoscopist, and surgeon at different settings in a staged approach.

PREPROCEDURAL PLANNING AND PATIENT PREPARATION

Pertinent radiographs are reviewed for procedural planning. The degree of bile duct dilatation helps to predict the level of difficulty in accessing the ductal system. Lateralizing of ductal dilatation helps direct the needle access to either the right or left lobe. A hilar tumor will require both a right intercostal and left subxiphoid approach to demonstrate both ductal systems because of lack of communication between the systems. Left hepatic lobe access is warranted in the patient with ascites because there is less risk of ascites leakage after the procedure when compared with right intercostal access. The presence of a metallic coronary O-ring in the right abdomen may indicate that the hepatic surgeon placed the marker on the efferent limb of the jejunum when creating a Roux-en-Y biliary enteric anastomosis. This will facilitate percutaneous biliary access as described below.

The patient is kept in a fasting state for 4 hours prior to PTC. Prothrombin time (PT), partial thromboplastin time (PTT), and platelet counts are measured. Coagulation and platelet abnormalities are corrected to as near normal as possible with the use of vitamin K, fresh frozen plasma, and platelets. Antibiotics are administered intravenously.

The patient is transferred to the interventional radiology suite and placed on an angiography table. Use of an image intensifier with rotational capability contributes to the safety and success of the procedure and limits the radiation dose to the patient and radiologist. The patient is prepped and draped from the right midaxillary line to the left midclavicular line between the levels of the nipples and umbilicus. This provides access to the right and left hepatic lobes.

Optimal analgesia is required for all percutaneous liver access procedures. Conscious sedation is routinely administered. An intercostal nerve block with a long-acting anesthetic is performed for right-sided hepatic access procedures. A dedicated interventional radiology nurse closely monitors the patient's vital signs. General anesthesia is used for all pediatric patients and for those adults whose pain is not adequately controlled with conscious sedation.

TECHNIQUE FOR PERCUTANEOUS ACCESS TO THE RIGHT HEPATIC LOBE

The right intercostal approach to the biliary tree is the most commonly used access to the liver. The most inferior right intercostal space is chosen that will allow a 22-gauge, 15-cm-long needle to enter the liver capsule at the junction of its middle and lower thirds of the liver. An intercostal nerve block is performed by injecting a long-acting anesthetic at the level of access and at one level above and below the access site. Local infiltration of the skin with anesthetic is also performed. Injecting a local anesthetic drug into the pleural space (interpleural block) has been found to reduce the amount of pain during and after percutaneous access to the liver but increases the rate of pneumothorax for the procedure (6).

The needle is directed toward the left axilla and stopped when it is superimposed over the midportion of the vertebral bodies on fluoroscopy. The needle pass is made during shallow breathing. Exaggerated respiratory excursions during needle passes will result in a serpiginous access tract, creating problems for guidewire and catheter advancement. Iodinated contrast material diluted to 50% concentration is injected through the needle while the needle is slowly retracted. Once the needle tip enters a duct, a 0.018-inch guidewire is passed through the needle and into the bile duct. This is then exchanged for a 3 French catheter with sideholes. The biliary system is gently evacuated and a sample of bile is sent to the microbiology laboratory for culture and sensitivity. The least amount of contrast required for diagnostic cholangiography is then injected. Injecting too much contrast into the potentially infected biliary tree may result in sepsis.

Coaxial dilatation is performed to 6F catheter size. Brief attempts are made to cross an obstruction if one is present. Care is taken to avoid unnecessary manipulation in an infected system. If the obstruction cannot be crossed within 5 minutes, an 8F drainage catheter is left in place above the obstruction and left to external drainage. The patient is brought back in 24 to 48 hours for repeat attempts. Once the obstruction is crossed, a drainage catheter can be placed with sideholes above and below the obstruction. This catheter can then be placed to internal drainage.

TECHNIQUE FOR PERCUTANEOUS ACCESS TO THE LEFT HEPATIC LOBE

The left lobe is most easily accessed under sonographic guidance. A 22-gauge, 15-cm-long needle is advanced from a left subxiphoid approach into the ventral duct of the left lobe. The needle is directed slightly cephalad and to the patient's right. The ventral duct of the left lobe is more favorable than the dorsal duct for drainage catheter placement because of its more superficial location. If the bile ducts are not dilated and cannot be seen on ultrasound, the radiologist can direct the needle toward the portal vein branches, which are always visible. This increases the likelihood of bile duct puncture because of the close anatomical relationship between bile ducts and portal vein branches. If the right biliary tree has already been accessed, the left bile ducts can be opacified by injecting air into the biliary tree from the right catheter. The air will rise into the ventrally located left bile ducts for identification and needle access under fluoroscopic guidance.

ALTERNATE METHODS FOR OPACIFYING THE BILIARY TREE

The gallbladder can also be used to opacify the biliary tree in patients with a nondilated biliary tree and an obstruction distal to the point at which the cystic duct joins the common hepatic duct. The patient is then placed in the Trendelenburg position so that gravity assists the flow of the dense injected contrast material into the intrahepatic bile ducts (7).

Occasionally the endoscopist will be able to cannulate the ampulla for cholangiography but will be unable to pass a stent in the biliary tree for drainage. They will then send the patient to the radiology department for percutaneous placement of a biliary drainage catheter. In this case, the endoscopist can leave a nasobiliary drainage catheter in place for the radiologist to use (8). When the patient is transferred to the interventional radiology suite, the radiologist injects contrast through the nasobiliary drainage catheter to opacify the biliary tree (Fig. 4.1). A 22-gauge, 15-cm needle is then advanced into a peripheral duct through either a right- or left-sided access.

It is sometimes necessary to define the site of bile duct leak in a patient who has sustained a bile duct tear during

(A)

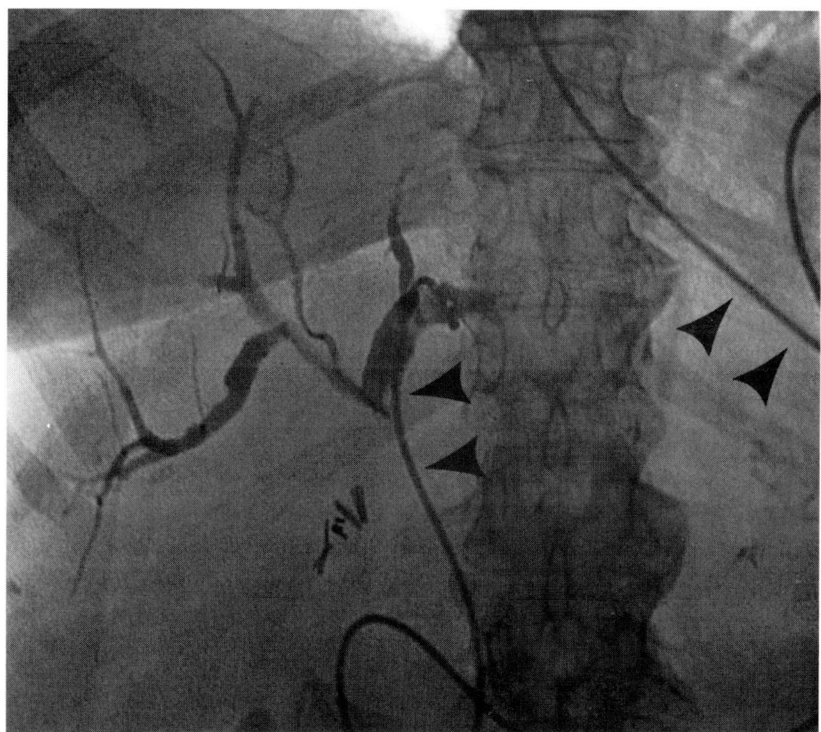

(B)

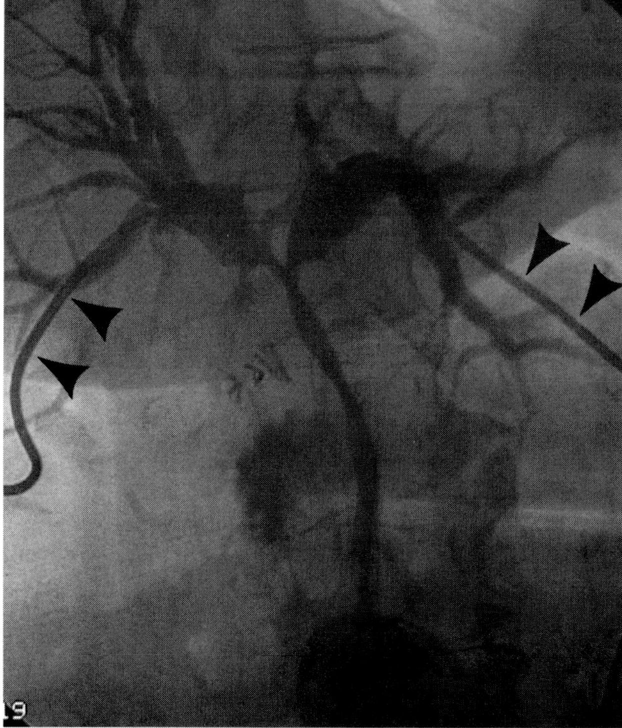

FIGURE 4.1. ***(A)*** *A nasobiliary drain (arrowheads) was placed by the endoscopist to facilitate percutaneous access to the bile ducts. Contrast injection opacifies the ducts for needle access.* ***(B)*** *Bilateral biliary drainage catheters (arrowheads) were placed, passing through the tumor at the bifurcation.*

trauma or operation (see Chapter 17). A surgically or radiologically placed drain is usually in place in the patient's biloma. The lacerated bile duct can sometimes be opacified in a retrograde fashion by injecting contrast into the biloma drainage catheter. Exaggerated respiratory excursions may increase the degree of success for this procedure.

When creating a biliary-enteric Roux-en-Y anastomosis, hepatic surgeons sometimes tack up a segment of the efferent limb to the anterior abdominal wall. A coronary O-ring is sewn to the efferent limb and marks the site of attachment of the loop of bowel to the wall (9). The radiologist accesses the efferent limb percutaneously using the O-ring as a target on fluoroscopy. A catheter is then advanced toward the biliary-enteric anastomosis for cholangiography. This method eliminates the need for transhepatic radiologic interventions and the possibility of hepatic injury.

COMPLICATIONS OF PERCUTANEOUS TRANSHEPATIC CHOLANGIOGRAPHY

Serious complications of percutaneous transhepatic cholangiography occur in 3% to 6% of patients (10). They include sepsis (most commonly), bile leakage into the peritoneal cavity or pleural space, and hemorrhage.

Sepsis and bile peritonitis are prevented by 1) adequate antibiotic coverage prior to instrumentation, 2) avoiding any aggressive interventions during the initial patient encounter, 3) aspirating the contents of the biliary tree as soon as it is accessed, and 4) injecting the biliary tree with an amount of contrast less than that of the bile aspirated.

Immediate or delayed bleeding can occur into the hepatic parenchyma, bile ducts, or peritoneal cavity. Bleeding can also occur onto the skin surface or through a drainage catheter tract if a catheter is left in place after PTC. Immediate hemorrhagic complications are made apparent by hypotension and tachycardia. Conscious sedation may mask any associated pain. Most bleeding is venous and self-limiting. Venous bleeding is avoided by abandoning transhepatic tracts that are demonstrated to cross large hepatic or portal veins.

Arterial hemorrhage can be catastrophic and must be treated immediately. A dreaded complication is a hepatic artery pseudoaneurysm, which can rupture days to months after PTC while the patient is at home. Arterial complications are decreased by avoiding the intercostal artery and by limiting bile duct access to the periphery of the liver, away from central major arteries.

Arterial complications are treated with percutaneous transcatheter embolization of the hepatic artery branch that has been injured. The hepatic artery is examined for the presence of transection, arteriovenous fistula formation, and pseudoaneurysm formation. The abnormal segment of the artery is embolized even if there is no active contrast extravasation from the abnormal site. Hepatic arterial embolization is discussed in Chapter 6.

In the patient with ascites, ascitic fluid may continue to leak from the percutaneous transhepatic access site after the needle is removed. This is seen most often in the patient with right-sided access, probably because this site is more dependent than the left lobe access with the patient recumbent. The ascites leak may be treated by placing a pursestring suture around the site of the leak. A tissue adhesive such as Dermabond can also be applied to the site while coapting the sides of the incision until the adhesive sets.

INTERPRETATION OF THE DIAGNOSTIC CHOLANGIOGRAM

At least three views of the biliary tree should be analyzed during cholangiography. The anterior, right anterior oblique, and left anterior oblique projections provide the most information. Newer angiography rooms have rotational angiography capabilities that acquire many projections of the biliary tree as the image intensifier describes an arc about the patient's abdomen. Overexposed or underexposed radiographs may mask bile duct abnormalities.

The Couinaud nomenclature for hepatic anatomy is generally used when interpreting a cholangiogram (see Chapter 1, Fig. 1.2). Its use is important for diagnosis as well as preoperative planning. This system describes eight distinct liver segments (11). Segment I is the caudate lobe. The left hepatic duct drains the left hemiliver and is formed by three individual tributaries draining segments II to IV. The right hepatic duct drains segments V to VIII. Two main tributaries, the right posterior sectorial duct and the right anterior sectorial duct form the right hepatic duct. The right posterior sectorial duct drains segments VI and VII. The right anterior sectorial duct drains segments V and VIII. The right anterior sectorial duct has a more vertical course than the right posterior sectorial duct. The right posterior sectorial duct passes behind the right anterior sectorial duct from the left side to join the right hepatic duct.

The most common bile duct anatomic variant involves the right posterior sectorial duct (11). The right posterior sectorial duct may join the right anterior sectorial duct from the right side. It may also join the left hepatic duct of the common hepatic duct directly. A triple confluence of the right posterior sectorial duct, right anterior sectorial duct, and the left hepatic duct may be seen also.

Biliary Obstruction

Most patients with biliary obstruction will have gross bile duct dilatation on abdominal CT, ultrasound, or MRCP. The ease of performing cholangiography increases with the degree of ductal dilatation seen on noninvasive studies. The lack of bile duct dilatation does not necessarily exclude the presence of an obstructing lesion. If clinical examination and laboratory tests suggest bile duct obstruction, the diagnosis should be pursued with cholangiography. Teplick et al. (12) performed PTC on 107 patients who had nondilated ducts. The cholangiogram was abnormal and showed poor emptying, stones, or strictures in 43% of the patients. Twenty-one percent of the patients had complications related to the PTC. Because the incidence of complications is higher and the success rate lower with PTC in patients without bile duct dilatation, ERCP should be attempted first in this group.

Primary Sclerosing Cholangitis

Primary sclerosing cholangitis (PSC) is a progressive fibrosis of the extrahepatic or intrahepatic bile ducts or both (see Chapter 19). The etiology of this disease is unknown. Ulcerative colitis is seen in 66% of the patients with PSC (13). Seventy percent of patients are male, and two-thirds are less than 45 years old (10). Patients with PSC have at least a 10% risk of developing cholangiocarcinoma.

Cholangiography typically demonstrates multiple short or long strictures of the ducts. The intrahepatic and extrahepatic ducts are involved in 68% to 89% of patients (Fig. 4.2). The extrahepatic ducts alone are involved in 3% and the intrahepatic ducts alone in 3% to 10% (10). There may be no dilatation of bile ducts proximal to the stricture because of fibrotic changes around the ducts. Outpouchings of the ducts may be seen between the strictures (Fig. 4.3). There may be areas of nonfilling of bile duct branches, giving the biliary tree a branchless appearance. Malignant degeneration of PSC is a difficult diagnosis to make. Marked ductal dilatation, worsening stricturing, and the presence of a polypoid mass on cholangiography suggest the progression to malignancy (14).

The primary differential diagnosis of PSC is diffuse sclerosing carcinoma of the bile ducts, which represents less than 10% of bile duct carcinomas (15). Diffuse metastatic disease to the liver can cause multiple strictures of the intrahepatic ducts without biliary dilatation.

Primary biliary cirrhosis can mimic PSC and is seen in middle-aged women. Recurrent biliary infections related to gallstones or surgical stricture produce similar findings. Sclerosing cholangitis can also be iatrogenic, occurring after infusion of chemotherapeutic agents through the hepatic artery (16).

Cystic Biliary Disease

The etiology of cystic biliary disease is unclear (see Chapter 16). The disorder may be related to anomalous drainage of

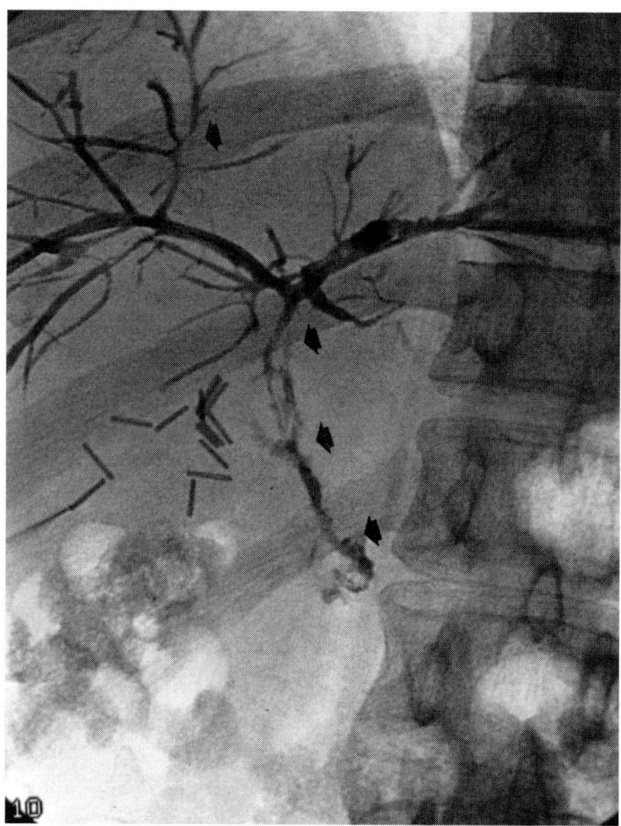

FIGURE 4.2. *Multiple strictures (arrows) due to primary sclerosing cholangitis involve the extrahepatic and intrahepatic bile ducts.*

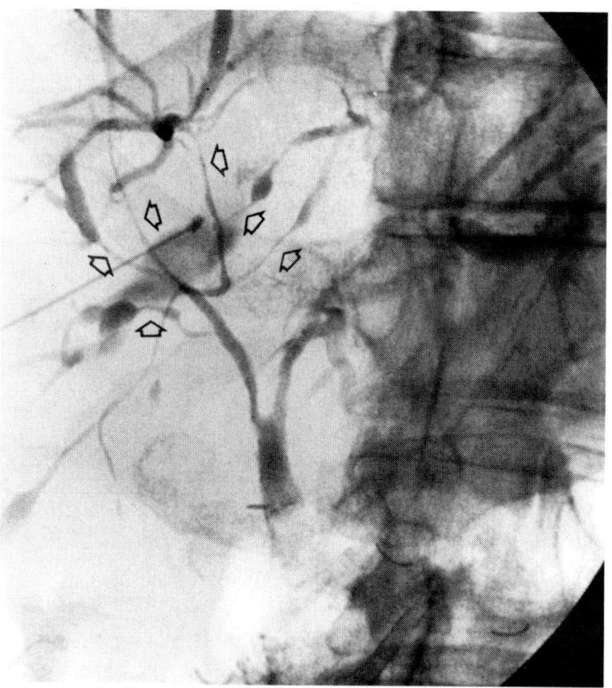

FIGURE 4.3. *Cholangiogram in a patient with primary sclerosing cholangitis demonstrates multiple long strictures (arrows) of the right hepatic ducts with areas of focal dilatation between the strictures.*

the pancreatic and biliary ducts and loss of the distal sphincter mechanism (17). The most commonly used classification system for biliary cystic disease is the Todani modification of the Alonso-Lej classification. This system describes five types of cysts (17). Type I is the most common (80% to 90%) and is a single cystic dilatation of the common hepatic duct, common bile duct, or both. Type II is a diverticulum of the common bile duct and accounts for 3%. Type III is a cystic dilatation of the common bile duct in the wall of the duodenum, accounting for 5%. Type IV is made up of multiple cysts involving the extrahepatic and/or intrahepatic ducts and accounts for 10% of cases. Type V is the variant known as Caroli's disease. Type V is commonly associated with congenital fibrosis and cysts outside of the liver.

Complications include biliary obstruction, hepatic abscess, cholangitis, and bile duct cancer. The risk of bile duct cancer is increased 20-fold in this patient group. It is unusual for gallstones to be found in association with biliary cystic disease.

Choledocholithiasis

Stones in the bile ducts either form there primarily or migrate there from the gallbladder. Primary bile duct stones are composed mainly of calcium bilirubinate. Bile stasis, dietary factors, and bacterial or parasitic infection contribute to their formation, although their precise pathogenesis is unknown (18).

Single or multiple filling defects in the biliary tree characterize the presence of gallstones (Figs. 4.4 and 4.5). Because contrast may obscure gallstones in the biliary tree, the contrast should be diluted with normal saline for optimal visualization. Air bubbles or blood clots can obscure or mimic gallstones. Changing patient positioning while observing the filling defects under fluoroscopy helps to differentiate air bubbles from stones. The air bubbles seek an anterior location and coalesce with one another.

Blood clots are more difficult to differentiate from stones. Blood often enters the biliary tree during the puncture by the PTC needle. The suspected presence of blood clots requires repeating the cholangiogram in several days. The lytic properties of bile and the passing of clots through the drainage catheter will have cleared blood clots from the biliary tree during that time.

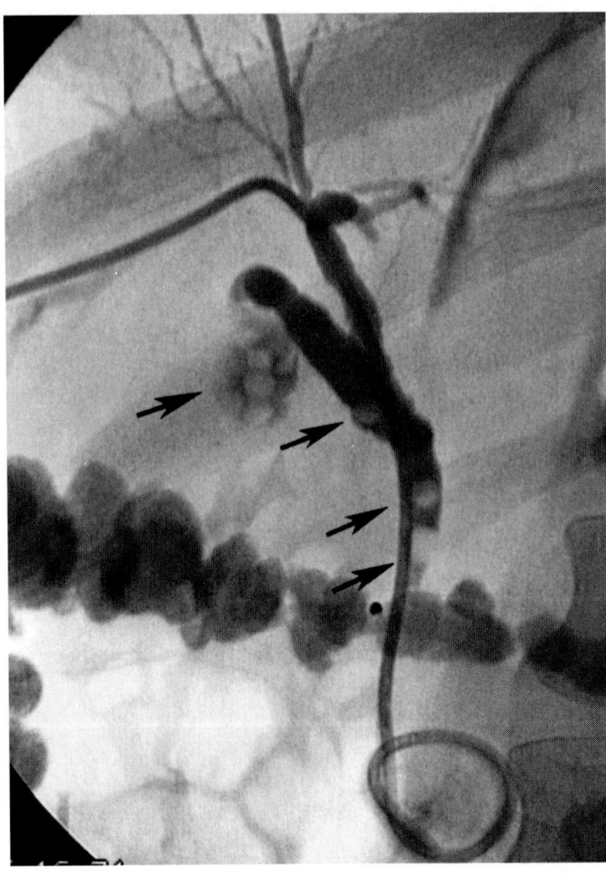

FIGURE 4.4. *Multifaceted gallstones (arrows) appear as filling defects throughout the gallbladder and bile ducts.*

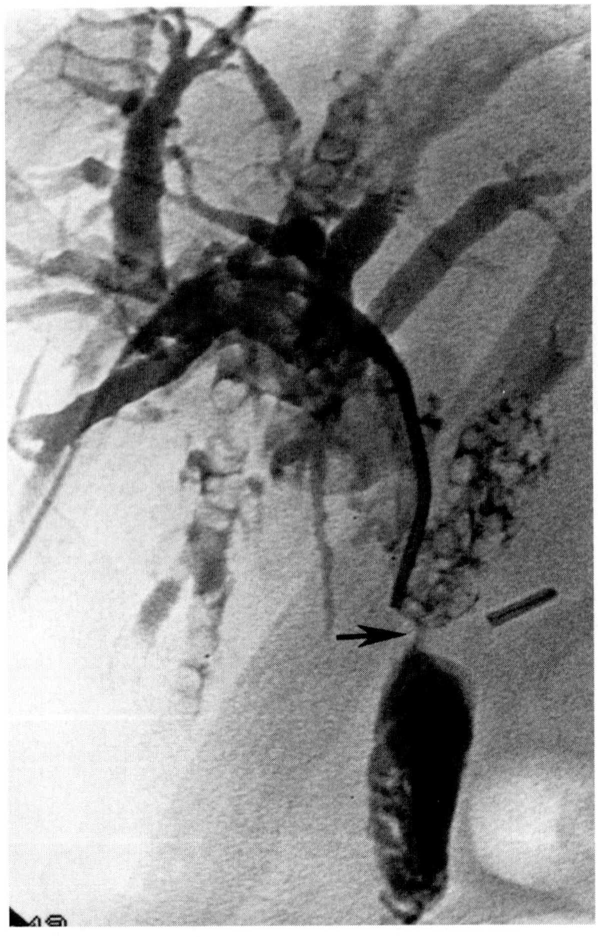

FIGURE 4.5. *Multifaceted gallstones appear as filling defects above a benign anastomotic stricture (arrow) which developed in a patient who underwent biliary-enteric bypass for a laparoscopic cholecystectomy bile duct injury.*

Gallstones sometimes become impacted within the bile ducts. In this form, they can be mistaken for a polypoid tumor (15). Manipulation with a stone extraction basket or balloon may help differentiate between the two entities.

Mirizzi's syndrome occurs when a gallstone lodges in the cystic duct or gallbladder neck and causes extrinsic compression of the common bile duct. The compression usually occurs at the lateral aspect of the common bile duct (19). The patient develops jaundice because of common bile duct obstruction.

Benign Biliary Strictures

Greater than 90% of benign biliary strictures are the result of surgical trauma, most commonly cholecystectomy (20) (see Chapter 17). Surgical strictures may be caused by duct ligation or clipping, as is seen with emergency maneuvers to control massive bleeding. They can also result from thermal injury or injury to the small arteries that run within the common bile duct wall (20). Transection of the duct interrupts the delicate arterial blood supply to the ducts. This may be the reason for ischemia and stenosis sometimes seen with biliary-enteric bypass operations (Fig. 4.6). Torsion of the bile duct may also occur following choledochojejunostomy (Fig. 4.7).

Benign biliary strictures are a common problem following orthotopic liver transplantation and occur in 3% to 22% of the patients (21) (see Chapter 18). The etiology of anastomotic strictures in this group is not well understood. Postoperative fibrosis and possibly ischemia are felt to be the causes. Prolonged cold ischemic time, hepatic artery thrombosis, surgical interruption of the peribiliary arterial plexus, and chronic rejection are potential causes of nonanastomotic biliary strictures in the transplanted liver (21) (Figs. 4.8 and 4.9).

Postoperative benign strictures are usually short and have an abrupt change in caliber at the site of abnormality. There is ductal dilatation above the stricture. Intrahepatic abscesses may be present. A longer stricture should raise the suspicion of malignancy (10).

Nonsurgical causes of benign biliary obstruction include gallstone erosion into the main bile duct, pericholedochal abscess, blunt trauma, compression by pseudoaneurysm or pseudocyst, and pancreatitis (Figs. 4.10 and 4.11).

Malignant Biliary Strictures

Distinguishing between malignant and benign strictures is difficult (see Chapter 2). Although certain cholangiographic features described in this section may suggest the presence of a malignant stricture, these features are not specific. Clinical information and results of noninvasive radiologic tests such as CT, MRI, and ultrasound may help to confirm a diagnosis of malignancy. CT, MRI, and ultrasound provide information about liver tissue surrounding the intrahepatic ducts and organs that surround the extrahepatic ducts. Results of these imaging modalities may be inconclusive, in which case a biliary biopsy may be helpful. Biliary biopsy techniques are discussed in Chapter 6.

Cholangiocarcinoma is a slowly growing tumor that usually presents in the sixth decade of life (see Chapter 20). Patients present at a younger age if the tumor is found in association with other diseases that predispose to cholangiocarcinoma, such as primary sclerosing cholangitis and choledochal cyst disease.

Cholangiocarcinoma presents as long or focal bile duct strictures. It spreads through local extension along the bile ducts or into the liver substance (10). The distal left or right main bile ducts and the common hepatic duct are the most common sites of involvement (Fig. 4.12). The tumor occurs

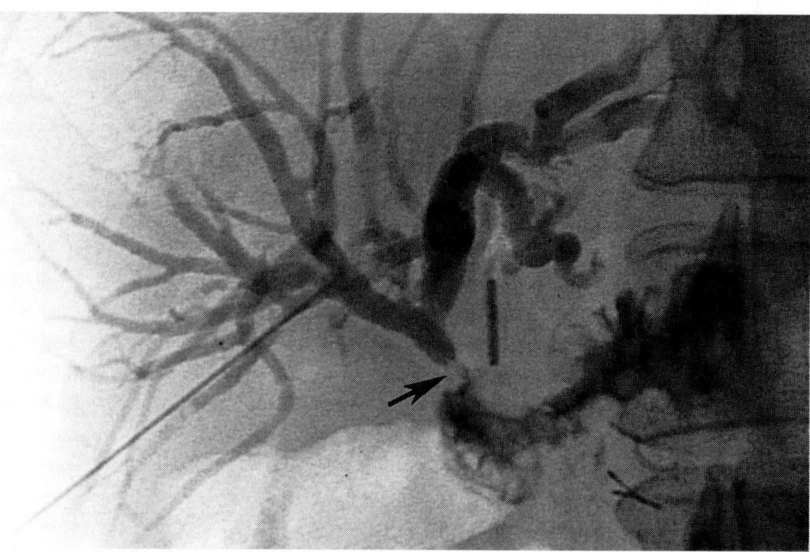

FIGURE 4.6. *A benign focal anastomotic stricture (arrow) is present in a patient who underwent biliary-enteric bypass for pancreatic cancer.*

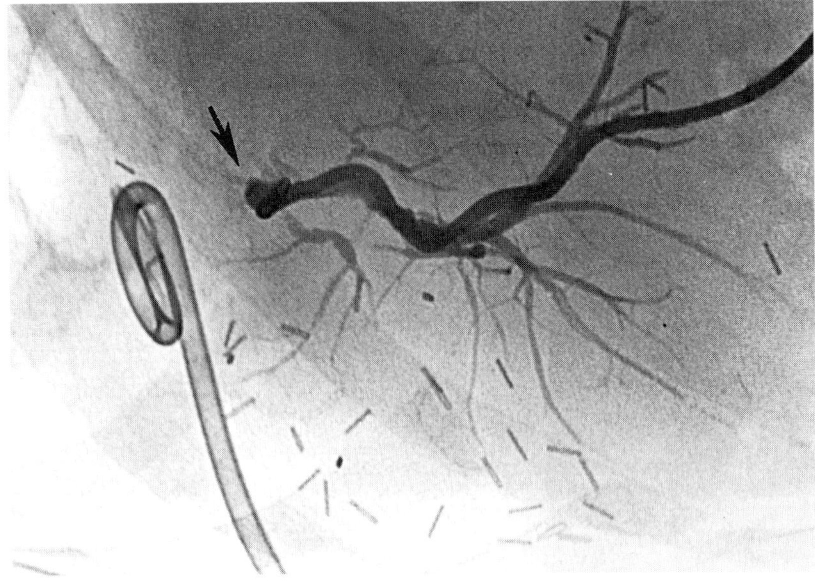

(A)

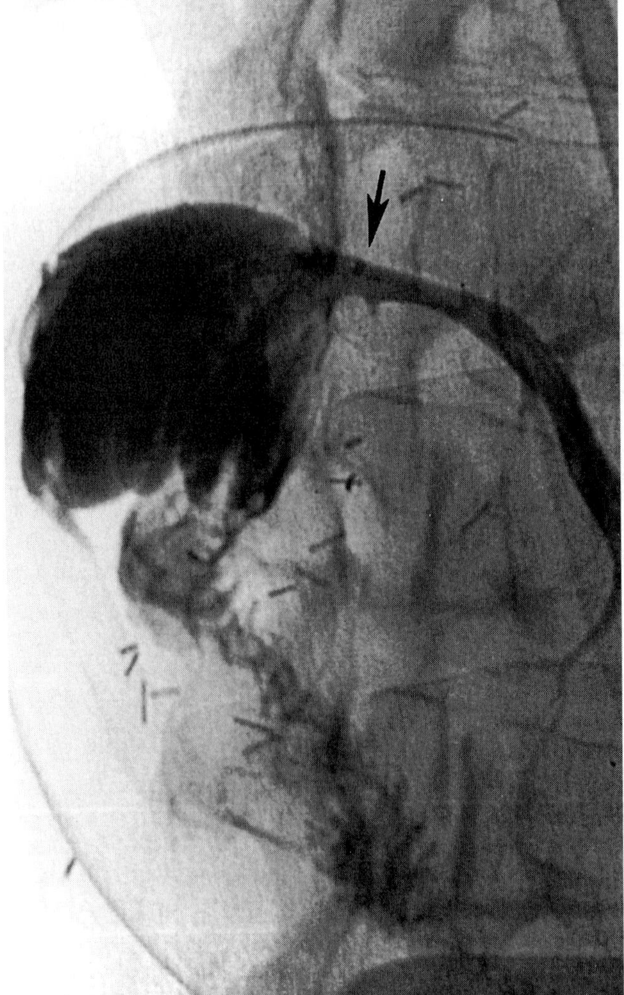

(B)

FIGURE 4.7. ***(A)*** *Postoperative cholangiogram following biliary-enteric anastomosis in a patient who underwent hepatic trisegmentectomy for metastatic colon cancer. Torsion has occurred at the anastomosis causing obstruction (arrow) of the bile duct.* ***(B)*** *The biliary-enteric anastomosis (arrow) is widely patent following revision of the anastomosis.*

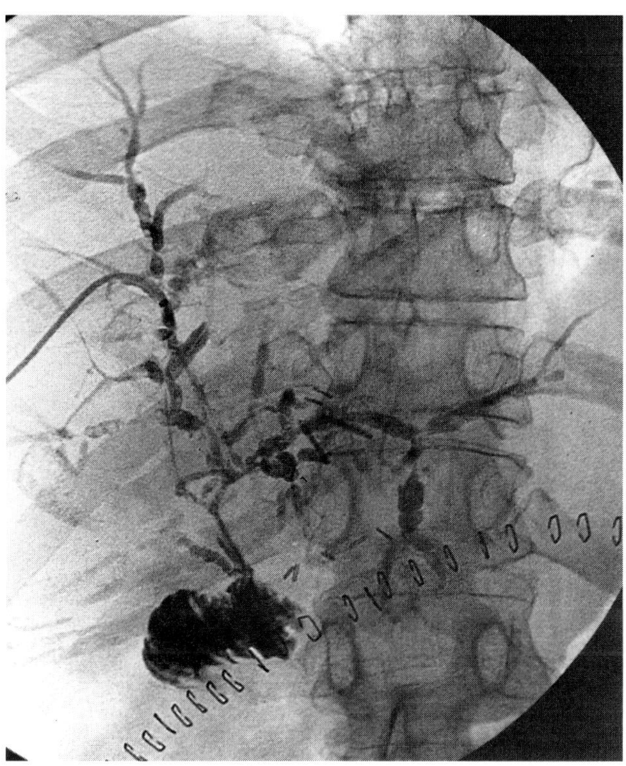

FIGURE 4.8. *Multiple focal ischemic strictures following orthotopic liver transplantation.*

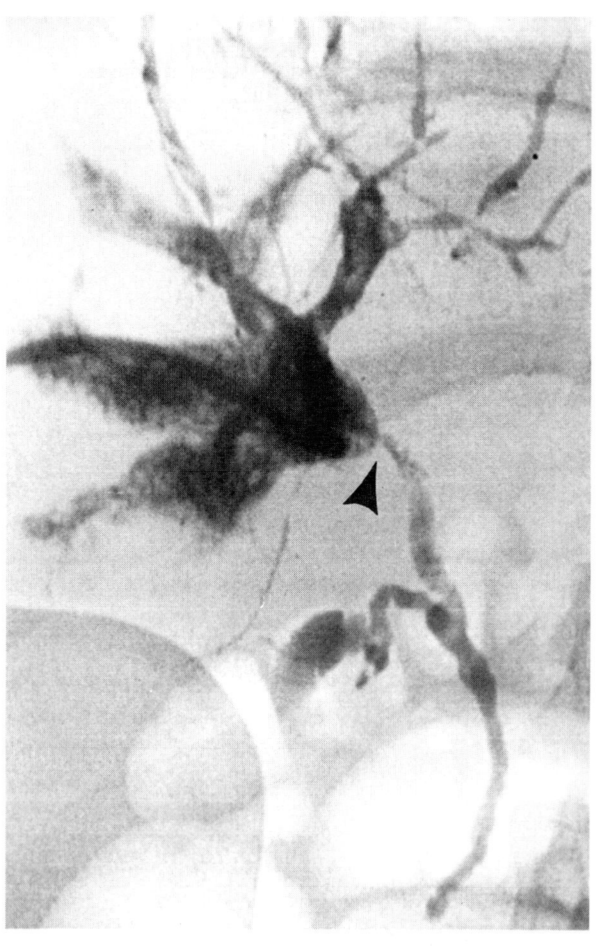

FIGURE 4.9. *Ischemic stricture (arrowhead) involving a branch of the right hepatic duct following orthotopic liver transplantation for primary sclerosing cholangitis. There is gross dilatation of the bile ducts above the stricture and a large amount of debris within the ducts.*

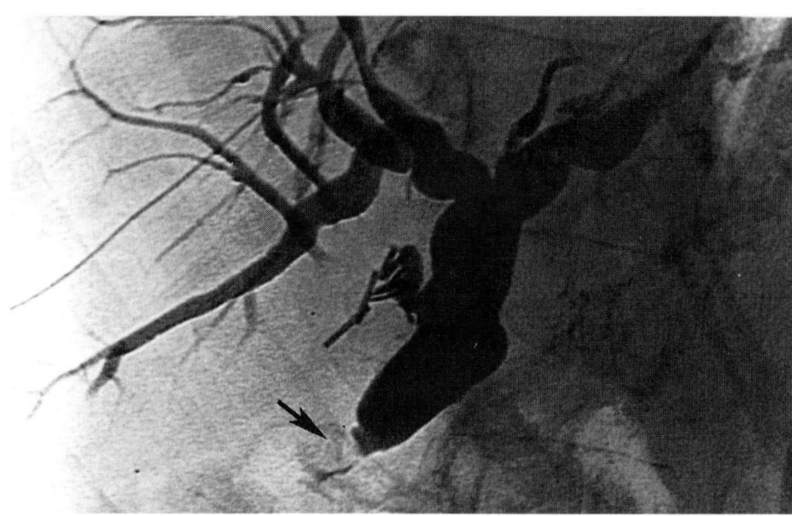

FIGURE 4.10. *Obstruction of the common bile duct (arrow) secondary to chronic pancreatitis.*

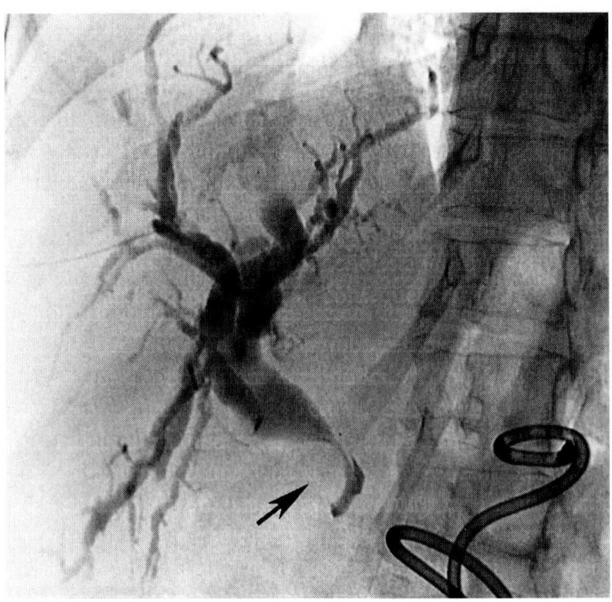

FIGURE 4.11. *A pancreatic pseudocyst causes obstruction (arrow) of the common bile duct by extrinsic compression.*

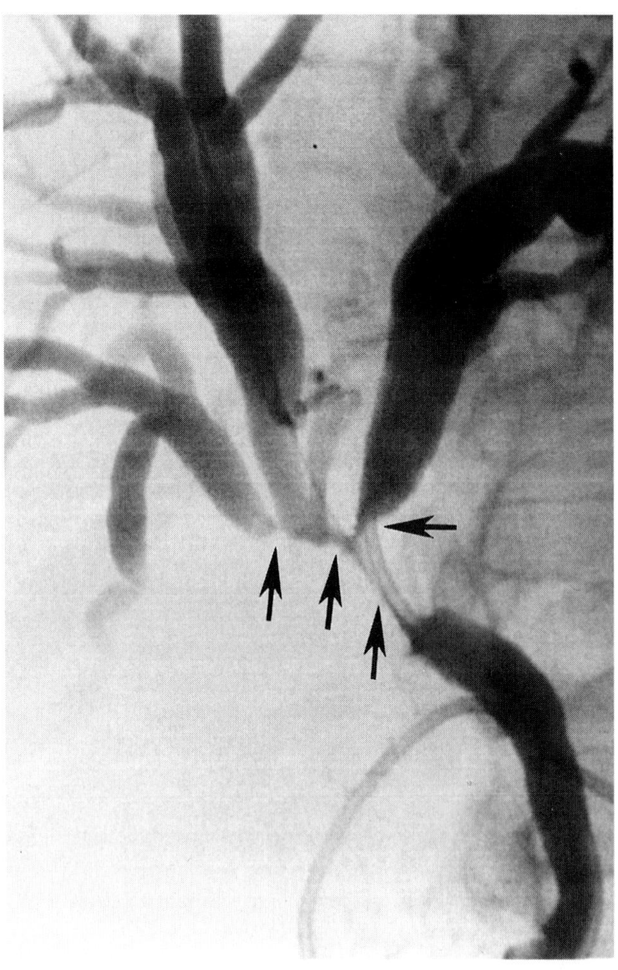

FIGURE 4.12. *A cholangiocarcinoma causes a malignant stricture (arrows) of the common hepatic duct, left main hepatic duct, and the first two divisions of the right hepatic duct.*

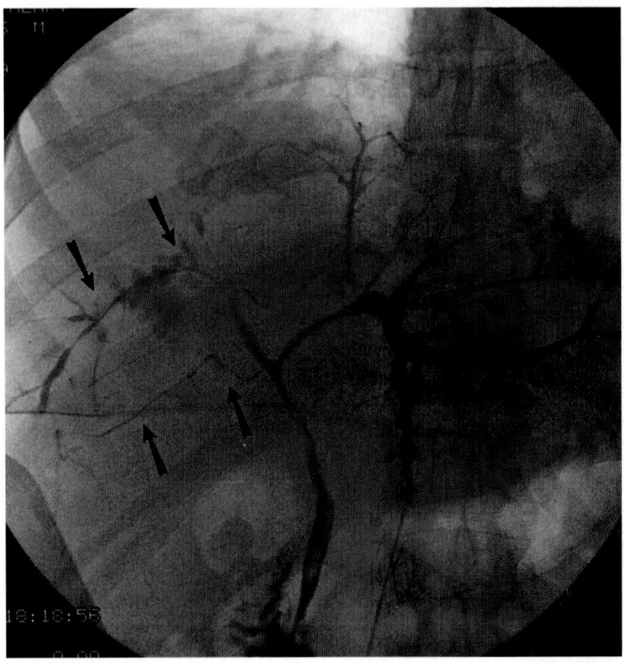

FIGURE 4.13. *Diffuse cholangiocarcinoma causes multiple strictures of the right intrahepatic ducts (arrows), left hepatic duct, and common hepatic duct.*

at the junction of the left and right main hepatic ducts in 20.5% to 45.5%, the common bile duct in 33% to 40.5%, and the cystic duct in 6% (10). The differential diagnosis for intrahepatic ductal involvement of cholangiocarcinoma includes PSC and liver metastases (Fig. 4.13). Pancreatic carcinoma, ampullary carcinoma, and chronic pancreatitis should be considered when the disease is confined to the distal common bile duct.

Gallbladder carcinoma occurs more frequently in females and usually presents in the sixth and seventh decades of life (see Chapter 14). Choledocholithiasis is found in 80% of the patients (10). Direct extension of the tumor is common and sometimes causes jaundice by obstructing the common hepatic duct (Fig. 4.14). The other common form of tumor spread is lymphangitic.

Pancreatic carcinoma is the fourth leading cause of cancer death in the United States. It is the most common cause of malignant biliary obstruction in patients in their sixth decade of life or older. Pancreatic cancer causes compression and obstruction of the mid to distal common bile

(A)

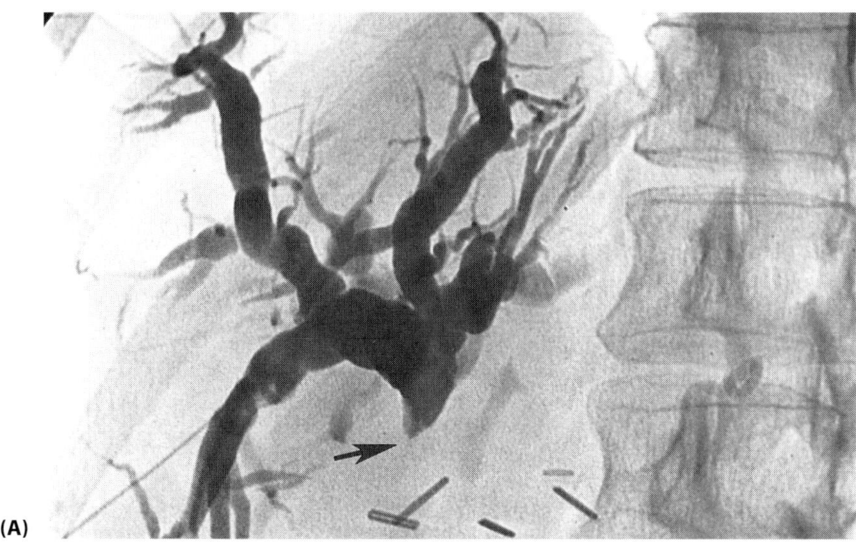

(B)

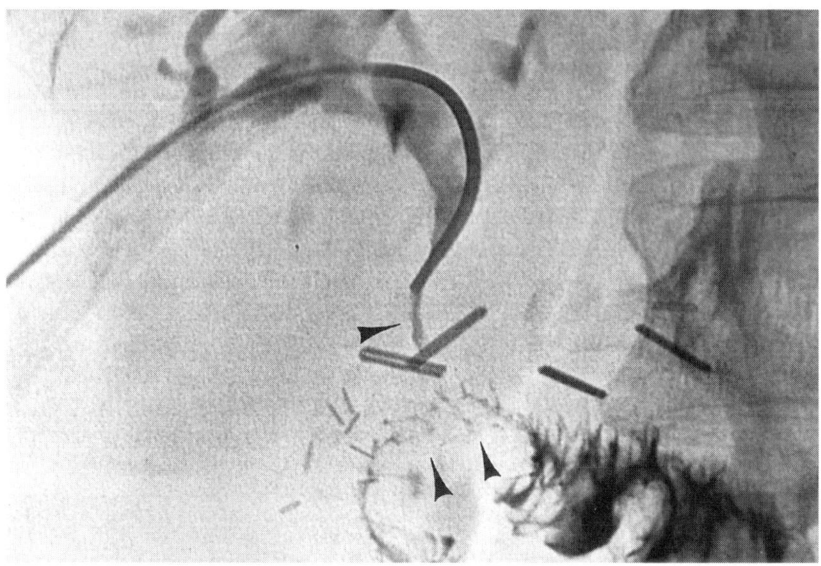

FIGURE 4.14. ***(A)*** *This patient with metastic adenosquamous carcinoma of the gallbladder had a surgical biliary-enteric bypass which is now obstructed by tumor involving the common hepatic duct.* ***(B)*** *A small amount of contrast passes through the biliary-enteric anastomosis showing marked thickening of the jejunal folds caused by tumor invasion (arrowheads).*

duct (Fig. 4.15). The contrast column passing through the tumor is typically irregular, with a "rat tail" appearance. Narrowing is usually concentric. The site of obstruction may have a nipple-like appearance (10). The proximal bile ducts are usually dilated.

Most patients with ampullary carcinoma present in the sixth and seventh decades of life. Ampullary carcinoma on cholangiography appears as an irregular filling defect located in the distal most portion of the common bile duct.

Metastatic disease from other organs causes biliary obstruction when it involves the hepatic hilum, periportal lymph nodes, or peripancreatic lymph nodes (Figs. 4.16, 4.17, and 4.18). Direct extension of tumor from adjacent organs, such as the stomach, may also cause biliary obstruction (Fig. 4.19). Tumor encasement can cause irregularity and displacement of the contrast column on cholangiography. Portal lymph nodes replaced by tumors may produce extrinsic compression of the contrast column.

Bile Leaks

Most bile leaks are iatrogenic and occur following cholecystectomy, partial liver resection, or orthotopic liver transplantation (see Chapters 17, 18). Uncomplicated bile leaks, such as cystic duct leak and duct of Luschka leak following cholecystectomy, usually respond to biliary decompression with an endoscopic stent (22). More extensive bile duct injuries require surgical biliary enteric reconstruction in the form of a Roux-en-Y anastomosis. Percutaneous methods can sometimes be used to treat a complex bile duct injury without surgery. More often, percutaneous interventions are performed prior to surgical repair to aid in identification of the bile ducts intraoperatively.

ERCP will demonstrate the abnormal bile duct in most cases of bile leak. PTC becomes necessary when a bile leak is occurring above a clipped or ligated common bile duct or when a common bile duct is transected and the

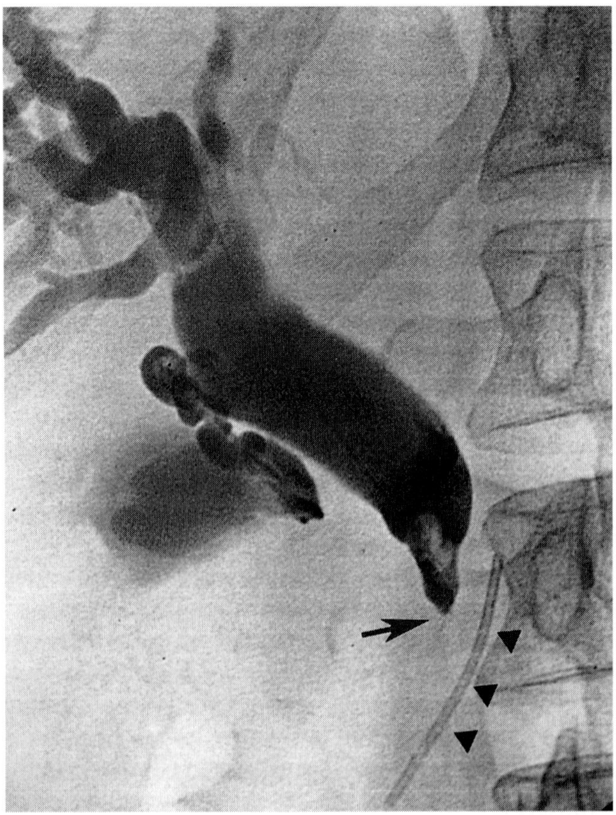

FIGURE 4.15. *Pancreatic carcinoma has caused complete obstruction (arrow) of the distal common bile duct. An occluded endoscopically placed stent (arrowheads) is present.*

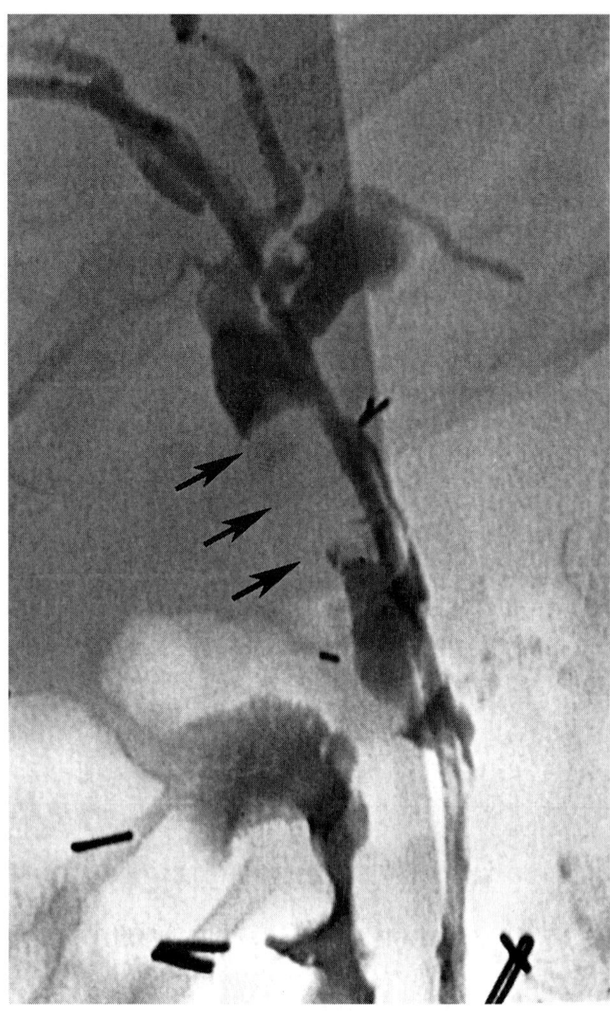

FIGURE 4.16. *Pancreatic carcinoma metastasis to a portal lymph node (arrows) causes obstruction of the common hepatic duct.*

intrahepatic ducts cannot be opacified in a retrograde fashion.

Patients with a bile leak will usually have the biloma drained percutaneously first under CT or sonographic guidance. Successful repair of the bile leak requires careful review of all intraoperative and postoperative cholangiograms and knowledge of normal and variant bile duct anatomy. This is especially important in cases where an aberrant bile duct has been inadvertently divided and no longer communicates with the remainder of the biliary tree (23). Cholangiography of the main biliary tree in such a case may lead the observer to believe that the entire biliary tree is intact.

PTC is difficult in cases of bile duct leak because of the small caliber of the decompressed bile ducts. Successful needle access to the decompressed bile ducts may require many needle passes, increasing the risk of vascular injury. The decompressed bile ducts can more easily be found by injecting the biloma drain with contrast and observing for retrograde flow of contrast into the torn bile duct (see Chapter 6). Once a peripheral branch of the torn bile duct is identified, the duct can be accessed with a needle for subsequent catheterization and diagnostic cholangiography. If this method of duct opacification fails, ultrasound can be used to direct needle passes into the portal region, increasing the chances of successful needle access to a decompressed bile duct (23). The opacified biliary tree must be examined in multiple projections to be certain that all ducts are accounted for. Occluding the torn bile duct with a balloon occlusion catheter during contrast injection prevents rapid egress of contrast into the biloma, allowing maximal duct opacification. The length of intact bile duct above the tear must be demonstrated if biliary enteric reconstruction is planned. Partial tears of large ducts or complete tears of small ducts may respond to biliary diversion techniques, either percutaneous or endoscopic (see Chapter 6).

SUMMARY

Until noninvasive imaging methods improve, iodinated contrast injection into the biliary tree will remain the gold standard for assessing the bile ducts. Although ERCP

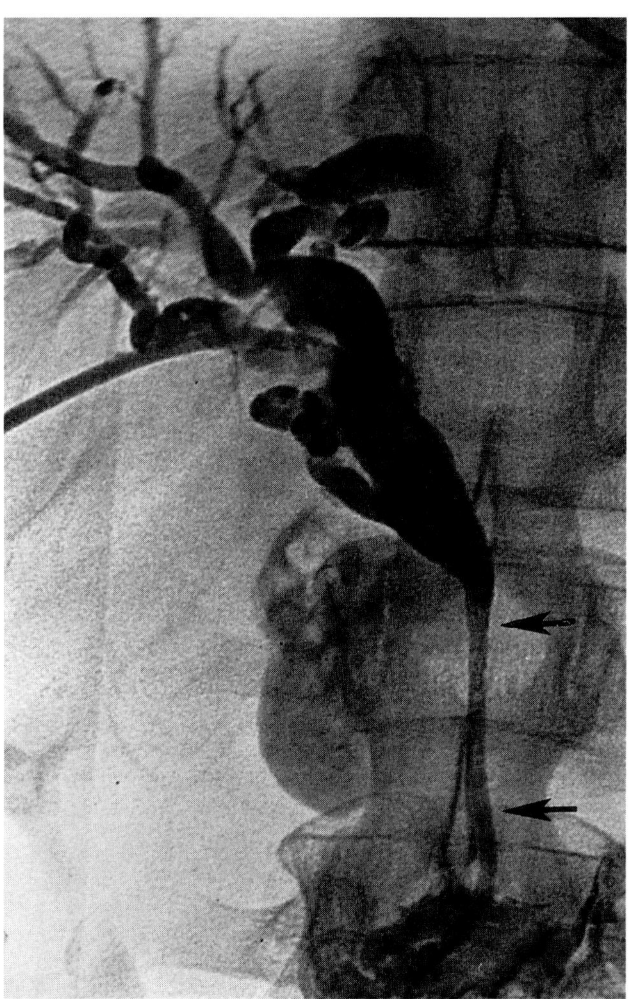

FIGURE 4.17. *Obstruction of the common bile duct (arrows) secondary to pancreatic carcinoma.*

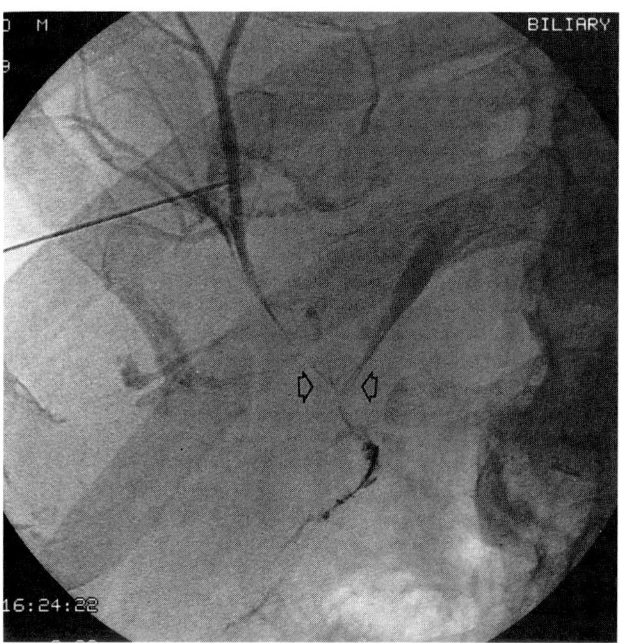

FIGURE 4.18. *Recurrent pancreatic cancer causes stricturing of the biliary bifurcation (arrows) following Roux-en-Y biliary-enteric anastomosis.*

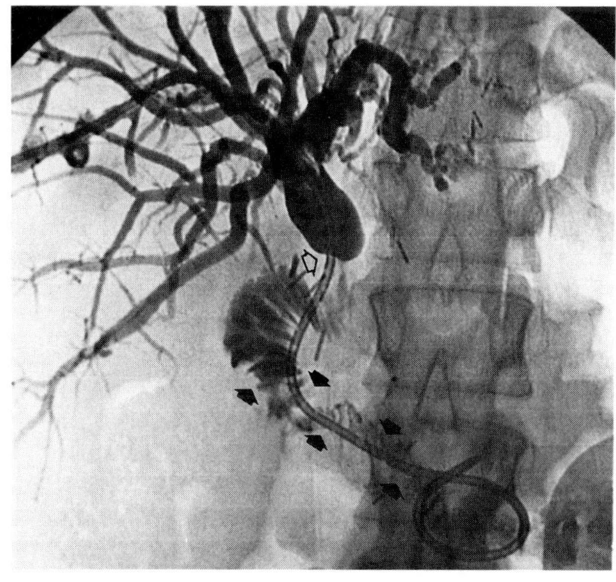

FIGURE 4.19. *Local recurrence of gastric cancer involves the common bile duct and duodenum. There is complete occlusion of the distal common bile duct (open arrow) and duodenum (closed arrows).*

is a safer method for opacifying the bile ducts, there are several situations in which PTC should be used as a primary diagnostic tool. The risks of sepsis and hemorrhage can be minimized by using sound interventional techniques.

SUGGESTED READINGS

Burke DR, Lewis CA, Cardella JF, et al. Quality improvement guidelines for percutaneous transhepatic cholangiography and biliary drainage. Society of Cardiovascular and Interventional Radiology Quality improvement guidelines for image-guided percutaneous biopsy in adults: Society of Cardiovascular & Interventional Radiology Standards of Practice Committee. J Vasc Interv Radiol 1997;8:677–81. This article provides an excellent overview of the indications, success rates and complication rates of PTC and PBD.

Gazelle G, Lee M, Mueller P. Cholangiographic segmental anatomy of the liver. Radiographics 1994;14:1005–13. This article discusses the normal and variant anatomy of the biliary tree essential for interpretation of cholangiograms.

Shlansky-Goldberg R, Weintraub J. Cholangiography. Semin Roentgenol 1997;32:150–60. This article discusses the technique of PTC and the cholangiographic findings in various biliary diseases.

REFERENCES

1. Burke DR, Lewis CA, Cardella JF, Citron SJ, Drooz AT, Haskal ZJ, et al. Quality improvement guidelines for percutaneous transhepatic cholangiography and biliary drainage. Society of Cardiovascular and Interventional Radiology Quality improvement guidelines for image-guided percutaneous biopsy in

adults: Society of Cardiovascular & Interventional Radiology Standards of Practice Committee. J Vasc Interv Radiol 1997;8:677–81.
2. Burckhardt H, Muller W. Versuche uber die punktion der gallenblase und ihre rontgendarstellung. Deutsche Zeitschrift fur Chirurgie 1921;162:168–97.
3. Huard P, Do-Xuan-Hop. La ponction transhepatique des canaux biliaires. Bull Soc med-chir. Indochine 1937;15:1090.
3a. Carter RF, Saypol GM. Transabdominal cholangiography. JAMA 1952;148: 235–238.
4. Arner O, Hagberg S, Seldinger S. Percutaneous transhepatic cholangiography. Surgery 1962;52:561–71.
5. Okuda K, Tanikawa K, Emura T, Kuratomi S, Jinnouchi S, Urabe K, et al. Nonsurgical, percutaneous transhepatic cholangiography—diagnostic significance in medical problems of the liver. Dig Dis 1974;19:21–37.
6. Therasse E, Choiniere M, Soulez G, et al. Percutaneous biliary drainage: clinical trial of analgesia with interpleural block. Radiology 1997;205:663–8.
7. van Sonnenberg E, D'Agostino H, Casola G. Interventional gallbladder procedures. Radiol Clin North Am 1990;28:1185–90.
8. Mergener K, Suhocki P, Enns R, et al. Endoscopic nasobiliary drain placement facilitates subsequent percutaneous transhepatic cholangiography. Gastrointest Endosc 1999;49:240–2.
9. McPherson S, Gibson N, Collier N, et al. Percutaneous transjejunal biliary intervention: 10-year experience with access via Roux-en-Y loops. Radiology 1998;206:665–72.
10. Kadir S. Cholangiography. In: Kadir S, ed. Diagnostic angiography. Philadelphia: W.B. Saunders, 1986:642–78.
11. Gazelle G, Lee M, Mueller P. Cholangiographic segmental anatomy of the liver. Radiographics 1994;14:1005–13.
12. Teplick S, Flick P, Brandon J. Transhepatic cholangiography in patients with suspected biliary disease and nondilated intrahepatic bile ducts. Gastrointest Radiol 1991;16:193–7.
13. MacCarty RL, LaRusso NF, Wiesner RH, Ludwig J. Primary sclerosing cholangitis: findings on cholangiography and pancreatography. Radiology 1983; 149:39–44.
14. MacCarty R, LaRusso N, May G, et al. Cholangiocarcinoma complicating primary sclerosing cholangitis: cholangiographic appearances. Radiology 1985; 156:43–6.
15. Shlansky-Goldberg R, Weintraub J. Cholangiography. Semin Roentgenol 1997; 32:150–60.
16. Pien EH, Zeman RK, Benjamin SB, et al. Iatrogenic sclerosing cholangitis following hepatic arterial chemotherapy infusion. Radiology 1985;156:329–30.
17. Meyers W, Jones R. Choledochal cysts. In: Meyers W, Jones R, eds. Textbook of liver and biliary surgery. Philadelphia: JB Lippincott Company, 1990:312–18.
18. Roston A, Lichtenstein D, Brooks D, Carr-Locke D. Choledocholithiasis. In: Pitt H, Carr-Locke D, Ferrucci J, eds. Hepatobiliary and pancreatic disease. Boston: Little, Brown, 1995:199–210.
19. Clement A, Lowman R. The roentgen features of the Mirizzi syndrome. Am J Roentgenol 1965;94:480–3.
20. Rossi P, Salvatori F, Bezzi M, et al. Percutaneous management of benign biliary strictures with balloon dilation and self-expanding metallic stents. Cardiovasc Intervent Radiol 1990;13:231–9.
21. Petersen BD, Maxfield SR, Ivancev K, et al. Biliary strictures in hepatic transplantation: treatment with self-expanding Z stents. J Vasc Interv Radiol 1996;7:221–8.
22. Neidich R, Soper N, Edmundowicz S, et al. Endoscopic management of bile duct leaks after attempted laparoscopic cholecystectomy. Surg Laparosc Endosc 1996;6:348–54.
23. Suhocki PV, Meyers WC. Injury to aberrant bile ducts during cholecystectomy: a common cause of diagnostic error and treatment delay. Am J Roentgenol 1999;172:955–9.

Section

2

Therapeutic Approaches and Techniques of the Biliary Tree and Gallbladder

Chapter

5

Endoscopic Diagnosis and Treatment of Disorders of the Biliary Tree and Gallbladder

KEVIN MCGRATH JOHN BAILLIE

ENDOSCOPIC RETROGRADE CHOLANGIOPANCREATOGRAPHY AND ENDOSCOPIC ULTRASOUND

Endoscopic retrograde cholangiopancreatography (ERCP) and endoscopic ultrasound (EUS) have become major tools in the investigation and treatment of disease of the biliary tree and gallbladder. ERCP evolved rapidly from a purely diagnostic technique into a therapeutic one with the development of endoscopic sphincterotomy (independently reported by Kawai and Classen in 1974). The development of large channel therapeutic duodenoscopes allowed endoscopists to place endoprostheses of 10 French gauge and larger in the biliary tree starting around 1980. Since that time, diagnostic and therapeutic ERCP have greatly evolved to allow us to treat a wide spectrum of biliary and pancreatic disorders. Such sophistication demands well-trained, experienced endoscopists to ensure that these procedures are applied appropriately and with the least morbidity. As judged by the complication rate, ERCP is the most dangerous procedure routinely performed by endoscopists.

Although ERCP remains the gold standard for investigating the biliary tree and pancreatic ductal system, it is just one of a growing number of imaging modalities available to us. These range from relatively noninvasive, such as abdominal ultrasound, computed tomography (CT), and magnetic resonance cholangiopancreatography (MRCP), to percutaneous transhepatic cholangiography (PTC), which is the most invasive procedure of all.

A rapidly evolving technique of particular interest to endoscopists is endoscopic ultrasound (EUS). Using specially modified endoscopes with ultrasound probes attached to the tip, high-resolution ultrasound images can be obtained of the wall of the bowel as well as adjacent organs and tissues. Using linear array technology, directed fine-needle aspiration (FNA) can be performed using EUS for target guidance. This has greatly increased our ability to target and diagnose lesions in the extrahepatic bile duct and pancreas. The depth of penetration (in millimeters) of the ultrasound image is inversely proportional to the image resolution, with adjustments being possible through changing probe frequencies. Special small ("mini") probes are available for insertion through large endoscope instrument channels to assess otherwise inaccessible areas, such as the inside of esophageal strictures and the biliary tree. The fine needle used for aspiration can also be used to inject local anesthetic and steroid solution (e.g., bupivacaine and triamcinolone) into the celiac nerve plexus to control pancreatic pain, in a procedure called chemolysis (neurolysis). As with ERCP, EUS requires procedure-specific supervised training. Given the need to learn EUS anatomy, there is a long learning curve. At present, there are very limited opportunities in the United States to train in this technique, and the procedure is largely confined to teaching hospitals and large regional centers of excellence.

General Indications for ERCP and EUS

Tables 5.1 and 5.2 outline the diagnostic and therapeutic indications for ERCP and EUS.

Patient Preparation

Informed consent—preferably in writing—should be obtained prior to all endoscopic procedures. The discussion has to be particularly detailed in the case of ERCP, given its complexity and potentially life-threatening complications (e.g., pancreatitis, bleeding, perforation). Similarly, EUS with FNA or chemolysis is an invasive procedure with potential risks that the patient must understand and agree to accept.

Table 5.1. Diagnostic indications (biliary) for ERCP

Choledocholithiasis*
Biliary strictures*
Malignancy of the biliary tree (cholangiocarcinoma) (including brushing)*
Presurgical and postsurgical evaluation of the biliary tree (selected cases)*
Detection of congenital abnormalities (e.g., choledochal cysts)*
Detection of cystic duct and gallbladder pathology*
Evaluation of space-occupying lesions in the liver
Evaluation of unexplained liver function test abnormalities
Manometry of the sphincter of Oddi

* Also an indication for EUS.

Table 5.2. Therapeutic indications (biliary) for ERCP

Choledocholithiasis
Extraction of cystic duct and (rarely) gallbladder stones
Dilation and stenting of benign and malignant strictures
Stenting of ampullary tumors
Decompression in sphincter of Oddi dysfunction/papillary stenosis
Removal of intra-biliary foreign bodies (e.g., parasites)
Treatment of bile leaks

There is a great deal of variation in the quoted morbidity and mortality of ERCP. Many of these data are based on old surveys and require updating in light of improved technology and procedural skills. The morbidity of ERCP is generally quoted to be in the range of 3% to 10%, with mortality ranging from 0.1% to 1.0% (1–3). A recent prospective study of complications of biliary sphincterotomy at the time of ERCP found an overall complication rate of 9.8% with a procedure related mortality of 0.4% (4). Particular risk factors for complications included suspected sphincter of Oddi dysfunction, the presence of liver cirrhosis, and performance of so-called precut papillotomy.

As patients are almost always sedated for ERCP and EUS, particular attention has to be paid to prior or existing medical problems that may affect the type of sedation given. Those patients who have previously exhibited intolerance of conscious sedation require general anesthesia. Most children tolerate ERCP and EUS better with general anesthesia of short duration than they do when intravenous sedatives are given.

Antibiotic Coverage

There are no data to support the routine use of prophylactic antibiotics in patients undergoing ERCP. Although the data supporting antibiotic prophylaxis against cholangitis in patients with known biliary obstruction, suspected choledocholithiasis, biliary leaks, and so on are scant, most endoscopists give antibiotics in these situations. The antibiotic(s) used must penetrate bile well. At Duke University Medical Center, we used to use a combination of ampicillin and gentamicin, substituting vancomycin in penicillin-sensitive patients. This prophylaxis is not suitable for patients with renal impairment, and is quite expensive. These days we tend to substitute Unasyn or a broad-spectrum cephalosporin. If a complication such as a contained or free perforation of the biliary tree is suspected during or after ERCP or EUS with FNA, antibiotic coverage should be broadened to include an agent active against anaerobic bacteria (e.g., metronidazole).

The effect of antibiotics depends on tissue concentration; simply injecting antibiotics into the biliary tree has no useful effect against the organisms that cause cholangitis. Although most endoscopists are using parenteral antibiotics, there are data to suggest that oral ciprofloxacin may be equally effective (5). We recommend collection of bile for culture and sensitivity determination when sepsis is suspected or known to be present (e.g., from positive blood cultures).

Contrast Allergy

It has been the practice of endoscopists for many years to administer antihistamines and steroids as prophylaxis against contrast allergy in patients undergoing ERCP. This is controversial: there are scant data supporting this practice (6). Although the routine use of low osmolality, nonionic contrast media has been advocated, there are insufficient data to support this approach. Nonionic contrast media are expensive and therefore should be reserved for patients with a documented history of major allergic reactions to iodinated contrast agents. Even then it is not clear that severe contrast reactions can be prevented by steroid prophylaxis. In our unit, we give three doses of prednisone 20 mg at 6 P.M., midnight, and 6 A.M. the night before/the morning of the procedure.

Difficult Anatomy

In experienced hands, cannulation of the bile duct and pancreatic duct can be achieved in the vast majority of ERCP cases attempted. An expert endoscopist will usually have a biliary cannulation success rate exceeding 90%. However, the endoscopic approach to the biliary tree (and pancreas) can be rendered difficult or impossible by surgical rearrangement (e.g., Billroth-II gastrectomy reconstruction) or strictures (e.g., post-bulbar in the duodenum) (Fig. 5.1). Similarly, EUS can be rendered difficult or impossible by anatomic problems. Perforations related to EUS are very rare, but those that have been reported are typically in the setting of "blind dilation" of an esophageal stricture.

THE NORMAL CHOLANGIOGRAM

Injection of radiographic contrast medium into the biliary tree through the main papilla (Fig. 5.2) provides excellent

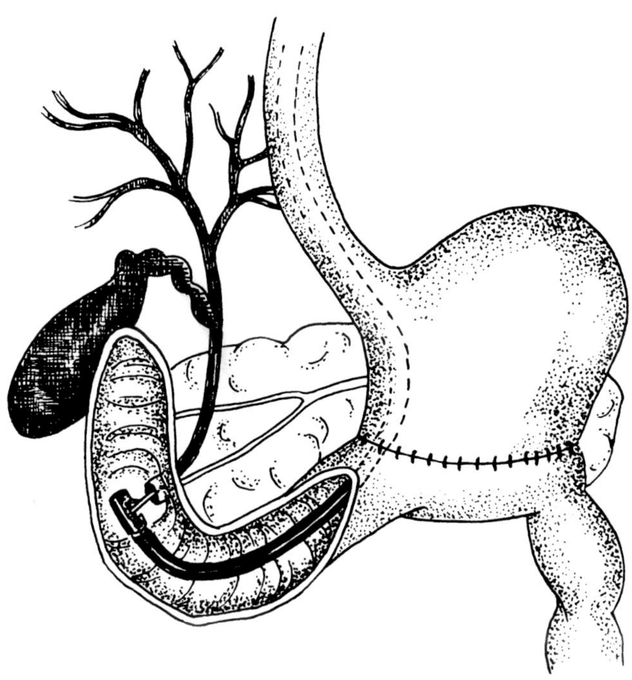

FIGURE 5.1. *Post-Billroth II gastrectomy surgical anatomy, with retrograde access to the duodenal papilla for ERCP.*

anatomic detail. In the majority of cases, the following structures can be identified: the common bile duct (CBD), the common hepatic duct, the cystic duct leading to the gallbladder, the gallbladder itself, the liver hilum with right and left main intrahepatic ducts, and secondary and tertiary ducts leading from these. Due to the patient's prone position during ERCP, the left intrahepatic ducts are usually filled preferentially and good visualization of the right system may require repositioning or the use of an occlusion (balloon) technique. Care must be taken not to "overinterpret" gallbladder findings when the gallbladder is opacified during ERCP; it is easy to miss small stones or polyps, especially when using dense contrast.

When assessing the biliary anatomy, endoscopists need to be aware of variability, including high and low "take off" of the cystic duct from the extrahepatic biliary tree. The upper limit of normal diameter for the CBD (measured by convention in the mid-duct) is 7 mm. However, it is not uncommon for elderly patients to have gross dilatation of the bile duct without clear pathology. Release of bile into the duodenum is not continuous but regulated by the activity of the sphincter of Oddi, a ring of smooth muscle at the level of the ampulla of Vater. So dysfunction may be associated with a syndrome of recurrent biliary pain with or without abnormal liver function tests and/or dilatation of the bile duct. In most individuals, the CBD is joined by the main pancreatic duct at the ampulla, where they share a final common channel into the duodenum. In patients with pancreas divisum, however, the main (dorsal) pancreatic duct empties into the duodenum through the minor duodenal papilla.

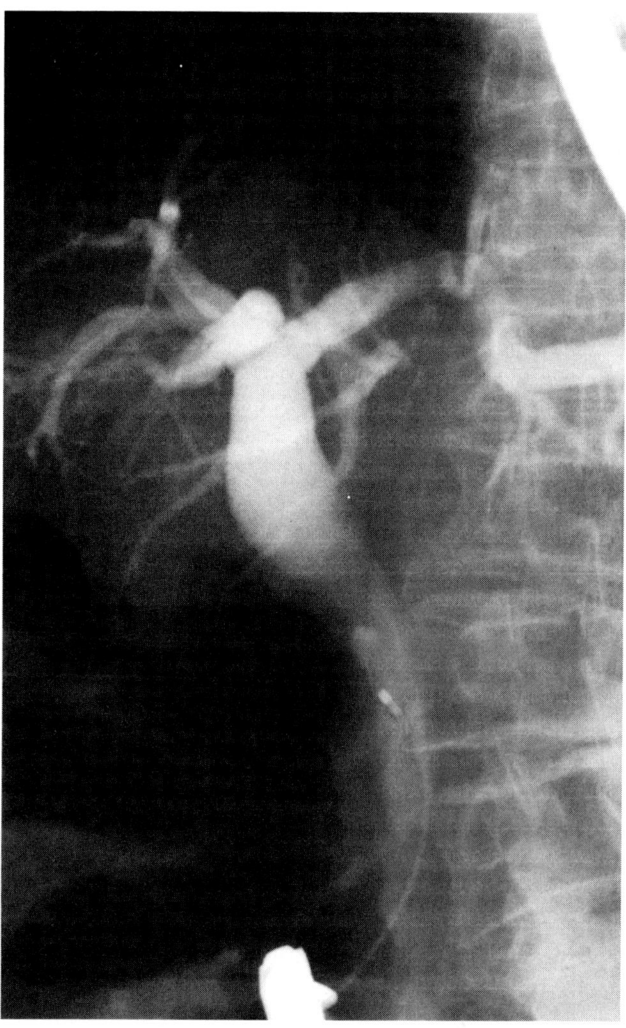

FIGURE 5.2. *Cholangiography (at ERCP) in a patient with post-Billroth II anatomy.*

CHOLELITHIASIS

Large stones and a gallbladder packed with small stones may be identified easily when that organ fills with contrast during ERCP. However, as previously noted, ERCP is not a particularly sensitive way to detect cholelithiasis. As we shall discuss, EUS is proving to be a much more sensitive tool in the hunt for gallbladder stones and other disorders. The management of stones in the biliary tree has been one of the success stories of ERCP. Approximately 20 million Americans have gallstones and around a half million cholecystectomies are performed annually in the United States. Symptoms relating to gallstones are a common cause of hospital admission, with estimated direct health costs exceeding $2 billion annually.

There are two basic types of gallstone: cholesterol stones and pigment stones (the latter divided between black stones and brown pigment stones). Cholesterol gallstones account for 75% to 80% of gallstones in the United States. They are most commonly found in middle-aged females, overweight individuals, and patients with ileal disease or following small bowel resection. Pigment stones are composed principally of calcium bilirubinate, phosphate, and carbonate salts. They are associated with chronic bacterial or parasitic infections (brown stones) or chronic hemolysis (black pigment stones). Gallstones usually form within the gallbladder. The majority of individuals with gallstones are asymptomatic. However, acute cholecystitis can develop when a stone lodges in the neck of the gallbladder or in the cystic duct. Patients who have had a prior episode of biliary colic have a 60% to 70% chance of developing recurrent gallstone-related problems. Removal of the gallbladder (these days, typically by the laparoscopic route) is now recommended for this group of patients.

Transabdominal ultrasound reportedly has a sensitivity of over 95% for diagnosing gallbladder stones (7). Given the high prevalence of disease and the excellent sensitivity of conventional ultrasound, it is unlikely that EUS will ever play a major role in diagnosing cholelithiasis. However, the number of symptomatic patients with normal transabdominal ultrasound exams is still significant. The major question is whether their symptoms are really biliary in origin and, if so, are they related to "microlithiasis" not detected by standard ultrasound.

EUS findings of cholelithiasis are based on at least one of three criteria:

1. Stones greater than 2 mm with associated acoustic shadowing (Fig. 5.3).
2. Sludge, defined as mobile, low amplitude echoes that layer in the most dependent part of the gallbladder lumen without acoustic shadowing.
3. "Microlithiasis" (or "minilithiasis"), defined as mobile, 1 to 2 mm hyperechoic foci without acoustic shadowing.

It has been suggested that cholesterol or bilirubinate crystal detection in bile aspirates may be helpful in identifying patients with cholelithiasis who have negative ultrasound findings. However, the sensitivity of bile microscopic examination is approximately 70% (7,8). There is a very small body of literature that suggests the combination of EUS and stimulated drainage of bile is accurate in predicting the presence of sludge and/or microlithiasis (9,10). The finding of biliary sludge or microlithiasis is more sensitive than microscopic bile examination in the detection of cholelithiasis. Additionally, EUS is more sensitive than abdominal ultrasound for detecting sludge and small stones. These small studies further demonstrate symptom relief or resolution after cholecystectomy in patients with positive tests. However, flawed scientific design and methodology makes it difficult to draw solid conclusions (11).

Currently, there are three clinical situations in which EUS is recommended for diagnosing cholelithiasis. The first scenario is idiopathic acute pancreatitis with negative TUS examinations. Amouyal et al. (12) studied 44 nonalcoholic patients with idiopathic acute pancreatitis. In 29 patients, biliary lithiasis was confirmed by surgery, ERCP, or microscopic examination. In 28 of these 29 patients, EUS demonstrated the presence of minilithiasis (microlithiasis) in the gallbladder. The second indication for EUS involved the evaluation of obese subjects with biliary colic and a nega-

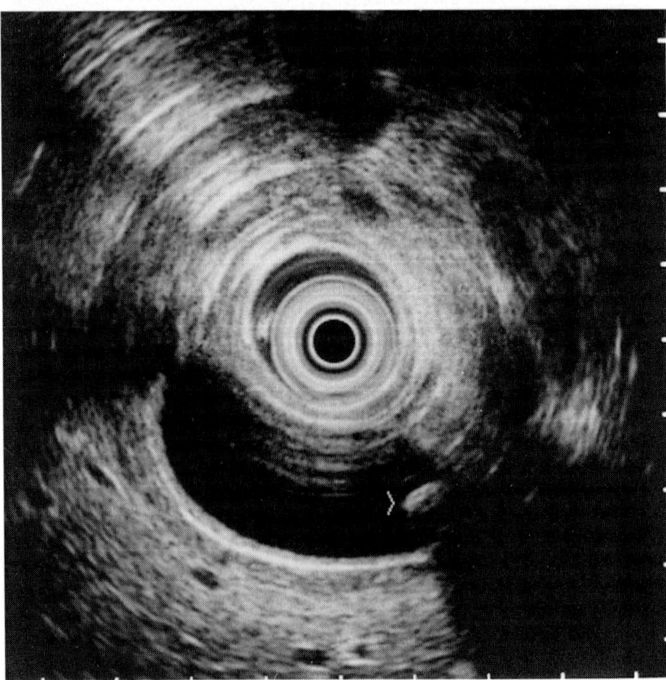

FIGURE 5.3. *Cholelithiasis: Hyperechoic focus with post-acoustic shadowing within the gallbladder consistent with cholelithiasis, as imaged by EUS.*

tive transabdominal ultrasound exam. The sensitivity of conventional transabdominal ultrasound is low in this population. Pieken et al. (13) reported their experience in which EUS revealed cholelithiasis in three obese subjects who had negative ultrasound examinations. The third clinical situation concerns patients with successive negative ultrasound examinations who have typical biliary colic or cholangitis. The sensitivity and specificity of EUS in the diagnosis of "minilithiasis" not detected by conventional ultrasound were 96% and 86%, respectively, in Amouyal's study (12).

In certain patients a guidewire can be advanced through the cystic duct into the gallbladder at ERCP. This can be used to place a nasocystic drain. There have also been reports of removing gallstones through the cystic duct after balloon dilation. These procedures are technical tours de force; in everyday ERCP practice, however, there is hardly ever an indication to perform such procedures.

CHOLEDOCHOLITHIASIS

EUS

Bile duct stones (choledocholithiasis) complicate gallstone disease in up to 20% of patients (14). These stones can cause cholangitis and pancreatitis. ERCP and intraoperative cholangiography (IOC) are considered to be the gold standards in the diagnosis of choledocholithiasis. However, the accuracy of that diagnosis is dependent on the operator's expertise. Technical problems—such as air bubbles injected into the biliary tree—may cause erroneous diagnosis of choledocholithiasis, and small stones can be missed. The sensitivity of ERCP for diagnosing choledocholithiasis is reported to be in the range of 79% to 95%, with specificity in the range of 92% to 98%. Overall, the accuracy of ERCP for diagnosing bile duct stones may be as high as 97% (15,16). The incidence of pancreatitis and cholangitis associated with diagnostic ERCP (i.e., without sphincterotomy) is 3% to 6% (17,18). If sphincterotomy is performed, the complication rate increases to 9.8% (4). Liver function test abnormalities correlate poorly with the actual presence of a common bile duct stone, although nomograms are available that can predict the presence or absence of choledocholithiasis based on the nature of the liver function tests and bile duct diameter (19).

Transabdomial ultrasound is the least expensive and invasive imaging test available to look for choledocholithiasis, and should therefore be performed first. Despite a high specificity (95%), the sensitivity of ultrasound is low, ranging from 20% to 80% in the literature (20–26). The presence of small stones or a nondilated bile duct lowers the sensitivity of ultrasound. In addition, most calculi settle in the intrapancreatic portion of the distal CBD, a location that is particularly troublesome to image using transabdominal ultrasound. CT also has limitations in the diagnosis of choledocholithiasis, especially when the diameter of the stones is less than the thickness of the CT "slices." Although the specificity of CT for detecting choledocholithiasis is over 95%, the sensitivity is poor, ranging from 23% to 85% (20–25,27). The combined overall accuracy rate of identifying choledocholithiasis is only 71% (15).

Recently, EUS has emerged as a highly accurate way to evaluate the extrahepatic bile duct. The distal intrapancreatic CBD can be visualized reproducibly from the second portion of the duodenum, whereas the proximal CBD and the common hepatic duct are viewed from the duodenal bulb. The CBD can be completely inspected in 96% to 100% of cases (25,26,28). However, anatomic limitations such as post-Billroth II gastrectomy reconstruction and significant stenoses may preclude the use of EUS to examine the extrahepatic bile duct. The sensitivity and specificity of EUS in the diagnosis of choledocholithiasis are said to be 88% to 96% and 96% to 100%, respectively (Fig. 5.4). Unlike transabdominal ultrasound and CT, EUS is able to detect calculi regardless of stone size or bile duct diameter (25). This has been confirmed in numerous studies, where the diagnostic accuracy of EUS for choledocholithiasis was approximately 95% (15,29–32). In direct comparison, EUS was more sensitive (96%) and specific (100%) than ultrasound (63% and 95%) and CT (71% and 97%), respectively. EUS compares favorably with ERCP in detecting choledocholithiasis, without statistical difference in sensitivity and specificity. The overall accuracy is also similar: 94% for EUS and 97% for ERCP (15,16).

Magnetic resonance cholangiopancreatography (MRCP) has recently shown promise in the diagnosis of pancreatic and biliary disorders. Its sensitivity ranges from 71% to 100% (33). In a rare comparative study, the overall accuracy of EUS versus MRCP for the diagnosis of choledocholithiasis was 97% versus 82%, respectively (34). However, there is concern that MRCP has difficulty detecting small stones in a thin bile duct; one study revealed a sensitivity of only 40% in this particular subgroup (35). We expect that the sensitivity of MRCP for detecting small bile duct stones will increase with operator experience and technologic development. At present, many are limiting their use of MRCP to those patients in whom conscious sedation is contraindicated, or those with altered or distorted anatomy that would preclude successful ERCP or EUS evaluation.

What is the role of EUS in identifying choledocholithiasis? It is as accurate as ERCP with a high negative predictive value, which means that ERCP will be unnecessary if stones cannot be seen at EUS. The impressive safety profile of EUS (complication rate of less than 1 : 2000) and an extremely low failure rate compare favorably with ERCP, with its 5% to 10% morbidity and significant failure rate in inexperienced hands (36,37). There is increasing interest in "risk stratification" when deciding on preoperative investigation of gallstone patients (Fig. 5.5).

Transabdominal ultrasound should be the first line study, given its low cost, relative safety, and high specificity. In patients with predicted high risk of having choledocholithiasis, preoperative ERCP is appropriate for stone

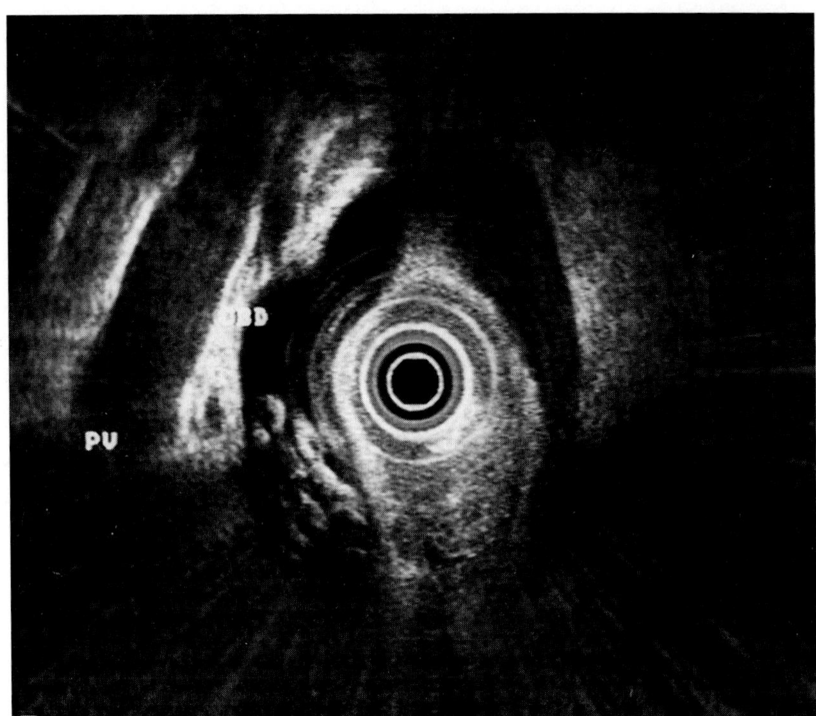

FIGURE 5.4. *Choledocholithiasis: Multiple hyperechoic foci with post-acoustic shadowing seen within the distal common bile duct (CBD = common bile duct; PV = portal vein).*

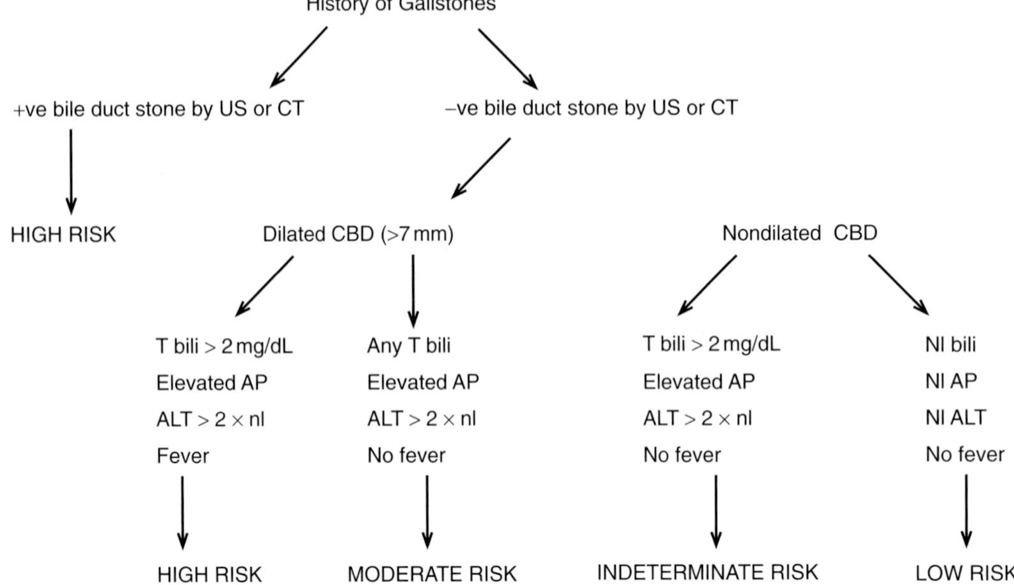

FIGURE 5.5. *Determination of risk groups for choledocholithiasis (US = ultrasound; CT = computed tomography; CBD = common bile duct; T bili = total [serum] bilirubin; AP = alkaline phosphatase; ALT = alanine aminotransferase). (Modified from Canto et al. EUS vs ERCP for diagnosis of choledocholithiasis. Gastrointest Endosc 1998;47:38–447.)*

identification and recovery. In patients whose risk of choledocholithiasis is considered moderate, indeterminate, or low, it is more cost-effective to employ preoperative EUS, with ERCP being reserved for those positively identified with stones. Low risk patients are expected to have choledocholithiasis in 2% to 3% of cases; therefore, it is acceptable to proceed to surgery without a preoperative study and manage the patient expectantly afterward (38). EUS may be the test of choice to evaluate pregnant women and patients with contrast allergy for choledocholithiasis, as EUS avoids exposure to ionizing radiation and contrast media.

ERCP

Most CBD stones form within the gallbladder and migrate into the bile duct. However, de novo formation of stones within the biliary tree can occur both before and after cholecystectomy. Patients with periampullary diverticula are at increased risk of developing CBD stones (Fig. 5.6). Possibly this is due to sphincter of Oddi dysfunction caused by the presence of the diverticulum, bacterial overgrowth within the diverticulum (encouraging colonization of the adjacent bile duct), or a combination of both. In countries where biliary parasites (e.g., *Fasciola, Ascaris, Clonorchis*) are common, the eggs and dead organisms form a nidus for stone formation. As previously stated, chronic hemolysis predisposes to biliary pigment stone formation.

Bile duct stones predispose to infection (cholangitis), obstruction (jaundice with or without cholangitis), and gallstone (biliary) pancreatitis. Acute cholangitis is a medical emergency, which has a high mortality rate when untreated (39). The classic Charcot's triad is comprised of pain, jaundice, and fever. When hypotension and confusion are added (evidence of systemic infection), this becomes the pentad of Reynolds.

One of the most important roles of the ERCP endoscopist is to relieve biliary obstruction caused by stones (choledocholithiasis). If the stone(s) cannot be removed, effective biliary drainage must be established by endoscopic, radiologic, or, if necessary, surgical means. As any ERCP may lead to a therapeutic procedure, ERCP endoscopists must be trained and skilled in techniques for biliary decompression.

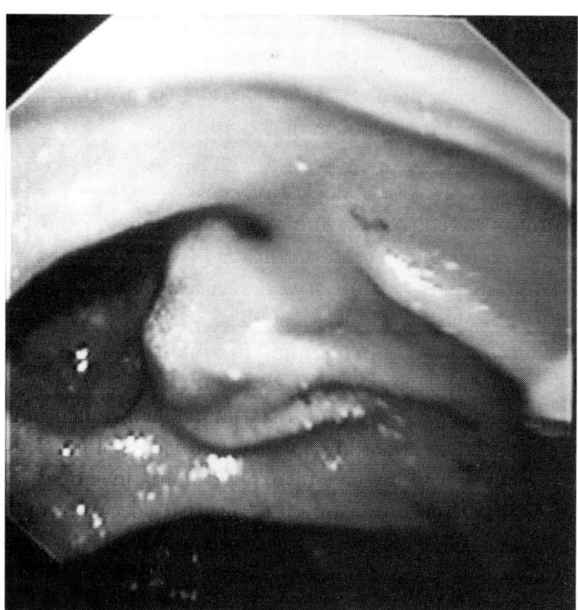

FIGURE 5.6. *Periampullary diverticulum. These predispose the patient to choledocholithiasis and can make ERCP quite difficult by altering the position of the duodenal papilla relative to the duodenoscope.*

Sphincterotomy

Endoscopic sphincterotomy (ES) revolutionized the management of CBD stones. Prior to the introduction of ES in 1974, CBD stones had to be removed surgically by an open procedure that carried a not inconsiderable morbidity. The current endoscopic approach to CBD stones is successful in at least 90% of cases in skilled hands, with morbidity and mortality rates that compared favorably with surgery in similarly expert hands. ES can be performed with a mortality less than 0.5% and a procedure-related morbidity less than 10% (4).

ES is the most invasive procedure routinely performed by gastrointestinal endoscopists. A sphincterotome is a modified cannula with an exposed wire at the distal end through which electric current is transmitted. The sphincterotome is inserted into the bile duct and short bursts of current are applied to incise the roof of the ampulla (including the sphincter of Oddi). A variety of less controlled techniques—described as "precut papillotomy"—have been developed to access the biliary tree in cases of anatomic difficulty (Fig. 5.7). Precut techniques carry significant morbidity and should only be used by experts for therapeutic access to the biliary tree.

In Freeman et al.'s study (4), 9.8% of patients undergoing ES had complications, including pancreatitis (5.4%), bleeding (2%), cholangitis (1%), and perforation (<0.5%). The incidence of late complications of biliary sphincterotomy in studies with extended follow-up (5 to 10+ years) ranges from 10% to 24% (40). These late complications include stenosis of the sphincterotomy site, recurrent choledocholithiasis, and cholangitis. This rate of complications compares favorably with the results of surgical exploration and drainage of the CBD. Most of the late complications of ERCP can be managed by endoscopic therapy.

Stone Extraction after Sphincterotomy

Following successful ES, removal of CBD stones can be achieved in 80% to 95% of patients. Although small stones may pass spontaneously after sphincterotomy, it is unwise to rely on this occurring. A variety of endoscopic balloons and basket catheters are available to retrieve stones. Forceful extraction against resistance should be avoided, as this risks traumatic extension of the sphincterotomy incision. Occasionally, a stone will be trapped in a basket in the bile duct such that it cannot be removed or disengaged. In the past, this was a very serious problem that sometimes required surgery to resolve. Nowadays we have an over-the-catheter lithotripsy system that uses a cranking device to pull the wires of the basket against and into a metal over-

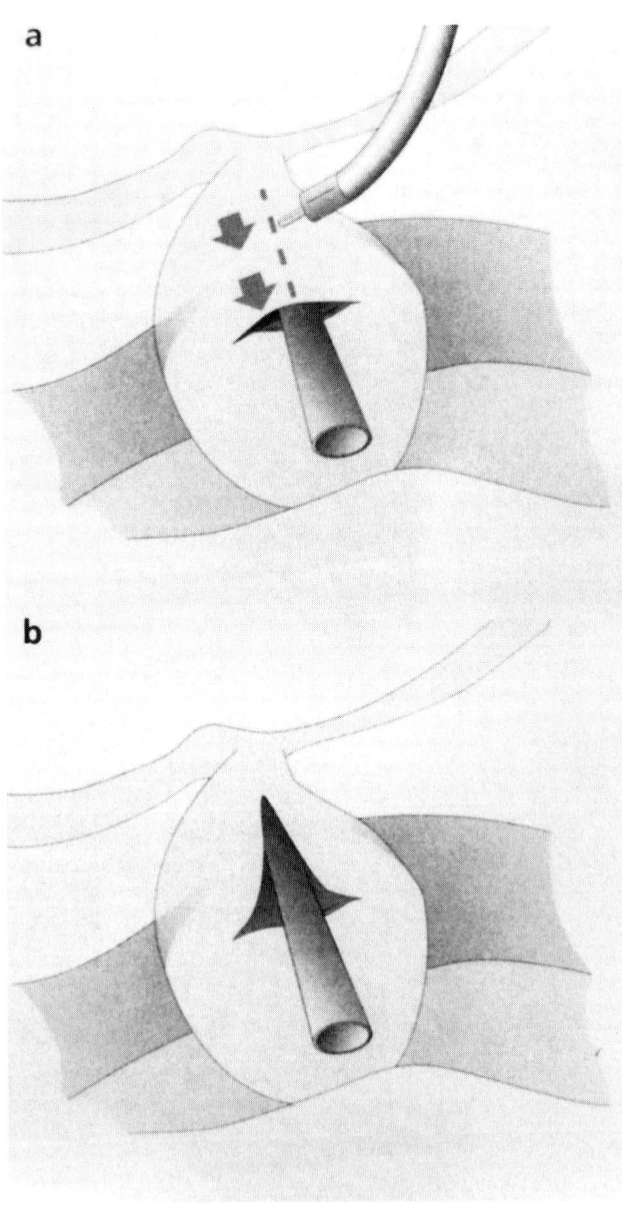

FIGURE 5.7. *Precut papillotomy over a stent.* ***(a)*** *Using a needle knife papillotome, the bile duct is deroofed over a prepositioned endoprosthesis (stent). This is a useful technique when there are technical difficulties in achieving a standard biliary sphincterotomy.* ***(b)*** *When opening has been created, the stent is removed.*

sleeve. Either the stone or the basket breaks, resolving the problem.

Stone Extraction through the Intact Papilla

Although sphincterotomy is frequently used to enlarge the opening to the CBD for stone extraction, it has been demonstrated that small stones can be removed safely through the intact papilla using balloon or basket catheters. This avoids the immediate and late complications of sphincterotomy, which are particularly likely in the presence of a nondilated bile duct. It is desirable to preserve the biliary sphincter, especially in young patients. MacMathuna et al. (41) demonstrated the use of balloon dilation to allow large stones (up to and exceeding 20mm) to be removed from the CBD without sphincterotomy. They dubbed this procedure "balloon sphincteroplasty." Stone extraction without sphincterotomy can cause significant edema of the papilla and make it difficult to remove all the stone fragments and debris. When the papilla is already swollen, as in gallstone pancreatitis with an obstructing calculus, ES may be necessary to improve biliary drainage, so balloon dilation has its limitations. A multicenter prospective, randomized trial of ES versus balloon sphincteroplasty [X] revealed a three times higher incidence of pancreatitis in the balloon group, and two of the patients in the balloon group died of severe pancreatitis complicating the procedure. This sobering study has greatly reduced enthusiasm for balloon sphincteroplasty as a first-line technique for stone recovery (DiSario, personal communication).

Difficult Bile Duct Stones

CBD stones that exceed 15mm in diameter present difficulties for retrieval as they will not easily pass through a standard sphincterotomy site. Smaller stones may present difficulty when they are located proximal to a bile duct stricture or in a tortuous, dilated bile duct (where they may be difficult to capture in a basket). Intrahepatic stones present particular difficulty, due to their inaccessibility. A variety of techniques are available to facilitate the removal of biliary stones, including mechanical lithotripsy (42), contact lithotripsy (electrohydraulic [43], laser [44]), extracorporeal shockwave lithotripsy (45), and chemical dissolution. By using one or more of these techniques, almost all biliary calculi can be removed.

Mechanical Lithotripsy

Mechanical lithotriptors consist of a reinforced basket with a mechanical cranking device (Fig. 5.8). After the stone is captured within the wires of the basket, the proximal end of the cable is attached to a crank. This is tightened to close the basket wires around the stone, breaking it by mechanical forces. Modern mechanical lithotriptors are highly effective, with success rates of 75% to 100% being reported (46).

Electrohydraulic Lithotripsy

Electrohydraulic lithotripsy (EHL) has been employed for many years by urologists, who use it to fragment stones in the urinary bladder, renal pelvis, and ureters. This technology has been adapted for use through percutaneous tracks into the liver and retrogradely into the bile duct through a choledochoscope. In EHL, rapid conversion of a liquid into its gaseous form results in sudden volume expansion, creating a shock wave that fractures the stone. Once suitably small fragments have been created (this is usually a rapid process), conventional stone retrieval techniques are used to

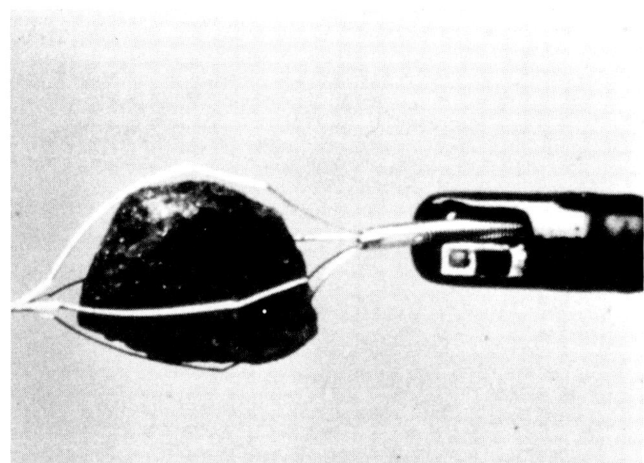

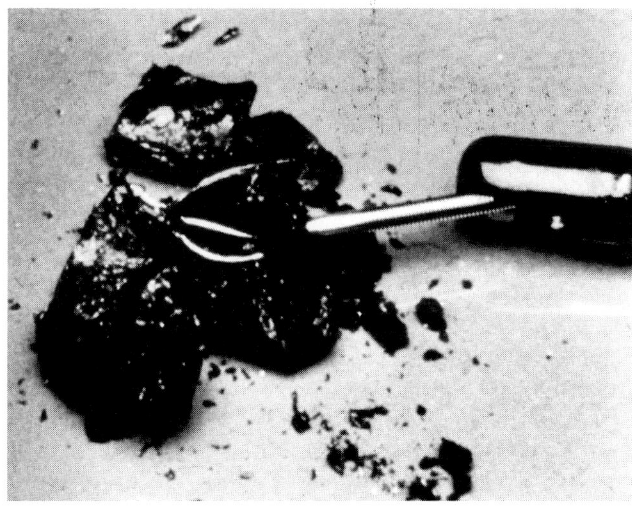

FIGURE 5.8. *Mechanical lithotripsy (crushing basket) for bile duct stones. The stones are crushed by the wires of a specially hardened basket catheter.*

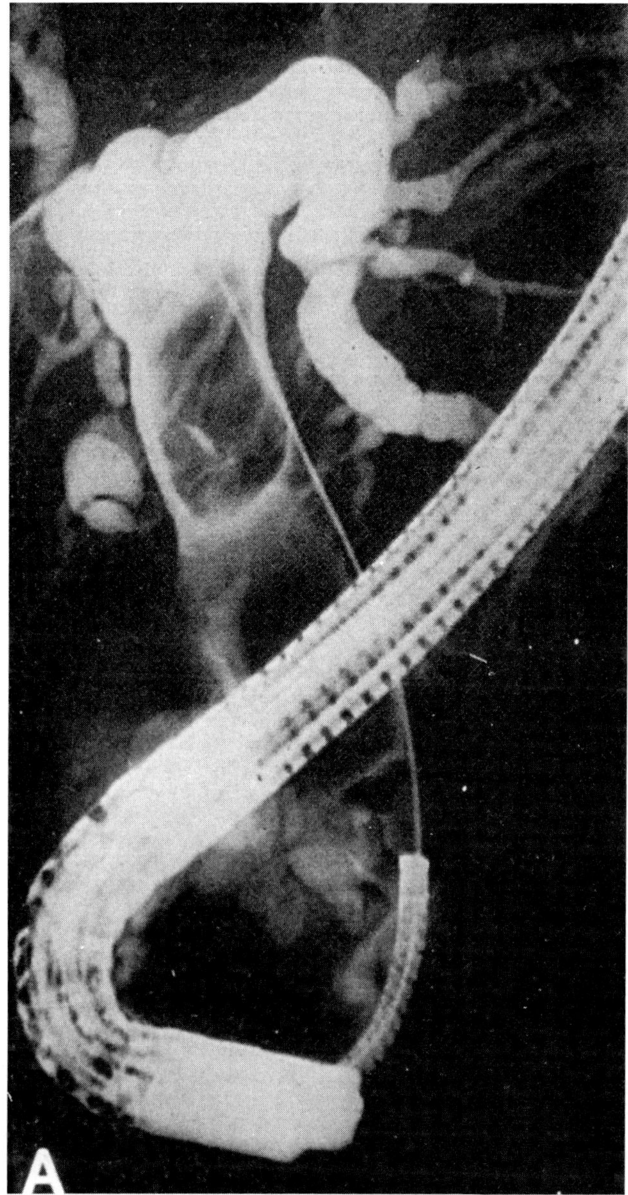

FIGURE 5.9. *Laser lithotripsy for bile duct stones. The laser "light guide" is advanced into bile duct using a thin caliber choledochoscope advanced through a large channel duodenoscope.*

complete duct clearance. Overall, EHL is safe and effective, with success rates reported to be around 80%. However, equipment costs and the need for a second, well-trained endoscopist to handle the choledochoscope limit this technique to a small number of specialist centers.

Laser Lithotripsy

Laser energy can be used to fragment bile duct stones in a mechanism similar to that of EHL (i.e., the creation of a shock wave from a burst of energy at the stone surface). A pulsed laser that emits discrete bursts of energy, usually at a frequency of around 10 Hz, is required. For this, a tunable dye laser is ideal. The laser light guide (fiber) is brought in contact with the stone after passing through the instrument channel of a choledochoscope (Fig. 5.9). To reduce the risk of collateral damage to the bile duct wall, so-called smart lasers have been developed, incorporating automated stone detection (i.e., they will not fire unless in contact with a stone).

Although laser lithotripsy of bile duct stones can be very effective, it is also very expensive. The equipment is costly, delicate, and requires frequent maintenance. As with EHL, several operators are needed. For these reasons, laser lithotripsy is not widely available.

Extracorporeal Shockwave Lithotripsy

Extracorporeal shockwave lithotripsy (ESWL) of CBD stones is another adaptation of technology first developed by urologists. ESWL was pioneered in Europe for the treatment of gallbladder stones. However, it is also useful for managing difficult bile duct stones, especially when contact methods of fragmentation are unavailable or have failed. ESWL procedures for CBD stones are usually carried out under fluoroscopy, with contrast being injected through a nasobiliary drain placed at the time of ERCP (Fig. 5.10) or percutaneous catheter. Some ESWL machines use ultrasound rather than fluoroscopy for targeting.

Although ESWL is no longer in widespread use for the treatment of gallbladder stones (having been superseded by laparoscopic cholecystectomy), many centers still have ESWL available for urologic use. The gastroenterologist can usually borrow time on the ESWL machine to treat the occasional patient with difficult biliary calculi.

Chemical Dissolution

Dissolving bile duct stones by infusing chemical agents through a nasobiliary drain or percutaneous catheter is an attractive concept, but in practice the results have been disappointing. The earliest dissolution agent used was mono-octanoin, a fatty acid derivative, which was infused over a 5 to 8 day period (47). The dissolution rates for pure cholesterol stones were in the range of 40% to 60%, but the treatment often had to be discontinued due to patient intolerance of the agent (e.g., nausea, abdominal cramps, diarrhea) or the nasobiliary tube.

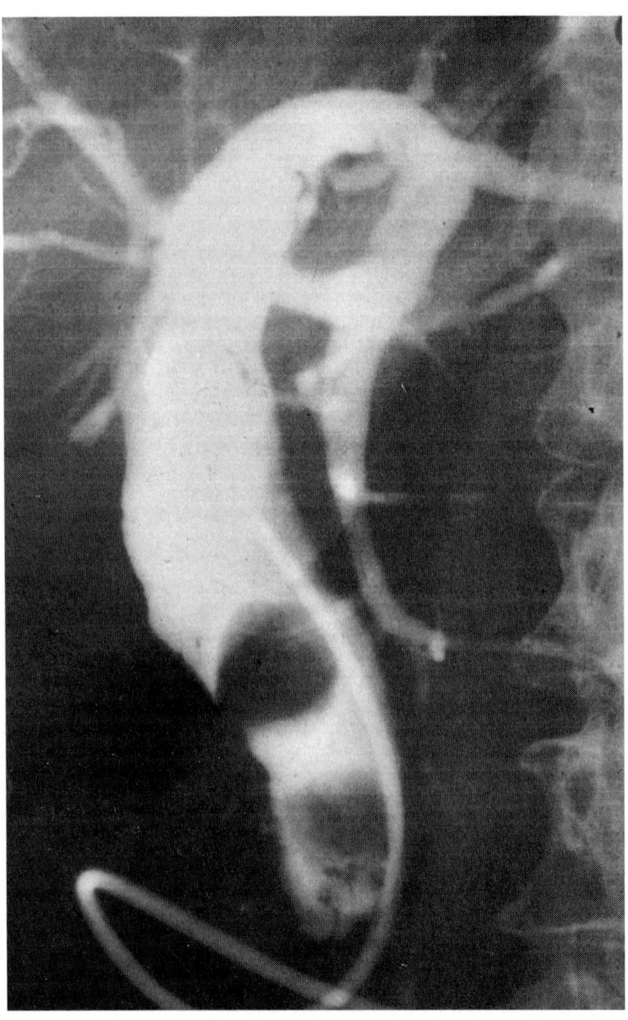

FIGURE 5.10. *Nasobiliary cholangiogram. Using an endoscopically placed nasobiliary tube, contrast injection reveals several large filling defects (stones) in the common bile duct.*

Mono-octanoin is not suitable for mixed stones, which comprise a significant proportion of CBD stones. When methyltert-butyl ether (MTBE) was being evaluated for treating cholesterol stones in the gallbladder, there was interest in modifying this to deal with CBD stones. Unfortunately, it proved impossible to reliably contain this volatile and toxic agent within the bile duct. MTBE leaking from the bile duct into the duodenum can cause a severe duodenitis; if enough ether is absorbed, it causes profound sedation and a variety of unpleasant systemic effects (e.g., hemolysis). For this reason, MTBE is not being used in the biliary tree to dissolve stones.

The search continues for an agent that will reliably disaggregate mixed bile duct stones but none has been identified so far.

Stents for Stones

When endoscopic techniques fail to completely clear the bile duct of stones, good biliary drainage must be established before finishing the procedure. An endoscopic prosthesis (stent) should be placed in the bile duct to prevent biliary obstruction and its sequel, cholangitis (Fig. 5.11). Thereafter, the patient may be brought back for a further procedure when local edema or bleeding has settled, or referred to an expert in another hospital. Ursodeoxycholic acid therapy may be a useful adjunctive treatment. As many elderly, frail patients are poor candidates for repeated endoscopy, biliary stents have been used for the long-term management of some bile duct stones. On the whole, this is a successful strategy; however, a recent large prospective study from Amsterdam suggests that long-term stenting is not without risk (e.g., cholangitis) (48).

ERCP in Relation to Laparoscopic Cholecystectomy

Laparoscopic cholecystectomy is now widely available as the first-line treatment for symptomatic choledocholithiasis. This has affected the practice of biliary endoscopists in a number of ways. When laparoscopic cholecyslectory was first introduced, endoscopists saw many patients with iatrogenic bile duct injuries and cystic duct leaks. This early rush of complications reflected the learning curve of surgeons performing this laparoscopic procedure. Although laparoscopic cholecyslectory-related biliary problems have greatly diminished, endoscopists still see them from time to time.

Common Bile Duct Stones It has been necessary to develop an algorithm for the management of suspected or proven bile duct stones in patients undergoing laparoscopic cholecyslectory (Fig. 5.12). There are ample data in the sur-

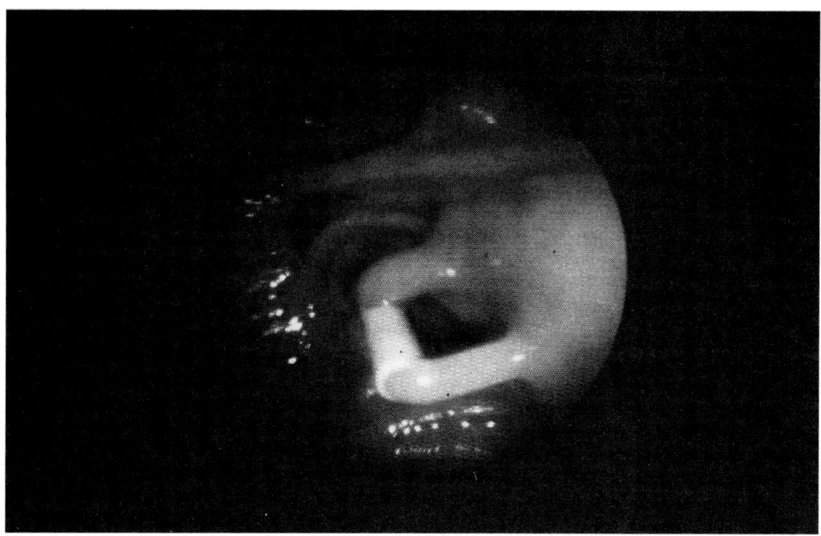

FIGURE 5.11. *Biliary stent placed to palliate stone obstruction. In this case, pus is seen coming out of the stent. This patient had cholangitis and septicemia causing a severe coagulopathy, a contraindication for biliary sphincterotomy.*

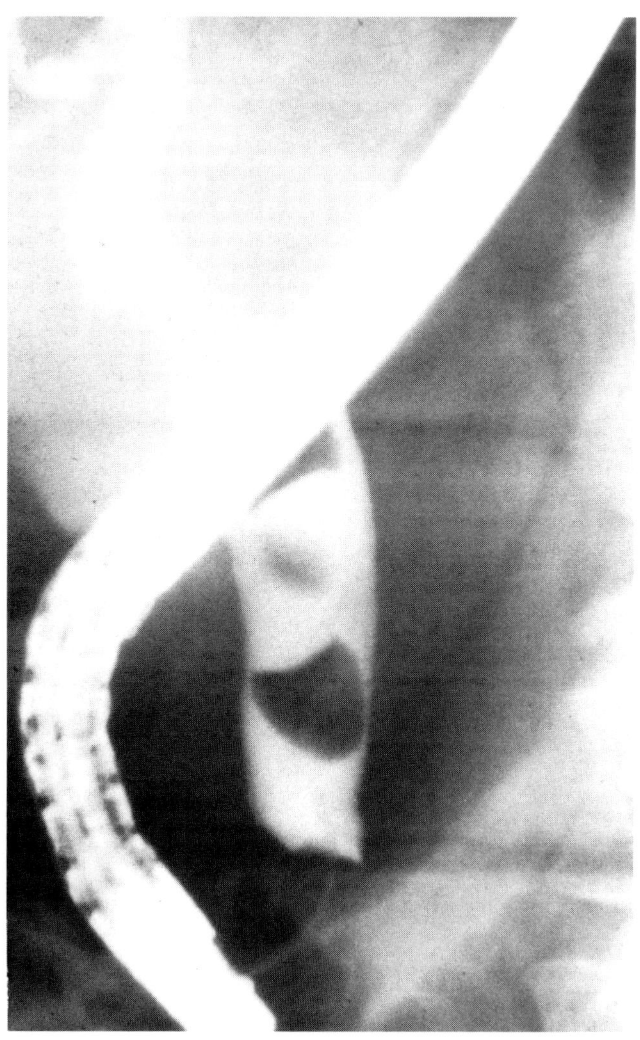

FIGURE 5.12. *Choledocholithiasis (common bile duct stones). ERCP showing bile duct stones.*

gical literature to allow stratification of patients with cholelithiasis into low (<5%), medium, and high (>20%) risk for having choledocholithiasis. The risk factors include cholestatic liver function tests, jaundice, dilated bile duct on ultrasound (with or without stones seen), and cholangitis. Interestingly, recent pancreatitis is not a reliable predictor of choledocholithiasis, as small stones that cause pancreatitis tend to pass spontaneously. Some surgeons request ERCP prior to laparoscopic cholecyslectory to assess the bile duct for stones and, if necessary, remove them. This strategy allows the surgeon to plan a single procedure: should the endoscopist fail to cannulate the bile duct or remove stones that have been seen, the surgeon can perform an intraoperative cholangiogram (IOC) or, where appropriate, convert a laparoscopic to an open procedure to deal with bile duct stones.

In our opinion, routine ERCP before laparoscopic cholecyslectory cannot be justified (49). The yield of bile duct stones is low in the absence of risk factors and ERCP exposes patients to the risk of complications, some of which can be severe. ERCP should not be used solely to define biliary anatomy, as there is no evidence that prior knowledge reduces the risk of operative complications. As evidenced by existing published studies (50–52), patients who have biliary (gallstone) pancreatitis with biliary obstruction (jaundice, cholangitis) may benefit from early ERCP and sphincterotomy (or stenting) to decompress the biliary tree. This is a select subgroup of patients in which ERCP before laparoscopic cholecyslectory is justified. Also, in patients in whom there is genuine doubt about the likely success of ERCP (e.g., after Billroth-II gastrectomy), a preoperative study may be justified to plan subsequent management. The preferred management for suspected choledocholithiasis in the absence of progressive jaundice or cholangitis is to proceed with laparoscopic cholecyslectory and have IOC performed. Those few patients found to have stones by IOC can have ERCP and duct clearance before leaving the hospital, usually the day after surgery.

Clearly, the current use of ERCP in relation to laparoscopic cholecyslectory is greatly influenced by the skill of the individual endoscopist and by the willingness and ability of the surgeon to perform IOC.

Bile Duct Leaks Bile leaks most commonly follow gallbladder surgery but can result from ductal injury related to blunt or sharp trauma or iatrogenic injury (e.g., liver biopsy). A patient who develops abdominal pain and low-grade fever soon after laparoscopic cholecyslectory requires investigation for a possible bile leak or other complication of the surgery (53). Cross-sectional imaging (e.g., CT or ultrasound) may detect a localized collection of bile (biloma) or sometimes bile lying free in the peritoneal cavity. Any significant collection of bile needs to be drained percutaneously or (when peritonitis is present) surgically. Although radionuclide scans (e.g., HIDA) may suggest or confirm the presence of a bile leak, cholangiography is necessary to define the leak site. ERCP is the preferred approach in most centers, percutaneous transhepatic cholangiography (PTC) being reserved for patients who have failed endoscopic access or who have leaks from inaccessible areas of the liver (e.g., sequestered segments).

The vast majority of bile duct leaks seen by biliary endoscopists arise from the cystic duct stump (Fig. 5.13). Injuries to the common hepatic duct, hilum, or intrahepatic ducts can cause leaks that are less straightforward to define. Particularly if a segment or even lobe of the liver has been sequestered, a combination of percutaneous cholangiography and CT scanning may be necessary to identify the lesion. As the bile ducts are usually not dilated when a leak has occurred, PTC in this setting is technically quite challenging, and requires the services of a skilled vascular radiologist.

When a cystic duct leak is identified at ERCP, placing a stent across the duodenal papilla is usually adequate therapy. Routinely performing ES is unnecessary; although effective, it exposes the patient to some additional risk. Sphincterotomy should be reserved for patients with mechanical obstruction at the papilla (e.g., obstructing stone or true papillary stenosis). The length of the stent probably has little to do with whether the bile fistula closes. It is probably sufficient to place a stent that is just long enough to bridge the duodenal papilla, thereby reducing transpapillary pressure. We tend to leave these stents in place from 2 to 4 weeks, by which time most bile leaks have resolved.

Persistent bile leaks are often an indication for PTC to look for unexpected accessory or aberrant bile ducts. It is rare for any patient with a bile duct leak to require surgery to deal with it, although sometimes the leak site is so large that it will not close spontaneously (e.g., avulsed cystic duct stump). The published results of endoscopic management of bile duct leaks suggest that this is a largely successful and cost-effective management strategy (54,55). Drastic injuries to the bile duct—such as transection—result in leaks that cannot be managed effectively by endoscopic or percutaneous means. These require surgery for bile duct repair. Bile leaks may occur after liver transplantation, especially when the biliary anastomosis is fashioned over a T-tube. When the T-tubes are removed, the patients may leak from the fistulous track. Endoscopic therapy is usually successful, although our experience has been that stents or drains have to be left in place much longer than in non-immunocompromised patients to guarantee healing of the leak. Breakdown of the biliary anastomosis after liver transplantation is usually ischemic and requires surgery.

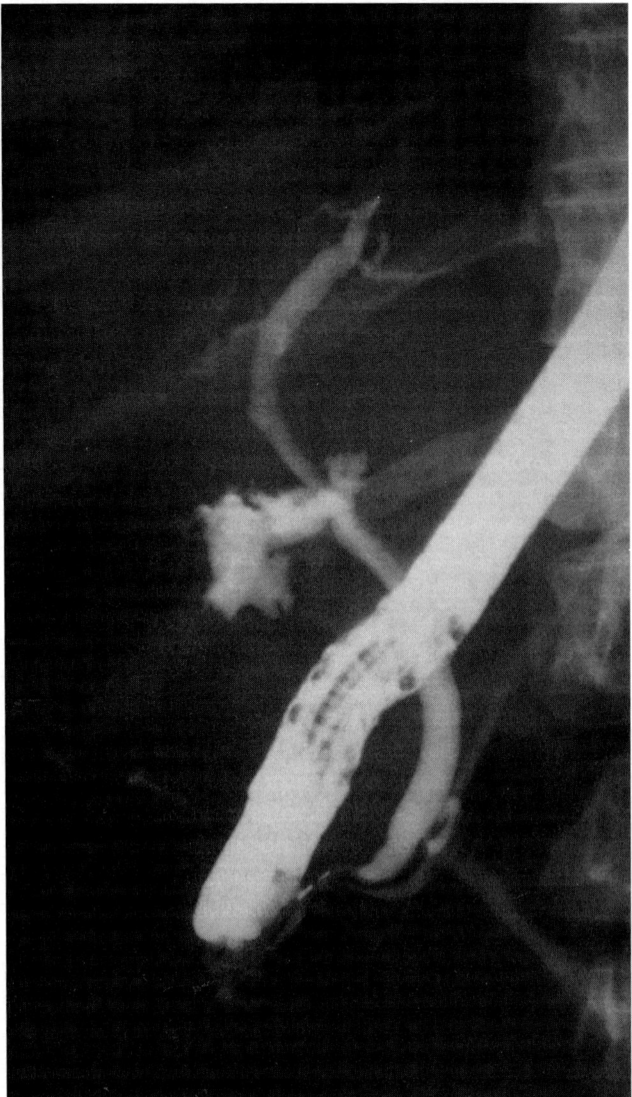

FIGURE 5.13. *Cystic duct stump leak. The little white "cloud" in the center of the image is contrast medium extravasating from the cystic duct stump at ERCP.*

Postsurgical Biliary Strictures A detailed discussion of postsurgical bile duct strictures and their potential endoscopic management is beyond the scope of this chapter. However, iatrogenic injury at the time of cholecystectomy is probably the commonest cause of benign bile duct stricture (56) (see Fig. 5.11). Postsurgical strictures are not uncommon after orthotopic liver transplantation, particularly at the site of the biliary anastomosis. Complete transection of a bile duct is a catastrophic injury that declares itself within days. Lesser degrees of ductal injury (short of transection) may result in early or late strictures. Many of these injuries result from trauma to the local vasculature, causing ischemic injury. Other causes of bile duct strictures such as chronic pancreatitis, pancreatic pseudocysts or stones in the gallbladder neck, or cystic duct (Mirizzi's syndrome) (Fig. 5.14) need to be considered (Table 5.3).

The first step in evaluating a benign biliary stricture is to make sure that it is truly benign. If there is any doubt about this, endoscopic brush cytology should be performed, with a CT scan to look for an adjacent mass that might indicate malignancy. If the stricture is in the extrahepatic bile duct or at the bifurcation (hilum) (Fig. 5.15), it is justifiable to attempt endoscopic or percutaneous radiologic dilation with or without stenting. Strictures (especially when multiple) involving the smaller intrahepatic bile ducts are not amenable to these interventions. Once accessible benign biliary strictures have been dilated, we like to stent them and leave the stent in place for 3 to 6 months.

A biliary stricture that persists beyond two dilations and stent exchanges is unlikely to resolve spontaneously, at which point surgical intervention (e.g., diversion procedure) should be considered in suitable patients. Especially in the setting of iatrogenic injury, early reconstructive surgery may be preferable to a prolonged trial of endoscopic dilation and stenting. Patients with persistent or progressive "benign" strictures should be carefully monitored for the development of malignancy, especially in primary sclerosing cholangitis (Chapter 19).

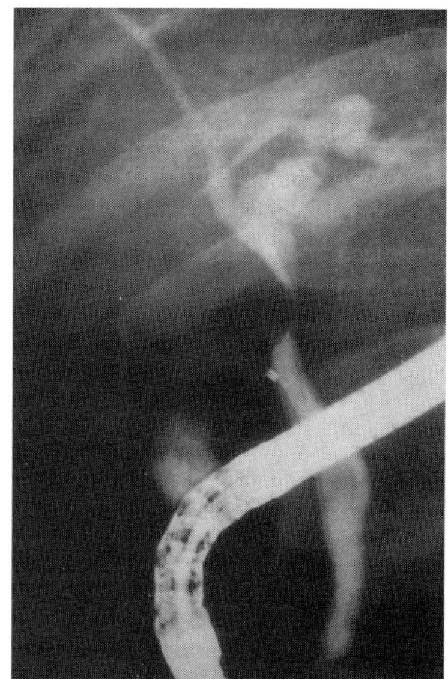

(A)

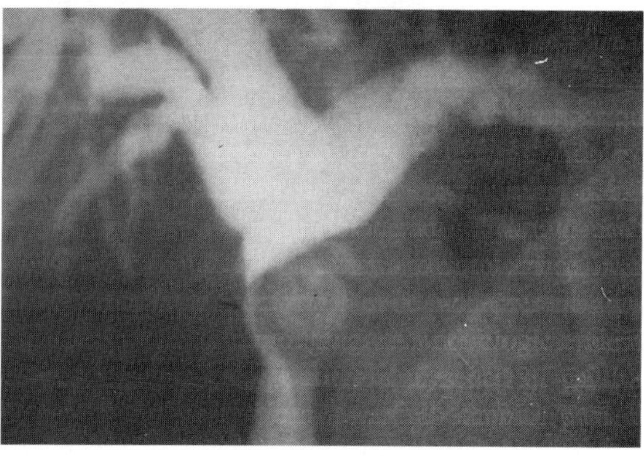

(B)

FIGURE 5.14. *Mirizzi's syndrome.* ***(A)*** *Smooth stricture at level of common hepatic duct caused by extrinsic pressure from a stone lodged in the cystic duct or neck of the gallbladder.* ***(B)*** *Faint calcification reveals the presence of a stone adjacent to common hepatic duct.*

GALLBLADDER LESIONS

Conventional ultrasound is commonly performed when cholelithiasis is suspected. With the frequent use of ultrasound, a number of polypoid lesions of the gallbladder can be discovered. It can be quite difficult to differentiate small (<20 mm) polypoid lesions using standard low frequency ultrasound. In addition, overlying bowel gas and body habitus can interfere with ultrasound imaging. By using high frequency probes and close proximity to the gallbladder, EUS has proved itself useful for investigating suspected gallbladder polyps seen on transabdominal ultrasound.

The gallbladder can generally be imaged from either the duodenal bulb or the gastric antrum. Cholesterol polyps are the most common polypoid lesions occurring in the gallbladder; they are generally less than 10 mm in diameter and appear as echogenic pedunculated masses without associated acoustic shadowing (57–59). Larger cholesterol polyps may appear heterogeneous or hypoechoic on ultrasound, making differentiation from adenocarcinoma challenging. Accurate imaging is required, as some

Table 5.3. Causes of benign bile duct strictures

- **Congenital**
- **Acquired**
  trauma (operative/nonoperative)
  sclerosing cholangitis
  liver transplantation
  chronic pancreatitis
  pancreatic pseudocysts
  Mirizzi's syndrome
  vascular indentation
  congenital hepatic cysts

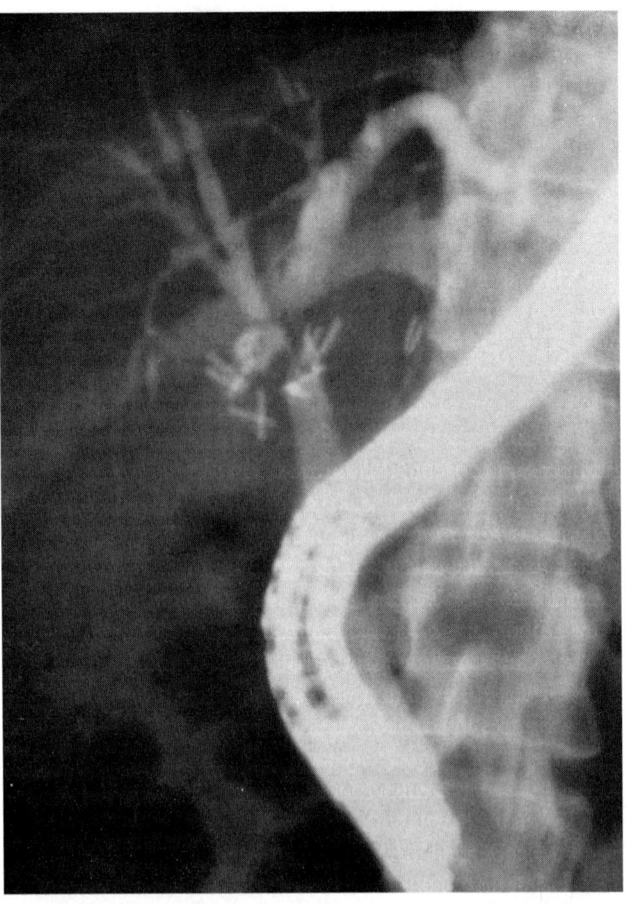

FIGURE 5.15. *Postsurgical hilar bile duct stricture. Note the surgical clips (linear densities) at the level of the obstruction. This injury often requires surgical repair.*

small polypoid carcinomas of the gallbladder can be resected for cure.

The differential diagnosis of polypoid lesions of the gallbladder includes cholesterol polyps, adenomyomatosis, adenoma, and adenocarcinoma. Cholesterol polyps are characterized at EUS as tiny echogenic spots 1 to 5 mm in diameter (60) or as an aggregation of echogenic spots with or without echopenic areas (61). Larger cholesterol polyps (>10 mm) tend to show echopenic areas. Adenomyomatosis is characterized by a sessile, solid, echoic mass with anechoic spots (microcysts) and/or "comet tail artifact." The microcysts and comet tail artifact represent dilated Rokitansky-Aschoff sinuses and intramural calculi, respectively. Adenoma and adenocarcinoma appear as echogenic or echopenic masses without the aggregation of echogenic spots, microcysts, or comet tail artifact (62,63).

Using these criteria, EUS has been shown to be the superior imaging modality for distinguishing between polypoid lesions of the gallbladder. In a Japanese study, EUS and transabdominal ultrasound correctly distinguished between various polypoid lesions in 97% and 71% of patients, respectively (61). The EUS findings specific for cholesterol polyps and adenomyomatosis are considered pathognomonic. Polypoid lesions without these findings are indicative of adenoma or adenocarcinoma. Sessile lesions with a nodular or irregular surface suggest malignancy. It can still be very difficult to differentiate between adenoma and adenocarcinoma, however. EUS is recommended for further differentiation of polypoid gallbladder lesions when standard ultrasound shows no finding consistent with cholesterol polyp or adenomyomatosis.

The normal thickness of the gallbladder wall is 3 mm or less in patients without calculous disease. With acute cholecystitis, the mean gallbladder wall thickness increases to 9 mm, whereas in chronic cholecystitis, the mean thickness is 6 mm (62). Gallbladder wall thickening is nonspecific and has been reported in renal disease, heart disease, hypertension, hypoproteinemia, hypoalbuminemia, hepatitis, ascites, alcoholic liver disease, myeloma, and as a normal variant. In chronic cholecystitis, the thickened gallbladder wall retains its normal multilayered appearance as viewed with EUS. Indeed, EUS adds little to the investigation of a thickened gallbladder wall, unless gallbladder cancer is considered a possible diagnosis.

The integrity of the gallbladder wall is a key factor in the diagnosis of depth of invasion of gallbladder cancer. The normal gallbladder wall generally appears as a two- or three-layer structure by EUS; however, this interpretation is controversial. Currently, the consensus is that the inner hypoechoic layer includes the mucosa, muscularis propria, and the fibrous layer of the subserosa. The outer hyperechoic layer represents the serosa. Hence, even if the outer hyperechoic layer appears intact, cancer invasion can still extend beyond the muscularis propria.

EUS can detect gallbladder tumors with a sensitivity of greater than 90% (63); the loss of the multiple-layer pattern of the gallbladder wall is considered to be the most specific finding in the diagnosis of gallbladder cancer. However, accurate staging by depth of invasion proves difficult and may be possible only in selected cases. In a surgically referenced series, the accuracy rate for EUS was 77% when invasions as far as the muscularis propria and subserosa were classified into a single category (64). As the majority of patients with gallbladder cancer present with advanced disease, EUS evaluation will likely add little to surgical exploration and management.

CHOLANGIOCARCINOMA

EUS

Bile duct cancer, cholangiocarcinoma (Table 5.4), is rare, with an estimated 2000 to 3000 new cases annually in the United States (see Chapter 20). These lesions can be intrahepatic, perihilar (bifurcation to cystic duct origin), or distal extrahepatic (CBD) (65). These cancers are challenging to detect, with small (<20 mm) tumors being especially problematic for TUS and CT imaging. The detection rate for small carcinomas approaches 100% using EUS and ERCP (66). ERCP with biopsy and cytologic brushing is the most sensitive and specific way to diagnose and localize malignancy of the biliary tree; however, it cannot offer staging information, such as the extent of tumor invasion (67). Given the proximity of the extrahepatic bile duct to the duodenum, EUS can visualize bile duct tumors and provide useful staging information that can help determine appropriate treatment (Fig. 5.16).

The distal CBD is best viewed by EUS from the descending duodenum at the level of the ampulla. The more proximal CBD and common hepatic duct can be viewed from the duodenal bulb. In general, EUS cannot reliably image the bifurcation of the right and left main intrahepatic ducts. However, one author reports very accurate staging of Klatskin tumors using EUS (68). The extrahepatic bile duct is seen as an anechoic ductal structure with a two-layered wall: an internal hypoechoic layer and an external hyperechoic layer. An interface hyperechoic echo is occasionally demonstrated just inside the internal hypoechoic later, simulating a three-layered wall. The inner hypoechoic layer includes the mucosa, the fibromuscularis, and the fibrous layer of the serosa. The outer hyperechoic layer corresponds to the subserosal fatty tissue, the serosa, and the interface echo between the serosa and the surrounding organs (67,69,70).

Staging of bile duct cancer is done according to the TNM (tumor/node/metastasis) classification. EUS is highly accurate for assessing the tumor stage of extrahepatic bile duct tumors, with accuracy rates of 81% to 85% when compared to surgery (66,67,70). Given the extremely thin wall layers of the bile duct, and the fact that they can frequently be obscured in the setting of inflammation, it can be quite difficult to distinguish between T1 and T2 lesions. Fortunately, the differentiation between these tumor stages usually does not influence therapeutic management. In contrast, vascular invasion or gross invasion into adjacent organs will likely alter treatment. EUS is capable of distinguishing T3 from T1 and T2 lesions with an 88% accuracy (69). The nodal staging of cholangiocarcinoma with EUS has an accuracy of 53% to 81% (66,67,70). These studies used solely radial array echoendoscopes to differentiate between benign and malignant lymph nodes; cytologic sampling via FNA

Table 5.4. Malignant tumors of the biliary tree

- **Primary**
  cholangiocarcinoma
  hepatoma
  gallbladder carcinoma
- **Secondary**
  pancreatic tumors, including adenocarcinoma/lymphoma
  metastatic malignancy

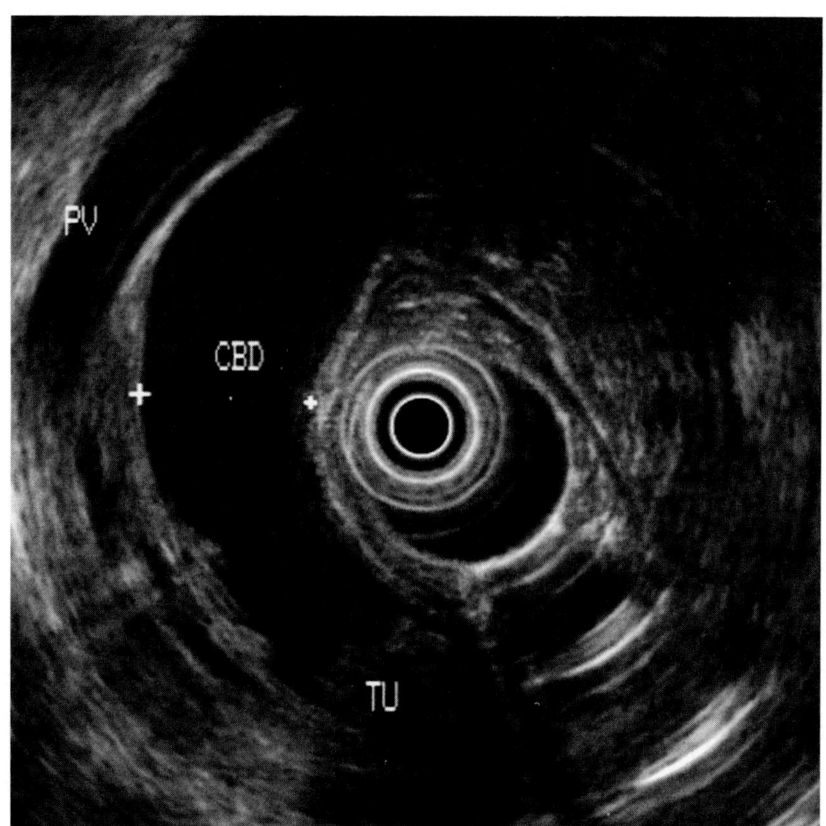

FIGURE 5.16. *EUS reveals a hypoechoic mass lesion in the distal CBD consistent with cholangiocarcinoma versus (intra)ampullary carcinoma (CBD = common bile duct, diameter 18 mm; TU = tumor; PV = portal vein).*

was not employed, which would have increased the diagnostic accuracy.

Intraductal ultrasonography (IDUS) uses selective cannulation of the bile duct with a 6 French gauge, high frequency (20 Mhz) mini-probe. This technique requires fluoroscopy, but enables examination of the entire extrahepatic bile duct and the right and left hepatic ducts. The main advantage of this technique is that staging can be performed during the initial diagnostic and/or therapeutic ERCP. Additionally, IDUS can assess portal vein invasion at the liver hilum and invasion of the right hepatic artery. It is difficult to image the liver hilum with EUS; in one study, bile duct tumors were inadequately visualized at this site (71). IDUS may be more accurate in assessing pancreatic parenchymal invasion by bile duct cancer than EUS (72). IDUS cannot be performed if the mini-probe cannot cross the malignant bile duct stricture. It also cannot reliably distinguish between T1 and T2 tumor stages. As stated, the differentiation of T3 from T1 or T2 tumors is most important as this affects management. In comparing the accuracy of EUS (88%) and IDUS (80%), there does not appear to be a significant difference in the ability of these techniques to identify tumor stage (73).

Malignancy Affecting the Biliary Tree

Malignancies resulting in bile duct strictures can be divided into primary and secondary (see Chapters 2 and 20). Primary malignancies are those arising from biliary epithelium or closely adjacent tissues, including cholangiocarcinoma, hepatoma, and gallbladder cancer. Secondary malignancies cause biliary strictures by extrinsic compression of the bile ducts; they include pancreatic tumors (e.g., adenocarcinoma and lymphoma) and metastatic malignancy (e.g., of the colon, breast, or bronchus). As the management of each type of these malignancies is unique, a vigorous effort must be made to identify the tissue of origin. A minority of tumors causing biliary strictures are amenable to surgical resection, but it is important to identify these cases as removal of the tumor may be the patient's only hope for cure or prolonged survival. Staging of such tumors includes CT scanning with or without portography and hepatic arteriography. Vascular encasement or invasion is often (but not always) evidence of unresectability.

Although curative resection may be impossible, surgery for biliary and sometimes gastric bypass provides useful palliation in carefully selected cases. In patients with distal bile duct strictures, laparoscopic biliary and gastric bypass may be an option. The gallbladder should not be used for biliary bypass if the tumor is within 2 cm of the cystic duct take-off, as tumor ingrowth will quickly occlude this and the patient will become jaundiced again (74). Endoscopic and percutaneous stenting procedures remain the mainstay of palliation for malignant biliary obstruction.

Imaging

Many radiologic techniques are available to study the biliary tree, including transabdominal ultrasound, CT, MRI, arteriography, and, most recently, EUS and positron emission tomography (PET) (see Chapter 3). ERCP and PTC are direct techniques for accessing and imaging the bile ducts, and offer the potential for cytologic diagnosis and palliative treatment (e.g., biliary drainage using stents or drains). A detailed discussion of the relative merits of all these imaging modalities is beyond the scope of this review. However, a combination of techniques (e.g., CT + ERCP, or MRI + PTC) will provide a higher diagnostic yield in most cases than a single technique used alone. Patients with complex hilar strictures may be best served by PTC and external biliary drainage (usually bilateral); using this access, expandable metallic stents can be placed for palliation of unresectable tumors (75). Local irradiation (brachytherapy) can be applied to suitable bile duct tumors using iridium-192 sources advanced over a percutaneously placed guidewire (76).

Tissue Sampling

Brush Cytology

Using an endoscopic brush, malignant cells can be scraped from the surface of biliary tumors for cytologic examination (Fig. 5.17). Foutch (77) reviewed the world literature on this subject and reported an overall sensitivity for brush cytology of 59%, with higher sensitivity in cholangiocarcinoma than in pancreatic head adenocarcinoma (see Chapters 2 and 20). Repeated brushing may increase the cytologic yield. Lee et al. (78) evaluated endoscopic bile duct brush cytology, stratifying samples into benign, low-grade, and high-grade dysplasia. Overall, the finding of dysplasia had a 37% sensitivity and a 100% specificity for bile duct cancer. The combination of brush cytology, FNA, and forceps biopsy has a greater sensitivity (around 80%) than any single modality alone (79).

Fine-Needle Aspiration and Forceps Biopsy

Howell et al. (80) reported a 61% sensitivity (16 of 26 patients) for endoscopic FNA of malignant bile duct strictures. Kubota et al. (81) found a sensitivity of 81% for transpapillary stricture biopsy in 43 patients with pancreatic and bile duct cancer (Fig. 5.18). Nimura et al. (82) have reported high diagnostic yield (>85%) for cholangiocarcinoma using forceps biopsy by the percutaneous route. Percutaneous FNA under radiologic guidance has very variable results but an acceptably low complication rate. Sherman et al. (83) performed "triple sampling" on 127 patients with the Geenen cytology brush, the Howell aspiration needles (two thrusts), and endobiliary forceps biopsy (three to four bites). The overall sensitivity was 71%.

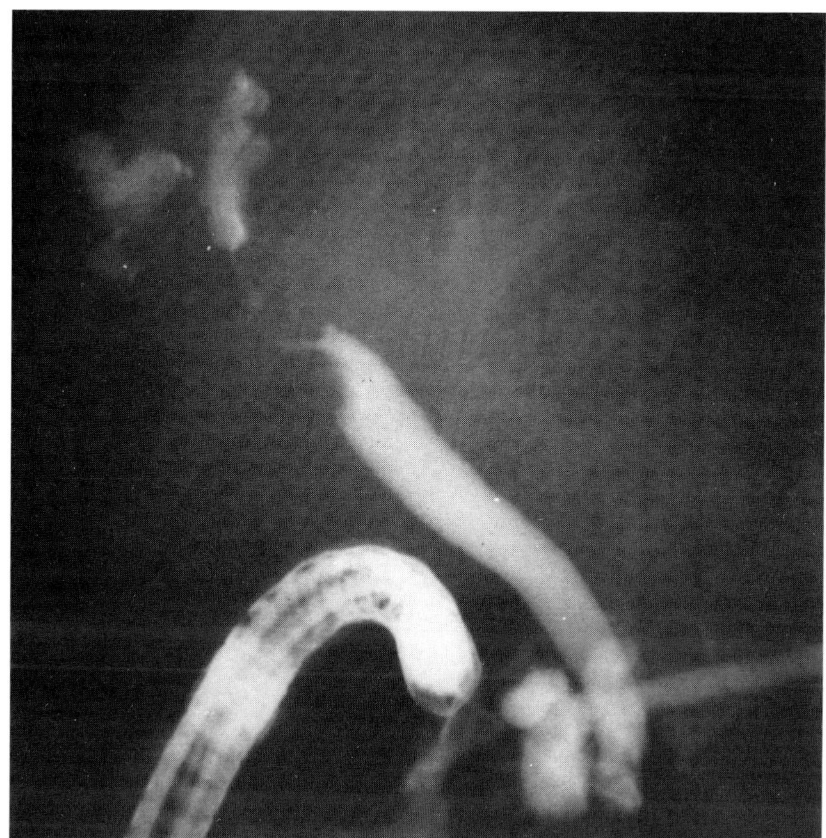

FIGURE 5.17. *A suitable case for cytologic brushing. This cholangiogram reveals a tight hilar stricture as the cause of obstructive jaundice.*

Molecular Markers

"Ploidy" refers to the DNA content of cells. The association between aneuploidy and malignant transformation makes evaluation of the ploidy status of biopsy samples potentially useful. Two techniques that can evaluate DNA content of cells are flow cytometry and absorptive cytometry; the latter requires a much smaller tissue sample and appears to be superior for diagnosing cancer. Patients with aneuploidy appear to have a shortened survival when compared to those whose cells have diploid DNA content (84). Mutations in the k-*ras* oncogene have been reported in 75% to 100% of pancreatic cancers (85). Tada et al. (86) noted a high incidence of *ras* gene mutations in bile duct cancers. The mutation occurs at the codon 12 position. The role of this mutation in the genesis of cholangiocarcinoma is uncertain. Other mutations that have been described in pancreatic and biliary cancers include the p53 mutation and loss of integrity of chromosomes 5 and 17 (87,88). Recently, there has been great interest in the enzyme telomerase as a marker of malignant transformation in pancreatic and bile duct cancer (89). Studies evaluating the role of telomerase assay in this setting are ongoing.

Staging of Bile Duct Tumors

The TNM classification is being used increasingly to categorize cholangiocarcinoma into four stages: stage I is limited to the mucosa, stage II has periductal invasion but without nodal disease or metastases, stage III has regional lymph nodes involved, and stage IV involves adjacent structures and/or distant metastases (see Chapters 2 and 20). Malignancies of the bile duct are also classified according to their location. Upper 1/3 tumors involve the common hepatic duct and confluence, middle 1/3 tumors arise from the common bile duct between the cystic duct and the upper border of the duodenum, and lower 1/3 tumors arise from the common bile duct between the upper border of the duodenum and the ampulla of Vater.

For endoscopists, the Bismuth classification (90) is helpful: type I tumors are located within the common hepatic duct, type II involve the right and left main hepatic ducts, and type III involve the secondary intrahepatic bile ducts (IIIA, the right ones; IIIB, the left ones) (Chapter 20, Fig. 20.2). A more advanced stage, where both right and left ducts are involved, is sometimes referred to as type IV.

The following findings on imaging studies commonly indicate lack of resectability (91):

1. Bilateral intrahepatic bile duct spread or multifocal disease
2. Involvement of the main trunk of the portal vein
3. Involvement of both branches of the portal vein or bilateral involvement of the hepatic artery and portal vein

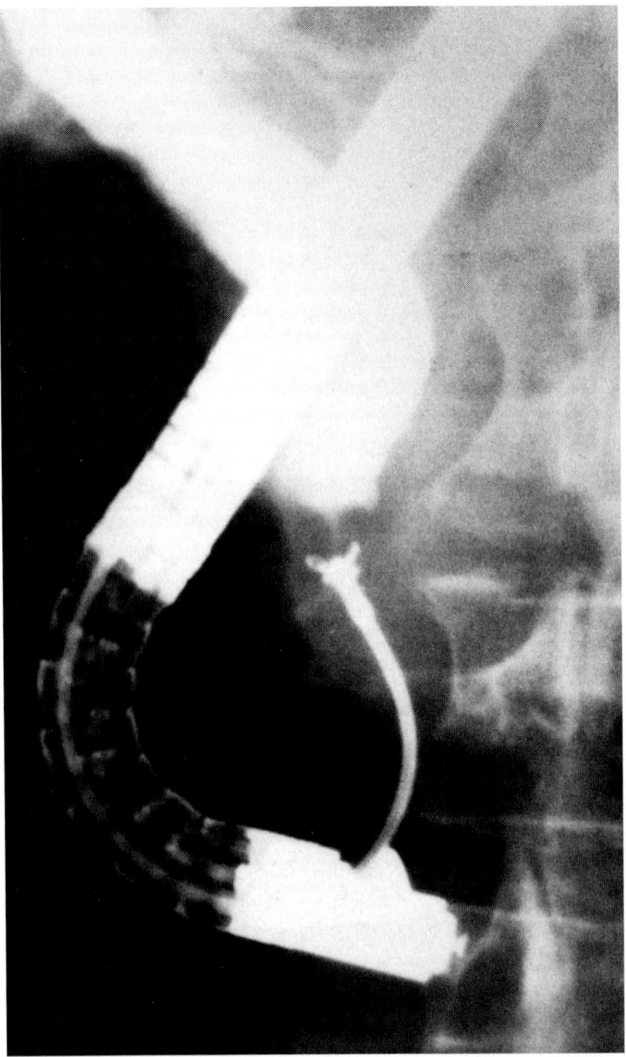

FIGURE 5.18. *Transpapillary forceps biopsy of a malignant mid-CBD stricture.*

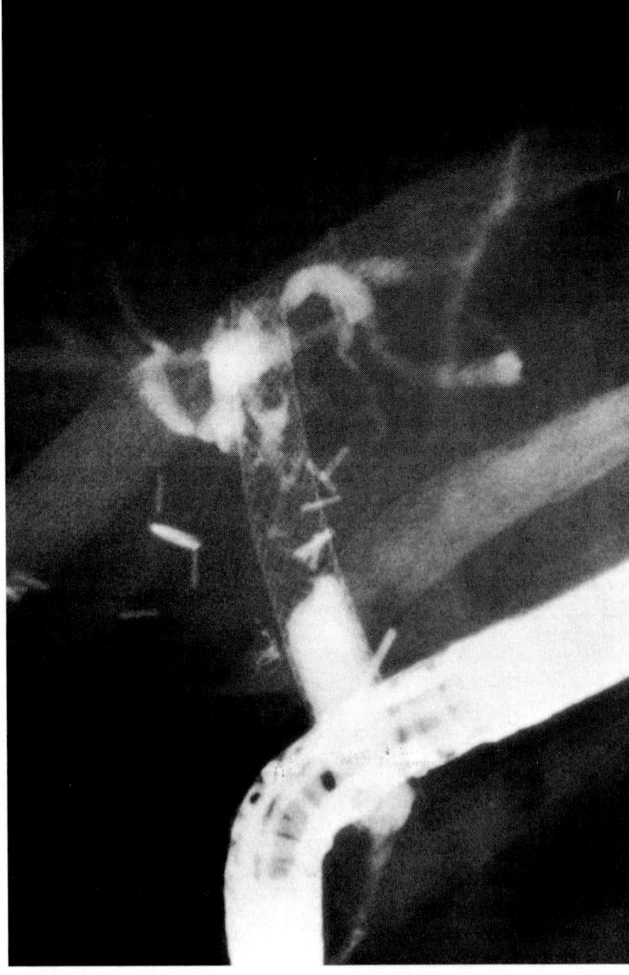

FIGURE 5.19. *Biliary metal mesh stent (Wallstent) occluded by tumor ingrowth.*

4. Vascular involvement on one side of the liver with extensive bile duct involvement on the other.

Biliary Stenting

Endoscopic stenting is now a well-established form of palliative treatment for malignant biliary obstruction. Hilar strictures are much more difficult to bridge than more distal ones. Two prospective, randomized trials have compared plastic and metal endoprostheses for distal biliary obstruction (92,93). In one study, overall survival was the same; however, the medium time to stent occlusion was longer for metal stents (33% after 273 days) than for plastic ones (54% after 123 days). The second study showed occlusion rates for metal stents of 22% and 43% for plastic during the lifetime of the patient. Patients stented for hilar obstruction suffer recurrent jaundice and cholangitis more frequently than those with other sites of obstruction.

A distinct advantage of the percutaneous approach in hilar malignancy is the ability to place two stents simultaneously through the right and left biliary systems. This can also be done endoscopically, but it is a technical tour de force. Bilateral placement of metal mesh stents has become common for palliating unresectable hilar bile duct tumors. Unfortunately, these metal mesh stents have a tendency to occlude due to tumor ingrowth (Fig. 5.19). When these stents block, it is sometimes possible to relieve the obstruction by advancing a plastic stent endoscopically through the metal stent lumen.

The choice of palliation used for patients with unresectable cholangiocarcinoma depends on the overall condition of the patient and his or her expected survival time. Comparison of surgical, endoscopic, and radiologic palliation of distal common bile duct strictures shows comparable survival and quality of life.

CONDITIONS COVERED ELSEWHERE IN THIS BOOK

Sclerosing Cholangitis

Primary and secondary sclerosing cholangitis are chronic cholestatic disorders of the biliary tree characterized by diffuse inflammatory stricturing of the intrahepatic and/or extrahepatic bile ducts (94). Endoscopists have an important role to play in the diagnosis and management of these conditions, especially as primary sclerosing cholangitis carries risk of malignant transformation. For a detailed discussion of sclerosing cholangitis, see Chapter 19.

Choledochal Cysts

These congenital cystic dilatations of the intrahepatic and extrahepatic biliary tree are rare, but the biliary endoscopist should be aware of them, because they present unique diagnostic and management challenges (95). For a detailed discussion of choledochal cysts, see Chapters 16 and 23.

SUGGESTED READINGS

Mallery S, Van Dam J. Advances in diagnostic and therapeutic endoscopy. Med Clin North Am 2000;80:1059–83.

Pickuth D, Spielmann RP. Detection of choledocholithiasis: comparison of unenhanced spiral CT, US and ERCP. Hepatogastroenterology 2000;47: 1514–7.

Rosch T, Schusdziarra V, Born P, et al. Modern imaging methods versus clinical assessment in the evaluation of hospital in-patients with suspected pancreatic disease. Am J Gastroenterol 2000;95:2261–70.

Wallace MB, Hawes RH. Emerging indications for EUS. Gastrointest Endosc 2000; 52(Suppl):S55–60.

REFERENCES

1. Baillie J. Complications of endoscopy. Endoscopy 1994;26:185–203.
2. Aliperti G. Complications related to diagnostic and therapeutic endoscopic retrograde cholangiopancreatography. Gastrointest Endosc Clin North Am 1996;6:379–407.
3. Ostroff JW, Shapiro HA. Complications of endoscopic sphincterotomy. In: Jacobsen IM, ed. Diagnostic and therapeutic applications. New York: Elsevier, 1989:61–73.
4. Freeman ML, Nelson DB, Sherman S, et al. Complications of endoscopic biliary sphincterotomy. N Engl J Med 1996;335:909–18.
5. Leung JW, Libby ED, Morck DW, et al. Is ciprofloxacin effective in delaying biliary stent blockage? Gastrointest Endosc 2000;32:175–82.
6. Draganov P, Cotton PB. Iodinated contrast sensitivity in ERCP. Am J Gastroenterol 2000;95:1398–401.
7. Amouyal G, Amouyal P. Endoscopic ultrasonography in gallbladder stones. Gastrointest Endosc Clin N Am 1995;825–30.
8. Marks JW, Bonorris G. Intermittency of cholesterol crystals in duodenal bile from gallstone patients. Gastroenterology 1984;87:622–7.
9. Dill JE. Combined endoscopic ultrasound and stimulated biliary drainage in cholecystitis and microlithiasis—diagnoses and outcome. Endoscopy 1995;27: 424–7.
10. Dill JE. Symptom resolution or relief after cholecystectomy strongly correlates with positive combined endoscopic ultrasound and stimulated biliary drainage. Endoscopy 1997;29:646–8.
11. Coyle WJ, Lawson JM. Combined endoscopic ultrasound and stimulated biliary drainage in cholecystitis and microlithiasis: diagnosis and outcomes. Gastrointest Endosc 1996;44:102–3.
12. Amouyal P, Amouyal G, Levy P, et al. Value of endoscopic ultrasonography in the diagnosis of idiopathic acute pancreatitis (abstract). Gastroenterology 1994; 106:283–4.
13. Pieken SR, Feld R, Kasterberg D, et al. Role of endosonography in the diagnosis of gallstone disease in obese subjects (abstract). Gastroenterology 1992;104:A328.
14. Hermann RE. The spectrum of biliary stone disease. Am J Surg 1989;158: 171–3.
15. Canto MIF, Chak A, Stellato T, et al. Endoscopic ultrasonography versus cholangiography for the diagnosis of choledocholithiasis. Gastrointest Endosc 1998;47:439–48.
16. Norton SA, Alderson D. Prospective comparison of endoscopic ultrasonography and endoscopic retrograde cholangiopancreatography in the detection of bile duct stones. Br J Surg 1997;84:1366–9.
17. Cotton PB. Progress report: ERCP. Gut 1977;18:307–41.
18. Shimuzu S, Tada M, Kawai K. Diagnostic ERCP. Endoscopy 1994;26:88–92.
19. Onken J, Brazer S, Eisen G, et al. Accurate prediction of choledocholithiasis (abstract). Gastroenterology 1994;106:A20.
20. Panasen P, Partanen K, Pikkarainen P, et al. Ultrasonography, CT and ERCP in the diagnosis of choledochal stones. Acta Radiol 1992;33:53–6.
21. Wermke W, Schultz HJ. Sonographic diagnosis of bile duct calculi: results of a prospective study of 222 cases of choledocholithiasis. Ultraschall Med 1987;8: 116–20.
22. Cronan JJ. Ultrasound diagnosis of choledocholithiasis: a reappraisal. Radiology 1986;161:133–4.
23. Stott MA, Farrand PA, Guyer PB, et al. Ultrasound of the common bile duct in patients undergoing cholecystectomy. J Clin Ultrasound 1991;19:73–6.
24. Dong B, Chen M. Improved sonographic visualization of choledocholithiasis. J Clin Ultrasound 1987;15:185–90.
25. Sugiyama M, Atomi Y. Endoscopic ultrasonography for diagnosing choledocholithiasis: a prospective, comparative study with ultrasonography and computed tomography. Gastrointest Endosc 1997;45:143–6.
26. Chak A, Hawes RH, Cooper GS, et al. Prospective assessment of the utility of EUS in the evaluation of gallstone pancreatitis. Gastrointest Endosc 1999;49: 599–604.
27. Baron RL. Common bile duct stones: reassessment of criteria for CT diagnosis. Radiology 1987;162:419–24.
28. Aubertin JM, Levoir D, Bouillot JL, et al. Endoscopic ultrasound immediately prior to laparoscopic cholecystectomy: a prospective evaluation. Endoscopy 1996;28:667–73.
29. Shim CS, Joo JH, Park CW, et al. Effectiveness of endoscopic ultrasonography in the diagnosis of choledocholithiasis prior to laparoscopic cholecystectomy. Endoscopy 1995;27:428–32.
30. Denis BJ, Bas V, Goudot C, et al. Accuracy of endoscopic ultrasonography for diagnosis of common bile duct stones (abstract). Gastroenterology 1993;104: A358.
31. Napoleon B, Pujol B, Ponchon T, et al. Prospective study of the accuracy of echoendoscopy for the diagnosis of bile duct stones (abstract). Endoscopy 1994;26:422.
32. Salmeron M, Simon JF, Houdart R, et al. Endoscopic ultrasonography versus invasive methods for the diagnosis of common bile duct stones (abstract). Gastroenterology 1994;106:A357.
33. Barish MA, Yucel EK, Ferruci JT. Magnetic resonance cholangiopancreatography. N Engl J Med 1999;341:258–64.
34. de Ledinghen V, Lecesne R, Raymond JM, et al. Diagnosis of choledocholithiasis: EUS or magnetic resonance cholangiography? A prospective controlled study. Gastrointest Endosc 1999;49:26–31.
35. Guibard L, Bret PM, Reinhold C, et al. Bile duct obstruction and choledocholithiasis: diagnosis with MR cholangiography. Radiology 1995;197: 109–15.
36. Rosch T, Dittler HJ, Fockens P, et al. Major complications of endoscopic ultrasonography: results of a survey of 42,105 cases (abstract). Gastrointest Endosc 1993;39:341.
37. Cotton PB. ERCP and laparoscopic cholecystectomy. Am J Surg 1993;165: 474–8.
38. Palazzo L. Which test for common bile duct stones? Endoscopic and intraductal ultrasonography. Endoscopy 1997;29:655–65.
39. Leung JW, Chung SC, Sung JJ, et al. Urgent endoscopic drainage for acute suppurative cholangitis. Lancet 1989;1:1307–9.
40. Bergman JJGHM, Van der Mey S, Rauws EAJ, et al. Longterm follow-up after endoscopic sphincterotomy for bile duct stones in patients younger than 60 years of age. Gastrointest Endosc 1996;44:643–9.
41. MacMathuna P, White P, Clark E, et al. Endoscopic sphincteroplasty: a novel and safe alternative to papillotomy in the management of bile duct stones. Gut 1994;35:127–9.
42. Siegel JH, Ben-Zvi JS, Pullano WE. Mechanical lithotripsy of common duct stones. Gastrointest Endosc 1990;36:351–6.

43. Hixton LJ, Fennerty MB, Jaffee PE, et al. Peroral cholangioscopy with intracorporeal electrohydraulic lithotripsy for choledocholithiasis. Am J Gastroenterol 1992;87:296–9.
44. Cotton PB, Kozarek RA, Schapiro RH, et al. Endoscopic laser lithotripsy of large bile duct stones. Gastroenterology 1990;99:1129–33.
45. Sauerbruch T, Stern M. Fragmentation of bile duct stones by extracorporeal shock waves. A new approach to biliary calculi after failure of routine endoscopic measures. Gastroenterology 1989;96:146–52.
46. Shaw MJ, Mackie RD, Moore JP, et al. Results of a multicenter trial using mechanical lithotripter for the treatment of large bile duct stones. Am J Gastroenterol 1993;730–3.
47. Palmer KR, Hofmann AF. Intraductal mono-octanoin for the direct dissolution of bile duct stones: experience in 343 patients. Gut 1986;27:196–202.
48. Bergman JJGHM, Rauws EAJ, Tijssen JGP, et al. Biliary endoprostheses in elderly patients with endoscopically irretrievable common bile duct stones: report on 117 patients. Gastrointest Endosc 1995;42:195–201.
49. Baillie J. Treatment of acute biliary pancreatitis (editorial). N Engl J Med 1997; 336:286–7.
50. Neoptolemos JP, Carr-Locke DL, London NJ, et al. Controlled trial of urgent endoscopic retrograde cholangiography and endoscopic sphincterotomy versus conservative treatment for acute pancreatitis due to gallstones. Lancet 1988;2: 979–83.
51. Fan ST, Lai ECS, Mok FTP, et al. Early treatment of acute biliary pancreatitis by endoscopic sphincterotomy. N Engl J Med 1993;328:228–32.
52. Folsch U, Nitsche R, Ludtke R, et al. Early ERCP and papillotomy compared with conservative treatment for acute biliary pancreatitis. The German Study Group on Acute Biliary Pancreatitis. N Engl J Med 1997;336:237–42.
53. Doctor N, Dooley JS, Dick R, et al. Multidisciplinary approach to biliary complications of laparoscopic cholecystectomy. Br J Surg 1998;85:627–32.
54. Chow S, Bosco JJ, Heiss FW, et al. Successful treatment of post-cholecystectomy bile leaks using nasobiliary tube drainage and sphincterotomy. Am J Gastroenterol 1997;92:1839–43.
55. Barkun AN, Rezieg M, Mehta S, et al. Post-cholecystectomy biliary leaks in the laparoscopic era: risk factors, presentation and management. Gastrointest Endosc 1997;45:277–82.
56. Kozarek RA. Endoscopic techniques in the management of biliary tract injuries. Surg Clinic North Am 1994;74:883–93.
57. Price RJ, Stewart ET, Foley WD, et al. Sonography of polypoid cholesterolosis. Am J Roentgenol 1982;139:1197–8.
58. Jeffrey RB, Ralls PW. Sonography of the abdomen. New York: Raven Press, 1995.
59. Sugiyama M, Atomi Y, Kuroda A, et al. Large cholesterol polyp of the gallbladder: diagnosis by means of ultrasound and endoscopic ultrasound. Radiology 1995;196:493–7.
60. Matsumoto J. Endoscopic ultrasonography diagnosis of gallbladder lesions. Endoscopy 1998;30(suppl 1):A124–7.
61. Sugiyama M, Xiao-Yan X, Atomi Y, et al. Differential diagnosis of small polypoid lesions in the gallbladder: the value of endoscopic ultrasonography. Ann Surg 1999;229:498–504.
62. Cohan RH, Mahony BS, Bowie JD, et al. Striated intramural gallbladder lucencies in ultrasound studies: predictions of acute cholecystitis. Radiology 1987;164:31.
63. Inui K, Nakazawa S. Diagnosis of depth of invasion of gallbladder carcinoma with endosonography. J Jap Surg Soc 1998;99:696–9.
64. Mizuguchi M, Kudo S, Fukahori T, et al. Endoscopic ultrasonography for demonstrating loss of multiple-layer pattern of the thickened gallbladder wall in the preoperative diagnosis of gallbladder cancer. Eur Radiol 1997;7: 1323–7.
65. De Groen PC, Gores GJ, LaRusso NF, et al. Biliary tract cancers. N Engl J Med 1999;341:1368–78.
66. Mukai H, Yasuda K, Nakajima M. Tumors of the papilla and distal common bile duct: diagnosis and staging by endoscopic ultrasonography. Gastrointest Endosc Clin N Am 1995;5:763–72.
67. Mukai H, Nakajima M, Yasuda K, et al. Evaluation of endoscopic ultrasonography in the pre-operative staging of carcinoma of the ampulla of Vater and common bile duct. Gastrointest Endosc 1992;38:676–83.
68. Tio TL. Proximal bile duct tumors. Gastrointest Endosc Clin North Am 1995; 5:773–80.
69. Fujita N, Noda Y, Kobayashi G, et al. Staging of bile duct carcinoma by EUS and IDUS. Endoscopy 1998;30(suppl 1):A132–4.
70. Tamada K, Kanai N, Ueno N, et al. Limitations of intraductal ultrasonography in differentiating between bile duct cancer stage T1 and stage T2: in vitro and in vivo studies. Endoscopy 1997;29:721–5.
71. Tio TL, Cheng J, Wijers OB, et al. Endosonographic TNM staging of extrahepatic bile duct cancer: comparison with pathological staging. Gastroenterology 1991:100:1351–61.
72. Tamada K, Ido K, Ueno N, et al. Pre-operative staging of extrahepatic bile duct cancer with intraductal ultrasonography. Am J Gastroenterol 1995;90: 239–46.
73. Tamada K, Ueno N, Ichiyama M, et al. Assessment of pancreatic parenchymal invasion by bile duct cancer using intraductal ultrasonography. Endoscopy 1996;28:492–6.
74. Tarnasky PR, England RE, Lail LM, et al. Cystic duct patency in malignant obstructive jaundice. An ERCP-based study relevant to the role of laparoscopic cholecystojejunostomy. Ann Surg 1995;221:265–71.
75. Stoker J, Lameris JS, van Blankenstein M. Percutaneous metallic self-expandable endoprostheses in malignant hilar biliary obstruction. Gastrointest Endosc 1993;39:43–9.
76. Lai ECS, Tompkins RK, Roslyn JJ, et al. Proximal bile duct cancer. Ann Surg 1987;205:111–18.
77. Foutch PG. Diagnosis of cancer by cytologic methods performed during ERCP. Gastrointest Endosc 1994;40:249–52.
78. Lee JG, Leung JW, Baillie J, et al. Benign, dysplastic or malignant? Making sense of endoscopic bile duct brush cytology. Results in 149 consecutive patients. Am J Gastroenterol 1995;90:722–6.
79. Fogel EL, Sherman S. How to improve the accuracy of diagnosis of malignant biliary strictures. Endoscopy 1999;31:758–60.
80. Howell DA, Beveridge RP, Bosco JJ, et al. Endoscopic needle aspiration biopsy at ERCP in the diagnosis of biliary strictures. Gastrointest Endosc 1992;38: 531–5.
81. Kubota Y, Takaoka M, Tani K, et al. Endoscopic transpapillary biopsy for diagnosis of patients with pancreaticobiliary strictures. Am J Gastroenterol 1993; 88:1700–4.
82. Nimura Y, Shionoya S, Hayakawa N, et al. Value of percutaneous transhepatic cholangioscopy. Surg Endosc 1988;2:213–19.
83. Sherman S, Esher EJ, Pezzi JS, et al. Yield of ERCP tissue sampling of biliary striuctures by brush, forceps and needle aspiration methods (abstract). Gastrointest Endosc 1995;41:478.
84. Ryan MR, Baldarf MC. Comparison of flow cytometry for DNA content and brush cytology for detection of malignancy in pancreaticobiliary strictures. Gastrointest Endosc 1994;40:133–9.
85. Almoguera C, Sawicki M, Samara G, et al. Most human carcinomas of the exocrine pancreas contain mutant c-l-*ras* genes. Cell 1988;53:549–54.
86. Tada M, Omata M, Ohto M. High incidence of *ras* gene mutation in intrahepatic cholangiocarcinoma. Cancer 1992;69:1115–18.
87. Hurwitz M, Sawicki M, Samara G, et al. Diagnostic and prognostic markers in cancer. Am J Surg 1992;164:299–306.
88. Ding SF, Delanty JDA, Bowles L, et al. Loss of constitutional heterozygosity on chromosomes 5 and 17 in cholangiocarcinoma. Br J Cancer 1993;67: 1007–10.
89. Itoi T, Shinohara Y, Takeda K, et al. Detection of telomerase activity in biopsy specimens for diagnosis of biliary tract cancers. Gastrointest Endosc 2000;52: 380–6.
90. Bismuth H, Nakache R, Diamond T. Management strategies in resection for hilar cholangiocarcinoma. Ann Surg 1992;215:31–8.
91. Looser C, Stain SC, Baer HU, et al. Staging of hilar cholangiocarcinoma by ultrasound and duplex sonography. A comparison of angiography and operative findings. Br J Radiol 1992;65:871–7.
92. Krynim K, Wagner HJ, Pausch J, et al. A prospective, randomized, controlled trial of metal stents for malignant obstruction of the common bile duct. Endoscopy 1993;25:207–12.
93. Wagner HJ, Krynim K, Vakil N, et al. Plastic endoprostheses versus metal stents in the palliative treatment of malignant hilar biliary obstruction. A prospective and randomized trial. Endoscopy 1993;25:213–18.
94. Lee Y-M, Kaplan MM. Primary sclerosing cholangitis. N Engl J Med 1995;332: 924–33.
95. Todani T, Wanatabe Y, Narusue M, et al. Congenital bile duct cysts: classification, operative measures and review of 37 cases including cancer arising from choledochal cyst. Am J Surg 1977;134:263–9.

Chapter 6

Percutaneous Treatment of Diseases of the Biliary Tree and Gallbladder

Paul V. Suhocki

Percutaneous biliary interventions were first performed in the 1950s. They relied heavily on basic percutaneous biliary access techniques established in the 1930s (see Chapter 5). Remolar was the first to use the percutaneous biliary access tract in 1956 for external biliary drainage (1). Mondet used a T-tube sinus tract for gallstone extraction from the common bile duct in 1962 (2). Burhenne described a technique that would allow internal drainage of bile across an obstruction in 1974 (3). Ring modified the internal biliary drainage technique with a pigtail self-retaining catheter in 1979 (4).

Imaging capabilities and instrumentation have improved greatly since the early pioneering work. The current indications for percutaneous biliary access include 1) percutaneous biliary drainage or stent placement for biliary obstruction, 2) biliary diversion as a definitive treatment for bile leakage or as a step to operative treatment, 3) gallbladder drainage for the nonoperative candidate with cholecystitis, 4) percutaneous gallstone extraction or gallstone contact lithotripsy, 5) percutaneous access for brachytherapy for malignant bile duct obstruction, 6) percutaneous biliary biopsy, 7) transhepatic enteric access for jejunal feeding tube placement in the patient with a percutaneous biliary drain already in place (5), 8) percutaneous choledochocholedochostomy in the patient with intrahepatic benign bile duct obstruction (6), and 9) percutaneous choledochojejunostomy in the postoperative patient with an excluded aberrant bile duct and an existing Roux-en-Y limb (7).

PERCUTANEOUS ACCESS OF THE BILIARY TREE FOR BILIARY INTERVENTIONS

Percutaneous access to the biliary tree becomes necessary when a biliary obstruction or leak 1) fails to respond to endoscopic treatment, 2) is located at or above the biliary bifurcation where endoscopic therapy may be ineffective, 3) will be treated surgically and percutaneous biliary drainage catheters must be in place at the time of surgery to facilitate identification of the bile ducts, or 4) was in a favorable location to be treated endoscopically but ERCP was technically unsuccessful. ERCP (Chapter 4) can be unsuccessful when the endoscopist fails to 1) cannulate the ampulla because of unfavorable anatomy or tumor, 2) cross an obstruction or tear in the extrahepatic bile duct, or 3) pass the endoscope through the efferent limb of a biliary enteric bypass. When this occurs, the endoscopist attempts placing a nasobiliary tube before removing the endoscope. The patient is then transferred to the interventional radiologist for percutaneous cholangiography and biliary drainage. The radiologist injects contrast into the nasobiliary drain to opacify the biliary tree (Fig. 6.1). This greatly simplifies percutaneous needle access to the biliary tree for diagnosis and possibly intervention (8). Lower procedure time reduces the risk and radiation dose for the patient.

The risk of vascular injury during percutaneous biliary interventions is greatest in the central portion of the liver, where the vascular structures are the greatest in caliber. Therefore, the biliary tree is best entered through a peripheral bile duct. In this manner, all central instrumentation will be done within the confines of the biliary tree.

The technique for percutaneous needle access to the bile ducts of the left and right lobes was described in Chapter 4. Once a peripheral bile duct is accessed with a 22 gauge needle, the needle is replaced with a temporary 3 French drainage catheter. Most of the bile is aspirated from the biliary tree. This avoids overdistension of the infected biliary tree when injecting contrast into the biliary tree for cholangiography. Aspiration of bile also prevents spillage of bile into the peritoneal cavity during catheter exchanges and tract dilatation. Once the bile ducts are opacified, the

(A)

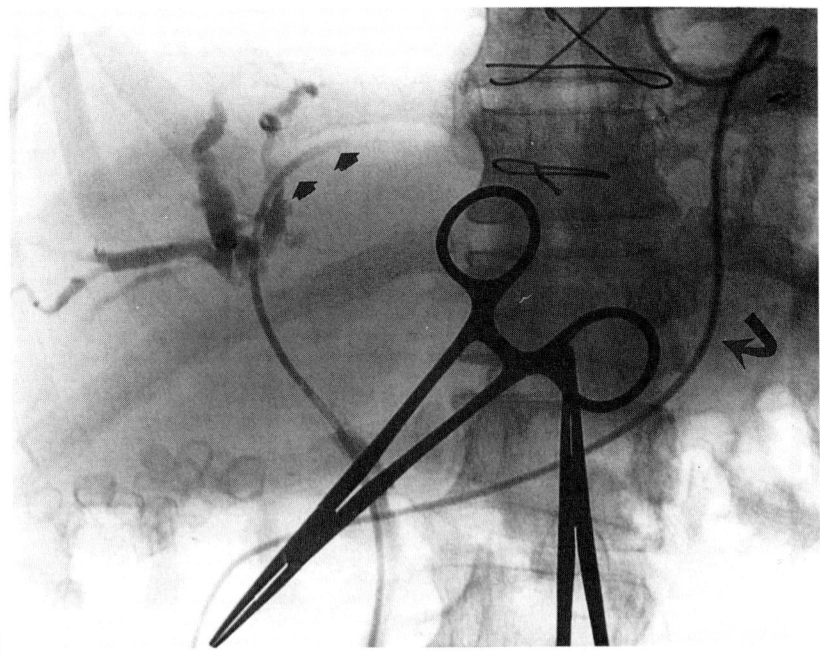

(B)

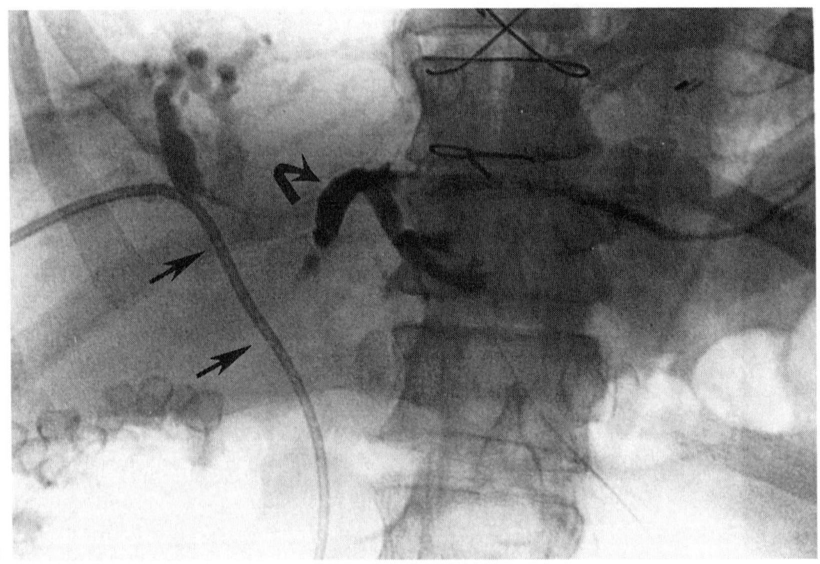

FIGURE 6.1. ***(A)*** *The tip of a nasobiliary drainage catheter (arrows) was passed into the right biliary tree in a patient with cholangiocarcinoma involving the biliary bifurcation.* ***(B)*** *The nasobiliary drain was used to opacify the biliary tree for facilitation of right-sided percutaneous biliary drainage (arrows). The noncommunicating left biliary system (curved arrow) was accessed under sonographic guidance. Multiple radiopaque gallstones fill the gallbladder.*

cholangiogram is analyzed for the presence of any bile duct abnormalities.

The percutaneous tract is then evaluated using a pullback contrast injection technique to see if a major vascular structure has been transgressed (9,10). A guidewire is left in place during this maneuver so as not to lose access to the biliary tree. The access is not used for biliary intervention if a major vessel has been transgressed. Once a favorable transhepatic tract is obtained, a curved tip catheter and guidewire are negotiated through sites of leak or obstruction. When the catheter reaches the intestine, it is replaced with an 8F percutaneous biliary drainage catheter. If an obstruction or tear cannot be passed, a straight or pigtail drainage catheter is placed above the abnormal site.

Left biliary drainage is necessary when a bifurcational occlusion prevents communication between the two ductal systems. A left-sided biliary drainage catheter is easier for patients to care for by themselves because of ease of access. It is also associated with less leakage of ascites around the catheter. Left biliary access is best performed under sonographic guidance (see Chapter 4).

The gallbladder can also be used as a portal of entry for interventions involving the common bile duct. Although the cystic duct is difficult to navigate, it may be used as an avenue for placement of an internal-external biliary drainage catheter (11). This method requires the obstructing lesion to be below the level of the cystic duct origin.

Once cholangiography is performed and an abnormality is identified, a drainage catheter is often placed. Aggressive interventions including balloon dilatation and biopsy are avoided during the first patient encounter to avoid biliary sepsis. There are three types of drainage catheters available for draining the biliary tree. An external drainage catheter is placed above an obstruction, draining bile externally into a bag. An internal-external drainage catheter lies within the biliary tree and intestine and traverses the obstruction. Bile can drain externally into a bag or internally into the bowel or both. An internal drain is more often referred to as a biliary endoprosthesis or stent. It has no external component. The biliary stent crosses the obstruction and drains bile internally only. It is usually placed endoscopically. Plastic removable stents must be exchanged periodically, usually every 3 months. This avoids occlusion from bile salts and bacterial colonization. Metallic stents are permanent devices. They are used almost exclusively for unresectable malignant occlusions and usually remain patent through the patient's lifespan. Ingrowth of a tumor will occasionally occlude the stent, requiring coaxial placement of another stent. Metallic endoprostheses can be placed either percutaneously or endoscopically.

The right internal jugular vein is an important portal of entry to the biliary tree in the patient with ascites and a malignant biliary occlusion (12) (Fig. 6.2). The curved needle is directed from the inferior vena cava into the middle hepatic vein, across liver parenchyma and into the dilated biliary tree. A metallic stent is then placed across the malignant occlusion through the access and the jugular venous catheter is removed.

Patients with ascites are at risk for ascites leakage around the percutaneous biliary drainage catheter. This is less of a problem with a drainage catheter placed via the left hepatic lobe rather than the right, possibly because of the right access being more dependent in the recumbent position. An ostomy bag can be placed temporarily around the catheter insertion site to collect ascitic fluid and prevent skin breakdown. To stop the leakage of ascites around the catheter, a T-fastener set can be used to retract the liver surface against the abdominal wall and seal off the tract from leaking (13). For patients in whom percutaneous access is given up after a biliary stent is placed, cyanoacrylate glue can be injected into a transhepatic tract to prevent leakage of ascites and bile at the end of the procedure (14).

DRAINING THE ISOLATED BILIARY SYSTEM

Occasionally a tumor, stricture, or surgical clip prevents passage of a percutaneous biliary drainage catheter from the left or right bile ducts into the intestine (Fig. 6.3). It then becomes necessary to divert bile externally from the isolated biliary tree. Long-term external drainage of bile complicates medical management with fluid and electrolyte loss. The bile can be rerouted back into bowel by connecting the drainage catheter externally to a T-tube (15), an internal-external percutaneous biliary drainage in the contralateral bile ducts (16,17), or a gastrostomy feeding tube (18). A communication between the isolated bile ducts and the internally draining ducts may also be created using a sharpened guidewire. This results in an intrahepatic choledochocholedochostomy (6).

An isolated left biliary tree can be drained directly into the stomach. This is done by transhepatic perforation of the left lobe of the liver into the lesser curvature of the stomach using fluoroscopic, endoscopic, and laparoscopic guidance. In a study of 35 patients who underwent hepaticogastrostomy, the mean patency rate was reported to be 234 days ± 252 (19). The reintervention rate was 14%. Complications included cholangitis (20%) and gastritis (12%).

PERCUTANEOUS TREATMENT OF BILE DUCT FISTULAS

Bile leaks following cholecystectomy are usually minor and arise from either the cystic duct stump or a transected bile duct in the gallbladder fossa (see Chapters 10, 17). Simple drainage of the bile collection usually causes the bile duct leak to seal spontaneously. Bile duct fistulas that traverse the diaphragm are rare but have been reported to resolve following drainage of the bilious pleural effusion (20).

Bile leaks that persist despite percutaneous drainage of the biloma usually seal following decompression of the biliary tree with an endoscopic stent or percutaneous biliary drainage catheter. If the bile leak does not respond to biliary decompression, the presence of a transected, noncommunicating aberrant bile duct should be suspected and sought out. Aberrant bile ducts, when present, are usually found in the right hepatic lobe. They usually drain into the extrahepatic ductal system within 30 mm of the cystic duct origin (21). A percutaneous biliary drainage catheter is placed in leaking aberrant bile and plans are made to treat the leak surgically with a biliary-enteric anastomosis. The presence of a percutaneous biliary drainage catheter in the aberrant duct facilitates intraoperative identification of the aberrant bile duct by both palpation and visualization of the catheter. Transected aberrant bile ducts can sometimes be treated percutaneously (Fig. 6.4). Percutaneous creation of a choledochojejunostomy has been described in a patient with a transected aberrant bile duct that was excluded from a Roux-en-Y choledochojejunostomy at the time of operation (7) (Fig. 6.5).

If bile continues to leak from a peripheral branch of a normal biliary tree following biliary decompression, the biliary cutaneous fistula can be sealed percutaneously. This can be done by injecting either a viscous preparation of 60% ethanol (Ethibloc) or isobutyl-2-cyanoacrylate (IBCA) (22) into the fistula tract. Transhepatic tracts have also been successfully closed with N-butyl-2-cyanoacrylate (14).

A persistent biliary-cutaneous fistula is a common biliary complication following orthotopic liver transplantation. It is seen in 7% to 35% of patients following T-tube removal (23). Goodwin et al. (23) demonstrated a significantly

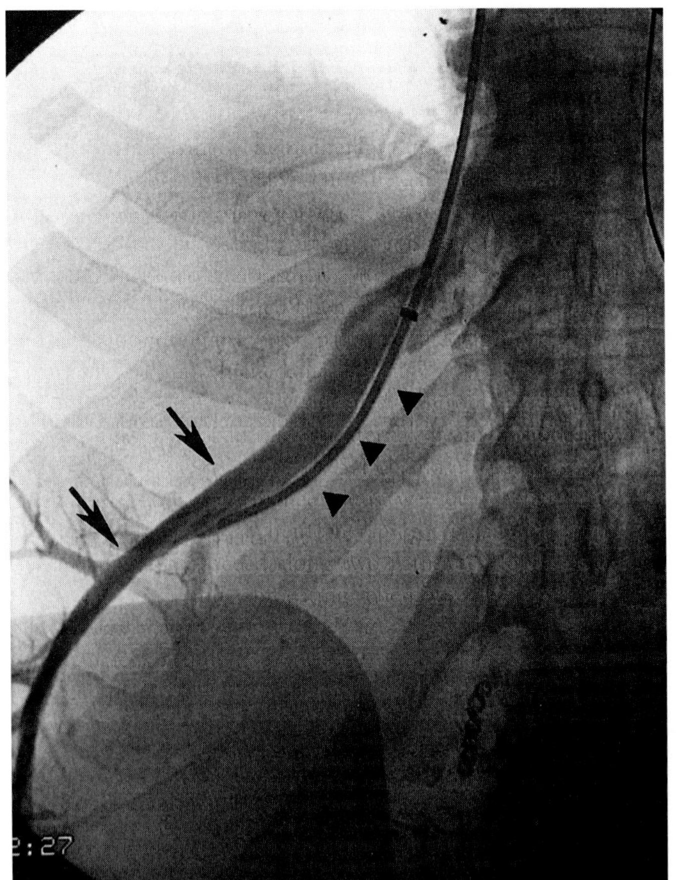

(A)

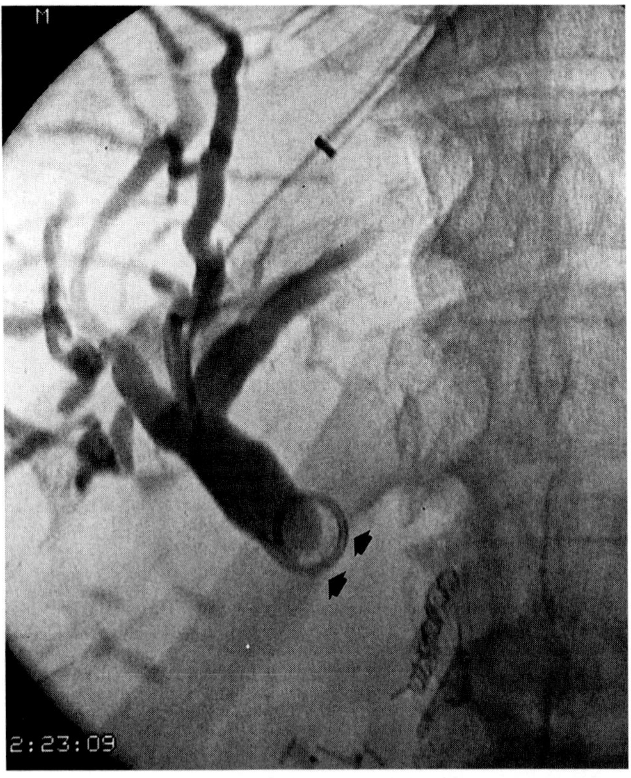

(B)

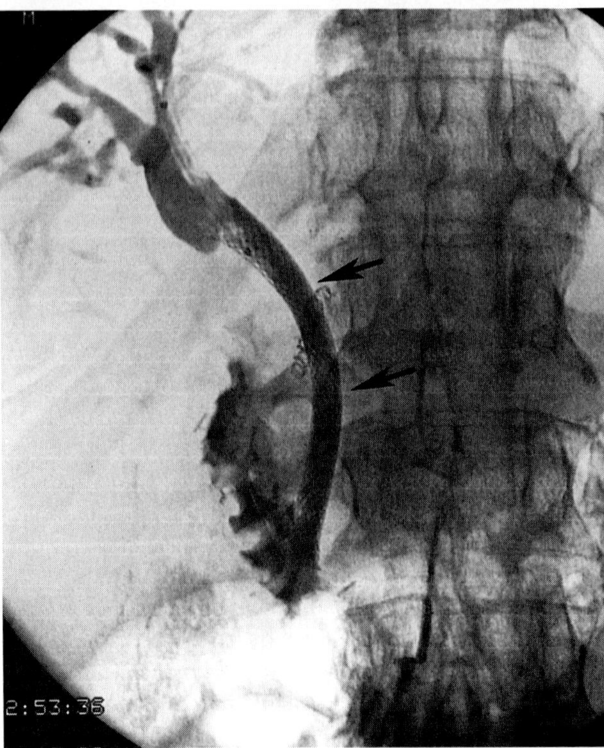

(C)

FIGURE 6.2. ***(A)*** *Transjugular access to the liver was used to avoid ascites complications in a patient with metastatic colon cancer with common bile duct obstruction and malignant ascites. A curved needle (arrowheads) was passed into the middle hepatic vein (arrows) through a vascular sheath placed in the right internal jugular vein.* ***(B)*** *A pigtail catheter (arrows) was advanced from the hepatic vein into the biliary tree after a communication between the two structures was created with the curved needle. There is complete obstruction of the common bile duct by tumor.* ***(C)*** *A biliary Wallstent (arrows) was placed across the malignant obstruction and into the duodenum. The venous access was then removed.*

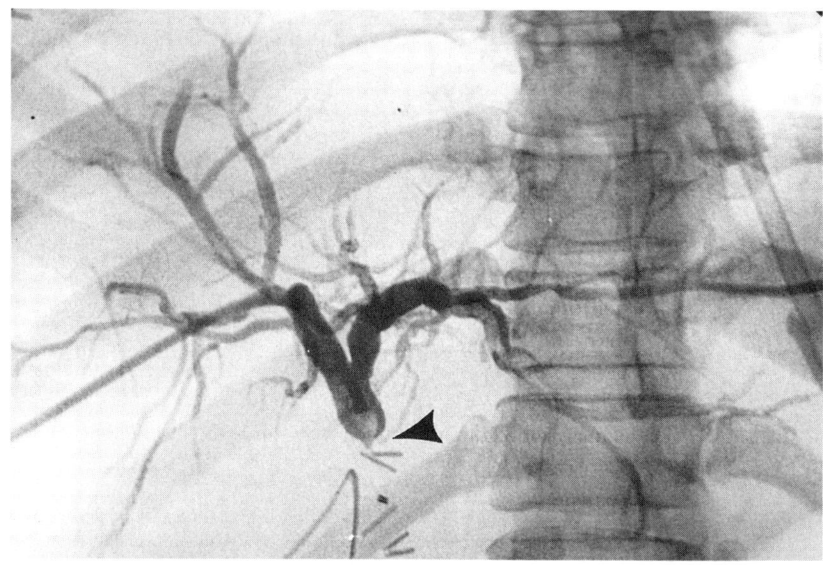

(A)

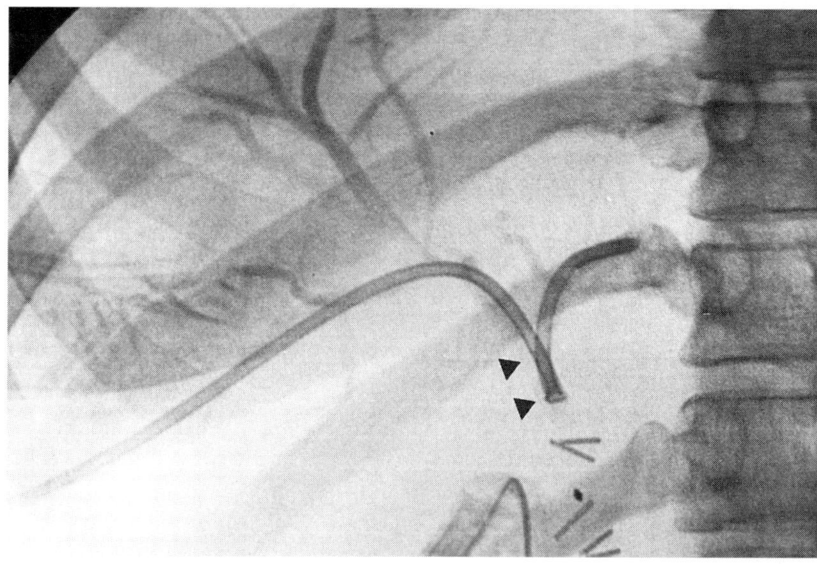

(B)

FIGURE 6.3. ***(A)*** *A vascular clip was placed on the common hepatic duct during laparoscopic cholecystectomy, causing complete obstruction of the duct (arrowhead).* ***(B)*** *A percutaneous biliary drainage catheter (arrowheads) was placed in the biliary tree to facilitate intraoperative identification of the biliary bifurcation for biliary enteric anastomosis.*

decreased incidence of bile peritonitis following a modification of the T-tube removal technique. They replaced the tube with a small caliber multiple sidehole catheter under fluoroscopic guidance. The catheter was gradually retracted over a 2 to 3 day period while bile drained externally into a bag. In a group of 363 patients, bile peritonitis was seen in 8.6% of the patients who had their T-tube removed with the modified technique. Bile peritonitis was seen in 19.5% of the control patients who had the T-tube removed in a conventional manner.

USE OF A METALLIC ENDOPROSTHESIS FOR THE TREATMENT OF BILIARY STRICTURES

The metallic stent has become a frequently used permanent endoprosthesis for the treatment of unresectable malignant biliary obstruction over the last decade. The Wallstent is the most commonly used stent for this purpose. Other stents include the self-expanding Z stent and the AVE stent. Patients prefer a metallic stent because it eliminates the need for periodic replacement of an internal-external biliary drainage catheter. The stent also eliminates the discomfort and cosmetic problems associated with a drainage catheter that exits the skin.

Metallic stents that are 8 or 10 mm in diameter are used for treatment of biliary obstruction. The struts of the stent become incorporated into the bile duct epithelium. Metallic stents can be placed across a malignant biliary obstruction either endoscopically or percutaneously (Fig. 6.6). When placed percutaneously, the biliary system is accessed in the manner described above. Once the malignant biliary occlusion is traversed with a catheter and guidewire, an 8F vascular sheath is placed at the skin access site. An angioplasty balloon catheter is used to balloon

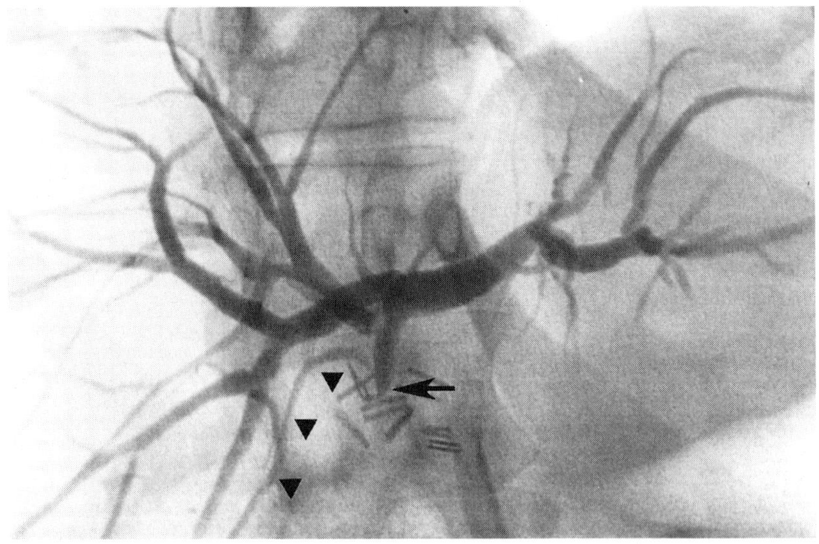

(A)

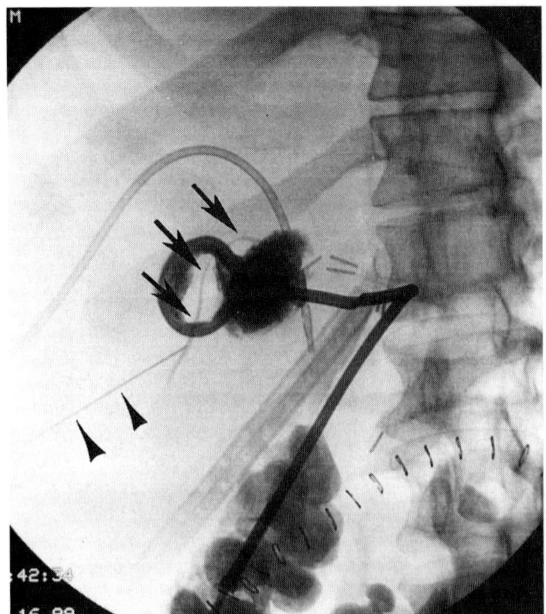

(B)

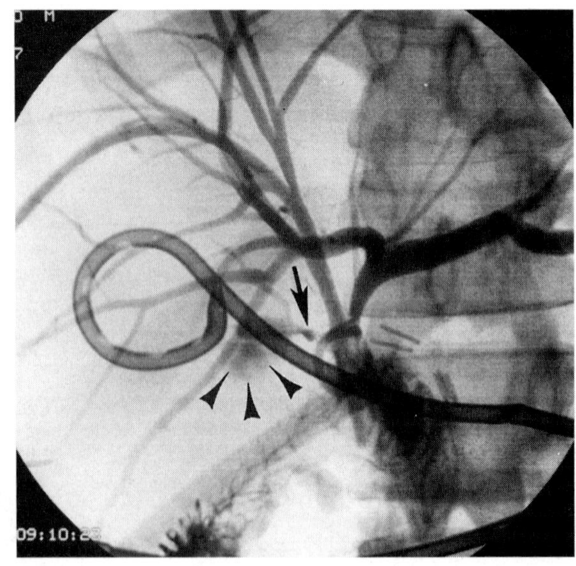

(C)

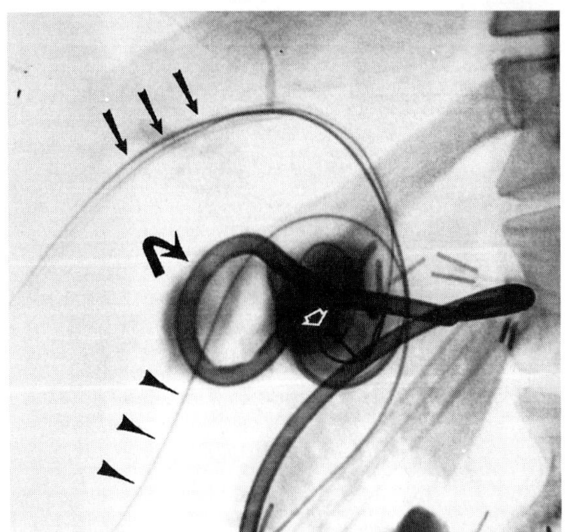

(D)

FIGURE 6.4. ***(A)*** *Cholangiogram following laparoscopic cholecystectomy shows several vascular clips obstructing the common hepatic duct (arrow). Note the low lying aberrant right hepatic bile duct (arrowheads) entering the common hepatic duct near the clipping injury.* ***(B)*** *A subhepatic biloma developed following repair with biliary-enteric bypass. Contrast injection of the biloma drain demonstrated retrograde filling of the aberrant right hepatic duct (arrows) that had been divided and was excluded from the anastomosis. A needle (arrowheads) was passed percutaneously into the opacified aberrant duct for access. A percutaneous biliary drainage catheter lies in the intact portion of the biliary tree that is unopacified.* ***(C)*** *Contrast injection of the intact biliary tree shows exravasation of contrast from the stump of the aberrant right hepatic duct (arrow) into the biloma (arrowheads).* ***(D)*** *A rendezvous procedure was performed from both sides of the aberrant bile duct tear to connect the duct remnants. A wire (arrowheads) was passed percutaneously from the aberrant right hepatic duct into the biloma. A snare (arrows) was passed from the intact biliary tree into the stump of the aberrant bile duct and into the biloma. Inside the biloma, the snare (white open arrow) was used to pull the wire from the aberrant right hepatic bile duct into the main biliary tree. A large biloma drain (curved arrow) is present.*

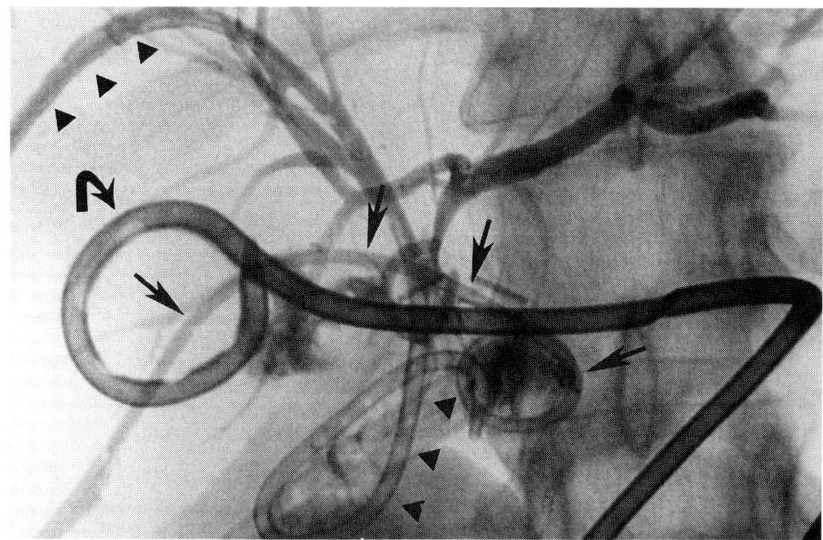

(E)

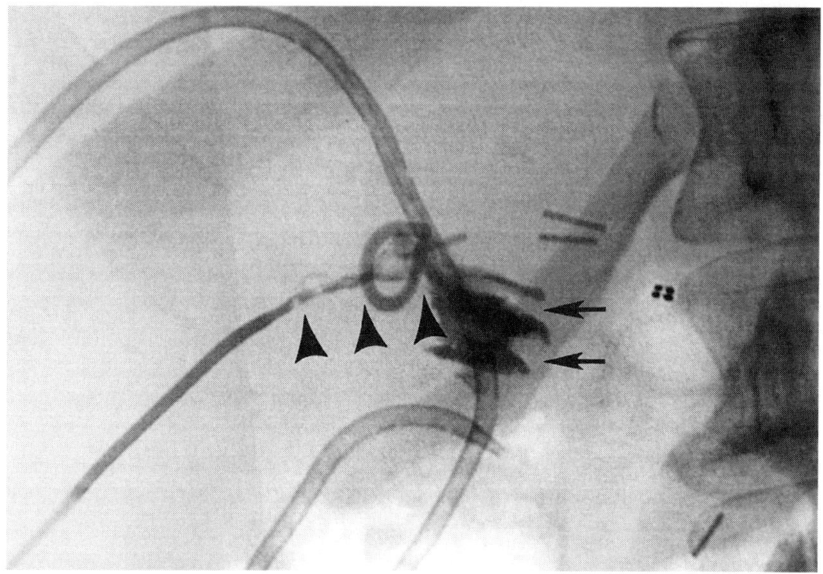

(F)

FIGURE 6.4. *continued*
***(E)** Following tract dilatation, an 8F biliary drainage catheter (arrows) was passed from the aberrant right hepatic bile duct, across the tear, into the main biliary tree and jejunum. A large biloma drain (curved arrow) and biliary drainage catheter (arrowheads) in the intact biliary tree are also seen. **(F)** Twelve weeks later, contrast injection through a catheter in the aberrant right hepatic duct demonstrates no exravasation from the previous site of tear. There is prompt flow of contrast from the bile duct into the jejunum.*

dilate the malignant obstruction to 8 to 12mm in diameter. A stent is then deployed across the obstruction under fluoroscopic guidance. The Wallstent is kept above the ampulla whenever possible, to avoid reflux of intestinal contents into the biliary tree. Balloon dilation of the stent is usually necessary to fully expand it. Bilateral biliary Wallstent placement is required for tumors at or near the biliary bifurcation (Fig. 6.7).

Sludge or tumor ingrowth may cause early stent occlusion (Fig. 6.8). Lammer et al. (24) reported a 272-day median stent patency in 52 patients who had a Wallstent placed for malignant biliary obstruction. Mean follow-up was 217 days (range 3 to 1321 days). The reocclusion rate was 19%, requiring repeat stent placement. These results were favorable when compared to 49 patients in the same study who had a 12F plastic stent with a 2.5-mm diameter lumen placed for malignant biliary obstruction. Median stent patency for that group was 96 days, with a 27% reocclusion rate. The 30-day mortality rate was significantly lower (10%) in the group with metallic stents compared to the group with plastic stents (24%).

Because of the high reocclusion and reintervention rate associated with ingrowth of granulation tissue through the struts of the metallic stent, the stent is not widely used for treatment of benign biliary strictures. Hausegger et al. (25) reported the results of Wallstent placement in 20 patients with benign biliary strictures. Median primary patency was 32 months ± 8.7 during a mean 31.2-month follow-up (range 3 to 78 months). Wallstents coated with polyurethane have not yielded better patency rates than uncovered stents. In a separate study, Hausegger reported the placement of polyurethane-coated Wallstents (26). During the mean follow-up period of 5 months (range 15 days to 24 months), there was a 37% reocclusion rate. The patency rate of self-

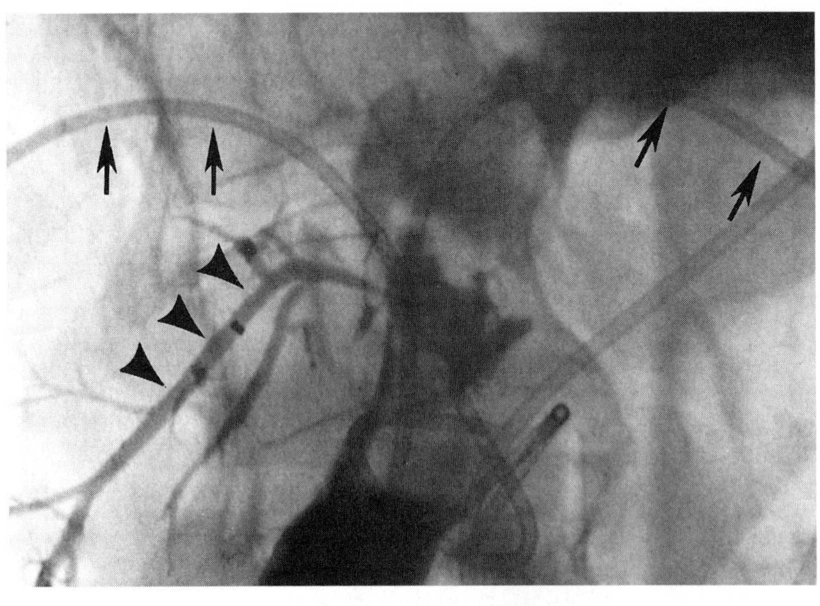

(A)

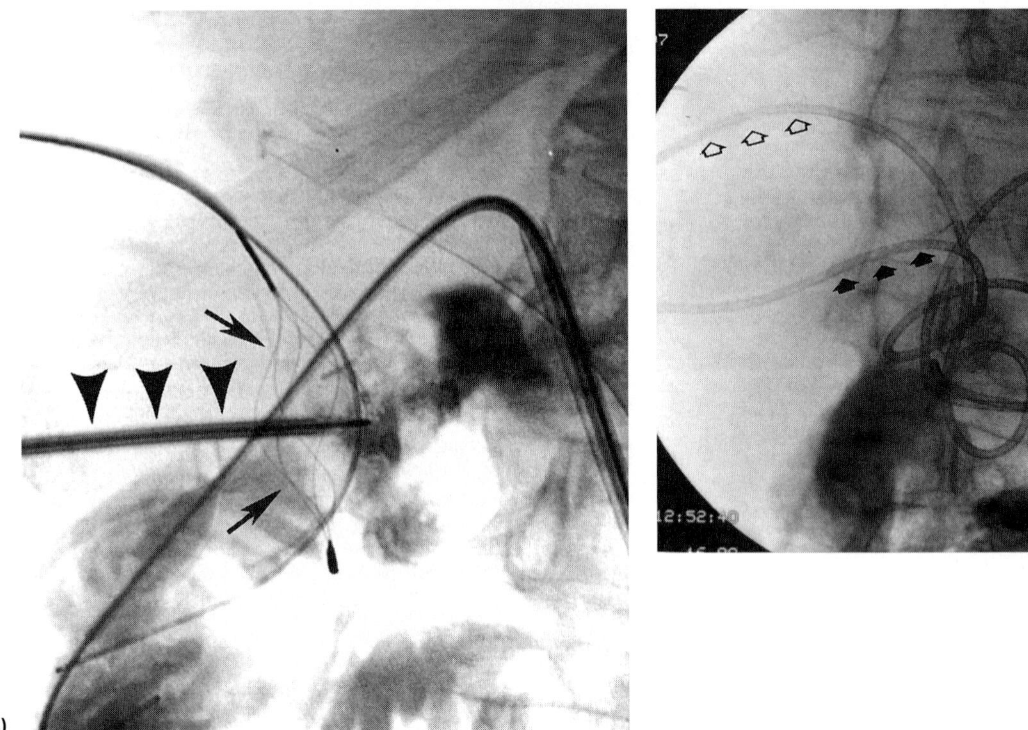

(B)

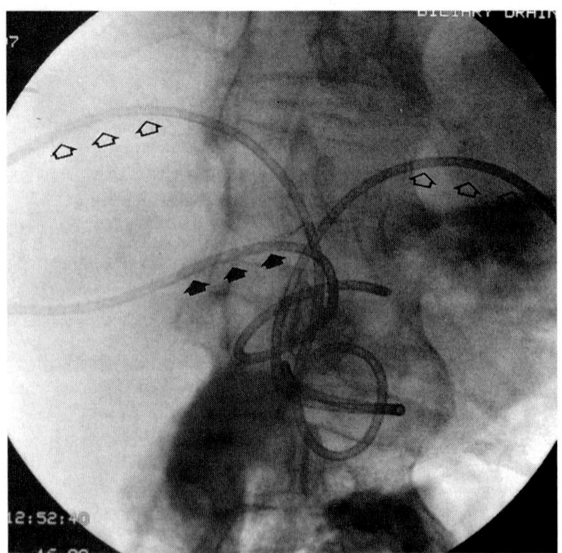

(C)

FIGURE 6.5. ***(A)*** *Contrast was injected into a biloma drain in a patient who had undergone biliary-enteric anastomosis for laparoscopic cholecystectomy bile duct injury. Contrast from the biloma fills an aberrant right hepatic duct (arrowheads) that was excluded from the anastomosis. Two percutaneous biliary drainage catheters (arrows) lie within the intact left and right hepatic ducts that are not opacified.* ***(B)*** *A helical stone extraction basket (arrows) was passed into the jejunum through the intact right hepatic duct into the jejunum. A sharpened guidewire (arrowheads) was passed from the aberrant bile duct through the wall of the jejunum, using the basket as a target.* ***(C)*** *Following tract dilatation, an 8F catheter (closed arrows) was placed, passing from the aberrant right hepatic duct into the jejunum. This catheter was placed to external drainage for 6 weeks, allowing healing of the percutaneous choledochojejunostomy to take place. Bilateral biliary drainage catheters (open arrows) are present in the intact biliary tree.*

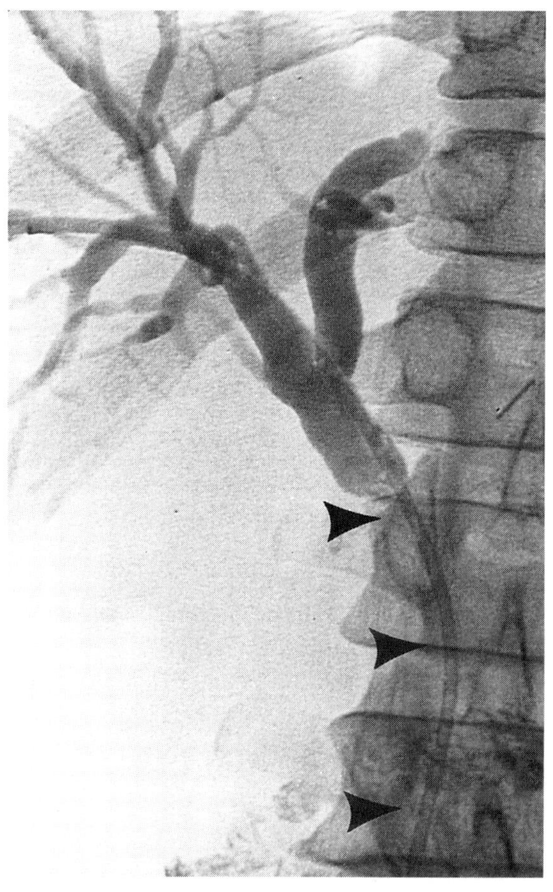

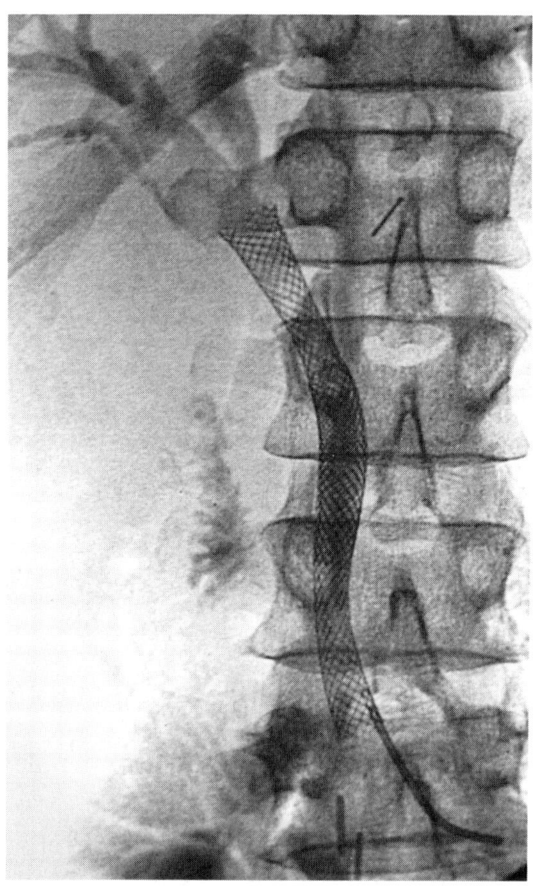

FIGURE 6.6. ***(A)*** *The common hepatic duct and common bile duct are completely obstructed by portal lymph node metastases (arrowheads) from gastric cancer.* ***(B)*** *A 10-mm diameter biliary Wallstent was placed across the tumor between the proximal portion of the common hepatic duct and duodenum.*

expanding Z stents in benign strictures is more favorable. Maccioni et al. (27) reported a patency rate of 68% in a group of 17 patients who received Z stents, with a mean follow-up of 37 months.

BILIARY BIOPSY

It is not always possible to differentiate between benign and malignant biliary strictures on cholangiography (see Chapter 2). Several biliary biopsy techniques have been developed to obtain cells from the stricture for cytologic analysis. Kurzawinski et al. (28) performed a review analysis of the sensitivity and specificity of these techniques for the diagnosis of biliary tract stricture. They reported sensitivities and specificities of 50% to 66% and 93% to 100% for brush cytology, 42% to 67% and 100% for fine-needle aspiration cytology, 30% to 73% and 100% for bile cytology, and 30% to 100% and 100% for endobiliary biopsy forceps.

The Simpson atherectomy catheter is a percutaneous tool that can be used when repeated biopsy attempts yield negative results. The device was originally designed for percutaneous removal of peripheral arterial atheroma. It has a cylindrical blade that shaves off layers of cells and compacts the specimen in a canister for easy removal. Schechter et al. (29) reported the results of 19 Simpson atherectomy catheter shave biopsies in 18 patients who had previous negative brush biopsies (n = 18). Seven of the patients also had negative percutaneous needle biopsies. A histologic diagnosis was obtained in 15 of the 19 biopsies (sensitivity 79%) and included cholangiocarcinoma (n = 7), pancreatic carcinoma (n = 5), metastatic carcinoma (n = 2), and primary sclerosing cholangitis (n = 1). Two transient but significant hemorrhages occurred, one of which required transfusion.

GALLBLADDER INTERVENTIONS

Percutaneous drainage of the gallbladder is indicated for the patient who is unable to undergo emergent operation for

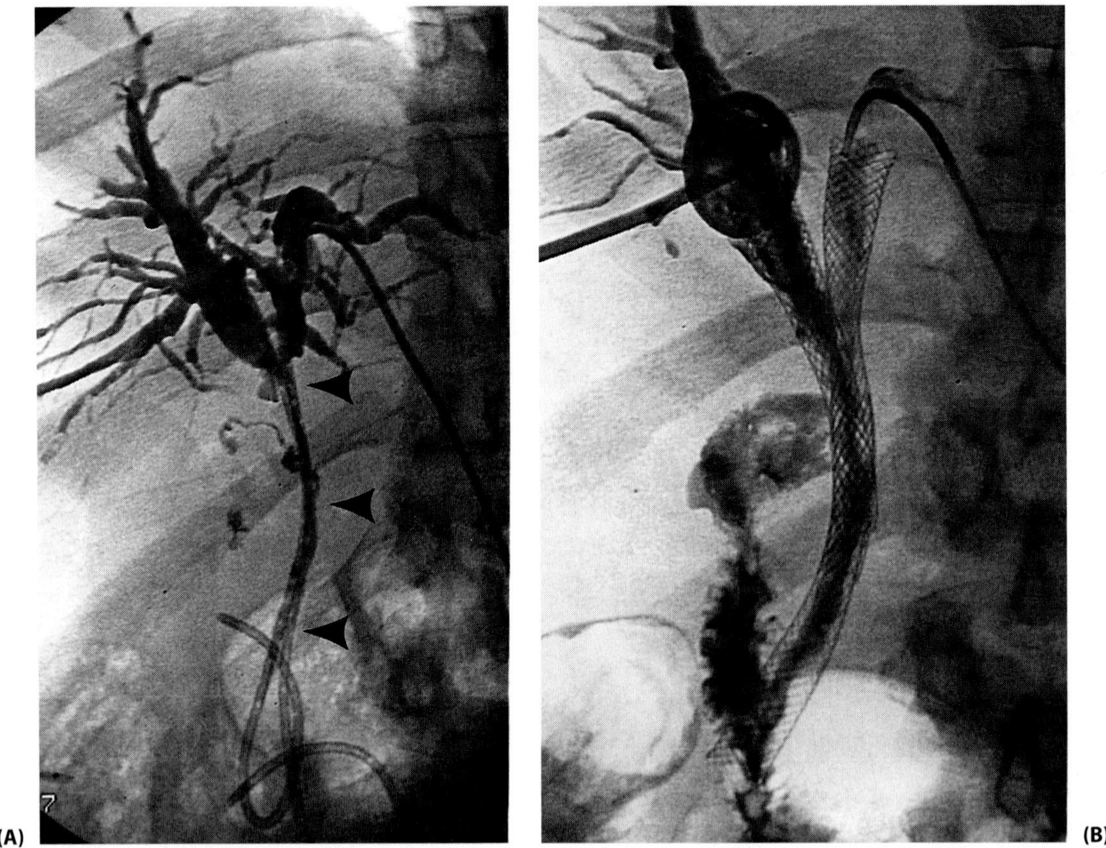

FIGURE 6.7. ***(A)*** *The biliary bifurcation, common hepatic duct, and common bile duct are obstructed by metastatic pancreatic cancer (arrowheads).* ***(B)*** *Bilateral 10-mm biliary Wallstents were simultaneously placed side by side in the common hepatic and common bile duct, extending from the duodenum into the left and right main hepatic ducts.*

acute cholecystitis because of serious comorbidities or being hemodynamically unstable (see Chapter 12). Aspiration of bile from the gallbladder for diagnosing infection is useful only if the results are positive (30). False-negative results of bile aspiration are common (31). Therefore, a gallbladder drain is often empirically placed in patients in whom all other sources of infection have been ruled out. This typically occurs in the intensive care patient who has acalculous cholecystitis and whose radiologic imaging findings are nonspecific. Lee et al. (32) reported a series of 24 patients who had persistent unexplained sepsis and nonspecific findings on gallbladder sonography. Fourteen patients (58%) responded to percutaneous cholecystostomy. Their white blood cell count decreased and they were weaned off vasopressors. Gallbladder drainage is also an effective treatment for spontaneous gallbladder perforation and iatrogenic bile leak (33).

Prior to gallbladder instrumentation, the patient's radiologic images are reviewed. The gallbladder size and any interposed bowel loops in the needle path are noted. The distance from the gallbladder to the anterior skin surface is usually 5 cm (34). The shortest route from the skin to gallbladder usually requires passage of the catheter through 1 cm of liver tissue. Passing the needle through the window of liver tissue also stabilizes the guidewire during tract dilatation and limits the amount of bile leakage around the catheter into the peritoneal cavity.

Gallbladder drainage is most easily performed under sonographic guidance with a needle guide. The procedure is performed in the interventional radiology suite. Coagulation abnormalities are first corrected and antibiotics are administered. An 18-gauge needle is advanced into the gallbladder below the costal margin during quiet respiration. Once the needle tip is confirmed to be inside the gallbladder, fluoroscopic guidance is used to advance a guidewire into the gallbladder. The needle is removed and the tract is dilated to 8F. An 8F pigtail drainage catheter is placed. The catheter is placed to Jackson Pratt bulb drainage. Diagnostic cholecystography is performed after the gallbladder has been drained for 24 to 48 hours (Fig. 6.9). This delay avoids bacteremia caused by tube injection with contrast.

Gallbladder drainage is sometimes performed in the intensive care unit for the patient who is too unstable to be transported to the radiology department. A portable ultrasound unit is used for this life-saving procedure. Portable fluoroscopy, when available, helps ensure safe drainage tube placement.

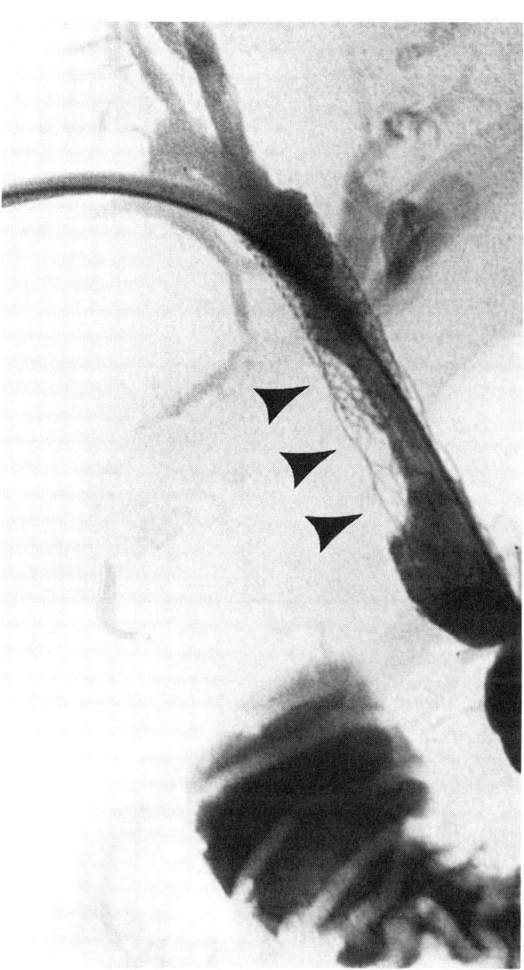

FIGURE 6.8. *Tumor ingrowth (arrowheads) has caused occlusion of a metallic biliary stent in a patient with cholangiocarcinoma.*

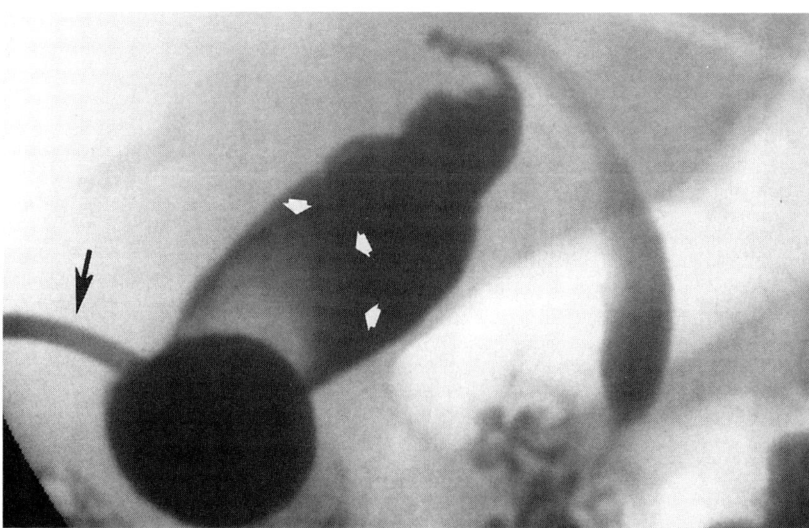

FIGURE 6.9. *A percutaneous drainage catheter (black arrow) was placed in an infected gallbladder containing a large gallstone (white arrows). Contrast flows through the cystic duct into the common bile duct, which is free of stones.*

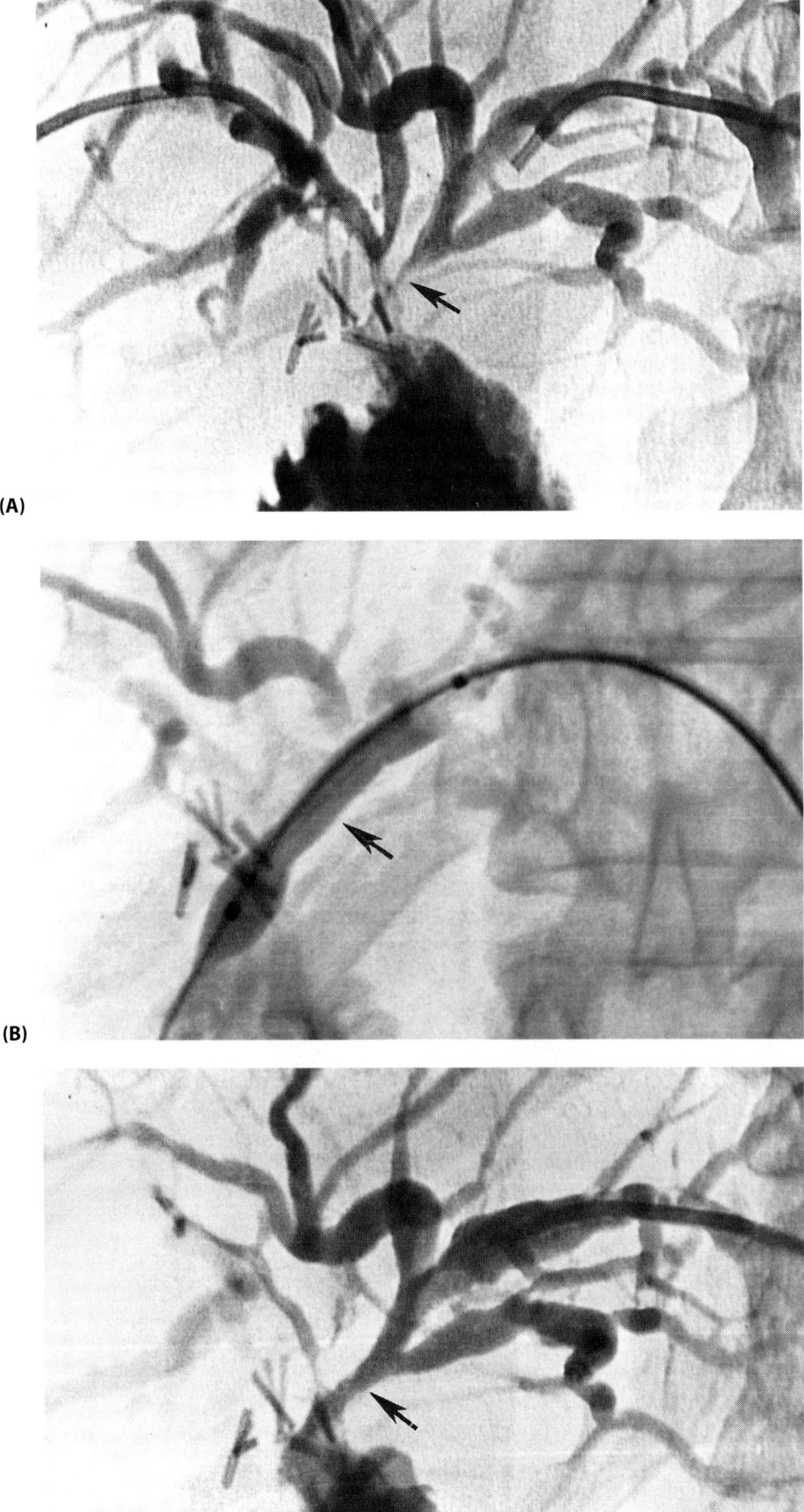

FIGURE 6.10. ***(A)*** *Biliary strictures (arrow) developed in the left and right main hepatic ducts following biliary-enteric anastomosis performed for a bile duct injury that occurred during laparoscopic cholecystectomy.* ***(B)*** *The left main bile duct was balloon (arrow) dilated to 10-mm diameter.* ***(C)*** *There is improvement in the appearance of the left main bile duct (arrow) following balloon dilatation.*

Complications of gallbladder interventions include vagal reactions, hypotension, bile peritonitis, secondary infection, and catheter dislodgement (30). The procedure is safer than surgery for controlling gallbladder sepsis in the acutely ill high-risk patient. There were no procedure-related deaths in a series of 322 patients who underwent gallbladder drainage (35).

After gallbladder drainage, the catheter is left in place until cholecystectomy is performed. If stones are present and the patient will never be an operative candidate, the tube remains in place for the life of the patient. It is exchanged every 3 months. In patients with acalculous cholecystitis, the tube may be removed after contrast injection confirms patency of the cystic duct and common bile duct. The tract should be allowed to mature for 6 weeks before removing the catheter. This prevents leakage of bile into the peritoneal cavity following tube removal.

Although there had been much interest in percutaneous removal of gallstones from the gallbladder and radiologic gallbladder ablation, this interest has waned. Gallstones have been removed from the gallbladder by extraction with a basket, methyl tert-butyl ether (36), and extracorporeal shock wave lithotripsy (37). However, a 50% recurrence rate of gallstones over 5 years was reported in patients whose gallbladder was preserved following stone removal (38).

Several investigators have reported ablating the gallbladder mucosa using liquid sclerosing agents such as ethanol, tetracycline, hot contrast material, morrhuate sodium, cyanoacrylate-nitrocellulose, and trifluoroacetic acid (39–41). These agents cause either complete or partial obliteration of the gallbladder mucosa and lumen. It is essential that the cystic duct be occluded when using these agents to prevent injury to the biliary tree. Becker et al. (42) reported the use of percutaneous bipolar radiofrequency electrocoagulation to ablate the cystic duct prior to gallbladder ablation.

Although gallbladder ablation may seem to be an attractive alternative to surgical removal of the gallbladder, it is not clear what becomes of the gallbladder mucosal remnant over time. Some authors have suggested that there could be an increased risk of gallbladder carcinoma after these procedures (43). The technique of chemical gallbladder ablation has not gained widespread clinical use.

PERCUTANEOUS MANAGEMENT OF BENIGN BILIARY STRICTURES

The treatment of choice for primary benign biliary strictures is surgical repair, which has a success rate of 78% to 88% (44). The most successful surgical repair is a Roux-en-Y choledochojejunostomy (see Chapter 17). Secondary surgical repairs have a success rate of 61% because of periductal scarring and progressive shortening of the bile duct (44).

Percutaneous balloon dilatation of the stricture provides a safe alternative to repeat surgery in patients who develop a recurrent benign biliary stricture at the surgical anastomosis (Fig. 6.10). The biliary tree is accessed transhepatically as described in Chapter 4. Intrahepatic and extrahepatic duct strictures are balloon dilated to 8 to 10 mm diameter. Strictures at the biliary enteric anastomosis are dilated to 10 to 12 mm diameter. An 8F drainage catheter is left in place across the dilated stricture for 2 to 4 weeks. Rossi et al. (44) reported a success rate of 68% for percutaneous balloon dilatation of strictures in 47 patients with a mean 23 months follow-up.

Focal biliary strictures have the lowest recurrence rate following balloon dilatation. Longer or multifocal strictures may not respond to balloon dilatation. They usually require chronic indwelling biliary drainage catheters. As mentioned earlier in this chapter, metallic stents are not widely used to treat benign biliary strictures because of a high reocclusion rate. However, the stent may have a role in treatment of a benign stricture in the transplanted liver. In liver recipients who are not candidates for surgical treatment of a stricture, placement of a stent allows the percutaneous drainage catheter, a source of infection in this group of patients, to be removed (see Chapter 18). Petersen et al. (45) used the Z stent to treat 12 strictures that developed in eight patients following orthotopic liver transplantation. Four of the eight patients did not require reintervention at the follow-up examination after 31 months (mean). The other four patients required repeat percutaneous or endoscopic interventions to maintain stent patency during follow-up.

MANAGEMENT OF HEMOBILIA RELATED TO BILIARY INTERVENTIONS

Hemorrhagic complications during biliary interventions are avoided by accessing only peripheral bile ducts. A fourth order branch duct above the common hepatic duct is a desirable target (46). This avoids injury to large central branches of the portal vein and hepatic artery. Most bleeding associated with a biliary intervention is venous. It occurs when the PBD passes through a portal or hepatic vein. Bleeding occurs around or through the tube. This problem is corrected by proper positioning of the PBD so that the sideholes are located completely within the biliary tree and not in surrounding veins. If a venous bleed cannot be treated in this manner, the PBD is removed and the parenchymal tract is embolized with gelfoam pledgets. A new PBD is then placed using a new access site.

Arterial bleeding is a more worrisome and potentially fatal complication. This occurs when a hepatic artery branch is punctured during PBD. An arterial transection, pseudoaneurysm, or arteriovenous fistula can be created. As with venous complications, bleeding is usually seen through or around the PBD with arterial injuries. An intrahepatic hematoma may also develop. Untreated arterioportal venous fistulae may result in portal venous hypertension. Untreated arteriohepatic venous fistulae may cause high output cardiac failure.

Contrast injection of a PBD is usually unrevealing when an arterial injury has occurred. Emergent angiography should be performed and the radiologist should plan to embolize the injured vessel when one is found. An arterial branch is usually involved, in which case the main hepatic arteries can be spared from embolization. If the arteriogram is normal, the PBD should be removed over a guidewire and the arteriogram repeated. This maneuver releases the tamponade effect of the drainage catheter on the injured vessel and usually discloses the bleeding site. When an abnormal site is seen, the catheter is advanced into the artery and coils are deployed to bridge the site of injury. Acute hepatic failure because of hepatic artery embolization is rare but may occur in the presence of advanced cirrhosis or portal vein occlusion.

Occasionally, the radiologist will tear the intercostal artery during a biliary intervention. Bleeding into the pleural space or the chest wall results. When this occurs, emergent angiography is performed and the catheter is advanced from the aorta into the injured intercostal artery. Coils are deposited on each side of the injury to avoid continued bleeding from both the aortic and internal mammary supplies to the intercostal artery.

SUMMARY

Percutaneous interventions add a host of alternatives for the patients with biliary tract disorders. These procedures can be performed in isolation or in conjunction with surgical or endoscopic procedures. Good technique and knowledge of hepatic anatomy are essential for the safe performance of these procedures. Percutaneous radiologic management of complications is usually possible.

SUGGESTED READINGS

Rossi P, Salvatori FM, Bezzi M, Maccioni F, Porcaro ML, Ricci P. Percutaneous management of benign strictures with balloon dilation and self-expanding metallic stents. Cardiovasc Intervent Radiol 1990;13:231–239. This article compares surgical treatment with percutaneous alternatives for benign biliary strictures.

Wu SM, Marchant LK, Haskal ZJ. Percutaneous interventions in the biliary tree. Semin Roentgenol 1997;32:228–245. This article provides a general overview of currently available percutaneous biliary procedures.

REFERENCES

1. Remolar J, Katz S, Rybak B. Percutaneous transhepatic cholangiography. Gastroenterology 1956;31:39–46.
2. Burhenne H. The history of interventional radiology in the biliary tract. Radiol Clin North Am 1990;28:1139–44.
3. Burhenne H. Nonoperative roentgenologic instrumentation techniques of the postoperative biliary tract: treatment of biliary stricture and retained stones. Am J Surg 1974;128:111–17.
4. Ring E, Husted J, Oleaga J, Freiman D. A multihole catheter for maintaining longterm percutaneous antegrade biliary drainage. Radiology 1979;132:752–4.
5. Suhocki P, Matsumoto A, Potter J, Barth K. Percutaneous transhepatic feeding tube: an alternate method for enteral alimentation. J Interv Radiol 1990;5:65–7.
6. Workman M, Suhocki P, Meyers W, Branch M. Percutaneous transhepatic choledochocholedochostomy in the management of the postoperative patient. J Vasc Interv Radiol 1998;9:359–62.
7. Suhocki P, Clavien P. Percutaneous creation of a choledochojejunostomy between an excluded aberrant bile duct and a Roux-en-Y limb. AJR Am J Roentgenol 1999;172:655–7.
8. Mergener K, Suhocki P, Enns R, et al. Endoscopic nasobiliary drain placement facilitates subsequent percutaneous transhepatic cholangiography. Gastrointest Endosc 1999;49:240–2.
9. Goodwin S, Stainken B, McNamara T, Yoon H. Prevention of significant hemobilia during placement of transhepatic biliary drainage catheters: technique modification and initial results. J Vasc Interv Radiol 1995;6:229–32.
10. Goodwin S, Bansal V, Greaser LI, et al. Prevention of hemobilia during percutaneous biliary drainage: long term followup. J Vasc Interv Radiol 1997;8:881–3.
11. Vingan H, Wohlgemuth S, Bell J. Percutaneous cholecystostomy drainage for the treatment of acute emphysematous cholecystitis. AJR Am J Roentgenol 1990;155:1013–14.
12. Ring E, Gordon R, LaBerge J, Shapiro H. Malignant biliary obstruction complicated by ascites: transjugular insertion of an expandable metallic endoprosthesis. Radiology 1991;180:580–1.
13. Hayashi N, Sakai T, Kitagawa M, et al. Application of gastrointestinal suture anchor to prevent pericatheter fluid leakage in percutaneous biliary drainage. J Vasc Interv Radiol 1996;7:555–6.
14. Cekirge S, Akhan O, Ozmen M, et al. Malignant biliary obstruction complicated by ascites: closure of the transhepatic tract with cyanoacrylate glue after placement of an endoprosthesis. Cardiovasc Intervent Radiolol 1997;20:228–31.
15. Kaude J, Weidenmier C, Agee O. Decompression of bile ducts with the percutaneous transhepatic technique. Radiology 1969;93:69–71.
16. Hoevels J, Lundeerquist A, Ihse I. Percutaneous transhepatic intubation of bile ducts for combined internal-external drainage in preoperative and palliative treatment of obstructive jaundice. Gastrointest Radiol 1978;3:23–31.
17. Becker C, Fache J, Gibney R, Burhenne H. External-internal cross connection for bilateral percutaneous biliary drainage. AJR Am J Roentgenol 1987;149:91–2.
18. Morita S, Matsumoto S, Soejima T, et al. Biliary drainage: conversion of external to internal drainage. Radiology 1988;167:267–8.
19. Soulez G, Therasse E, Olkiva V, et al. Left hepaticogastrostomy for biliary obstruction: long term results. Radiology 1997;204:780–6.
20. Feld R, Wechsler R, Bonn J. Biliary-pleural fistulas without biliary obstruction: percutaneous catheter management. AJR Am J Roentgenol 1997;169:381–3.
21. Moosman D, Coller F. Prevention of traumatic injury to the bile ducts. Am J Surg 1951;82:132–43.
22. Gorich J, Rilinger N, Sokiranski R, et al. Percutaneous transhepatic embolization of bile duct fistulas. J Vasc Interv Radiol 1996;7:435–8.
23. Goodwin SC, Bittner CA, Patel MC, et al. Technique for reduction of bile peritonitis after T-tube removal in liver transplant patients. J Vasc Interv Radiol 1998;9:986–90.
24. Lammer J, Hausegger KA, Fluckiger F, et al. Common bile duct obstruction due to malignancy: treatment with plastic versus metal stents. Radiology 1996;201:167–72.
25. Hausegger K, Kugler C, Uggowitzer M, et al. Benign biliary obstruction: is treatment with the Wallstent advisable? Radiology 1996;200:437–41.
26. Hausegger K, Thumher S, Bodendorfer G, et al. Treatment of malignant biliary obstruction with polyurethane-covered Wallstents. AJR Am J Roentgenol 1998;170:403–8.
27. Maccioni F, Rossi M, Salvatori FM, et al. Metallic stents in benign biliary strictures: three-year follow-up. Cardiovasc Intervent Radiol 1992;15:360–6.
28. Kurzawinski T, Deery A, Davidson BR. Diagnostic value of cytology for biliary stricture. Br J Surg 1993;80:414–21.
29. Schechter MS, Doemeny JM, Johnson JO. Biliary ductal shave biopsy with use of the Simpson atherectomy catheter. J Vasc Interv Radiol 1993;4:819–24.
30. van Sonnenberg E, D'Agostino H, Casola G. Interventional gallbladder procedures. Radiol Clin North Am 1990;28:1185–90.
31. McGahan J, Walter J. Diagnostic percutaneous aspiration of the gallbladder. Radiology 1985;155:619–22.
32. Lee MJ, Saini S, Brink JA, et al. Treatment of critically ill patients with sepsis of unknown cause: value of percutaneous cholecystostomy. AJR Am J Roentgenol 1991;156:1163–6.
33. vanSonnenberg E, D'Agostino H, Casola G, et al. Gallbladder perforation and bile leakage: percutaneous treatment. Radiology 1991;178:687–9.

34. Warren L, Kadir S, Dunnick N. Percutaneous cholecystectomy: anatomic considerations. Radiology 1988;168:615–16.
35. Malone D, Burhenne H. Advantages and disadvantages of the newer "interventional" procedures for the treatment of cholecystolithiasis. Hepatogastroenterology 1989;36:317–26.
36. Allen M, Borody T, Bugliosi T, et al. Rapid dissolution of gallstones by methyl tert-butyl ether: preliminary observations. N Engl J Med 1985;312:217–20.
37. Ferruci J. Biliary lithotripsy 1989. AJR Am J Roentgenol 1989;153:15–22.
38. Lanzini A, Jazrawi R, Kupfer R, et al. Gallstone recurrence after medical dissolution: an overestimated threat? J Hepatol 1986;3:241–6.
39. Gerajdman G, O'Toole K, Logerfo P, et al. Transcatheter sclerosis of the gallbladder in rabbits: a preliminary study. Invest Radiol 1985;20:393–8.
40. Remley K, Cubberley D, Watanabe A, et al. Systemic absorption of gallbladder sclerosing agents in the rabbit. A preliminary study. Invest Radiol 1986;21:396–9.
41. Salomonowitz E, Frick M, Simmons R, et al. Obliteration of the gallbladder without formal cholecystectomy. A feasibility study. Arch Surg 1984;119: 725–9.
42. Becker C, Burhenne H. Percutaneous ablation of the cystic duct and gallbladder: experimental and early clinical results. Radiol Clin North Am 1990;28:1277–87.
43. Blenkinsopp W. Comparison of tetradecyl sulfate of sodium with other sclerosants in rats. Br J Exp Pathol 1986;49:197–201.
44. Rossi P, Salvatori F, Bezzi M, et al. Percutaneous management of benign biliary strictures with balloon dilation and self-expanding metallic stents. Cardiovasc Intervent Radiol 1990;13:231–9.
45. Petersen BD, Maxfield SR, Ivancev K, et al. Biliary strictures in hepatic transplantation: treatment with self-expanding Z stents. J Vasc Interv Radiol 1996;7:221–8.
46. Harris V, Kopecky K, Harman J, Crist D Percutaneous transhepatic drainage of the nondilated biliary system. J Vasc Interv Radiol 1993;4:591–5.

Chapter 7

Radiation Therapy for Disease of the Biliary Tree and Gallbladder

Rachel H. Chou   Catherine G. Lee   Mitchell S. Anscher

HISTORY OF RADIATION THERAPY

In 1895, the x-ray was discovered by Wilhelm Conrad Roentgen of Germany, a professor at the Institute of Physics in the University of Wurzburg (1). The next year, Professor Antoine Henri Becquerel of France discovered natural radioactivity when working with uranium. This was followed by the discovery of radium, another radionuclide, by Madam Marie Curie of France in 1898 (1). During this same time period, in the United States, Thomas A. Edison of New Jersey, Professor W.F. Magie of Princeton, and E.P. Thompson of New York investigated the ability of the newly discovered roentgen ray to induce fluorescence in various combinations of substances and explored its potential clinical use (1).

During the early days after discovery of the roentgen ray, later called the x-ray, various researchers investigated its possible therapeutic effects. Without any significant knowledge regarding the properties of the newly discovered x-ray, it is believed that E.H. Grubbe of Chicago first applied roentgen rays to a patient with carcinoma of the breast on January 29, 1896, and to a case of lupus vulgaris the next day (1). In Europe, in February 1896, Dr. Voigt reported a case of a patient with nasopharyngeal carcinoma whose pain was relieved by treatment with roentgen rays; however, he never published his report. Dr. V. Despeignes of Lyon, France, was credited with having been the first to publish on the therapeutic application of roentgen rays to a patient with gastric carcinoma in July 1896 (2).

Thereafter, many investigators in both the United States and Europe began to use x-rays to treat various malignant and nonmalignant diseases. Because of the low energy and limited penetration of x-rays in the early years, only cutaneous lesions and other superficial malignant diseases were treated. Some investigators tried to apply the x-ray to treat more deeply situated tumors within the body, though they reported side effects, especially radiation-induced "dermatitis." In 1902, C.E. Skinner was the first investigator to report on "The x-ray treatment of intra-abdominal and other deeply located malignant growths" (3). In his report, he described 33 cases of such "deep cancer." Other investigators proposed the direct implantation of radioactive sources into deep seated tumors (referred to as brachytherapy); however, this approach was not used in the treatment of biliary malignancies until later in the 20th century (1).

In the early 20th century, the effects of radiation delivered to the hepatobiliary region were largely unknown; however, there were early reports on irradiation of the hepatobiliary region in various animal models. Inflammation, congestion, edema, hemorrhage, and necrosis of epithelium were observed (5). These were followed by two reports on changes in the human hepatobiliary region caused by irradiation: in 1921, Wetzel published on necrosis of the liver following x-ray therapy for gastric cancer; and in 1924, Case and Warthin reported on three cases in which x-ray was used for treating malignancies in the upper gastrointestinal region (4,5). From the gross examination and histopathologic studies of the autopsies, they concluded that the epithelium of the biliary tract, especially the smaller ducts, could be injured by irradiation. They further characterized the injury as "vacuolation, swelling, and necrosis of the epithelial cells of the ducts, and by a slow and atypical regeneration" eventually resulting in "biostasis and hemorrhage." It was nearly 20 years later that Warren described the effects of radiation on normal tissue, including the gallbladder and biliary region, with similar findings (6).

It was not until the 1950s that radiotherapy became more commonly used in the treatment for malignancy of the gallbladder and biliary tract, collectively called the extrahepatic bile duct (EHBD) system, as it was then that sources of higher energy such as cobalt 60 and, later, linear accelerators became widely available (7). These high energy x-ray sources permitted the delivery of therapeutic radiation doses at depth, while sparing the superficial structures.

Early reports of radiotherapy for gallbladder and bile duct cancer focused on its use in the palliative setting, with an occasional cure reported (8–13). In 1972, Krain reviewed over 1800 cases of gallbladder and EHBD carcinoma from the California tumor registry and reported that 24% of patients had received radiotherapy during the course of their disease (9). Green et al. and Hudgins et al. reported on the palliative benefit of radiation therapy in treating bile duct carcinoma, as evidenced by the relief of jaundice, tumor shrinkage, and, rarely, tumor disappearance (10,11). Kopelson and colleagues also described similar successful palliation with radiotherapy; in their series, 92% of patients were significantly palliated by irradiation (12). Pilepich and Lambert also reported occasional long-term disease-free survival following external beam irradiation and suggested that radiotherapy may contribute to the cure of EHBD carcinoma (13).

TOLERANCE OF THE HEPATOBILIARY TREE, LIVER, AND SURROUNDING STRUCTURES TO RADIATION

When using radiotherapy for treating malignancy, one must respect the radiation tolerance of the particular organ and its surrounding structures. Tolerance depends upon many factors, including volume of tissue irradiated, the dose per fraction, the use of chemotherapy, and other coexisting conditions such as diabetes. The dose-limiting organs, when irradiating the hepatobiliary tree, are the liver parenchyma and bile ducts, kidneys, small bowel, stomach, distal esophagus, and spinal cord. Rubin and colleagues described the therapeutic use of assigning a certain percentage risk of complication, based upon the fractionation, treatment volume, and the cumulative radiation dose (14). The data are derived empirically and are not based on formal dose escalation studies. The minimal tolerance dose is defined as TD 5/5, representing the radiation dose which results in a 5% severe complication rate within 5 years after irradiation. TD 50/5 is defined as having 50% or more probability of developing severe complication within 5 years after treatment. Table 7.1 summarizes radiation tolerances of various organs (15).

In general, the whole liver should receive less than 30 Gy (grays) at 1.8–2.0 Gy per fraction over 3 to 4 weeks with the potential risk of liver toxicity rising when the total liver dose exceeds 40 Gy (16). However, recent studies using three-dimensional conformal radiotherapy (3D-CRT), a technique that allows deposition of a very high dose to only a small field while sparing the surrounding tissues, have shown that partial liver can tolerate much higher doses than

Table 7.1. Normal tissue tolerance to irradiation (with fractionated dose of 1.8 Gy/day)

Structure	TD 5/5[a] (Gy)	TD 50/5[a] (Gy)
Whole liver	30	40
Partial liver	see text	—
Bile duct	60	—
Duodenum	50	60
Small bowel	50	60
Esophagus	60	75
Stomach	50	55
Kidney	23	28
Spinal cord	50	60

[a] TD 5/5 represents the radiation dose which results in a 5% severe complication rate within 5 years after irradiation. TD 50/5 is defined as having 50% or more probability of developing severe complication within 5 years after treatment.

previously believed (17–20). The investigators from University of Michigan have reported that less than 33% of the "normal" liver can be safely treated with 3D-CRT at 66.0–72.6 Gy in 1.5–1.65 Gy twice a day fractionation and 34% to 66% of the liver can be irradiated to 48–52 Gy (8) in the same fashion, with "normal" liver being the portion of the liver not occupied by tumor (19–20). Tolerance of the bile duct is thought to be 60 Gy in 30–33 fractions, including the intrahepatic bile duct, when the dose is targeted to a small volume only (16).

When kidneys are included in the treatment fields, a minimum of two-thirds of a single functional kidney should be excluded from the field to reduce the risk of irreversible renal complications. Strictly speaking, renal dose is limited to 15–18 Gy at standard time dose fractionation, much lower than its TD 5/5, to avoid irreversible damage. Tolerance of the spinal cord, small intestine, and stomach is 45–50 Gy of external beam radiotherapy (EBRT) in 1.8–2.0 Gy per fraction, depending upon the volume and dose-fractionation.

Increasing use of brachytherapy and intraoperative radiotherapy (IORT) also gives us more understanding of the radiation tolerance of the upper abdominal organs. IORT delivers a single large dose of radiotherapy in the operating room while the extent of tumor and surrounding normal tissues are fully visualized. Figure 7.1 demonstrates the use of IORT with an electron treatment cone "docking" in the tumor bed in the operating suite. Electrons are typically used for IORT rather than photons because of the rapid dose fall-off with distance, resulting in much less dose to the surrounding normal critical structures. Intraluminal transcatheter brachytherapy allows the delivery of radioactive sources such as Ir-192 to the tumor through a percutaneous transhepatic biliary drainage (PTBD) tube under fluoroscopic guidance or through catheters which are placed in

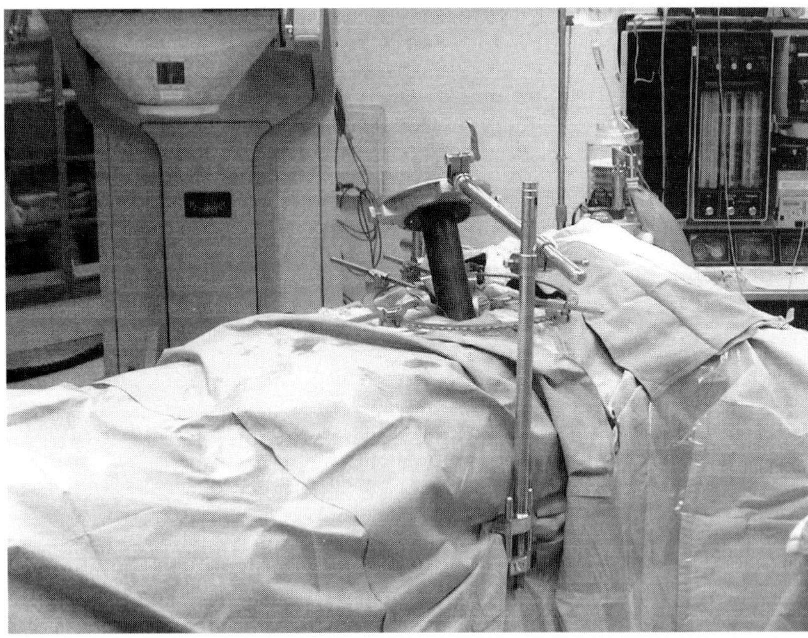

FIGURE 7.1. *The use of intraoperative radiotherapy with an electron treatment cone "docking" in the tumor bed in the operating suite. The cone will be connected to the linear accelerator for treatment. (Courtesy Joe Hsu, M.D., Department of Radiation Oncology, University of California at San Francisco.)*

the tumor bed during surgery. Figure 7.2 depicts the placement of intraluminal Ir-192 seeds via a PTBD tube. Both IORT and brachytherapy can be used to attain higher doses without exceeding normal tissue tolerances, as the dose fall-off with distance is quite rapid with either electrons or Ir-192, in contrast to high energy photons used for EBRT. Iwasaki et al. (21) have shown that the incidence of complications from IORT is minimized if the dose is 20 Gy or less in one fraction. Buskirk et al. (22) also recommend that Ir-192 catheter brachytherapy boost be limited to under 20–30 Gy when combined with EBRT of 45–50 Gy in 25–28 fractions.

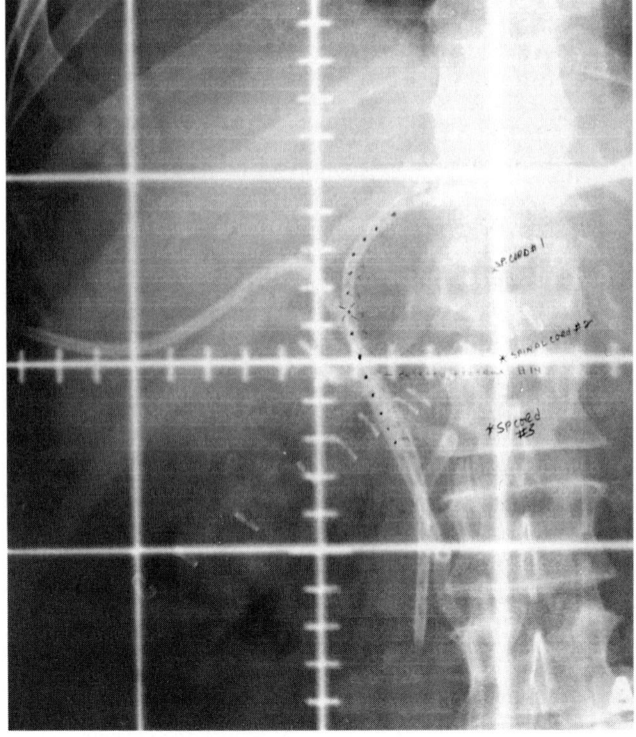

FIGURE 7.2. *Placement of intraluminal Ir-192 seeds via a percutaneous transhepatic biliary drainage catheter. The pencil marks are used to locate the seeds within the catheter.*

THE PROBLEM OF LOCAL TUMOR CONTROL

Patients with primary carcinoma of the gallbladder and bile duct cancer are rarely, if ever, cured with any treatment modality other than surgical resection. However, the majority of patients have locally infiltrative disease with only 20% to 30% of patients being resectable at presentation. Of those who undergo a "curative" resection, at least 50% experience a locoregional recurrence (12). Furthermore, most patients die secondary to locoregional disease progression resulting in biliary obstruction, eventual sepsis, and liver failure. Therefore, the majority of patients with gallbladder and biliary carcinomas are only benefited by palliative treatment, consisting of the establishment and ongoing management of biliary drainage. Survival is poor: 2 to 3 months for patients who receive medical management, 6 to 12 months for those who undergo surgical palliation, and 12 to 22 months for those patients that are resected. Five-year survival remains dismal at less than 10% (16).

ANATOMY AND ROUTE OF SPREAD WITH REGARD TO RADIATION THERAPY PLANNING

For radiation therapy planning, it is important to include all potential areas of local spread either by direct extension or by metastases to lymph nodes, as local progression or relapse is the major mode of failure for carcinomas of the gallbladder and bile duct. In patients with cancer of the gallbladder, hepatic involvement by direct extension or satellite nodules via venous drainage into the portal vein is very common, ranging from 51% to 67% (23). Obstruction of the common and cystic ducts by local extension is also frequent. Peritoneal seeding is seen in 20% of patients with gallbladder cancer (23). Lymphatic drainage is initially to the cystic or hiatal lymph nodes, and then to the superior pancreaticoduodenal nodes to the celiac axis, and eventually to the superior mesenteric or aortic system. In 2011 cases of 41 combined series, regional lymph nodes were involved in 42% of patients at exploration and 50% at autopsy; retroperitoneal lymph nodes were involved in 23% and 26%, respectively (23).

Similarly, local spread to adjacent organs by direct extension and by metastasis to draining lymph nodes are also very common for bile duct carcinomas, especially intrahepatic cholangiocarcinoma. The initial lymphatic drainage is to the porta hepatis and to the celiac axis. Peritoneal seeding is seen in fewer than 10% of patients with bile duct cancer (23). Other distant metastatic sites include lung and bones.

TREATMENT OF GALLBLADDER AND BILE DUCT TUMORS WITH RADIOTHERAPY: RADIATION DOSE RESPONSE

Mittal et al. (24) have observed a radiation dose response in gallbladder and biliary cancer. The patients who received radiation doses greater than or equal to 45 Gy had longer median survivals than those receiving less than 45 Gy. Mahe et al. (25) and Hayes et al. (26) also suggest a radiation dose response for bile duct carcinoma; the median survival in patients treated with curative intent and palliative intent (i.e., radiation doses ≥42 Gy vs. ≤35 Gy) was 22 and 10 months, respectively, in Mahe's series, and 12.8 and 2 months in the Hayes series, respectively (25,26). The results, however, are very likely to be confounded by the extent of disease at presentation and patient's overall medical conditions. Both factors could easily influence the physician's decision regarding curative versus noncurative treatment.

A dose response is, however, more convincingly suggested by Alden and colleagues from Thomas Jefferson University Hospital. Patients in their study who were treated to a combined dose of EBRT and Ir-192 brachytherapy of more than 55 Gy or less than 55 Gy had a median survival of 24 months and 6 months, with 2-year survival rates of 48 and no survivors, respectively (27). Furthermore, the authors noted the lengthening of the median survival with increasing irradiation dose; the median survival is 4.5, 9, 18, 25, and 24 months for the groups of greater than 45 Gy, 45–54 Gy, 55–65 Gy, 66–70 Gy, and greater than 70 Gy, respectively. However, none of the studies were randomized, so the outcome could have easily influenced by patient selection bias.

Postoperative Radiotherapy

Because of the high locoregional recurrence rate, even in the setting of a potentially curative resection, multiple studies have explored the role of postoperative radiotherapy. Although no randomized comparisons have been conducted, most nonrandomized studies have demonstrated a survival advantage with the addition of postoperative RT after either a complete or incomplete resection. Kopelson et al. (12) noted that 3 of 13 patients who received irradiation with curative intent following surgery had a longer average survival (31.9 months), compared with the entire cohort (12.7 months). Treadwell and Hardin reviewed 41 cases of gallbladder carcinoma, reporting a similar benefit of adjuvant radiation therapy (RT) following surgery at one year (28). Twenty-six patients underwent surgery alone and 15 patients received adjuvant RT or chemotherapy. The investigators observed longer survivals in patients who received adjuvant treatment; however, the benefit of improved survival disappeared at 2 years.

Recently, the EORTC (European Organization for Research and Treatment of Cancer) retrospectively reviewed 112 patients with Klatskin tumors (tumors at the bifurcation of common hepatic duct) treated at seven centers, and found statistically improved survivals in patients receiving resection and postoperative radiotherapy versus those with resection only (median survivals of 19 versus 8.3 months). The 3-year survival rates for postoperative irradiation versus surgery alone group were 31% and 10%, respectively (29).

Cameron et al. (30) also reported similar findings from Johns Hopkins Hospital. In this series of 96 patients with proximal cholangiocarcinoma treated surgically, 41% underwent curative resection, 14% had noncurative resections, and 45% underwent palliative stenting. Sixty-six percent of patients received postoperative RT. Patients with gross total resection or major debulking surgery had increased survival versus those in the stented group. The 1-, 3-, 5-, and 10-year survivals in the resected group were 66%, 21%, 8%, and 4%, respectively, and these values were superior to those in the stented group of 27, 6, none, and none, respectively. Longer survival was seen in those stented patients who underwent RT versus those treated with stent only. The actuarial survival at 2 years in the stented plus RT and stented-only groups were 10% and none, respectively. A survival difference was also noted between patients treated with resection alone compared to those who also received adjuvant postoperative RT. The actuarial survival rates at 5 years in the adjuvant RT versus resection alone groups were 16% and none, respectively. The difference, however, did not reach statistical significance secondary to the small number of patients. All three of the 5-year survivors in the resection group received postoperative radiotherapy.

Pitt et al. (31), also from Johns Hopkins Hospital, later reported a follow-up prospective nonrandomized study of perihilar cholangiocarcinoma and concluded that postoperative radiotherapy does not improve survival, in contrast to their previous observations. In this study, 50 patients who underwent resection or palliative decompression without distant metastases and with a Karnofsky Performance Status of 60 or more were considered eligible for postoperative RT. The decision as to whether to deliver RT was based on patient preference, after evaluation by the radiation oncologists. The mean dose in the group of patients who received adjuvant RT after curative resection was 54 Gy and 51 Gy for the palliative surgery plus RT group. Radiotherapy was given as either EBRT only or EBRT plus Ir-192 implant. In the group undergoing curative resection, there was no difference in median survivals between the patients who did or did not receive RT (20 vs. 20 months). There was also no statistically significant difference in median survival between the palliative surgery and the palliative surgery plus RT patients (8 vs. 12.5 months). However, there were several major flaws in the study. Most importantly, the cohort population is very small, and therefore the study did not have the power to detect a significant difference between treatment groups. In this study, 31/50 patients underwent a complete or partial tumor resection, and the remaining 19 patients underwent palliative surgical procedures. Fourteen of 31 resected patients and 9 of the 19 palliative patients received postoperative radiotherapy. Of those 14 patients who received adjuvant RT after curative resection, the investigators did not specify the extent of surgery (i.e., gross total resection vs. partial resection). This distinction is important as many studies in the literature have observed a survival difference between these two groups. Furthermore, more patients in the radiation group had a higher percentage of known surgical and pathological adverse features, including vascular invasion, hepatic extension, and lymphatic involvement. In addition, the RT protocol varied among the resected patients. Eight of the 14 resected patients received EBRT plus Ir-192 brachytherapy, and the remaining 6 patients received EBRT alone. Thus, no conclusions as to the benefit, or lack thereof, from postoperative RT can reasonably be drawn from this study. A summary of these studies is compiled in Table 7.2.

Table 7.2. Outcomes following surgery for biliary cancers with or without postoperative radiotherapy (RT)

Author	N	RT	RT Dose (Gy)	Median Survival (months)	3-Year Survival (%)	Local Control (%)
Kopelson (12)	13	Yes	38–72.25	12.7[a]	—	15
Treadwell (28)	15	Yes	10–45	—	47[b]	—
	26	No	—	—	27[b]	—
Gonzalez (29)	95	Yes	10–80	19	31	—
	17	No		8.3	10	—
Cameron (30)	63	Yes	50–80	—	21	—
	33	No		—	0	—
Pitt (31)	23	Yes	51–54[c]	20[d]	—	—
	27	No		20[d]	—	—

[a] 31.9 months for patients treated with a curative intent.
[b] 1-year survival rate.
[c] Mean dose.
[d] Patients treated with a curative intent.

Radiotherapy for Unresectable Disease

For patients with unresectable disease, further palliative therapy after biliary bypass has been shown to prolong survival. Farley et al. (32) reported on 103 patients in which the 3-year survival was 9% for the entire cohort. In this study, the univariate analysis showed a survival advantage for those patients who had additional palliative therapy such as radiotherapy ($P < 0.01$), though the details were not given. Grove et al. (33) also noted a survival advantage for those unresected patients without metastatic disease who received RT versus those who did not (12.2 vs. 2.2 months, median survival) (33). Veeze-Kuijpers et al. (34) reported a 14% 2-year survival and 10-month median survival in 42 patients with unresectable EHBD carcinoma who received the EBRT with or without an Ir-192 implant boost. They noted that patients undergoing debulking surgery followed by RT had a longer median survival than those receiving radiation alone (15 vs. 8 months). A summary of studies regarding unresectable disease is listed in Table 7.3.

Table 7.3. Results of radiotherapy (RT) for unresectable biliary cancers

Author	N	RT	RT Dose (Gy)	Medial Survival (months)	3-Year Survival (%)	Local Control (%)
Farley (32)	103	Yes[a]	—	—	9%	—
Grove (33)	19	Yes	12.6–64.0	12.2	—	—
	9	No	—	2.2	—	—
Veeze-Kuijpers (34)	42	Yes	30–65	10	14%[b]	—

[a] In some patients but details not given.
[b] 2-year survival rate.

Intraluminal Transcatheter Brachytherapy

Despite the addition of EBRT, most patients with gallbladder and bile duct cancer still die of disease due to local progression and obstruction of the biliary tree. Newer modalities of radiotherapy such as intraluminal brachytherapy have been used alone or in conjunction with EBRT in treating gallbladder and biliary carcinoma. The advantage of intraluminal brachytherapy is that a high radiation dose can be administered to the tumor with a rapid fall-off of the dose at a short distance from the source, thus sparing adjacent normal tissues. Doses of 20–30 Gy at 10 Gy per day are typically prescribed at a distance of 0.5 cm to 1 cm from the iridium source, in conjunction with EBRT of 45–50.4 Gy in 25–28 fractions.

Since the original report by Fletcher and co-workers describing the use of intraluminal brachytherapy with Ir-192, multiple series have demonstrated the feasibility of using brachytherapy alone or in combination with EBRT for treating gallbladder and bile duct cancer (22,26,27,29,30,34–39). Although there are no randomized trials comparing combined EBRT plus brachytherapy with either modality alone, there is a suggestion of improved median survival among patients treated with combined treatment. Combined EBRT and intraluminal brachytherapy can also provide good to excellent palliation (25,40,41). In fact, long-term survivals for resected patients with the use of such aggressive treatment with EBRT and transcatheter brachytherapy boost have been reported. Foo et al. (38) reported the Mayo Clinic experience in which 24 patients with unresectable EHBD cancer were treated with EBRT doses of 50.4 Gy in 28 fractions and a brachytherapy boost of 20 Gy delivered at 1-cm radius (the median implant duration was 42 hours). The median survival for all patients was 12.8 months and 5-year survival was 14%. Three patients were still alive at the time of the report at 10 years, 6.9 years, and 8.2 years after diagnosis.

Buskirk and co-workers have shown that of those patients treated with "curative intent," only those who received "specialized" boosts (Ir-192 implant or IORT) in addition to EBRT or those who underwent total or subtotal excision in addition to EBRT experienced survival longer than 18 months (42). They also noted that patients who received an Ir-192 boost or IORT experienced lower rates of local failure than those who received EBRT alone (± 5-fluorouracil chemotherapy). Fields et al. (39) have described 20 patients treated with curative intent; those who received an Ir-192 implant in addition to EBRT exhibited an improved survival when compared to those patients who received EBRT alone (median survival of 15 vs. 7 months). Montemaggi and coworkers have likewise concluded that the addition of intraluminal RT after biliary drainage prolongs survival (41).

Combining EBRT with intraluminal brachytherapy has also been shown to extend stent patency in the unresectable palliative setting. Eschelman et al. (43) have prospectively described a mean metal stent patency of 19.5 months and a mean survival of 22.6 months in 11 patients with cholangiocarcinoma. Their mean stent patency compared favorably with the surgical literature on stenting alone following malignant biliary obstruction (mean stent patency, ranging 5 to 10 months). Patients with biliary obstruction due to metastasis also had a mean stent patency of 4.8 months and a mean survival of 5.3 months, following Ir-192 implant with or without EBRT or chemotherapy. The results for metastatic disease were similar but not superior to the surgical literature and the authors partially attributed this to their underlying advanced disease at the time of treatment.

The most commonly used intraluminal brachytherapy is low dose rate brachytherapy, typically delivering doses of 0.4–0.6 Gy/hour at 0.5 to 1.0 cm, using Ir-192 sources. A PTBD tube placement is necessary for the delivery of intraluminal brachytherapy. Prior to loading of the active sources, a PTBD catheter is typically changed over a wire for a larger 10 French Ford stent which is more conducive to loading and accommodating the Ir-192 implant. Dummy sources are first inserted to aid in the treatment planning. Active sources are then loaded and accuracy of their final placement is confirmed by orthogonal films. Dose calculations are performed and sources remain in place an approximate length of time to deliver the prescribed dose. Following unloading of the implant, the Ford stent is again changed out over a wire for a PTBD catheter and the patient is typically discharged to home the same day.

High dose rate brachytherapy which delivers over 0.2 Gy/minute using a higher activity Ir-192 source has also been explored recently in treating gallbladder and bile duct cancer. Fritz and colleagues reported improved survival in 30 unresectable biliary cancer patients treated with combined EBRT and intraluminal high dose rate Ir-192 brachytherapy. The actuarial survival was 34% at 1 year, 18% at 2 and 3 years, and 8% at 5 years (44).

Although there are no randomized data to indicate improved survival with radiotherapy in unresectable disease and patient selection bias may influence the nonrandomized results, the retrospective data from multiple studies suggest that improved survival is the case. The addition of intraluminal radiotherapy to EBRT appears to be beneficial, probably because of the relatively high dose of RT delivered to the primary tumor along the bile ducts, where the highest volume of gross disease exists. Table 7.4 summarizes the outcomes of the above studies.

Intraoperative Radiotherapy

IORT allows the delivery of a single high dose of irradiation to the target in the operating room while sparing the surrounding normal tissues. The most commonly used radiation source for IORT is an electron beam, chosen for its rapid dose fall-off with distance. IORT theoretically has advantages over intraluminal brachytherapy, as small bowel, stomach, duodenum, and other normal structures can be displaced during the procedure, thus sparing these tissues. The typical IORT dose is 12–20 Gy in 1 fraction, generally delivered in conjunction with EBRT of 45–50.4 Gy in 25–28 fractions.

The potential role of IORT in the treatment of bile duct cancer was first reported by Japanese physicians. Iwasaki et al. (21) were among the first to report on the use of IORT alone or in conjunction with EBRT in 20 patients with bile duct cancer. IORT combined with noncurative resections showed a superior 2-year survival rate of 17%, comparing favorably to 9% after noncurative resection alone. Deziel and co-workers reviewed the Rush-Presbyterian experience in 9 patients with localized unresectable or partially resected proximal biliary tract cancer and described a median survival of 13 months for use of IORT with or without EBRT (45). They noticed that the survival was comparable to the 13 contemporaneous patients treated with EBRT with or without Ir-192 brachytherapy at their institution. Busse et al. (46) also reported similar results for 15 (12 primary, 3 recurrent) patients treated with IORT with or without EBRT. The median survival of the 12 patients with primary cancer was 14 months, with disease controlled in the porta hepatis in 5 of the 10 patients who could be evaluated. The three patients with recurrent disease were still alive at 2, 9, and 11 months at the time of their report. Monson et al. (47) also described similar positive results from the Mayo Clinic with IORT for unresectable cholangiocarcinoma in 13 patients, who had a median survival of 16.5 months. The results of IORT studies are also summarized in Table 7.4.

Intrahepatic Cholangiocarcinoma

A review of the literature reveals no significant survival difference between intrahepatic and extrahepatic bile duct cancer stage for stage and the treatment philosophy is essentially the same. Altaee et al., at Kings College in London, reported the same median survival of 12 months for 42 patients with intrahepatic cholangiocarcinoma and for 70 patients with perihilar bile duct cancer (48). Chen et al. (49) from Taiwan reviewed 20 patients with intrahepatic cholangiocarcinoma who underwent curative or palliative surgery followed by intraluminal brachytherapy and chemotherapy. The median survival was 20.5 months; four patients lived more than 3 years and one patient was still alive at 5 years. The seemingly improved survival was felt to be due to early diagnosis in 80% of patients.

Table 7.4. Outcome of external beam radiotherapy plus boost (intraoperative radiotherapy or brachytherapy for biliary cancers

Author	N	Boost (I/B)[a]	Median Survival (months)	5-Year Survival (%)	Local Control (%)
Foo (38)	24	B	12.8	14	—
Buskirk (42)	17	I/B	—	30–43[b]	67–70[c]
	17	No	—	12	47
Fields (39)	8	B	15	—	—
	12	No	7	—	—
Montemaggi (41)	12	B	14	—	—
Eschelman (43)	11	B	22.6[d]	—	—
Fritz (44)	30	B	—	8	—
Iwasaki (21)	20	I	—	17[e]	—
	41	No	—	9[e]	—
Deziel (45)	9	I	14	—	50
Busse (46)	12	I	14	—	50
Monson (47)	13	I	16.5	—	50

[a] Boost technique: I = IORT, B = brachytherapy, I/B = some patients received IORT while others received brachytherapy.
[b] 18-month survival rate, 30% = brachytherapy, 43% = IORT.
[c] 67% with IORT and 70% with brachytherapy.
[d] 2-year survival rate with non-curative resections.
[e] Mean survival.

Radiosensitization with Chemotherapy

The role of chemotherapy alone or in combination with radiation therapy for gallbladder and bile duct carcinoma remains unclear. A number of studies have reported the use of various combinations of chemotherapy in conjunction with RT with or without surgery. However, the number of patients who received chemotherapy was too small to draw any meaningful conclusions. Despite small numbers of patients who received various combinations of chemotherapy, preliminary results are encouraging.

Minsky and co-workers reported an aggressive combined modality treatment for biliary carcinoma in 12 patients using EBRT, brachytherapy boost, and concurrent 5-fluorouracil (5-FU) and mitomycin-C chemotherapy with or without a curative resection (36,37). Five patients had a surgical decompression and the remaining seven had a biopsy or subtotal resection of the tumor. The median survival was 17 months and the overall 4-year actuarial survival was 36%. Four patients had no evidence of disease at 16, 30, 40, and 64 months, respectively. Alden and colleagues described a similar aggressive approach in 19 patients with EHBD cancer using EBRT, brachytherapy, and chemotherapy (5-FU alone or in combination with Adriamycin or mitomycin-C) (27). They observed a 2-year survival rate of 30%. In an early study, Kopelson et al. (12) also showed the feasibility and potential benefit of chemotherapy in addition to radiation. A summary of these studies is listed in Table 7.5.

Table 7.5. Concurrent chemoradiotherapy for biliary carcinomas

Author	N	Chemotherapy Media	4-Year Survival (months)	Survival (%)
Minsky (36, 37)	12	5-FU + mitomycin-C[a]	17	36
Alden (27)	19	5-FU[b]	—	30[c]
Kopelson (12)	13	5-FU	12.7	—

[a] 5-FU = 5-fluorouracil.
[b] 5-FU alone or in combination with adriamycin or mitomycin-C.
[c] 2-year survival rate.

Preoperative Radiotherapy

Because of the high risk of locoregional recurrence, despite multimodality treatment with surgery, radiation with or without chemotherapy, and the low percentage of potentially resectable patients, novel treatment approaches to improve the local control and survival of gallbladder and biliary carcinoma are being explored. At Duke University Medical Center, we have treated marginally resectable and resectable cases of EHBD cancer with preoperative chemoradiotherapy with EBRT and 5-FU via continuous infusion, or an oral derivative of 5-FU which mimics a continuous infusion, followed by attempted resection with or without low dose rate intraluminal brachytherapy boost with Ir-192. The preliminary results (unpublished data) appear to be encouraging when compared to historical data in the postoperative adjuvant setting. This approach allows adjuvant therapy to be delivered in a timely fashion to all patients deemed appropriate, potentially shrinking the tumor and sterilizing microscopic disease that has spread along the bile duct mucosa or submucosa and lymph nodes. In addition, it allows a period of observation to ensure that metastases are not occurring at such a rapid rate as to render resection unbeneficial.

We have treated five patients with radiographically resectable cholangiocarcinoma with neoadjuvant 5-FU and EBRT. All patients underwent staging laparoscopy prior to chemoradiation. Two of six patients underwent Whipple resections; one had a pathologic complete response and is alive without evidence of cancer 7.5 months after diagnosis. The other resected patient had residual disease and died of unrelated causes 23 months after diagnosis. At autopsy, local residual disease was found. Of the remaining three patients, one underwent exploratory laparotomy; a palliative biliary bypass was performed, as she was found to have liver metastases. One patient continued to decline and never underwent surgery. He is alive with disease 11 months after diagnosis. One patient has just begun chemoradiation.

New Modalities

Other modalities including liver transplantation in addition to the combined modality treatment have been described by Flickinger et al. (50). Among 12 patients with gallbladder or biliary cancer who underwent orthotopic liver transplantation following EBRT to the tumor and regional lymph nodes with or without Ir-192 or chemotherapy, 2 were still alive at 50 months.

Charged particles such as protons and helium ions have also been explored in the treatment of gallbladder and biliary cancers. In contrast to photons, the energy deposition patterns resulting from these charged particles are highly localized due to the absorption of majority of their energy at the end of their track range, the so-called Bragg peak. The dose unit of charged particles is the Gray Equivalent (GyE). Figure 7.3 compares the energy deposition patterns of 15 MV photons, 9 MeV electrons, 30 MeV neutrons, 160 MeV protons, and Ir-192 seeds.

Schoenthaler and co-workers at the University of California at San Francisco retrospectively reviewed their experience of 129 patients with EHBD carcinoma (51). Sixty-two patients were treated with surgery alone, and of these, 24% underwent gross total resection. The remaining surgery-only patients underwent debulking, biopsy, or decompression alone. Sixty-seven patients received adjuvant radiotherapy, 45 with conventional EBRT and 22 with charged particles of helium and/or neon. They defined patients who were treated with curative intent to include those who underwent a gross total resection or received greater than 45 Gy or 45 GyE after any surgical procedure. In total there were 50 patients treated with curative intent

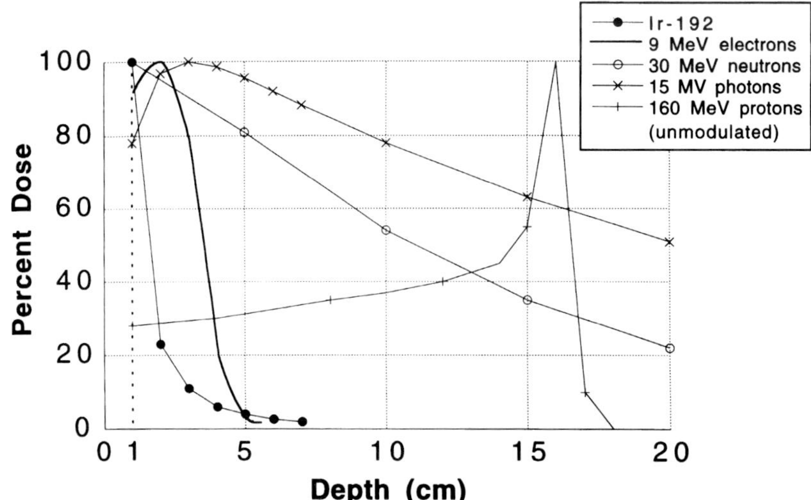

FIGURE 7.3. *Relative dose deposition as a function of depth for Ir-192 seeds, 9 MeV electrons, 30 MeV neutrons, 15 MV photons, and 160 MeV protons. (Courtesy Mike Munley, Ph.D., Department of Radiation Oncology, Duke University Medical Center, Durham, NC.)*

in the surgery alone group, 35 in the surgery plus conventional RT group, and 18 in the surgery plus charged particle group. Five patients in the conventional RT group also received Ir-192 brachytherapy. The authors observed a survival difference in patients undergoing gross total resection versus those receiving debulking or decompression only. They noted that patients with microscopic residual disease had increased median survival with adjuvant irradiation, most markedly after charged particle therapy ($P = 0.0005$), but also with conventional RT ($P = 0.01$). Patients with gross residual disease had a less marked but still statistically significant improved survival after irradiation ($P = 0.05$ for conventional RT and $P = 0.04$ for charged particle RT). The median survival with surgery alone, surgery plus conventional RT, and surgery plus charged particle was 6.5, 11, and 14 months for the entire group, respectively, and 16, 16, and 23 months for patients treated with curative intent, respectively ($P = 0.008$).

I-131 anti-CEA antibody has also been used in treating biliary cancers. Stillwagon et al. (52) reported a median survival of 13.6 months in 24 unresectable patients with intrahepatic cholangiocarcinoma following whole liver irradiation of 21 Gy in 7 fractions, doxorubicin, cisplatin, and I-131 anti-CEA antibody. However, no patient survived more than 2 years after the treatment.

Other innovative radiotherapy modalities including hyperfractionated EBRT and 3D-CRT are being explored. Preliminary reports from the University of Michigan Medical Center at Ann Arbor are very encouraging (17–20). A total of 22 patients with hepatobiliary cancers treated with concurrent intrahepatic arterial fluorodeoxyuridine and twice daily 3D-CRT of either 48 or 66 Gy (depending on the volume of liver irradiated) at 1.5–1.65 Gy per fraction, had a median survival of 16 months with an actuarial 4-year survival of 20%. The overall freedom from hepatic progression at more than 2 years was about 50% (20). The studies appear to be promising, especially in treating biliary carcinoma with a significant intrahepatic ductal component.

TREATMENT RECOMMENDATIONS

At Duke University Medical Center, postoperative chemoirradiation with a 5-FU–based regimen (usually delivered by protracted venous infusion or an oral derivative of 5-FU) and a combination of EBRT with or without an Ir-192 implant is generally offered to patients with resected tumors of the gallbladder and bile duct. EBRT is generally delivered via anterior–posterior opposed fields or multiple shaped fields using CT treatment planning with 6–15 MeV photons. Figure 7.4 is a simulation film of EBRT for proximal bile duct cancer and Figure 7.5 demonstrates an example of 3D-CRT and associated dose-volume histograms (DVHs) in treating biliary cancers. The DVHs reveal the volume of tumor or surrounding normal tissues/organs receiving a specified radiation dose level. A PTBD catheter must be in place to deliver a brachytherapy boost. Doses are individually tailored to the patient, but a combined RT dose of ≥ 50–55 Gy for microscopic and ≥ 60–65 Gy for gross disease is generally given; the weighting of dose between the EBRT and the Ir-192 implant is individualized. The chemotherapy is often delivered during both the implant and the EBRT for radiosensitization.

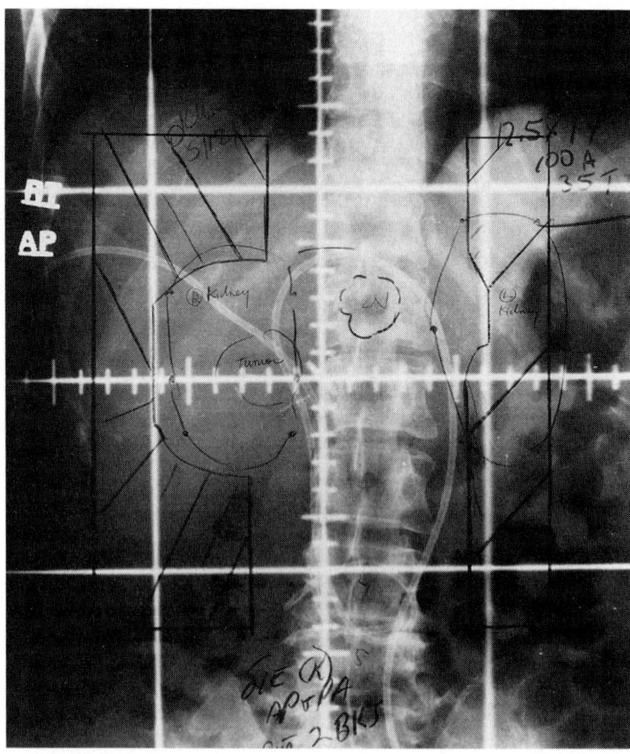

FIGURE 7.4. *External beam anterior–posterior opposed (AP/PA) two-field technique for proximal bile duct adenocarcinoma. The AP/PA fields include the tumor mass and the nodal area at risk. Note the outlines of kidneys and the attempt to exclude the majority of left kidney.*

For patients with unresected disease, primary chemoirradiation is generally offered at our institution. Typically, 20–30 Gy, at 10 Gy/day, is prescribed to 0.5 cm in tissue via an Ir-192 implant and another 45–55 Gy (at 1.8 Gy/day, 5 days/week) is delivered via EBRT. At times, all of the RT is delivered via an Ir-192 implant, and in those cases, the dose delivered is in the neighborhood of 40–50 Gy, at 10 Gy/day, at 0.5 cm in tissue. The 5-FU–based chemotherapy is delivered during the EBRT and the Ir-192 implant for radiosensitization.

METASTASIS TO THE HEPATOBILIARY SYSTEM

For hepatobiliary metastases secondary to other primary cancers, irradiation is generally used for symptomatic relief of pain and obstructive symptoms. Two-thirds of patients

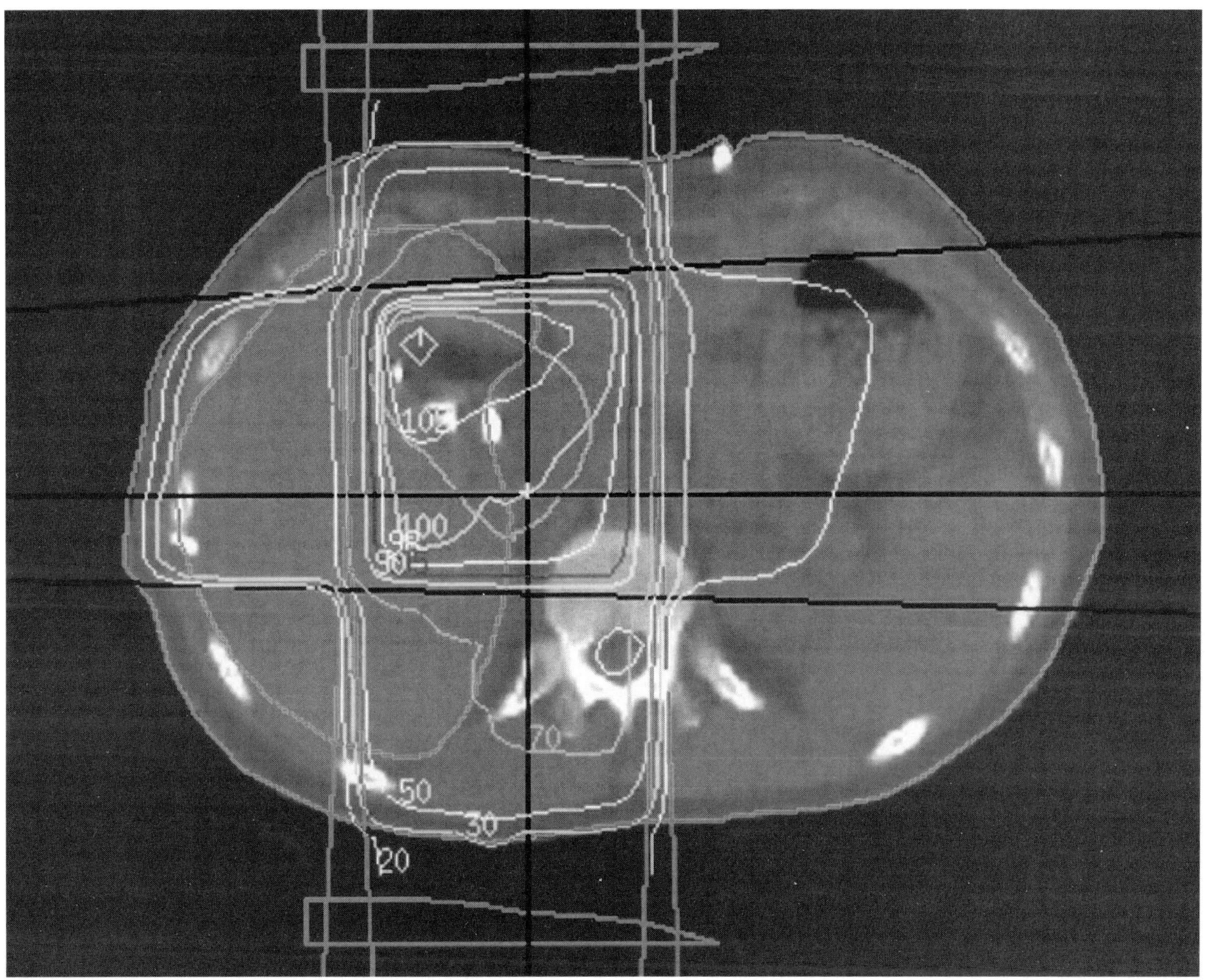

(A)

FIGURE 7.5. *Three-dimensional conformal radiotherapy (3D-CRT) for proximal common bile duct adenocarcinoma and associated dose-volume histograms (DVHs) for the tumor and its adjacent critical organs. The numbers correspond to the normalized dose percentage and the volume encompassed for irradiation. (Courtesy Mike Munley, Ph.D., Department of Radiation Oncology, Duke University Medical Center, Durham, NC.)* ***(A)*** *Transverse plane of 3D-CRT at the central axis.*

typically have some relief of pain and obstructive signs and symptoms such as pruritus and jaundice, though many of these patients require stenting as well. The most commonly used palliative RT dose to the whole liver is 21 Gy in 7 fractions. Small portions of the liver or extrahepatic biliary tract can be palliatively irradiated to a much higher dose as in definitive cases; however, the dose must be individualized. Doses ranging from 30 Gy in 10 fractions to 60 Gy in 30–33 fractions have been used.

OTHER RARE MALIGNANCIES OF GALLBLADDER AND BILE DUCT SYSTEM

Rare malignancies of the gallbladder and bile duct such as anaplastic carcinoma, squamous cell carcinoma, and adenocanthoma are generally treated in the same fashion as adenocarcinoma, though data are lacking. Sarcoma is exceedingly rare and the prognosis is poor in spite of treatment.

Lymphoma of the gallbladder and bile duct is rare and is generally treated with a combined modality approach with chemotherapy and low-dose irradiation. Surgery is not generally necessary. The typical radiation dose is 25–40 Gy (at 1.8–2 Gy/fraction, 5 days/week), usually given with chemotherapy, depending upon the stage and histology of the disease.

TOXICITIES AND COMPLICATIONS

Acute toxicities of EBRT include potential nausea, vomiting, anorexia, skin irritation, distal esophagitis, gastritis,

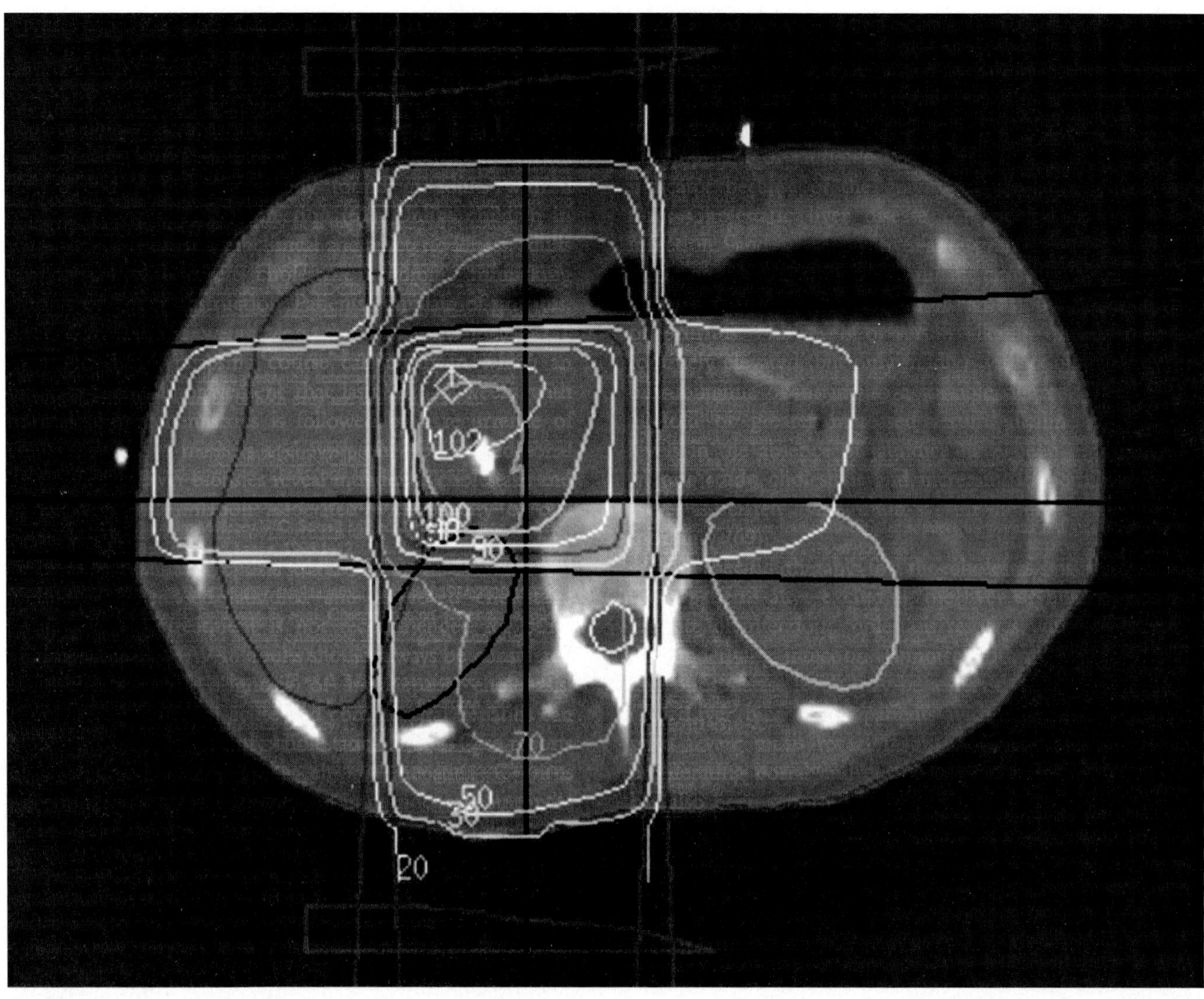

(B)

FIGURE 7.5. *(B) Transverse plane of 3D-CRT at the level of kidneys.*

duodenitis, fatigue, weight loss, asymptomatic elevated liver function tests (usually alkaline phosphatase), and mild immunosuppression. These generally resolve after the completion of treatment. Late complications secondary to RT for EHBD or intrahepatic bile duct carcinomas are difficult to define, but certainly do occur. They include gastrointestinal bleeding (especially duodenal), biliary fibrosis and duct stricture, cholangitis, hepatitis, and small bowel obstruction. There are several reasons why complications are difficult to precisely define: many patients do not survive long enough to exhibit them; some signs and symptoms that indicate complications are nonspecific and may also be seen secondary to tumor progression (i.e., gastrointestinal bleeding, biliary fibrosis and stricture, cholangitis, and hepatitis); and most of these patients have undergone numerous therapeutic interventions, many of which have common complications.

Nevertheless, with external doses of greater than 55 Gy when treating gallbladder and biliary carcinoma, at least 30% to 50% of patients will develop complications such as duodenal hemorrhage, ulceration, and obstruction (16). Care must be taken to respect dose tolerances of surrounding structures (see Table 7.1). When using EBRT of 45–50 Gy in 1.8–2.0 Gy per fraction combined with the brachytherapy boost, significant gastrointestinal complications, especially bleeding and ulceration, have been reported (22,26, 42). Therefore it is important to limit the brachytherapy dose to 20–30 Gy or less when combined with a curative EBRT dose of 45–50.4 Gy. In addition, it is important to ensure that the implant does not pass distal to the ampulla, to reduce the risk of resultant bleeding. When using IORT, Iwasaki et al. (21) have also described significant hepatic artery injury when IORT doses in excess of 20 Gy were used.

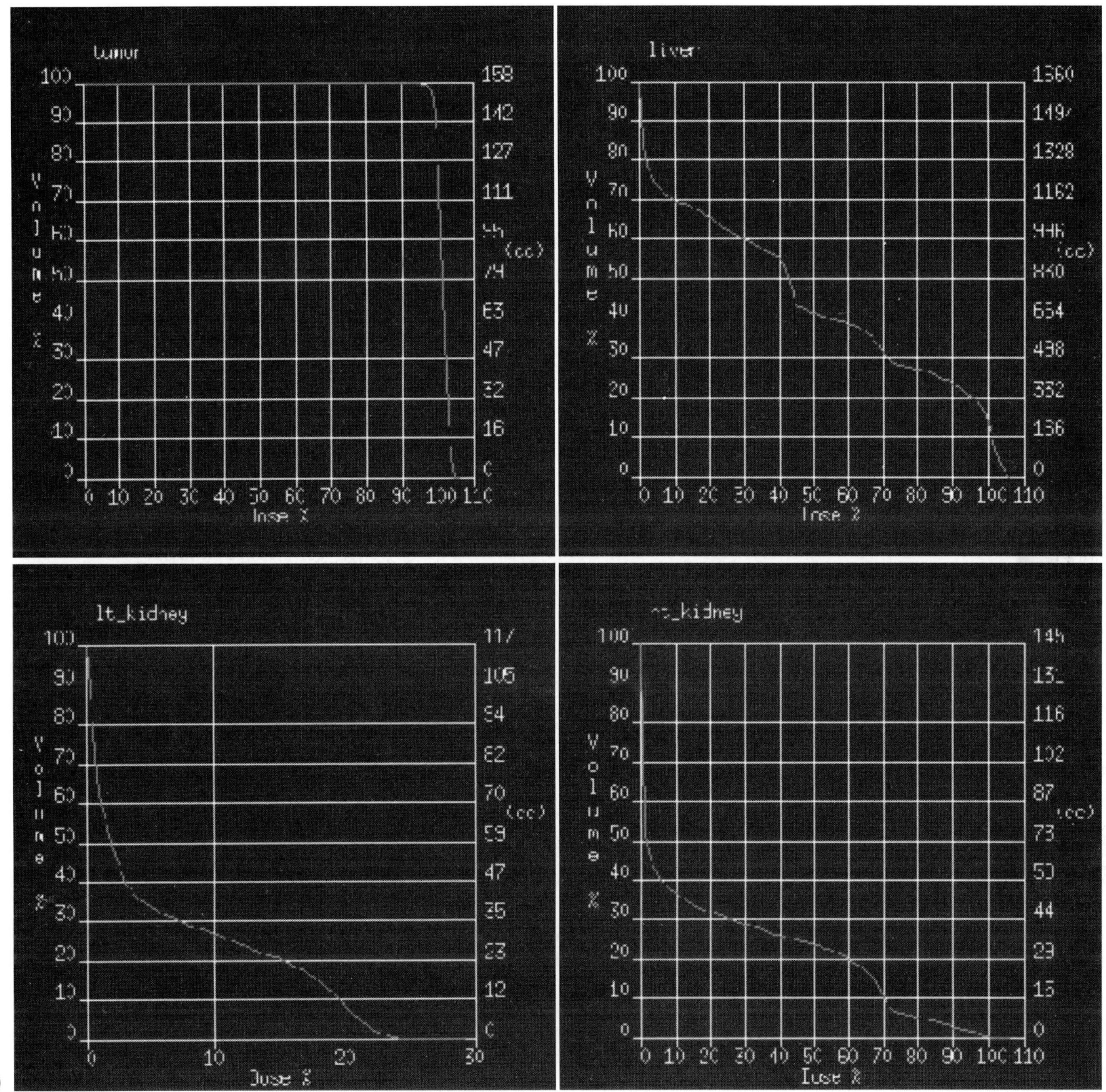

(C)

FIGURE 7.5. ***(C)*** *DVHs for the tumor and its surrounding normal organs/tissues.*

CONCLUSIONS AND FUTURE DIRECTIONS

Gallbladder and bile duct cancer continues to frustrate physicians with its overall poor prognosis, requiring newer and more innovative treatment techniques to be investigated. Surgery, when feasible, remains the treatment of choice. Most patients who undergo resection are found to have pathologically poor prognostic factors (lymphovascular invasion, positive lymph nodes, positive margins, etc.), and are often selected to receive adjuvant irradiation. It appears that RT (with or without chemotherapy) decreases the risk of locoregional recurrence, and possibly increases the survival of patients. It also appears that those patients who receive chemotherapy in addition to RT have improved survival over those who received RT alone, probably due to radiosensitization by the chemotherapy. An aggressive multimodality approach should be used in patients who are potentially resectable by combining surgery, intraoperative radiotherapy, and/or brachytherapy with Ir-192 and EBRT with concurrent chemotherapy. For unresectable cancers, combined modalities with maximum surgical debulking, EBRT, IORT, brachytherapy, and chemotherapy should also be used when possible. Newer modalities such as preoperative chemoradiation therapy, hyperfractionated radiotherapy, 3D conformal radiotherapy, and intra-arterial hepatic chemotherapy may improve the survival and local control in the future.

Acknowledgements

We thank Diane Evans, Brenda Brooks, and other Duke Radiation Oncology secretarial staff for their assistance in preparation of this chapter.

SUGGESTED READINGS

Foo ML, Gunderson LL, Bender CE, Buskirk SJ. External radiation therapy and transcatheter iridium in the treatment of extrahepatic bile duct carcinoma. Int J Radiat Oncol Biol Phys 1997;39:929–35. A recent summary of aggressive multimodality treatment for biliary cancer.

Gonzalez Gonzalez D, Gerard JP, Maners AW, et al. Results of radiation therapy in carcinoma of the proximal bile duct (Klatskin tumor). Semin Liver Dis 1990;10:131–41. A good summary of the radiation oncology literature for biliary cancer up to 1990, including the use of IORT.

Mould RF. A century of x-rays and radioactivity in medicine: with emphasis on photographic records of the early years. Philadelphia: Institute of Physics Publishing, 1993. A thorough review of the history of radiology since its original discovery in 1895, with excellent photographic records of the early years.

REFERENCES

1. Glasser O. The science of radiology. Springfield, IL: Charles C Thomas, 1933.
2. Despeignes V. Observation on a case of cancer of the stomach treated by roentgen rays. Lyon Med 1896;82:428.
3. Skinner CE. The x-ray treatment of intra-abdominal and other deeply located malignant diseases. Trans Am Roent Ray Soc 1903;142.
4. Wetzel E. Strahlentherapie. 1925;19:585.
5. Case JT, Warthin AS. The occurrence of hepatic lesions in patients treated by intensive deep roentgen irradiation. AJR Am J Roentgenol 1924;12:27–46.
6. Warren S. Effects of radiation on normal tissue. Arch Pathol 1942;34:749–87.
7. Webb S. The physics of three-dimensional radiation therapy: conformal radiotherapy, radiosurgery, and treatment planning. Philadelphia: Institute of Physics, 1993:355.
8. Del Regato JA, Spjut HJ. Cancer of the digestive tract. In: Ackerman LV, Del Regato JA, Spjut HJ, eds. Ackerman and Del Regato's cancer diagnosis, treatment, and prognosis. St. Louis: CV Mosby;1977:446–612.
9. Krain LS. Gallbladder and extrahepatic bile duct carcinoma. Analysis of 1,808 cases. Geriatrics 1972;27:111–17.
10. Green N, Mikkelsen WP, Kernen JA. Cancer of the common hepatic bile ducts—palliative radiotherapy. Radiology 1973;109:687–9.
11. Hudgins PT, Meoz RT. Radiation therapy for obstructive jaundice secondary to tumor malignancy. Int J Radiat Oncol Biol Phys 1976;1:1195–8.
12. Kopelson G, Harisiadis L, Tretter P, Chang CH. The role of radiation therapy in cancer of the extra-hepatic biliary system: an analysis of thirteen patients and a review of the literature of the effectiveness of surgery, chemotherapy and radiotherapy. Int J Radiat Oncol Biol Phys 1977;2:883–94.
13. Pilepich MV, Lambert PM. Radiotherapy of carcinomas of the extrahepatic biliary system. Radiology 1978;127:767–70.
14. Rubin P, Cooper R, Phillips TL, eds. Radiation biology and radiation pathology syllabus (Set RT 1: Radiation Oncology). Chicago: American College of Radiology, 1975.
15. Rubin P, Constine LS, Williams JP. Late effects of cancer treatment: radiation and drug toxicity. In: Perez CA, Brady LW, eds. Principles and practice of radiation oncology. 3rd ed. Philadelphia: Lippincott-Raven;1998:155–212.
16. Schoenthaler R. Hepatobiliary carcinomas. In: Leibel SA, Phillips TL. Textbook of radiation oncology. Philadelphia: Saunders, 1998:659–76.
17. Lawrence TS, Dworzanin LM, Walker-Andrews SC, et al. Treatment of cancers involving the liver and porta hepatis with external beam irradiation and intraarterial hepatic fluorodeoxyuridine. Int J Radiat Oncol Biol Phys 1991;20:555–61.
18. McGinn CJ, Lawrence TS. Clinical results of the combination of radiation and fluoropyrimidines in the treatment of intrahepatic cancer. Sem Rad Oncol 1997;7:313–23.
19. Robertson JM, McGinn CJ, Walker S, et al. Phase I trial of hepatic arterial bromodeoxyuridine and conformal radiation therapy for patients with primary hepatobiliary cancers or colorectal liver metastases. Int J Radiat Oncol Biol Phys 1997;39:1087–92.
20. Robertson JM, Lawrence TS, Andrews JC, et al. Long-term results of hepatic artery fluorodeoxyuridine and conformal radiation therapy for primary hepatobiliary cancers. Int J Radiat Oncol Biol Phys 1997;37:325–30.
21. Iwasaki Y, Todoroki T, Fukao K, et al. The role of intraoperative radiation therapy in the treatment of bile duct cancer. World J Surg 1988;12:91–8.
22. Buskirk SJ, Gunderson LL, Adson MA, et al. Analysis of failure following curative irradiation of gallbladder and extrahepatic bile duct carcinoma. Int J Radiat Oncol Biol Phys 1984;10:2013–23.
23. Vaittinen E. Carcinoma of the gall-bladder. A study of 390 cases diagnosed in Finland 1953–1967. Ann Chir Gynaecol Fenniae 1970;59:1–81.
24. Mittal B, Deutsch M, Iwatsuki S. Primary cancers of extrahepatic biliary passages. Int J Radiat Oncol Biol Phys 1985;11:849–54.
25. Mahe M, Romestaing P, Talon B, et al. Radiation therapy in extrahepatic bile duct carcinoma. Radiother Oncol 1991;21:121–7.
26. Hayes JK Jr, Sapozink MD, Miller FJ. Definitive radiation therapy in bile duct carcinoma. Int J Radiat Oncol Biol Phys 1988;15:735–44.
27. Alden ME, Mohiuddin M. The impact of radiation dose in combined external beam and intraluminal IR-192 brachytherapy for bile duct cancer. Int J Radiat Oncol Phys 1994;28:945–51.
28. Treadwell TA, Hardin WJ. Primary carcinoma of the gallbladder. The role of adjunctive therapy in its treatment. Am J Surg 1976;132:703–6.
29. Gonzalez Gonzalez D, Gerard JP, Maners AW, et al. Results of radiation therapy in carcinoma of the proximal bile duct (Klatskin tumor). Semin Liver Dis 1990;10:131–41.
30. Cameron JL, Pitt HA, Zinner MJ, et al. Management of proximal cholangiocarcinomas by surgical resection and radiotherapy. Am J Surg 1990;159:91–8.
31. Pitt HA, Nakeeb A, Abrams RA, et al. Perihilar cholangiocarcinoma. Postoperative radiotherapy does not improve survival. Ann Surg 1995;221:788–98.
32. Farley DR, Weaver AL, Nagorney DM. "Natural history" of unresected cholangiocarcinoma: patient outcome after noncurative intervention. Mayo Clin Proc 1995;70:425–9.
33. Grove MK, Hermann RE, Vogt DP, Broughan TA. Role of radiation after operative palliation in cancer of the proximal bile ducts. Am J Surg 1991;161:454–8.
34. Veeze-Kuijpers B, Meerwaldt JH, Mameris JS, et al. The role of radiotherapy in the treatment of bile duct carcinoma. Int J Radiat Oncol Biol Phys 1990;18:63–7.
35. Fletcher MS, Dawson JL, Wheeler PG, et al. Treatment of high bile duct carcinoma by internal radiotherapy with iridium-192 wire. Lancet 1981;2:172–4.
36. Minsky BD, Wesson MF, Armstrong JG, et al. Combined modality therapy of extrahepatic biliary system cancer. Int J Radiat Oncol Biol Phys 1990;18:1157–63.
37. Minsky BD, Kemeny N, Armstrong JG, et al. Extrahepatic biliary system cancer: an update of a combined modality approach. Am J Clin Oncol 1991;14:433–7.
38. Foo ML, Gunderson LL, Bender CE, Buskirk SJ. External radiation therapy and transcatheter iridium in the treatment of extrahepatic bile duct carcinoma. Int J Radiat Oncol Biol Phys 1997;39:929–35.
39. Fields JN, Emami B. Carcinoma of the extrahepatic biliary system—results of primary and adjuvant radiotherapy. Int J Radiat Oncol Biol Phys 1987;13:331–8.
40. Johnson DW, Safai C, Goffinet DR. Malignant obstructive jaundice: treatment with external-beam and intracavitary radiotherapy. Int J Radiat Oncol Biol Phys 1985;11:411–16.

41. Montemaggi O, Costamagna G, Dobelbower RR, et al. Intraluminal brachytherapy in the treatment of pancreas and bile duct carcinoma. Int J Radiat Oncol Biol Phys 1995;32:437–43.
42. Buskirk SJ, Gunderson LL, Schild SE, et al. Analysis of failure after curative irradiation of extrahepatic bile duct carcinoma. Ann Surg 1991;215:125–31.
43. Eschelman DJ, Shapiro MJ, Bonn J, et al. Malignant biliary duct obstruction: long-term experience with Gianturco stents and combined-modality radiation therapy. Radiology 1996;200:717–24.
44. Fritz P, Brambs H-J, Schraube P, et al. Combined external beam radiotherapy and intraluminal high dose rate brachytherapy on bile duct carcinomas. Int J Radiat Oncol Biol Phys 1994;29:855–61.
45. Deziel DJ, Kiel KD, Kramer TS, et al. Intraoperative radiation therapy in biliary tract cancer. Amer Surg 1988;54:402–7.
46. Busse PM, Stone MD, Sheldon TA, et al. Intraoperative radiation therapy for biliary tract carcinoma: results of a 5-year experience. Surgery 1989;105:724–33.
47. Monson JRT, Donohue JH, Gunderson LL, et al. Intraoperative radiotherapy for unresectable cholangiocarcinoma—the Mayo Clinic experience. Surg Oncol 1992;1:283–90.
48. Altaee MY, Johnson PJ, Farrant JM, Williams R. Etiologic and clinical characteristics of peripheral and hilar cholangiocarcinoma. Cancer 1991;68:2051–5.
49. Chen M, Jan Y, Wang C, et al. Clinical experience in 20 hepatic resections for peripheral cholangiocarcinoma. Cancer 1989;64:2226–32.
50. Flickinger JC, Epstein AH, Iwatsuki S, et al. Radiation therapy for primary carcinoma of the extrahepatic biliary system. An analysis of 63 cases. Cancer 1991;68:289–94.
51. Schoenthaler R, Phillips TL, Castro J, et al. Carcinoma of the extrahepatic bile ducts. The University of California at San Francisco Experience. Ann Surg 1994;3:267–74.
52. Stillwagon GB, Order SG, Haulk T, et al. Variable low dose rate irradiation (131I-Anti-CEA) and integrated low dose chemotherapy in the treatment of nonresectable primary intrahepatic cholangiocarcinoma. Int J Radiat Oncol Biol Phys 1991;21:1601–5.

Chapter

8

Surgery of the Biliary System

MARKUS SELZNER PIERRE-ALAIN CLAVIEN

The biliary tree was already identified in 1440 as a source of abdominal pain, but further knowledge and technical skills were necessary before the first therapeutic intervention could be attempted. In 1867 John Stough Bobbs (1) performed the first cholecystostomy in a patient with severe acute cholecystitis, and in 1882 Carl Langenbuch performed the first cholecystectomy in Berlin (2). A breakthrough was achieved in 1909, when Robert Dahl (3) described for the first time a technique of Roux-en-Y hepaticojejunostomy reconstruction to drain the biliary system in the presence of a stricture.

Knowledge of the anatomy is critical for any surgical approach to the biliary tree (see Chapter 1). The anatomy of the porta hepatis is highly variable, and the surgeon must be fully aware of these variations. About one-third of the patients have an atypical supply from the hepatic artery. In 16% of patients, the left hepatic artery is supplied by the left gastric artery; in 17% the right hepatic artery is supplied by the superior mesenteric artery; and in 5% of the patients both variations coexist. The biliary tree shows less variability. Nine percent of the patients have an aberrant common bile duct from the left hemiliver to the right bile duct. In another 6% of the cases an aberrant bile duct originates from the posterior right side of the liver to the left hepatic duct (4) (Fig. 8.1).

The goals of surgery of the biliary tree include 1) relief of obstructing jaundice, 2) prevention of recurrent obstruction and cholangitis, and 3) eradication of malignant tumors.

PREOPERATIVE CONSIDERATIONS

Surgical procedures of the biliary system range from simple bypass procedures to extensive resections including liver resection and pancreaticoduodenectomy. The type of procedure has to be selected according to the disease and the clinical condition of each patient. Patient age, cardiac and pulmonary diseases, and chronic liver diseases are significant risk factors for surgical interventions on the biliary system. These conditions have to be carefully assessed when planning an operative procedure.

The indications for preoperative percutaneous drainage of cholestasis are still under debate. Two prospective randomized trials reported in the early 1980s showed no benefit of preoperative drainage in patients with biliary obstruction (5,6). However, the results of these studies were influenced by the high rate of catheter-related complications. Today, the incidence of complications related to the percutaneous biliary drainage (PBD) has decreased. A newer retrospective study has indicated significant benefit of preoperative biliary drainage (7).

In our opinion, preoperative drainage of the biliary tree has several advantages. First, it decreases the swelling of the liver parenchyma, which facilitates the dissection and determination of the proximal limit of an intrahepatic tumor. Second, percutaneous cholangiogram allows excellent visualization of intrahepatic ducts (see the discussion of radiologic evaluation). Sludge and swelling of the bile ducts due to severe obstruction can mimic extensive disease, so effective decompression of the biliary tree is necessary to evaluate the exact location of a malignant stricture. We recommend a second percutaneous transhepatic cholangiogram (PTC) after normalization of the serum bilirubin to accurately evaluate the bile duct and determine the operative strategy (Fig. 8.2). Third, decompression of the dilated bile ducts increases the tolerance of the liver parenchyma to ischemic injury, and decreases the risk for postoperative liver failure (8). Finally, percutaneous catheters can be palpated during dissection of the hilum, which may facilitate difficult dissections. We routinely drain patients with an elevated

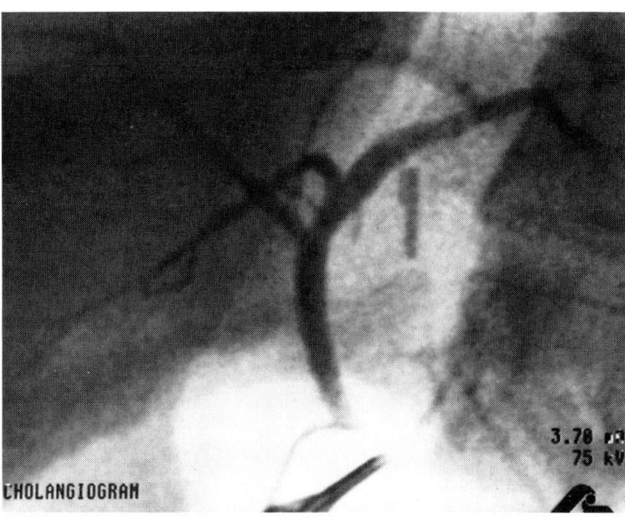

FIGURE 8.1. *Aberrant bile duct originating from the posterior right side of the liver to the left hepatic duct.*

bilirubin (>5 mg/dL) and consider major resection only when the bilirubin is below 2 mg/dL.

Perioperative antibiotic prophylaxis should be given 1 hour before the skin incision and 24 hours after surgery. We currently use 1 or 2 grams of cefazolin (Ancef). Recent prospective studies suggested that perioperative antibiotics have no beneficial effect if the procedure is restricted to a laparoscopic cholecystectomy (9,10).

Radiologic Evaluation

A clear visualization of the biliary tract is critical prior to surgery (see Chapters 3–5). Initial assessment of the biliary tree can be performed by ultrasound to identify dilatation of hepatic ducts, the level of an obstruction, and possible vascular encasement. The second step is a computed tomography (CT) scan or magnetic resonance imaging (MRI) to detect a tumor mass or metastases and to determine the involvement of the portal vein or hepatic artery. If the stricture is located below the bifurcation, then endoscopic retrograde cholangiopancreatography (ERCP) is the next diagnostic step. This allows an evaluation of the distal bile duct and often provides important information on the etiology of a ductal stricture. In contrast, in patients with high biliary strictures, percutaneous transhepatic cholangiography (PTC), with or without placement of biliary drains, is preferable.

It is important to recognize that biliary stasis and sludge can mimic advanced cancer stages. Therefore, patients with severe obstructive jaundice should be decompressed, and then reevaluated before making a final decision about resectability as highlighted above (see Fig. 8.1). Magnetic resonance cholangiopancreatography (MRCP) allows noninvasive evaluation of the biliary tree; it has great diagnostic potential and may replace other investigations in the future. However, at this point it is mostly used in children or in cases when an ERCP is not possible for anatomic reasons. Hepatic arteriography is no longer recommended as a routine procedure; we only perform this in selected cases, when the presence or absence of vascular encasement is unclear on CT or MRI.

Clinical Assessment

Bile duct resection for cholangiocarcinoma or gallbladder cancer is often combined with major liver resection. Therefore, patients should be carefully evaluated for the operative risk associated with major hepatic tissue loss. Underlying liver diseases, such as cirrhosis or severe steatosis, should be identified preoperatively, because they may represent a contraindication for surgery. Similarly, ongoing infection such as cholangitis or hepatitis should be addressed prior to surgery.

Patients with bile duct malignancies are often elderly and have accompanying pulmonary and/or cardiovascular risk factors. In a recent multivariate analysis (11), cardiovascular disease and cholangitis were identified as predominant risk factors for biliary surgery. In this study, patients with cardiovascular disease and cholangitis had, respectively, a five and eight times greater operative risk when compared to the general population.

Finally, patients with biliary strictures may present with frequent nausea and vomiting resulting in dehydration and malnutrition. Abnormalities in their electrolyte status should be corrected prior to surgery and preoperative tube feeding might be of benefit in selected patients.

BILE DUCT RESECTION FOR CHOLANGIOCARCINOMA

The operative strategy for cholangiocarcinoma differs for intrahepatic, hilar, and distal tumors. Intrahepatic cholangiocarcinomas are treated according to the principles of oncologic liver resection (12). This section focuses on strategies for the treatment of hilar and distal bile duct cancer.

Resection of Hilar Cholangiocarcinoma

Cholangiocarcinoma is a slow-growing cancer with a tendency for local invasion and late metastasis. The proximity of hilar cholangiocarcinoma to critical vascular structures inside the hepatoduodenal ligament often precludes resection, resulting in reported resectability rates between 20% and 50% (13–16). The wide range of resectability reported in the literature reflects the bias of patient referral to specialized centers and the difference in "aggressiveness" of surgical approaches among various groups. Improvements in hepatobiliary surgery during the last 10 years have allowed more aggressive strategies, including combined bile duct and major liver resection, sometimes associated with vascular resection and reconstruction.

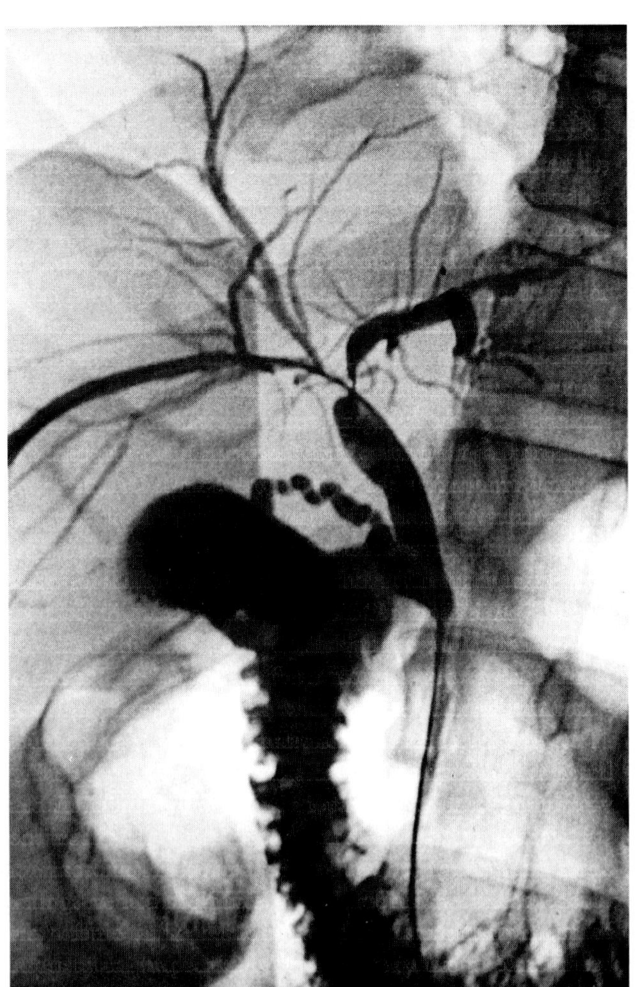

(A)

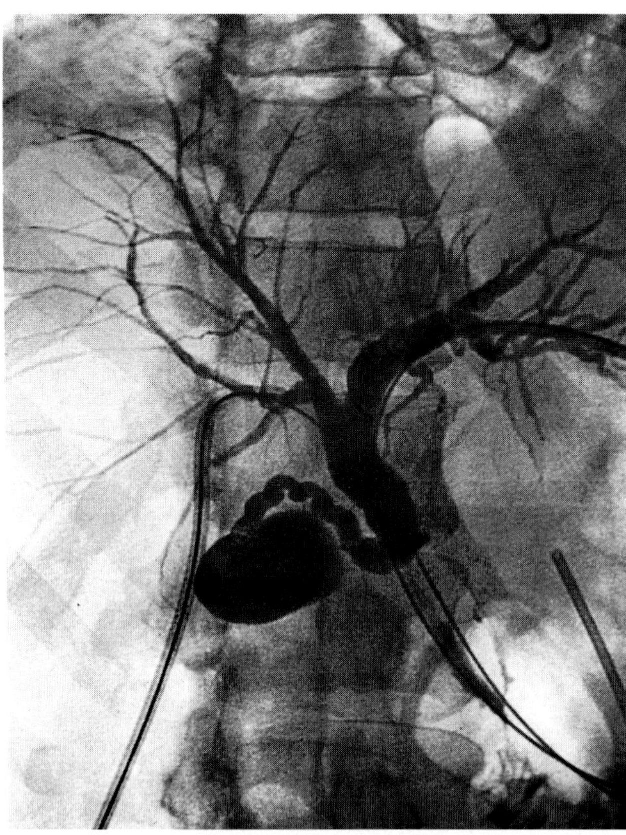

(B)

FIGURE 8.2. ***(A)*** *Preoperative cholangiography of a patient with severe biliary obstruction because of a cholangiocarcinoma. The radiologic evaluation suggests tumor involvement of segmental ducts of both sides.* ***(B)*** *Four weeks after percutaneous drainage, the reevaluation demonstrates that the tumor is limited to the bile duct confluence.*

Absolute contraindications for resection include 1) moribund patients with a significant increased operative risk, 2) massive infiltration of the main portal vein or hepatic artery, 3) vascular involvement of the left and right branches of the hepatic artery or portal vein, 4) involvement of one portal vein/hepatic artery branch with simultaneously major bile duct involvement of the contralateral side, and 5) bilateral hepatic or distant metastasis.

Indications for resection of cholangiocarcinoma with vascular involvement remain controversial. Nimura et al. (17) reported a 5-year survival of 41% and a perioperative mortality of only 8% in patients undergoing vascular resection and reconstruction for cholangiocarcinoma. Other studies have reported less favorable 5-year survival, less than 5% after resection of cholangiocarcinoma in the presence of vascular infiltration (18,19). The operative risk in each patient has to be balanced against the chance of complete tumor removal. The success of each surgical approach will be discussed in Chapter 20. One problem with interpreting published data is that curative resection is defined differently among various authors. Some surgeons classify a resection as noncurative in the presence of any lymph node involvement; others still consider the resection as curative if local lymph nodes are resected together with the primary cancer. For example, Sugiura et al. (14) found that regional lymph node involvement was not associated with decreased long-term survival in a series of 83 patients. In contrast, there is consensus that distant extrahepatic metastasis precludes curative surgery.

Some patients might benefit from noncurative resection. Two studies found improved survival and quality of life after noncurative resection compared to endoscopic or percutaneous drainage procedures alone (20,21). Similarly, Bismuth et al. (22) compared patients with noncurative resection and drainage procedures (biliary-enteric bypass and intubation of the bile ducts), and found a significant improvement of survival and quality of life after tumor resection compared to those receiving biliary drainage alone. Blumgart et al. (15) found that patients treated with palliative tumor resection spend 88% of their remaining time at home in good health compared to 6% of patients with palliative surgical drainage procedures.

The need for extensive resection depends on the localization of the tumor. The Bismuth classification is often used to describe tumor localization (Chapter 20). Bile duct resection alone is sufficient when the tumor is limited to the common bile duct without involvement of the bifurcation (stage I). More extensive procedures, often including liver resection, are necessary when the tumor involves the bifurcation (stage II). Caudate lobe (segment I) involvement in patients with bile duct cancer of the bifurcation or above has been reported in between 30% and 95% of cases (17,20,23), and the caudate lobe is a frequent cause of early recurrence. Therefore, the caudate lobe should always be removed if the tumor reaches the bile duct bifurcation. Sugiura et al. (14) have reported a significantly improved 5-year survival in patients treated with caudate lobe resection compared to patients treated with bile duct resection alone (46% vs. 12%).

Tumor progression beyond the second bifurcation on the left or right side (Bismuth IIIa or b) makes bile duct resection in combination with hemihepatectomy or extended hemihepatectomy necessary. Tashiro et al. (20) reported significantly improved 3-year survival for patients treated with combined liver and bile duct resection as compared to patients treated with local resection alone (37% vs. 20%). Although no randomized controlled studies are available comparing combined bile duct and liver resection with bile duct resection alone, most hepatobiliary surgeons recommend routine liver resection for proximal bile duct cancer (14,16,20,22,24,25). Advanced cases of cholangiocarcinoma (Bismuth IV) are not candidates for resection or transplantation in most centers, and have to be treated with supportive care only, or in the setting of experimental protocols.

Technical Approach

A number of surgeons perform laparoscopy prior to laparotomy in oncologic patients to exclude distant metastases or peritoneal disease. In addition, laparoscopic intraoperative ultrasound can be used to determine local invasion of the tumor (Chapter 20) and to exclude peritoneal metastases.

If laparoscopy fails to show advanced disease, the abdomen is opened by a bilateral transverse incision, which can be extended by an upper midline incision. The abdominal cavity is evaluated for metastases or distant lymph node involvement. Then the tumor is palpated to estimate its size and spread. The hepatoduodenal ligament is dissected and the structures isolated by vessel loops (Fig. 8.3).

The transection of the bile duct is the point of no return—to proceed the surgeon must be convinced that reconstruction of the biliary outflow can be performed. The common bile duct is transected above the second part of

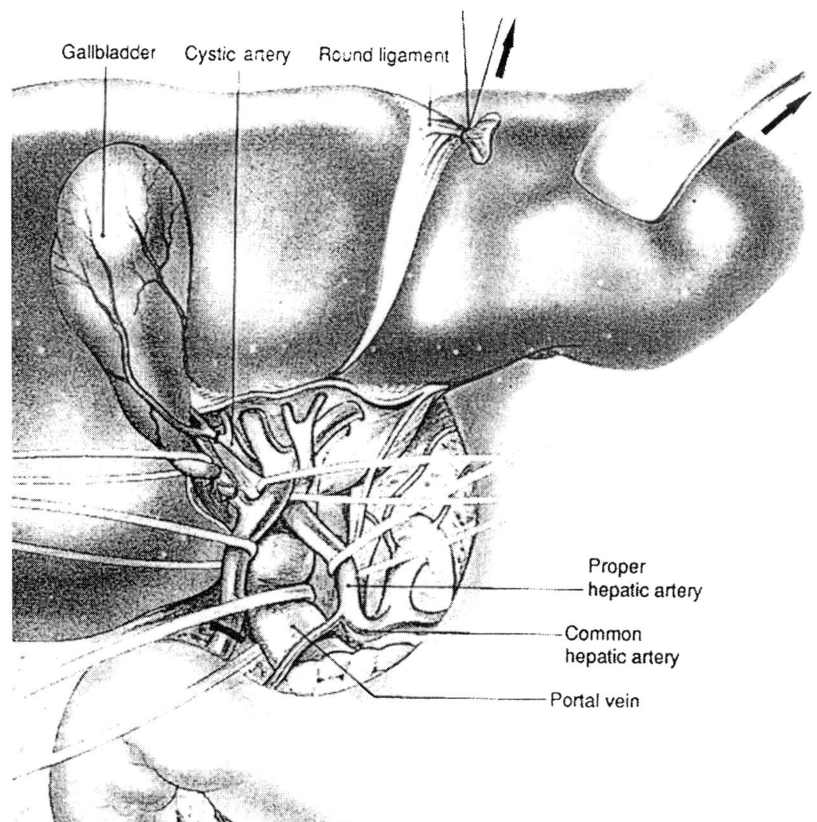

FIGURE 8.3. *Prior to the bile duct resection the structures of the hepatoduodenal ligament are isolated and marked with vessel loops.*

the duodenum (D2). The distal end is ligated and a segment of the proximal end is evaluated for the presence of tumor by frozen section. The bile duct is turned upward and then separated en bloc together with the lymphatic tissue from the portal vein and the hepatic artery. The hilus is isolated by elevation and lowering the hilus plate and dissecting along the bile duct (Fig. 8.4).

For the local resection of the bile duct, the left hepatic duct is exposed first. The left duct is marked with sutures and transected. The distal end of the duct is examined by frozen section to ensure tumor clearance. Then the duct is turned to the right side, followed by mobilization of the gallbladder and the right hepatic duct. The distal right duct is also marked with sutures and transected. The bile duct containing tumor is then removed en bloc.

Combined liver and bile duct resection is indicated if the tumor extends proximal to the bile duct bifurcation. The dissection of the common hepatic duct is as described above to the point of the dissection of the bile duct confluence. Whether left or right hemihepatectomy should be carried out depends on the tumor involvement on each side. If a left hemihepatectomy (segments II to IV) or extended left hemihepatectomy (segments II to VIII) is planned, the right main hepatic duct is dissected first, until the level of its segmental bifurcation. The duct is transected and the distal part pulled to the contralateral side. This allows access to the vessels of the porta hepatis, which can then be isolated and ligated according to the resection of liver parenchyma. If a right hemihepatectomy (segments V to VIII) or extended right hemihepatectomy (segments IV to VIII) is planned, the dissection starts with the left hepatic duct, which is transected and then pulled to the right side. In both cases liver resection is performed according to oncologic principles (e.g., tumor-free margin, anatomic resection) as described previously (12).

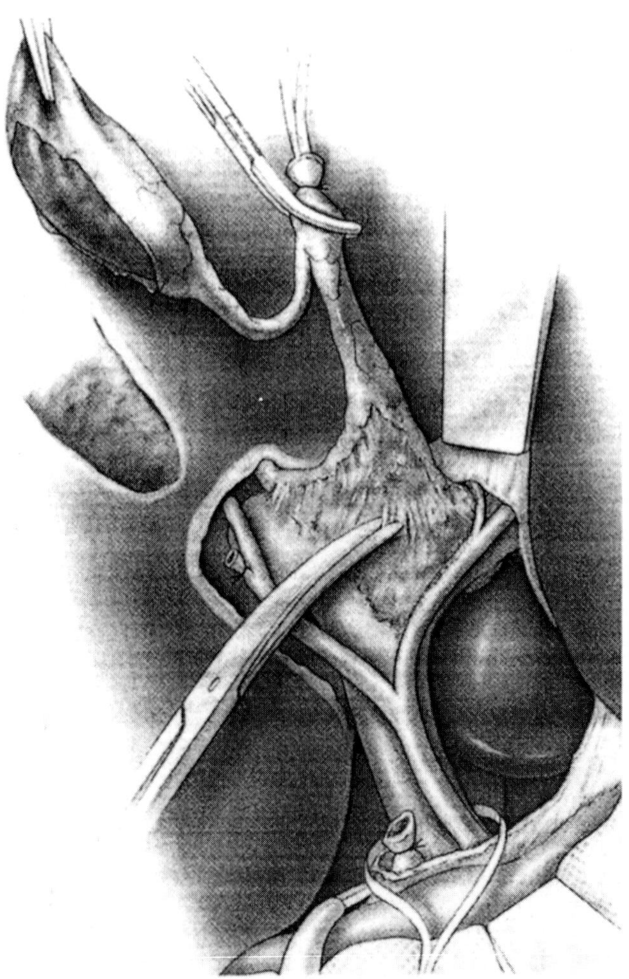

FIGURE 8.4. *After transsection the bile duct is elevated and separated from the hepatic artery and the portal vein.*

The caudate lobe is frequently involved in cholangiocarcinoma and should be removed if the tumor reaches the bifurcation. In most cases, caudate lobe resection is performed together with a left or right hemihepatectomy. Only in rare cases, when the tumor is strictly limited to the confluence, a caudate resection alone is sufficient. The resection of the caudate lobe can be difficult because of its close relation to the inferior vena cava (IVC). After complete mobilization of the liver from the diaphragm, the right liver is turned to the midline. Then the entire posterior liver is freed from the retrohepatic vena cava by dissecting the small hepatic veins. After mobilization of the liver from the retroperitoneum, the veins draining the caudate lobe can be transected at the anterior surface of the vena cava. Finally, the branches of the portal vein and the hepatic artery supplying the caudate lobe are dissected at the hilum. The vessels are found in the left portal triad just prior to the umbilical fissure. After completion of the vascular isolation, the caudate lobe can be resected. Caudate lobe resection in combination with left hemihepatectomy is technically less demanding and the caudate lobe can be simply transected with a stapler in most cases.

After resection of the bile duct with or without liver resection the biliary outflow is reconstructed with a biliary-enteric Roux-en-Y anastomosis, which is described in detail below in the section on reconstruction of the biliary outflow.

Resection of Cholangiocarcinoma of the Mid and Distal Common Bile Duct

Tumors of the common bile duct are less common than perihilar cholangiocarcinomas (see Chapter 20). As in hilar tumors, radical local tumor resection is the goal, and sometimes duodenopancreatectomy is necessary. The portal vein and hepatic artery are dissected and isolated with vessel loops. The common bile duct is transected proximal to the tumor and is evaluated for tumor cells. Tumors located close to the pancreas require a subtotal pancreaticoduodenectomy with or without partial gastrectomy. Reconstruction of the bile duct and pancreatic duct is then performed with a

Roux-en-Y anastomosis. The results of surgery for distal bile duct tumors are discussed in Chapter 20.

SURGERY FOR GALLBLADDER CANCER

The surgical approach to patients with gallbladder cancer depends on the general condition of the patient and the extent of the disease. Four different scenarios can be encountered in the clinical practice:

1. The tumor is found incidentally during cholecystectomy.
2. Limited gallbladder cancer is suspected preoperatively, and confirmed intraoperatively.
3. Extensive gallbladder cancer is found incidentally during surgery.
4. Extensive gallbladder cancer is diagnosed prior to surgery.

If gallbladder cancer is found incidentally during cholecystectomy, the operation should be limited to a simple cholecystectomy including a resection of the lymph nodes in the triangle of Calot. The patient with the specimen should be referred to a center with extensive experience in bile duct and liver surgery. Of importance, the tumor specimen should be carefully reviewed by an experienced pathologist to evaluate the degree of tumor infiltration. The surgical approach depends on the depth of tumor invasion into the gallbladder wall and major liver resection may be necessary.

If the tumor is limited to the mucosa (carcinoma in situ), a simple cholecystectomy is sufficient, offering excellent long-term survival (see Chapter 14). If the tumor infiltrates the muscularis propria without reaching the gallbladder serosa, an extended cholecystectomy (gallbladder resection plus wedge resection of the liver) is the therapy of choice. The hepatoduodenal ligament is dissected and the portal vein and hepatic artery are isolated by vessel loops as described for hilar bile duct tumors. Finally, the gallbladder plus a 1- to 3-cm wedge of the gallbladder bed are resected en bloc, together with the cystic duct. If the intraoperative cystic duct biopsy is positive for tumor, then resection of the choledochal and hepatic ducts and the surrounding lymphatic tissue has to be added to the procedure.

For gallbladder carcinoma found during or after a laparoscopic cholecystectomy, we recommend excising the port sites. In recent studies the incidence of port site metastases was found to be between 14% and 16% independent from the extent of the gallbladder cancer (26,27). In addition, in cases with gallbladder perforation during laparoscopic cholecystectomy, the reported incidence of port site metastases has been as high as 40%.

More extensive resections are indicated if the tumor extends beyond the gallbladder serosa. Extended right hemihepatectomy or central hepatectomy, including segments IV and V, together with a resection of the cystic duct, common bile duct, and the lymphatic tissue are often used to achieve tumor clearance. The prognosis and results of the different approaches are discussed in detail in Chapter 14.

If a curative resection is not possible due to a large tumor load or extensive involvement of the liver hilum, then surgery is not a therapeutic option. The prognosis of patients with unresectable gallbladder cancer is poor and the therapy should focus on supportive care. The results of each therapeutic approach mentioned above will be discussed in detail in Chapter 14.

RECONSTRUCTION OF THE BILIARY OUTFLOW

Adequate reconstruction of the biliary outflow is critical after resection of cholangiocarcinoma and sometimes after resection of a gallbladder cancer. Effective techniques of bypass procedures for unresectable malignant or benign strictures are also important. Endoscopic and percutaneous drainage procedures will be described in Chapters 5 and 6. In this section we focus on surgical procedures for biliary reconstruction.

The goal of biliary reconstruction is to relieve jaundice, prevent cholangitis, and avoid recurrent biliary stricture. A Roux-en-Y anastomosis is performed in most cases to ensure good blood supply of a wide mucosa-to-mucosa anastomosis between all transected bile ducts and a Roux-en-Y jejunum limb. Direct choledochocholedochostomy is frequently associated with recurrent stricturing and should only be used for biliary reconstruction during liver transplantation.

Although drainage of one side of the biliary tree is theoretically sufficient to relieve jaundice, the jejunal limb should drain all parts of the liver to prevent cholangitis. The principles of reconstruction are 1) identification of healthy bile duct mucosa proximal to the stenosis/transection, 2) preparation of a Roux-en-Y loop, usually 40 cm in length, and 3) direct mucosa-to-mucosa anastomosis. Whether a biliodigestive anastomosis should be stented by a drain remains controversial. As there is no proven benefit for stenting, we do not insert anastomotic stents.

The most common biliodigestive drainage procedure is the end-to-side hepaticojejunostomy. The Roux-en-Y jejunal limb is directly anastomosed to the hepatic bifurcation, draining both lobes of the liver. If a major hilum resection has been performed, the Roux-en-Y limb can also be anastomosed directly to segmental ducts (Fig. 8.5). Biliodigestive anastomoses are performed with absorbable monofilament sutures (e.g., PDS or Maxom 5.0). The sutures of the anterior layer are performed first prior to any attempt to place the posterior row. If more than one bile duct orifice is present, then all anterior row sutures have to be placed before any posterior ones can be placed. Each anterior suture is placed full thickness from the inside to the outside, from left to right. When the entire row has been placed, the anterior sutures are elevated and the corner sutures held tight (Fig. 8.6). Then the sutures of the posterior row are

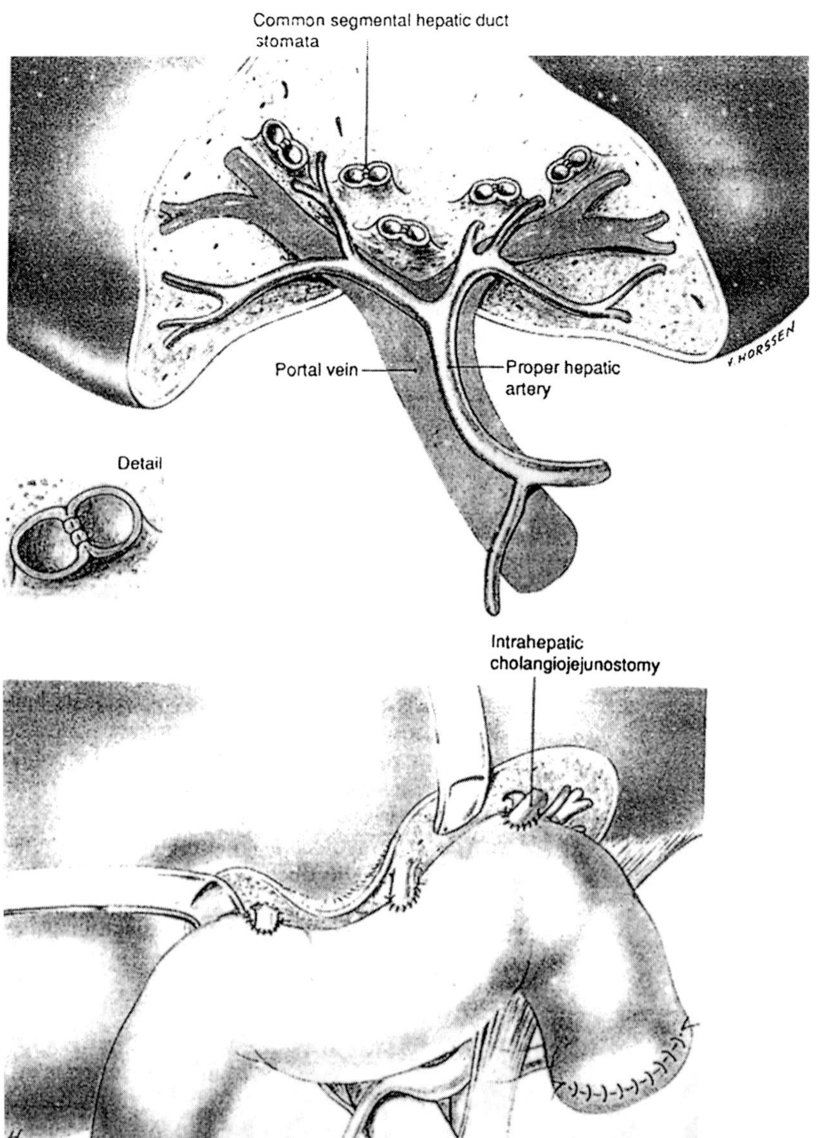

FIGURE 8.5. *The biliodigestive anastomosis is facilitated if small segmental ducts are sutured together and connected in one anastomosis.*

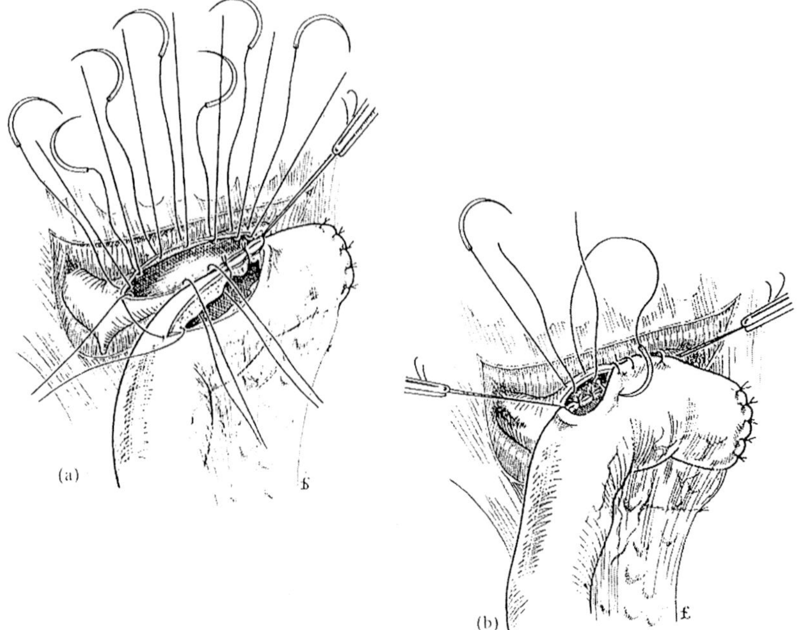

FIGURE 8.6. ***(a)*** *At first, the sutures of the anterior row are placed in full thickness and the sutures are elevated.* ***(b)*** *Then the posterior row is performed from the right side to the left side. Finally, the anterior row is completed.*

subsequently tied with the nodes outside or inside the lumen. Finally, the anterior row is completed by suturing the anterior jejunal side from the inside to the outside.

If the hepatic hilum is not accessible for the biliodigestive anastomosis then the left common hepatic duct is an adequate choice. The left main hepatic duct has a long horizontal extrahepatic course, which can easily be reached in most cases. Division of the ligamentum teres from the abdominal wall to the diaphragm is necessary. A solid tie has to be placed on the ligament to allow elevation and traction. Then the parenchymal bridge connecting the left lobe and the quadrate lobe is transected by diathermy. Glisson's capsule at the base of the quadrate ligament is dissected and the main left hepatic bile duct is exposed (Fig. 8.7). From this point, the dissection can be extended to the right side to include the confluence of the right hepatic duct in the anastomosis. A side-to-side anastomosis to a Roux-en-Y loop is performed as described above.

Most biliodigestive anastomoses can be performed by a hilum or left duct approach. If both options are not possible, then the round ligament approach is the next option. The ligamentum teres is divided and the parenchymal bridge between segment IV and the left lobe is transected. Then the liver is lifted up and the ligamentum teres stump is pulled downward (Fig. 8.8). The left base of the ligamentum teres is transected and the duct for segment III exposed above and behind the portal vein; a side-to-side anastomosis with a Roux-en-Y loop can be performed as was described above (see Fig. 8.7).

In 1949, Longmire described an approach to the segment II duct in the presence of extensive strictures of the left and right hepatic duct (12,28,29). The Longmire procedure is often less effective than the other methods, and involves liver resection with an increased risk of bleeding. The left lateral sector of the liver is mobilized. A clamp is placed across the left lateral segment next to the ligamentum teres. A wedge resection of the left lateral sector is performed exposing the ducts of segment II. Careful release of the clamp allows identification of the vessels, which are selectively ligated. The branches of the portal vein run in close proximity to the bile ducts and bleeding has to be controlled carefully without compromising the lumen of the ducts.

Occasionally, the right side of the liver has to be approached for drainage. A wedge resection of segments V or VI can be performed exposing the underlying ducts. Similarly, a cholecystectomy and incision of the gallbladder fossa has been described to expose the duct of segment V (29). However, with the advances of percutaneous transhepatic biliary drainage during the last decade, surgical drainage pro-

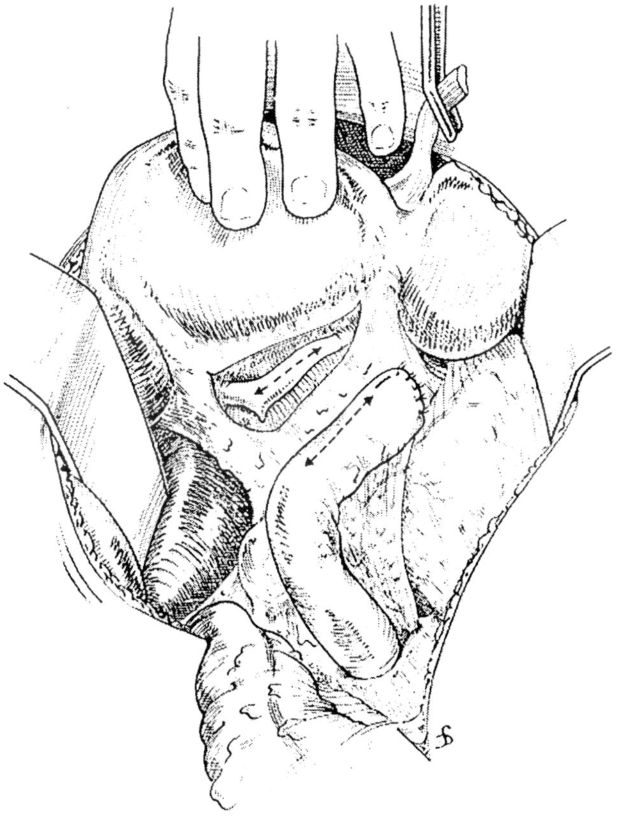

FIGURE 8.7. *The left hepatic duct is exposed after transection of the Glisson capsule at the base of the quadrate lobe. The horizontal extrahepatic course allows a wide Roux-en-Y anastomosis.*

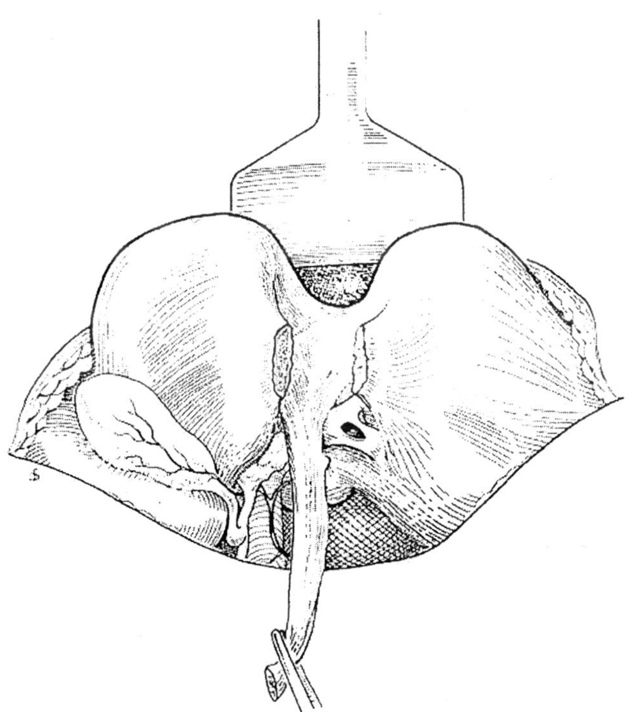

FIGURE 8.8. *The liver is pulled up and the ligamentum teres downwards. The duct of SIII can be approached by dissecting the left part of the base of the ligamentum teres. A side-to-side Roux-en-Y anastomosis can be performed.*

cedures using the segmental bile ducts are rarely performed today.

SUGGESTED READINGS

Blumgart LH. Hilar and intrahepatic biliary-enteric anastomosis. In: Blumgart LH, ed. Surgery of the liver and the biliary tree. 1st ed. Edinburgh: Churchill Livingstone, 1988:899–1515. This well-illustrated chapter describes in detail the different options and tricks for the reconstruction of the biliary tree.

Lygidakis NJ, Heyde MN. Surgical management of malignancies of the biliary tree. In: Lygidakis NJ, Tytgat GNJ, eds. Hepatobiliary and pancreatic malignancies. New York: Thieme, 1989:341–81. This chapter provides a well-illustrated description of the surgical approaches for cholangiocarcinoma.

Schlitt HJ, Meier PN, Nashan B, et al. Reconstructive surgery for ischemic-type lesions at the bile duct bifurcation after liver transplantation. Ann Surg 1999; 229:137–45. The authors evaluated their experience with biliary reconstruction after ischemic bile duct lesions. The different treatment options, complications and outcome are carefully analyzed.

REFERENCES

1. Bobbs J. Case of lithotomy of the gallbladder. Trans Med Soc Indiana 1868;18: 68–73.
2. Traverso W. Carl Langenbuch and the first cholecystectomy. Am J Surg 1976; 132:81–2.
3. Dahl R. Eine neue Operation der Gallenwege. Zentralbl Chir 1909;36:266–7.
4. Mizumoto R, Suzuki H. Surgical anatomy of the hepatic hilum with special reference to the caudate lobe. World J Surg 1988;12:2–10.
5. Hatfield ARW, Terblanche J, Fataar S, et al. Preoperative external biliary drainage in obstructive jaundice. Lancet 1982;23:896–9.
6. McPherson GAD, Benjamin IS, Hodgson HJF, et al. Pre-operative percutaneous transhepatic biliary drainage: the results of a controlled trial. Br J Surg 1984; 71:371–5.
7. Kawarada Y, Higashiguchi T, Yokoi H, et al. Preoperative biliary drainage in obstructive jaundice. Hepatogastroenterology 1995;42:300–7.
8. Takahashi K, Ogura Y, Kawarada Y. Pathophysiological changes caused by occlusion of blood flow into the liver during hepatectomy in dogs with obstructive jaundice. J Gastroenterol Hepatol 1996;11:963–70.
9. Dobay K, Freier D, Albaer P. The absent role of prophylactic antibiotics in low-risk patients undergoing laparoscopic cholecystectomy. Am Surg 1999;65: 226–8.
10. Higgins A, London J, Charland S, et al. Prophylactic antibiotics for elective laparoscopic cholecystectomy. Arch Surg 1999;134:611–14.
11. Larraz-Mora E, Mayol J, Martinez-Sarmiento J, et al. Open biliary tract surgery: multivariant analysis of factors affecting mortality. Dig Surg 1999;16: 204–8.
12. Selzner M, Clavien PA. Resection of liver tumors: special emphasis on neoadjuvant and adjuvant therapy. In: Clavien PA, ed. Malignant liver tumors: current and emerging therapies. Malden, MA: Blackwell Science, 1999:137–49.
13. Nakayama F, Miyazaki K, Naggafuchi K. Radical surgery for middle and distal thirds bile duct cancer. World J Surg 1988;12:60–3.
14. Sugiura Y, Nakamura S, Iida S, et al. Extensive resection of the bile ducts combined with liver resection for cancer of the main hepatic duct junction: a cooperative study of the Keio Bile Duct Cancer Study Group. Surgery 1994; 115:445–51.
15. Blumgart L, Benjamin I, Hadjis N, Beazley R. Surgical approaches to cholangiocarcinoma at confluence of hepatic ducts. Lancet 1984;14:66–9.
16. Stain S, Parekh D, Selby R. Tumors of the gallbladder and the biliary tract. In: Kaplowitz N, ed. Biliary disease. Los Angeles: Williams & Wilkins:725–38.
17. Nimura Y, Hayakawa N, Kamiya J, et al. Hepatic segmentectomy with caudate lobe resection for bile duct carcinoma of the hepatic hilus. World J Surg 1990;14:535–44.
18. Launois B, Terblanche J, Lakehal M, et al. Proximal bile duct cancer: high resectability rate and 5-year survival. Ann Surg 1999;230:266–75.
19. Klempnauer J, Ridder GJ, Werner M, et al. What constitutes long term survival after surgery for hilar cholangiocarcinoma? Cancer 1997;79:26–34.
20. Tashiro S, Tsuji T, Kanemitsu K, et al. Prolongation of survival for carcinoma at the hepatic duct confluence. Surgery 1993;113:270–8.
21. Tsuzuki T, Ueda M, Kuramochi S, et al. Carcinoma of the main hepatic junction: indications, operative morbidity and mortality, and long-term survival. Surgery 1990;108:495–501.
22. Bismuth H, Caistaing D, Traynor O. Resection or palliation: priority of surgery in the treatment of hilar cancer. World J Surg 1988;12:39–47.
23. Mizumoto R, Kawarada Y, Suzuki H. Surgical treatment of hilar carcinoma of the bile duct. Surg Gynecol Obstet 1986;162:153–8.
24. Pinson W, Rossi R. Extended right hepatic lobectomy, left hepatic lobectomy, and skeletonization resection for proximal bile duct cancer. World J Surg 1988;12:52–9.
25. Klempnauer J, Ridder G, Wasielewski R, et al. Resectional surgery of hilar cholangiocarcinoma: a multivariate analysis of prognostic factors. J Clin Oncol 1997;15:947–54.
26. Z'gragger K, Birrer S, Maurer C, et al. Incidence of port site recurrence after laparoscopic cholecystectomy for preoperatively unsuspected gallbladder carcinoma. Surgery 1998;124:831–8.
27. Lundberg O, Kristoffersson A. Port site metastases from gallbladder cancer after laparoscopic cholecystectomy. Results of a Swedish survey and review of published reports. Eur J Surg 1999;165:215–22.
28. Longmire W, Sandford M. Intrahepatic cholangiojejunostomy with partial resection of the liver. Surgery 1949;128:330–47.
29. Lygidakis N, Heyde M. Surgical management of malignancies of the biliary tree. In: Lygidakis N, Tytgat G, eds. Hepatobiliary and pancreatic malignancies. New York: Thieme, 1989:341–63.

Chapter 9

Laparoscopic Treatment for Diseases of the Biliary Tree and Gallbladder

STEVE EUBANKS ALEX GANDSAS

LAPAROSCOPIC CHOLECYSTECTOMY

Even though laparoscopic cholecystectomy is a relatively new procedure, it has been widely accepted as the treatment of choice for patients suffering from noncomplicated cholecystitis. Less postoperative pain, faster recovery, less disability, and better cosmesis are advantages of the laparoscopic approach when compared to open cholecystectomy.

Many developments and innovative ideas took place during the preceding 180 years that contributed to this new modality of treating patients. In 1806, Bozzini designed the *lichtliter* to perform cystoscopies. This apparatus was much bigger than current devices and the light source was a candle. In 1901, George Kelling of Dresden coined the term *coelioskope* to describe the technique that used a cystoscope to assess the effect of pneumoperitoneum in dogs (1). Some years later, in 1910, Hans Christian Jacobaeus published the first report of laparoscopy in humans (2). Technological advances were slow to develop, until 1963 with the introduction of a high flow insufflation device by Karl Semm.

Additional developments, including the Hopkins rod lens telescopes and videoscopic technology, enabled surgeons to work with a laparoscope using both hands and be assisted by team members who experienced the same view. This technological growth enabled Erich Mühe to perform the first laparoscopic cholecystectomy on September 12, 1985. But it was not until 1988 that this procedure was introduced to the United States by McKernan, Saye, Reddick, and Olsen (3).

Indications

The incidence of cholelithiasis is approximately 10% in the United States, of which 10% to 15% of patients will become symptomatic (4). The most frequent signs and symptoms are summarized in Table 9.1. Despite all of the different therapeutic options available to treat symptomatic gallstone disease—including oral dissolution therapy, extracorporeal shock wave lithotripsy, or methyl tert-butyl ether as contact dissolvent—the most effective cure is the removal of the gallbladder. The indications for laparoscopic cholecystectomy have not changed when compared to the open technique (Table 9.2). The relative indications are summarized in Table 9.3.

Whether diabetic patients suffering from asymptomatic gallstones should undergo selective cholecystectomy is not yet resolved. Patino et al. (5) support elective cholecystectomy in diabetic patients; however, Babineau et al. (6) concluded that asymptomatic gallstones in diabetic patients are not an indication for surgery. The prevalence of symptomatic gallstone disease in the diabetic patient population is approximately 15%, similar to that in nondiabetic patients, but the morbidity and mortality following an episode of cholecystitis are minimally higher among diabetic patients than nondiabetics (7).

Patients undergoing laparoscopic cholecystectomy have not shown an increase in mortality when the results are compared to those of the open technique (8). The incidence of common bile duct (CBD) injury, however, remains higher than for open cholecystectomy (Table 9.4).

Technique

General anesthesia is preferred for patients undergoing laparoscopic cholecystectomy. The patient is placed in a supine position and the operating surgeon usuall[illegible] the left side of the patient, with the assisting surg[illegible] right. The lithotomy position proposed by Persis[illegible] be used, with the surgeon standing between t[illegible]

Table 9.1. Symptoms of cholelithiasis

Biliary colic (right upper quadrant pain)
Fatty food intolerance
Bloating
Dyspepsia
Nausea
Vomiting

Table 9.2. Indications for laparoscopic cholecystectomy

Symptomatic cholelithiasis
Acute cholecystitis
Acalculous cholecystitis
Gallstone pancreatitis
Porcelain gallbladder
Polyps

Table 9.3. Relative indications for laparoscopic cholecystectomy

Asymptomatic diabetic women <60 years with gallstone disease
Immunosuppressed patients

Table 9.4. Injuries in open versus laparoscopic cholecystectomy (combined data)

	Open[a]	Laparoscopy[b]
Number of patients	42,974	5367
Mortality	0.17%	0.14%
CBD injury	0.2%	0.3%
Morbidity	14.7%	1.8%

[a] Open: Roslyn (8).
[b] Laparoscopy: Bailey (9), Schirmer (10), Cuschieri (11), Southern Surgeons Club (12), Spaw (13), Peters (14).

legs. The operating table should be adapted for fluoroscopic images if an intraoperative cholangiogram is sought. High-resolution monitors should be used facing the surgeon and the first assistant.

Prophylaxis against deep vein thrombosis is achieved by using sequential compression devices or subcutaneous heparin. Prophylactic antibiotics are not required for elective cholecystectomies and may increase the risk for bacteria resistance (15).

Once the patient is intubated and anesthetized, an orogastric tube and an indwelling urinary catheter are inserted with the aim of decompressing these organs to avoid injury while introducing the trocars and instruments. The skin is prepped from the mid-thorax to the groin, extended laterally to both posterior axillary lines. Pneumoperitoneum is achieved by two different techniques. A 1-cm incision is made below or into the umbilical scar to allow the insertion of a Veress needle. The intra-abdominal location is verified by observing a drop of normal saline solution flowing down the bore of the needle. The needle is then connected to carbon dioxide insufflator to achieve an intra-abdominal pressure of 15 mm Hg. This is followed by the insertion of a 10-mm (umbilical) trocar.

Alternatively, an open or Hasson technique is performed through a 1-cm incision within or near the umbilical scar and dissection is carried down through the subcutaneous tissue, the midline fascia, then the peritoneum. After entering the abdominal cavity, sutures are placed through the fascia layers to hold a 10-mm Hasson trocar in place.

Once the umbilical trocar or the Hasson cannula is placed, carbon dioxide flowing at a rate of 5 to 20 liters/minute is used to achieve pneumoperitoneum to a pressure of 12 to 15 mm Hg. This allows the insertion at 0 or 30 degrees of the laparoscope, and the abdomen is examined for comorbid pathology. Under direct vision, an additional trocar is inserted through the subxiphoid area, aiming toward the gallbladder. The location of this port is crucial, as its correct angulation to the biliary tree will provide an optimal position for dissection and manipulation. Additional trocars are inserted in the right mid-clavicular and anterior axillary line, 3 cm below the costal margin. These trocars should be at least 8 to 10 cm apart to avoid "sword fighting."

A grasper is inserted via the most lateral port to elevate the gallbladder fundus above the liver edge while another grasper is passed through the mid-clavicular port to retract the infundibulum in an inferior and lateral direction.

Dissection begins laterally at the infundibulum to expose the cystic duct and minimize the risk of injury to the biliary tree.

It is very important to keep the Calot's triangle opened by using lateral retraction of the gallbladder infundibulum. This maneuver allows a safe dissection for identifying the cystic artery and cystic duct. If the infundibulum is pulled laterally too hard, the CBD can be tented toward the cystic duct and therefore be exposed to injury. Furthermore, retraction of the infundibulum upward and/or medially will close the triangle, resulting in a CBD injury. At least 1 cm of well dissected cystic duct is necessary to place clips before dividing it or performing an intraoperative cholangiogram.

Caution should be exercised during electrocautery to avoid thermal injury to the biliary tree. The cystic duct is doubly clipped distal to the junction of the CBD before dividing the cystic duct with scissors. The same technique is applied to division of the cystic artery. A hook electrocautery is usually used to dissect the gallbladder from its attachments to the liver. The gallbladder or the liver should not be punctured, otherwise bile and/or stone spillage or bleeding, respectively, may occur. It is important to be aware that during this dissection an injury to the porta hepatis can occur and the plane of dissection must be maintained adjacent to the gallbladder wall. Before the gallbladder is completely excised, the liver bed should be examined for bleeding.

The dissection is then completed and the gallbladder retrieved via the umbilical or subxiphoid port incision. A specimen bag may be used to retrieve the organ, especially when an inflammatory process was involved, rupture or bile spillage occurred, or malignancy is suspected. It is occasionally necessary to open the gallbladder and manually remove the stones and bile at the skin edge. This will facilitate passage of the gallbladder through the 10-mm incision.

The 10-mm trocar is then returned to the abdominal cavity and the right upper quadrant is irrigated with saline solution and aspirated. The fascia at the 10-mm incision is closed with absorbable sutures to prevent port-site hernias.

Once they have recovered from anesthesia, patients are allowed to drink liquids and the diet is advanced according to patients' tolerance. Discharge usually takes place within the first 24 hours after surgery, and in many cases within 2 to 4 hours after surgery.

Contraindications

In patients known to be high risks for general anesthesia due to underlying cardiac or pulmonary disease, laparoscopic procedures should be planned with caution. Portal hypertension could become a serious problem due to the ascites or extreme bleeding from the collateral venous tributaries. Noncorrected coagulopathy may result in bleeding, impairing visualization, and increased risk for injury.

Although successful laparoscopic surgery in pregnant patients has been reported (16), special guidelines and careful patient selection should be considered (17). The effect of pneumoperitoneum on fetal outcome is still subject to investigation to determine the real adverse effect on the maternal–fetal well-being (18–19).

Complications of Laparoscopic Cholecystectomy

Complications of laparoscopic cholecystectomy can be divided into those occurring intraoperatively and those occurring postoperatively. Bile duct injuries and their management are discussed in depth in a separate chapter.

Intraoperative

Bleeding can occur at any time during the procedure, but transection of the superior epigastric artery or one of its branches during trocar insertion may result in a significant amount of bleeding. Control of port-site bleeding can be achieved by tilting the trocar temporarily to tamponade the bleeding vessel. Also, it can be ligated by using trocar site closure devices or by placing suture ligatures cephalad and caudal to the bleeding site (20). Sharp dissection should be used to divide adhesions or omentum attached to the liver; failure to do so will result in avulsion of the liver capsule with subsequent bleeding.

Bleeding that obscures anatomical structures may occur during dissection in Calot's triangle, resulting in a bile duct injury from blind clip placement.

There is usually adequate time to carefully identify the source of the bleeding so that precise control can be accomplished. Bleeding observed on the video monitor is magnified, so the actual blood loss is usually quite minimal. Occasionally it is helpful to insert a fifth port site so that the existing exposure of the bleeding site is maintained and an extra instrument can be inserted to grasp the bleeding vessel or to provide with suction and irrigation.

Bile spillage occurs approximately in 30% of all laparoscopic cholecystectomies (21–23). An enlarged gallbladder with signs of severe inflammation, edema, and thick walls may be very difficult to grasp and manipulate. Intraoperative decompression of the gallbladder is recommended to facilitate grasping and holding of the gallbladder. If the gallbladder wall is torn with subsequent bile and stone spillage, every effort should be made to retrieve all gallstones. Unretrieved stones have been shown to have a low complication rate, but 1% of patients may develop an intra-abdominal abscess (24,25). Additionally, fistulas from unretrieved gallstones have also been reported (26).

The role of laparoscopy in the management of carcinoma of the gallbladder is still controversial (27). As with any other malignancy, the disease stage will dictate the most appropriate treatment. For lesions confined to the mucosa and submucosa, simple cholecystectomy will suffice; however, a radical cholecystectomy should be performed if there is serosa involvement (28). Apparently the use of retrieval bags or a gasless technique has not prevented site-port metastasis or peritoneal seeding (29). Furthermore, although there is some evidence that laparoscopy may increase the incidence of local recurrence and abdominal wall spreading, the overall survival rate was similar to those patients undergoing an open procedure (30).

Thermal injury may result from excessive use of electrocautery or lasers. The effects of the heat transmitted to the tissue can damage small blood vessels, producing ischemia of the biliary tree. The subsequent postoperative stricture is not often recognized until months after the initial operation (31).

Postoperative Complications

Patients suspected of having a bile leak usually become symptomatic within the first week following laparoscopic or open cholecystectomy (32). Although most (87%) of the leaks presented in a study by Ramesh were noted in patients who underwent a laparoscopic procedure (33), the frequency of bile leakage in this group is decreasing as experience has been gained (34). Furthermore, the incidence of biliary leak has been high in laparoscopic cases that require open conversion, due to technical difficulties or the presence of edema and inflammation of the tissues (33% incidence of leak), when compared to those cases not converted (6.25%) (32).

The signs and symptoms of bile leak include abdominal pain (89%), fever (74%), peritonitis (81%), jaundice (43%), and nausea and vomiting (43%). Diagnostic studies have identified the cystic duct as the main source of bile leak (77%), followed by accessory ducts (15%) and the CBD (8%) (32). The approach to this problem should be multidisciplinary. The diagnosis is usually suspected based on clinical findings and supported by complementary studies. Ultrasound can detect a collection in 75% of the cases, and computed tomography (CT) scan in 95%. Endoscopic retrograde cholangiopancreatography (ERCP) may demonstrate the presence and site of leakage (80%) helping differentiate a simple fluid collection from a biloma (32). Although the hepatoiminodiacetic acid (HIDA) scan is also 80% successful in showing the leakage, ERCP is preferred because it not only serves as diagnostic tool, but also provides an adequate opportunity to render therapy.

Ryan et al. (35) have shown the effectiveness of endoscopic therapy by reducing the sphincter of Oddi pressure. This is achieved by placing biliary stents if the leak is small or using a combination stenting and endoscopic sphincterotomy for large leaks. Stents are left in place for an average period of 4 weeks. A cholangiogram is not routinely performed as part of the follow-up. Most abdominal fluid collections can be managed by percutaneous drainage alone (36). Persistent leaks may require surgical repair by laparoscopy or open procedures.

Cholangiography

Since the introduction of the intraoperative cholangiography (IOC) by the Argentinean surgeon Pedro Mirizzi in 1931 (37), the surgical community has been polarized regarding its indications. Those who support routine IOC contend that an image or a "road map" would allow the surgeon not only to document the presence of stones in the CBD (36) but also to identify the anatomy of the biliary tree, thus lowering the risk for injury (38). In addition, IOC is much more cost effective when compared to the postoperative endoscopic procedures necessary to diagnose and treat residual stones in the CBD (39). However, CBD stones found during IOC can be successfully managed by endoscopic maneuvers, avoiding the manipulation of the biliary tree during surgery (40). Many surgeons prefer to perform cholangiography in selective cases, based upon specific criteria such as a history of jaundice or pancreatitis, dilation of the CBD and cystic duct observed on ultrasound, or elevation of bilirubin and alkaline phosphatase (41).

The role of operative cholangiogram to prevent injuries is still somewhat controversial. Although there is inadequate data that demonstrates that IOC decreases the incidence of iatrogenic bile duct injuries, it may facilitate injury recognition during the operation. Whereas ductal injuries that are recognized during the initial operation can often be repaired primarily, delayed recognition may result in septic complications (42). Injuries can result despite performance of the cholangiogram. Aggressive cannulation of a difficult cystic duct may sever the posterior wall of the cystic duct or CBD (43). Further interpretation of the images by the surgeon may lead to an unrecognized injury or improper dissection and injury of the CBD after the IOC (36). Preoperative infusion cholangiogram avoids manipulation of the CBD to assess the biliary tree during the operation. However, this modality has not been proven to be safer than IOC; also, the incidence of allergic reaction is about 8% (44), so its use is not justified (45).

Technique

Calot's triangle is dissected and the cystic duct is identified. A distal clip is placed into the cystic duct–gallbladder junction. An incision is performed on the anterior wall using microscissors. Multiple cuts should be avoided, as this could result in complete transection of the duct. The opening is confirmed by documenting bile coming out of the duct.

At this time it is advisable to "milk" the cystic duct upward toward the gallbladder to retrieve any stones or debris that may exist in the lumen and make cannulation of the duct much more laborious.

A cholangiograsper is inserted via the mid-clavicular port holding a cholangiogram catheter or a 4 French ureteral catheter. Prior to insertion, the catheter should be flushed with normal saline. This catheter should never be forced into the duct, as this maneuver can result in a perforation or tear of the cystic duct or the CBD. If resistance is encountered, normal saline can be injected to distend the duct's lumen wall, thus facilitating the insertion into the cystic duct beyond the valves of Heister.

Once the catheter is in position, it is secured with the cholangiograsper. The scope and additional graspers are removed and the catheter is secured to the abdomen to avoid dislodging. Injected air bubbles have the appearance of stones and can mislead the surgeon. Dynamic real-time fluoroscopy is preferred to view the contrast injection.

Problems and Solutions for Laparoscopic Cholangiography

Difficult Cannulation

The valves of Heister are often responsible for difficult cannulation of the cystic duct. A hydrophilic guidewire can be used as a guide to facilitate catheter insertion.

Re-incising the cystic duct at a closer point to the CBD may help bypass the valves of Heister.

Air Bubbles

If radiolucent images consistent with air bubbles are noticed during cholangiogram, a reverse Trendelenburg position can help in making the correct diagnosis. Air bubbles will tend to float cranially while stones will remain in the distal CBD.

Excess of Contrast

Saturating the biliary tree with contrast material can impair visualization, making it difficult to identify small stones. Saline can be used to flush the CBD and make it possible to repeat the cholangiogram.

Nonvisualization of the Proximal Ducts

Contrast material can pass to the duodenum very rapidly, preventing visualization of the proximal ducts. Berci suggests the use of morphine and the Trendelenburg position to maximize CBD visualization (46). Another useful technique involves compressing the CBD with the shaft of a grasper while injecting the contrast material. Visualization of the proximal biliary tree is mandatory, and if it cannot be accomplished using the above technique, it must be assumed that the CBD has been mistaken for the cystic duct and cannulated.

Filling Defects

When the contrast material reveals well-rounded radiolucent images that are consistent with choledocholithiasis, the decision to proceed with either CD–CBDE (cystic duct CBD exploration) or CBDE (CBD exploration) will be based on the size of the biliary tree and any stones. This is discussed in more detail in the section on choledocholithiasis.

Accessory Duct of Luschka

If the gallbladder is noted to fill with contrast, despite adequate clip placement on the cystic duct at the junction with the Hartmann's pouch, an accessory duct of Luschka should be sought. Management of this variant involves the proper identification of the duct and ligation. Failure to do so can result in a postoperative biloma.

Hepatic Duct Injury

If only the cystic duct and the CBD are visualized in addition to a pool of contrast with no definite anatomy, injury to the hepatic duct from contrast extravasation should be suspected (see Chapter 17).

Hepatic Duct Obstruction

If the contrast material delineates the cystic duct, CBD, and part of the hepatic duct, there may be a partial obstruction of the common hepatic duct, possibly due to clip placement.

COMMON BILE DUCT STONES

The incidence of CBD stones found on routine cholangiography has been calculated to be approximately 10% to 20% (47). If selective cholangiography is performed based upon clinical history or laboratory or ultrasound findings, unexpected stones can be found in 3.5% to 4.0% (48).

When a positive cholangiogram has been obtained, the technique used to clear stones from the biliary tree will depend on many factors. Those familiar with advanced laparoscopic skills usually favor a laparoscopic common bile duct exploration (LCBDE), which allows for removal of the stones during the primary operation. In experienced hands, the morbidity and mortality of the LCBDE ranges from 5% to 10% and 0% to 2%, respectively (49–50). LCBDE and postoperative ERCP have similar morbidity (17% and 15%, respectively) and success rates (97% and 93%, respectively) in clearing the CBD (51–52). ERCP with sphincterotomy has a reported mortality rate of 1.5%. Specific complications associated with ERCP include pancreatitis (1.9%), perforation (1%), bleeding (3%), and sepsis (1.7%) (53). There are reports supporting laparoscopic cholecystectomy combined with preoperative ERCP (54) or perioperative endoscopic retrograde sphincterotomy (55,56) as an optional single-stage approach for patients suffering from choledocholithiasis. However, prospective studies are needed to determine the cost-effectiveness of this modality.

Intraoperative options for the management of choledocholithiasis are guided by the anatomy of the biliary tree, size of the stones, resources, and operator's laparoscopic skills. These options include:

- Transcystic CBD exploration
- Fluoroscopic bile duct wire basket stone retrieval
- Biliary balloon catheter stone retrieval
- Ampullary balloon dilatation
- Laparoscopic choledochotomy
- Choledochoscopy

Transcystic Common Bile Duct Exploration

Indications

The indications for transcystic CBD exploration (TCBDE) are an abnormal cholangiogram showing or suggesting choledocholithiasis; cystic duct larger than 4 mm merging into the hepatic duct at a straight angle; CBD stones less than 6 mm of diameter; CBD less than 6 mm; and/or minimal tissue edema. This technique is useful for the surgeon unfamiliar with advanced laparoscopic suturing techniques.

Contraindications

This procedure should not be performed by operators who are not familiar with the technique or when the stones are larger than 10 mm.

Technique

The cholecystectomy trocar configuration is usually sufficient for TCBDE. The cystic duct is dissected free of the surrounding tissues and medially toward the junction with the CBD. A small opening is made in the cystic duct with microscissors, and the cholangiogram is performed. Dilation of the cystic duct is achieved by inserting a floppy tipped, hydrophilic guidewire and advancing it into the CBD. A #5 Phantom balloon catheter is inserted over the guidewire and inflated to dilate the cystic duct no wider than the diameter of the CBD. The balloon is kept inflated for 3 minutes at 10 to 12 atmospheres of pressure.

If small stones (<2 mm) are noticed in the CBD, 1 mg of glucagon can be administered intravenously to relax the sphincter of Oddi; this is followed by flushing of the CBD with a small catheter, lavaging the stones into the duodenum. Clearance of the biliary tree should be verified with cholangiography. If larger stones are encountered, a small 3-mm diameter flexible choledochoscope can be inserted through the mid-clavicular port and negotiated into the CBD via the dilated cystic duct.

A four-wired basket (2.4F) can be used to retrieve stones no larger than 10 mm (57). It is recommended that the more proximal stones be captured initially to avoid pushing them up into the hepatic duct. With choledochoscope guidance, the basket is passed beyond the stone and is then opened, allowing the stone to be captured by applying small rotational movements. The scope and basket are withdrawn from the cystic duct as an entire ensemble. If the stone is impacted in the CBD, a Fogarty-type balloon catheter can be used to dislodge it by passing the catheter beyond the fixed point, inflating the balloon, and slowly retrieving the stone.

For stones larger than 10 mm, laser or hydraulic lithotripsy can be employed to achieve fragmentation (57).

The procedure is finished by performing a final cholangiogram documenting the biliary tree free of stones. A small cystic duct catheter is left in place and secured with an Endoloop. This will allow postoperative cholangiogram as well as percutaneous stone manipulation, if needed.

Fluoroscopic Bile Duct Wire Basket Stone Retrieval

The fluoroscopic bile duct wire basket stone retrieval technique is very useful for stones smaller than 3 mm and when the operator is unable to dilate the cystic duct. The Trocar positions are similar to those used for TCBDE. Following cholangiogram, all stones should be flushed from the CBD to the duodenum as described above. If repeat cholangiogram continues to show remaining stones, a 4F six-wire basket is carefully introduced into the CBD, not severing it during insertion. The catheter should be advanced up to the papilla into the duodenum. Its position is confirmed with fluoroscopy showing the catheter marker above the papilla. Catheter entrapment is the cause of bleeding and pancreatitis.

The basket is then opened and under fluoroscopic guidance the stone is engaged, applying a rotational movement to the basket while pulling out. If the stone is too big to pass the cystic duct, more pressure should be applied to the basket wires with the goal of fragmenting the stone. A cholangiogram is performed at termination of the procedure to verify ductal stone clearance.

Biliary Balloon Catheter Stone Retrieval

Biliary balloon catheter stone retrieval procedure is very useful when the intraoperative cholangiogram shows small stones and debris. A 4F balloon-tipped catheter is inserted into the cystic duct and into the CBD to the duodenum. The balloon is inflated and then the catheter is pulled back until the papilla is engaged. Confirmation of the catheter position is made with fluoroscopy. The balloon is then deflated and pulled 1 cm into the CBD. The balloon is once again inflated and pulled toward the cystic duct. Care should be taken not to lodge the stones into the hepatic duct. Once the biliary tree is clear a cholangiogram is repeated.

Ampulla Balloon Dilatation

Ampulla balloon dilatation is mostly used with cystic ducts that are too small to accommodate a choledochoscope. The goal is to increase the size of the sphincter of Oddi by means of balloon dilation (58). A 7-mm balloon catheter is inserted into the CBD via the cystic duct over a balloon-tipped guidewire. The catheter is positioned in such a way that the radio-opaque mark spans the sphincter of Oddi. The balloon catheter is inflated for 3 minutes up to a pressure of 12 atmospheres, after which it is deflated and the CBD is flushed with warm normal saline. A cholangiogram is repeated to assess the patency of the CBD. If there is a good passage of contrast to the duodenum, the cystic duct can be clipped or ligated with an Endoloop.

Laparoscopic Choledochotomy

The following situations indicate laparoscopic bile duct exploration via a choledochotomy:

- Failure of the transcystic approach
- Unfavorable anatomy with a tortuous cystic duct
- Multiple stones with dilated CBD (>8 mm)
- ERCP unavailable or has failed to extract impacted stones
- Intrahepatic stones that cannot be extracted through the cystic duct approach

Although laparoscopic bile duct exploration has a reportedly high rate of success—close to 97% stone extraction rate with 2% retained stones (50)—the procedure is quite demanding and should only be performed by those familiar with advanced laparoscopic techniques and intracorporeal suturing. Furthermore, if multiple stones are found on a significantly dilated CBD, the choledochotomy could be used to carry out a choledochoduodenostomy.

Contraindications

Laparoscopic bile duct exploration should not be performed by those who have poor operative skills or are unable to perform intracorporeal suturing. It should not be attempted when the CBD is too small (<8 mm).

Technique

The port configuration is similar to the one used to remove the gallbladder. A cholangiogram is obtained documenting the presence of stones in the biliary tree and their characteristics, as well as providing a road map of the anatomy. Once Calot's triangle is dissected, the cystic duct is clipped at the junction with the neck of the gallbladder. Following opening of the cystic duct, a cholangiogram is obtained. An intraoperative cholangiogram also helps reveal malignancy within the biliary tree in jaundiced patients (39). The gallbladder is not removed, as retracting it will aid in exposing the bilary tree.

The CBD is dissected from the surrounding tissues, exposing at least 5 mm of anterior surface. A 1-cm vertical incision is made very close to the duodenum if choledochoduodenostomy is anticipated (58).

Upon opening the CBD it is sometimes feasible to milk a single stone upward to the choledochotomy and remove it with graspers. A 7F choledochoscope is inserted and the CBD is irrigated and flushed distally. If impacted stones are found, a Fogarty catheter can be used to dislodge the stones and extraction should proceed with a 3F four-wire-basket. If the stones are still impacted and cannot be retrieved into the choledochotomy, stone fragmentation can be achieved with the use of an electrohydraulic or laser lithotripter.

Once the biliary tree has been cleared of stones, the scope can be easily passed to the duodenum, although this maneuver is discouraged. If the sphincter is found to be tight, then dilatation of the ampulla can be sought as described before with or without a laparoscopic anterograde sphincterotomy (59). A cholangiogram can be performed through the scope to document a clear passage of contrast to the duodenum. Following this, the choledochotomy is closed over an 8F to 10F T-tube (with crossbar trimmed) using absorbable material in an interrupted fashion or by primary closure leaving a transcystic duct catheter. It is necessary to decompress the biliary tree while performing primary closure of the CBD to avoid bile leak during the postoperative period. A Jackson Pratt drain is left in the subhepatic area.

Cuschieri et al. (60) recommend conversion when the procedure has taken more than 2 hours and there is no evidence of progress, when the surgeon is not trained in laparoscopic choledochoenterostomy, and when there is uncontrollable bleeding.

Patients are allowed to drink liquids during the immediate postoperative period and the diet is advanced the following day. The Jackson Pratt drain is removed on second postoperative day if it does not contain bile and drainage is below 30 mL/day. The transcystic catheter can be clamped once the output recorded is less than 300 mL/day. It should not be removed before 10 days to ensure a good fistulous tract. The T-tube is clamped after 10 days and left in place for 3 weeks. A cholangiogram is performed prior to its removal to assess the biliary tree and the passage of contrast into the duodenum.

Laparoscopic CBD exploration performed in a single setting has proved to be effective with good short-term results, low morbidity and mortality, and low incidence of retained stones (49–50) (Tables 9.5 and 9.6).

Siddique et al. (61) have recently published the largest study of endoscopic choledochoscopy use as an extension of ERCP for diagnostic and therapeutic purposes. They report that the diagnosis was made in 58% of patients with choledochoscopy, and that it provided unsuspected information in 29.5%. This technique was successful in treating 44.2% of patients.

Intraoperative Ultrasonography

After laparoscopic cholecystectomy became the gold standard for acute cholecystitis, surgeons realized that the lack of tactile sensation was a disadvantage, compared to the open procedure. This drawback must be compensated for with good visualization. Thus, this has been the perfect

Table 9.5. Outcome of laparoscopic common bile duct exploration

	Study	
	Dorman (50)	Paganini (49)
Success	97.5%	94%
Retained stones	3.5	2.0
Conversion rate	2.4	3.4
Morbidity	3.8	4.0
Mortality	0.6	0.6

Table 9.6. Complications following laparoscopic common bile duct exploration

Biloma	1.9
Hyperamylasemia	1.9
Port side infection	1.2
Umbilical hernia	0.6
Hemoperitoneum	1.9
Dyspepsia	15.0

scenario to reassess the role of routine IOC as a complementary tool to "show" what the surgeon could not "touch." While this debate continues today, laparoscopic ultrasound (LUS) technology has emerged as an important utensil in the armamentarium of any surgeon committed to advanced laparoscopy. When compared to IOC, LUS has proven to be less time consuming and provides the surgeon with images of the biliary tree before dissection. It can also provide information about the accuracy of arterial and venous structures (62). Another advantage of LUS is that it can recognize small (2 mm) stones that are not seen with IOC (63). LUS does not produce any radiation, so it can be performed several times during the same procedure.

Many studies have shown that LUS is less sensitive but more specific when compared to cholangiography in detecting CBD stones (Table 9.7). Infusing normal saline through the cystic duct increases the ultrasound sensitivity up to 100%, adding a dynamic view of the papilla while the fluid flows through the duodenum (64).

Technique

The same trocar position configuration for laparoscopic cholecystectomy is used. The ultrasound probe is introduced through the umbilical port. A 5-mm camera is placed in the lateral port. Around 100 to 200 mL of normal saline is instilled into the abdomen to enhance acoustic coupling. The examination starts by placing the probe on the anterior surface of the liver and visualizing both hepatic ducts as well as the common hepatic duct confluence. The probe is then moved below the liver edge at the most cephalad aspect of the hepatoduodenal ligament with the goal of identifying the portal vein, common hepatic duct, and hepatic artery. Finally, the ultrasound probe is positioned lateral to the duodenum to scan, through a duodenal window, the CBD, pancreas, and ampulla. While rigid probes are able to scan extrahepatic bile ducts in a transverse fashion, a mobile tip (flexible) ultrasound probe allows visualization of the CBD in a longitudinal fashion (65).

Among the major disadvantages of LUS is its inability to properly scan tissues if edema or excess adipose tissue exists (63). Undoubtedly, the learning curve for correct interpretation of ultrasound images is difficult. However, Barteau et al. (66) proposed the use of routine LUS in simple cases so that practitioners can become familiar with the technique. Skills developed during this period can be of enormous value during complex cases.

Table 9.7. Laparoscopic ultrasound compared to cholangiogram

	Ultrasound		Cholangiogram	
	Sensitivity	Specificity	Sensitivity	Specificity
Roethlin (63)	91%	100%	64%	100%
Thompson (64)	76.5%	100%	100%	96.7%
Birth (65)	83.3%	100%	100%	98.9%
Barteau (66)	71.4%	100%	92.8%	76.2%

REFERENCES

1. Litynski GS. Highlights in the history of laparoscopy: the development of laparoscopic techniques—a cumulative effort of internists, gynecologists, and surgeons. Frankfurt/Main: Barbara Bernert Verlag, 1996.
2. Jacobaeus HC. Ueber die Moeglichkeit die Zystoskopie bei Untersuchung seroeser Hoehlungen anzuwenden. Munch Med Wochenschr 1910;57:2090–2.
3. Reddick EJ, Olsen DO, Daniel JP, et al. Laparoscopic laser cholecystectomy. Laser Med Surg News 1989;7:38–40.
4. Friedman G. Natural history of symptomatic and asymptomatic gallstones. Am J Surg 1993;165:339–404.
5. Patino JF, Quintero GA. Cholelithiasis revisited. World J Surg 1998;22:1119–24.
6. Babineau TJ, Bothe Jr, A. General surgery considerations in the diabetic patient. Infect Dis Clin North Am 1995;9:183–93.
7. Del Favero G, Caroli A, Meggiato T, et al. Natural history of gallstones in non-insulin-dependent diabetes mellitus. A prospective 5-year follow-up. Dig Dis Sci 1994;39:1704–7.
8. Roslyn HJ, Binns GS, Hughes EF, et al. Open cholecystectomy: a contemporary analysis of 42,474 patients. Ann Surg 1993;218:129–37.
9. Bailey RW, Zucker KA, Flowers JL, et al. Laparoscopic cholecystectomy: experience with 375 consecutive patients. Ann Surg 1991;214:531–40.
10. Schirmer BD, Edge SB, Dix J, et al. Laparoscopic cholecystectomy: treatment of choice for symptomatic cholelithiasis. Ann Surg 1991;1:2–7.
11. Cuschieri A, DuBois F, Mouiel J. The European experience with laparoscopic cholecystectomy. Am J Surg 1991;161:358–87.
12. The Southern Surgeons Club. A prospective study analysis of 1518 laparoscopic cholecystectomies. N Engl J Med 1991;324:1073–8.
13. Spaw AT, Reddick EJ, Olsen DO. Laparoscopic laser cholecystectomy: analysis of 500 procedures. Surg Laparosc Endosc 1991;1:2–7.
14. Peters JH, Gibbons GD, Innes JT, et al. Complications of laparoscopic cholecystectomy. Surgery 1991;110:769–78.
15. Illig KA, Schmidt E, Cavanaugh J, et al. Are prophylactic antibiotics required for elective laparoscopic cholecystectomy? J Am Coll Surg 1997;184:353–6.
16. Pucci RO, Seed RW. Case report of laparoscopic cholecystectomy in the third trimester of pregnancy. Am J Obstet Gynecol 1991 Aug;165:401–2.
17. SAGES guidelines for laparoscopic surgery and pregnancy. Surg Endosc 1998;12:189–90.
18. Slim K, Canis M. Laparoscopic surgery and pregnancy. J Chir 1998;135:261–6.
19. Amos JD, Schorr SJ, Norman PF, et al. Laparoscopic surgery during pregnancy. Am J Surg 1996;171:435–7.
20. Cullen J. Laparoscopic cholecystectomy: avoiding complications. In: Scott-Conner CEH, ed. The SAGES Manual. Fundamentals of Laparoscopy and GI Endoscopy. New York: Springer-Verlag, 1999:137–42.
21. Assaff Y, Matter I, Sabo E, et al. Laparoscopic cholecystectomy for acute cholecystitis and the consequences of gallbladder perforation, bile spillage, and "loss" of stones. Eur J Surg 1998;164:425–31.
22. Kimura T, Goto H, Takeuchi Y, et al. Intraabdominal contamination after gallbladder perforation during laparoscopic cholecystectomy and its complications. Surg Endosc 1996;10:888–91.
23. Soper NJ, Dunnegan DL. Does intraoperative gallbladder perforation influence the early outcome of laparoscopic cholecystectomy?. Surg Laparosc Endosc 199;1:156–61.
24. Memon MA, Decik RK, Maffi TR, et al. The outcome of unretrieved gallstones in the peritoneal cavity during laparoscopic cholecystectomy. A prospective analysis. Surg Endosc 1999;13:848–57.
25. Schaefer M, Suter C, Kaliber CH, et al. Spilled gallstones after laparoscopic cholecystectomy. A relevant problem? A retrospective analysis of 10,174 laparoscopic cholecystectomies. Surg Endosc 1998;12:305–9.
26. Patterson EJ, Nagy AG. Don't cry over spilled stones? Complications of gallstones spilled during laparoscopic cholecystectomy: case report and literature review. Can J Surg 1997;40:300–4.
27. Razzetta F, Borgonovo G, Cagnazzo A, et al. Laparoscopic cholecystectomy and gallbladder cancer: a diagnostic and therapeutic dilemma. Eur J Surg Oncol 1997;23:84–5.
28. Bartlett DL, Fong Y, Fortner JG, et al. Long-term results after resection for gallbladder cancer. Implications for staging and management. Ann Surg 1996;224:639–46.

29. Sarli L, Costi R, Pietra N, et al. Incidental gallbladder cancer at laparoscopy: a review of two cases. Surg Laparosc Endosc Percutan Tech 1999;9:414–7.
30. Suzuki K, Kimura T, Ogawa H. Is laparoscopic cholecystectomy hazardous for gallbladder cancer?. Surgery 1998;123:311–14.
31. Davido FF, Pappas TN, Murray EA, et al. Mechanism of major biliary injury during laparoscopic cholecystectomy. Ann Surg 1992;215:196–202.
32. Barkum AN, Rezieg M, Mehta SN, et al. Post-cholecystectomy leaks in the laparoscopic era: risk factors, presentation and management. Gastrointest Endosc 1997;45:227–83.
33. Ramesh H. Postcholecystectomy bile leaks and their management. Gastrointest Endosc 1998;47:564–5.
34. Woods MS, Traverso LW, Kozarek RA, et al. Characteristics of biliary tract complications during laparoscopic cholecystectomy. Am J Surg 1994;167:27–33.
35. Ryan ME, Geenen JE, Lehman GA, et al. Endoscopic intervention for biliary tract complications during laparoscopic cholecystectomy. Am J Surg 1998;47:261–6.
36. MacFayden B Jr, Vecchio R, Ricardo AE, et al. Bile duct injury after laparoscopic cholecystectomy. Surg Endosc 1998;12:315–21.
37. Mirizzi P. Operative cholangiography. Surg Gynecol Obstet 1937;65:702–10.
38. Kullmann E, Borch E, Lindstrom J, et al. Value of routine intraoperative cholangiography in detecting aberrant bile duct injuries during laparoscopic cholecystectomy. Br J Surg 1996;83:171–5.
39. Sackier JM. Intraoperative cholangiography—routine. In: Arregui M, Fitzgibbons R Jr, Katkhouda N, et al., eds. Principles of laparoscopic surgery: basic and advanced techniques. New York: Springer-Verlag, 1995:129–38.
40. Talamini MA. Selective cholangiography. In: Arregui M, Fitzgibbons R Jr, Katkhouda N, et al., eds. Principles of laparoscopic surgery: basic and advanced techniques. New York: Springer-Verlag, 1995:139–42.
41. Csendes A, Burdiles P, Carlos Diaz J, et al. Prevalence of common bile duct stones according to the increasing number of risk factors present. A prospective study employing routine intraoperative cholangiography. Hepatogastroenterology 1998;45:1415–21.
42. Russell JC, Walsh SJ, Mattie AS, et al. Bile duct injuries, 1989–93. A state wide experience. Arch Surg 1996;131:382–8.
43. Flowers JL, Zucker KA, Graham SM, et al. Laparoscopic cholangiography, results and indications. Ann Surg 1992;215:209–16.
44. Shehadi WH, Giuseppe T. Adverse reactions to contrast media. Diag Radiol 1980;136:299–302.
45. Hammarstroem LE, Torsten H, Stridbeck H, et al. Routine preoperative infusion cholangiography versus intraoperative cholangiography at elective cholecystectomy: a prospective study in 995 patients. J Am Coll Surg 1996;182:408–16.
46. Berci G. Laparoscopic cholecystectomy: cholangiography. In: Scott-Conner CEH, ed. The SAGES manual. Fundamentals of laparoscopy and GI endoscopy. New York: Springer-Verlag, 1999:178–87.
47. Joyce WP, Keane R, Burke GJ, et al. Identification of bile duct stones in patients undergoing laparoscopic cholecystectomy. Br J Surg 1991;78:1174–6.
48. Phillips EH, Carroll BJ, Pearlstein AR, et al. Laparoscopic choledochoscopy and extraction of common bile duct stones. World J Surg 1993;17:22–8.
49. Paganini AM, Lezoche E. Follow up of 161 unselected consecutive patients treated laparoscopically for common bile duct stones. Surg Endosc 1998;12:23–9.
50. Dorman JP, Franklin ME, Glass JL. Laparoscopic common bile duct exploration via choledochotomy. An effective method of treatment of choledocholithiasis. Surg Endosc 1998;12:926–8.
51. Rhodes M, Sussmann L, Cohen L, et al. Randomised trial of laparoscopic exploration of the common bile duct versus postoperative endoscopic retrograde cholangiography for common bile duct stones. Lancet 1998;17;351:159–61.
52. Keeling NJ, Menzies D, Motson RW. Laparoscopic exploration of the common bile duct: beyond the learning curve. Surg Endosc 1999;13:109–12.
53. Cotton PB, Lehman G, Vennes J, et al. Endoscopic sphincterotomy complications and their management: an attempt at consensus. Gastrointest Endosc 1991;37:383–93.
54. Sarli L, Pietra N, Franze A, et al. Routine intravenous cholangiography, selective ERCP, and endoscopic cholecystectomy. Gastrointest Endosc 1999;50:200–8.
55. Basso N, Pizzuto G, Desdamona S, et al. Laparoscopic cholecystectomy and intraoperative indoscopic sphincterotomy in the treatment of cholecysto-choledocholithiasis. Gastrointest Endosc 1999;50:532–5.
56. Meyer C, Vo Huu Le J, Rohr S, et al. Management of common bile duct stones in a single operation combining laparoscopic cholecystectomy and perioperative endoscopic sphincterotomy. Surg Endosc 1999;13:874–77.
57. Carroll BJ, Fallas MJ, Phillips EH. Laparoscopic transcystic choledochoscopy. Surg Endosc 1994;8:310–14.
58. Gurbuz AT, et al. Laparoscopic choledochoduodenostomy. Am Surg 1999;65:212–14.
59. De Paula AL, Hashiba K, Bafutto M, et al. Laparoscopic antegrade sphincterotomy. Surg Laparosc Endosc 1993;3:147–60.
60. Cuschieri A, Kimber C. Common bile duct exploration via laparoscopic choledochotomy. In: Scott-Connor CEH, ed. The SAGES Manual. Fundamentals of laparoscopy and GI endoscopy. New York: Springer-Verlag, 1999:178–87.
61. Siddique I, Galati J, Ankoma V, et al. The role of choledochoscopy in the diagnosis and management of biliary tract diseases. Gastrointest Endosc 1999;50:67–73.
62. Roethlin MA, Schob O, Schlumpf R, et al. Laparoscopic ultrasonography during cholecystectomy. Br J Surg 1996;83:1512–16.
63. Roethlin MA. Laparoscopic ultrasound of the biliary tree. In: L Arregui ME, Fitzgibbons RJ Jr, Katkhouda N, et al., eds. Principles of laparoscopic surgery. New York: Springer-Verlag, 1995.
64. Thompson DM, Arregui ME, Tetik C. A comparison of laparoscopic ultrasound with digital fluorocholangiography for detecting choledocholithiasis during laparoscopic cholecystectomy. Surg Endosc 1998;12:929–32.
65. Birth M, Ehlers KU, Delinikolas H, et al. Prospective randomized comparison of laparoscopic ultrasonography using a flexible-tip ultrasound probe and intraoperative dynamic cholangiography during laparoscopic cholecystectomy. Surg Endosc 1998;12:30–6.
66. Barteau JA, Castro D, Arregui ME, et al. A comparison of intraoperative ultrasound versus cholangiography in the evaluation of the common bile duct during laparoscopic cholecystectomy. Surg Endosc. 1995;9:490–6.

Chapter 10

Medical and Innovative Therapies for Biliary Malignancies

MICHAEL A. MORSE

Malignancies of the biliary tree and gallbladder have remained a challenging area for medical oncologists because of the minimal to moderate chemosensitivity of these tumors and the complications associated with obstructive jaundice that increase the complexity and risks of medical therapy. Although for most patients, medical therapies remain palliative, they are an integral part of multimodality approaches that offer the promise of improved results in patients with initially unresectable disease. Newer approaches such as anti-angiogenic therapy, immunotherapy, and gene therapy may improve the results further in the future.

CHEMOTHERAPEUTIC APPROACHES TO BILIARY MALIGNANCIES

Chemotherapy has been integrated into the treatment of biliary malignancies in several different ways. For tumors not clearly resectable at presentation, there has been interest in preoperative (neoadjuvant) strategies using chemotherapy or chemotherapy combined with radiotherapy to induce enough tumor regression to permit a surgical resection. Because radiation is less effective in hypoxemic tissues and chemotherapy may not reach devascularized tissues, another benefit of preoperative treatment may be better delivery of therapeutic agents before surgery disrupts the vascular supply. Also, effective preoperative treatment may reduce the viability of any tumor cells released during surgical manipulations. Finally, the tolerance of patients to chemotherapy and radiation may be better prior to the major procedures required for tumor resection.

For tumors that have been resected, the risk of recurrence is high and may occur locoregionally or at distant sites. This has prompted interest in applying adjuvant chemoradiotherapy to reduce not only local recurrence, but also recurrence of micrometastases following surgery. Chemotherapeutic agents that act as radiosensitizers allow for augmentation of local control simultaneously with attempts to control distant metastases.

For locally advanced tumors with no hope for resection or for metastatic disease, chemotherapy or radiation may have a role in palliating symptomatic complications of biliary malignancies such as pain, biliary tract obstruction, and ascites. The goal of these treatments is to maximize survival or quality of life. Although these goals may be served by other modalities such as biliary stenting or narcotic analgesics, a short course of chemotherapy or radiation may reduce the need for other interventions or increase their effectiveness.

The delivery of chemotherapy to treat biliary malignancies may be accomplished by intravenous injections, protracted intravenous infusions, and regional (hepatic arterial) infusions. Single or multiple agents in combination may be given and chemotherapy may be combined with radiotherapy or immunotherapy. The discussions in the following sections separately focus on gallbladder and bile duct cancers and are subdivided into neoadjuvant and adjuvant therapy. Because most studies of palliative chemotherapy or chemoradiotherapy group gallbladder and biliary duct tumors, we will discuss palliative therapy in a single section.

NEOADJUVANT AND ADJUVANT CHEMOTHERAPEUTIC APPROACHES TO GALLBLADDER CANCER

Neoadjuvant Chemotherapy

Neoadjuvant chemotherapy or chemoradiotherapy has not been systematically studied for gallbladder cancer, partly due to the rarity of this cancer and partly due to the frequent need for an operative procedure to establish the diagnosis or provide palliation of obstructive symptoms. There are anecdotal reports of patients who received palliative chemotherapy or chemoradiotherapy and had a significant response permitting an attempted surgical resection. For example, a recent case report describes the use of intra-arterial chemotherapy (cisplatin [Platinol] 10 mg + 5-fluorouracil [5-FU], 250 mg/day/week, 5 times, and epirubicin 10 mg + 5-fluorouracil 250 mg/day/week, 3 times) through the hepatic artery and oral chemotherapy (UFT [uracil/ftorafur], 300 mg/day for 106 days) to induce a partial response in a woman with an unresectable gallbladder cancer. A curative resection (hepatopancreatoduodenectomy with regional lymph nodes dissection) was performed and the patient was still without evidence of disease at the 18-month follow-up examination (1). Another case report describes a complete clinical response of an unresectable gallbladder cancer with lymphadenopathy following repeated doses of intrahepatic arterial cisplatin, although disease was found at the time of a cholecystectomy (2).

For patients who appear to have localized, but unresectable, gallbladder cancer, we have employed either intrahepatic chemotherapy (with fluorodeoxyuridine [FUDR], doxorubicin, and cisplatin) or combined systemic chemotherapy (5-FU) with external beam radiation (see Chapter 7) and then performed restaging studies to determine whether an attempted resection was feasible. Given the small numbers of patients and the lack of agents with very high response rates, these individualized approaches to neoadjuvant therapy will continue to be necessary.

Adjuvant Therapy for Gallbladder Cancer

Because of the high risk of recurrence of resected biliary cancers, the use of adjuvant therapy is desirable, although there is limited data that demonstrate a prolongation of survival with chemotherapy. In a recent prospective, randomized clinical trial, mitomycin (Mutamycin) and 5-FU were administered to patients with resected pancreatic and biliary cancers (3). No overall benefit in survival was demonstrated except in the subgroup of patients with gallbladder cancer who had a 26% 5-year survival if they received chemotherapy and 14% if they did not. Confirmation of these results obtained by subgroup analysis is warranted.

In a nonrandomized study of 41 patients who underwent surgery for gallbladder cancers (4), 15 patients received postoperative "adjunctive" therapies which included radiotherapy for three, chemotherapy (5-FU, cyclophosphamide, steroids, or thiotepa) for 6, and chemotherapy and external beam radiation for six. Better survival was documented in the patients who received the postoperative therapy, but the precise role of the chemotherapy is uncertain.

For patients with completely resected gallbladder cancer with high risk features (invasion through the muscular layers, lymph node involvement, positive margins), we discuss on a case by case basis the administration of external beam radiotherapy with radiosensitizing doses of 5-FU (225 mg/m^2/day by continuous infusion).

NEOADJUVANT AND ADJUVANT CHEMOTHERAPEUTIC APPROACHES TO BILE DUCT CANCERS

Neoadjuvant Therapy

There are no reported prospective studies devoted specifically to neoadjuvant therapy of bile duct malignancies. Urego (5) reported a series of 61 patients with biliary tract tumors managed at the University of Pittsburgh. Twenty-three patients underwent an attempted curative surgical procedure including orthotopic liver transplant in 17. Preoperative chemotherapy (5-FU plus interferon-alpha) and external beam radiation was administered primarily to those listed for transplantation. Although multivariate analysis did not detect a significant association of survival with chemotherapy or radiotherapy, the long-term survivors had all received chemotherapy and radiation. A possible confounder was the fact that six of seven were recipients of orthotopic liver transplants as well.

As described above for gallbladder cancers and in Chapter 7, we offer combined 5-FU and external beam radiotherapy with or without Ir-192 brachytherapy to patients with unresectable biliary duct tumors. In those who have adequate tumor regression, surgical exploration is attempted.

Adjuvant Therapy for Biliary Tract Cancers

There are few studies evaluating chemotherapy alone as an adjuvant, postoperative therapy following attempted curative resections. As described above, no survival benefit has been observed in patients with resected pancreaticobiliary malignancies who received postoperative 5-FU and mitomycin except for the subgroup with gallbladder cancer (3). Most studies of postoperative adjuvant therapy for bile duct tumors have focused on radiotherapy, with chemotherapy used in only a few cases as a radiosensitizer. These studies are for the most part retrospective and contain a mixture of patients who had attempted curative resections and those with palliative procedures performed, making it difficult to derive firm conclusions. For a detailed discussion of these studies, see Chapter 7.

For patients with complete resections, we consider postoperative chemoradiotherapy on a case by case basis because there are retrospective studies that support (6) and refute (7) the benefit of postoperative radiotherapy. If a positive margin is found, and re-resection is not feasible, we offer external beam radiotherapy along with radiosensitizing doses of 5-FU by protracted continuous intravenous infusion, based on the suggestion in some studies that postoperative radiotherapy improves survival if positive margins are found (8).

CHEMOTHERAPY IN THE PALLIATIVE CARE OF PATIENTS WITH GALLBLADDER AND BILE DUCT TUMORS

Medical oncology approaches to the palliative care of patients with gallbladder cancer and cholangiocarcinoma are generally the same, and clinical trials in this area have usually not differentiated between the two types of tumors; therefore, we discuss them together here. For patients who are not candidates for curative resections, chemotherapy may provide a palliative benefit in biliary malignancies compared with best supportive care (9). In a randomized study of 5-FU and leucovorin versus best supportive care alone in patients with surgically noncurable pancreatic or biliary adenocarcinomas, the subgroup of 18 patients with biliary malignancies who received chemotherapy had a 6.5-month median survival compared with 2.5 months for the 19 patients in the best supportive care group. Although this difference did not reach statistical significance, the average quality adjusted survival was significantly better in the subgroup of biliary cancer patients who received chemotherapy.

Single Agent Chemotherapy

Because of the low frequency of biliary malignancies, there have been few trials of chemotherapy agents specifically devoted to these tumors (Table 10.1). In a compilation of 97 patients treated in several studies with various agents including 5-FU, mitomycin, and combination therapy, the partial response rate was 29% (10). More recently, a phase II study of mitomycin C (15 mg/m^2 every 6 weeks) reported 10% partial responses with a median duration of 6 to 8 months (11). Only 1 of 13 previously untreated patients had a partial response of 3 months' duration in a phase II study of cisplatin (12). No responses were observed following administration of paclitaxel at 200 mg/m^2 every 21 days in patients with unresectable or metastatic gallbladder and bile duct cancers (13).

One of the most tested agents is 5-fluorouracil (5-FU). In an early study, responses to 5-FU and the combinations of 5-FU and streptozocin, and 5-FU and lomustine, occurred in 11%, 12%, and 5%, respectively, of patients with gallbladder cancer, and in 8%, none, and 16% of patients with cholangiocarcinoma. There was no survival difference between the groups (14). For previously treated patients, only 6% responded to lomustine alone and none to streptozocin alone (14).

The modulation of 5-FU has also been tested. In a study of 5-FU, folinic acid (leucovorin), and hydroxyurea, 9 of 30 patients with gallbladder cancer had partial responses lasting 6.5 months. Eight other patients had stability of disease and the median overall survival was 8 months (15). An oral 5-FU analog, doxifluridine, plus oral folinic acid yielded a 16% response rate but it was of short duration (2 months) (16). In a study of 5-FU (750 mg/m^2/day by continuous infusion

Table 10.1. Palliative chemotherapy for biliary malignancies

Ref	Patient Group	Treatment	Response	Survival
10	BD 97 (compilation)	5-FU, MMC, FAM, 5-FU + lomustine	PR 29%	6–11 mo
11	GB 13, BD 16, both 1 untreated	MMC	PR 10% SD 30% combined	4.5 mo
12	GB 6 BD 7 untreated	cisplatin	PR 8% GB SD 54% combined	5.5 mo
13	GB 4 BD 11 untreated	paclitaxel	PR 0% MR 20% SD 13%	Not given
14	GB 53 Some pretreated	5-FU	PR 11%	21 wks
		5-FU + streptozocin	PR 12%	14 wks
		5-FU + lomustine	PR 5%	10 wks
	BD 34 Some pretreated	5-FU	PR 8%	26 wks
		5-FU + streptozocin	PR 0%	12 wks
		5-FU + lomustine	PR 16%	8 wks
15	GB 30	5-FU + LV + hydroxyurea	PR 30% SD 27%	8 mo
16	GB 10 BD 22 5 pretreated	doxifluridine + LV	PR 0% GB CR 5% BD PR 19% BD	8 mo combined
17	GB 10 BD 25 14 pretreated	5-FU + IFN-alpha	PR 25% GB MR 25% GB PR 38% BD MR 4% BD	12 mo combined
18	GB 8 BD 7	5-FU + cisplatin	PR 32% SD 47% combined	Not given
19	GB 4 BD 9	5-FU + LV + MMC	PR 0% GB PR 33% BD	22 wks combined
20	"biliary tract" 16	5-FU + cisplatin + MMC + MTX + LV	PR 25%	6 mo
21	GB 6 BD 11	5-FU + MTX + LV + epirubicin	PR 0% SD 83% GB SD 45% BD	8 mo GB 9 mo BD
22	GB 9 BD 12 2 pretreated	5-FU + epirubicin + cisplatin	PR 33% GB SD 22% GB PR 16% BD SD 42% BD	Not given
23	GB 19 BD 22	5-FU + cisplatin + doxorubicin + IFN-alpha	CR 5% GB PR 26% GB PR 9% BD	10.5 mo GB 18.1 mo BD
24	GB 10 BD 8	5-FU	0% PR combined	6.2 mo
	GB 10 BD 8	5-FU + doxorubicin + MMC	0% PR combined	6 mo

Abbreviations: 5-FU: fluorouracil, BD: bile duct cancers (intrahepatic and extrahepatic), CR: complete response, FAM: combination of fluorouracil, doxorubicin, and mitomycin-C, GB: gallbladder cancer, IFN: interferon, MMC: mitomycin-C, LV: leucovorin, MR, minor response, MTX: methotrexate, PR: partial response, SD: stable disease.

on days 1 to 5) and subcutaneous IFN-alpha-2b (5 MU/m^2 on days 1, 3, and 5 with cycles given every 14 days), there was a 34% partial response with a median survival of 12 months at the cost of mucositis in 20%, granulocytopenia in 14%, diarrhea in 9%, and dermatitis in 11% (17). Biliary decompression was performed as needed and patients were not treated until the bilirubin was less than 3.5 mg/dL.

Combination Chemotherapy

Combinations of chemotherapy have typically included 5-FU. In a study of 19 patients, 5-FU by continuous infusion and cisplatin (100 mg/m^2) resulted in six partial responses and nine patients with stable disease with a median survival of 10 months (18). A study of bolus 5-FU, folinic acid, and mitomycin-C reported 3 of 13 partial responses, but the median survival was only 22 weeks (19). A combination of 5-FU by continuous infusion, cisplatin, mitomycin-C, methotrexate, and folinic acid produced a 25% response rate with a 6-month median survival at the cost of severe toxicity (20). In another phase II study, no responses were observed with 5-FU, methotrexate, folinic acid, and epirubicin, but the median survival was 9 months (21). In contrast, the combination of 5-FU, epirubicin, and cisplatin gave 8 of 20 partial responses with a median duration of response of 20 months and an 11-month median survival (22). A response rate of 9% for cholangiocarcinomas and 35% for gallbladder cancers was recently reported in a study using the PIAF regimen consisting of cisplatin (80 mg/m^2 on day 1), IFN-alpha (5 MU/m^2 subcutaneously for 4 days), doxorubicin (40 mg/m^2 on day 1), and 5-FU (500 mg/m^2/day as a continuous infusion for 3 days) (23). Although it is difficult to compare phase II studies because of differences in the enrolled patient groups, it is intriguing that the cisplatin-containing regimens yielded the best results, despite a low response rate for single agent cisplatin. Nonetheless, there is no indication from randomized studies that combination chemotherapy is superior to single agents. 5-FU, doxorubicin, and mitomycin produced a similar median survival with similar toxicity compared with 5-FU alone in a combined group of previously untreated patients with biliary and pancreatic cancers (24).

Intrahepatic Arterial Chemotherapy

Because biliary cancers are frequently found confined to the liver, chemotherapy directed at the hepatic circulation may be a promising approach (Table 10.2). In a compilation of older studies using intrahepatic arterial FUDR, 5-FU, doxorubicin, or mitomycin, a 39% partial response rate in 38 patients was reported (10). In a Japanese study, hepatic artery infusion of cisplatin and 5-FU at a continuous low dose resulted in 5 (out of 8, 63%) partial responses with a median survival of 482 days (25). Attempted surgical resection was possible in three patients, one of whom was disease free at 52 months postoperatively. Patt and colleagues have developed an intrahepatic arterial version of the PIAF regimen for hepatomas and report initiation of a phase II study using this regimen for biliary malignancies (26). In a case of recurrent gallbladder cancer, intra-arterial cisplatin was followed by transcatheter arterial embolization and the tumor became undetectable (27). In a study of 27 patients with gallbladder cancer, intra-arterial mitomycin gave a 48% response rate and 14-month median survival (28).

Table 10.2. Palliative intra-arterial chemotherapy for biliary malignancies

Ref	Patient Group	Treatment	Response	Survival
10	BD and GB 38 (compilation)	FUDR, 5-FU, doxorubicin, MMC	PR 39%	Not given
25	GB 8	5-FU + cisplatin	PR 63%	Not given
27	GB 27	MMC	PR 48%	Not given

Abbreviations: 5-FU: fluorouracil, BD: bile duct cancers (intrahepatic and extrahepatic), FUDR: fluorodeoxyuridine, GB: gallbladder cancer, MMC: mitomycin-C, PR: partial response.

Table 10.3. Palliative chemoradiotherapy for biliary malignancies

Ref	Patient Group	Treatment	Response	Survival
29	GB 1 BD 7	5-FU bolus + LV + RT	Not reported	poorly tolerated
30[a]	BD 9	5-FU CI + RT	SD 44%	11.9 mo
31	GB 2 BD 10	5-FU + MMC + RT + brachyRT	Not reported	17 mo

[a] Whittington (30) included pancreatic cancer patients and did not break down the response data by tumor type.

Abbreviations: 5-FU: fluorouracil, BD: bile duct cancers (intrahepatic and extrahepatic), CI: continuous infusion, GB: gallbladder cancer, LV: leucovorin, MMC: mitomycin-C, RT: radiotherapy, SD: stable disease.

Palliative Chemotherapy with Radiotherapy

Palliation of biliary malignancies may be achieved by using chemotherapy to increase the radiosensitization of the tumor (Table 10.3). For details of radiotherapeutic strategies for palliation of biliary malignancies, see Chapter 7. Here we briefly discuss the combination of chemotherapy with radiotherapy for palliative purposes. Radiation therapy with 5-FU (350 mg/m^2 on days 1 to 5 and the last 5 days of radiation) modulated by folinic acid for pancreatic and biliary malignancies caused substantial toxicity, especially in the elderly and poor performance status patients (29); however, a protracted infusion of 5-FU concurrently with radiation therapy was more tolerable and 11 of 25 patients remained free of local progression following treatment (30).

In a study of 12 patients with locally advanced extrahepatic biliary system cancer, 5-FU and mitomycin were delivered at the beginning of radiation therapy (5000 cGy and a boost of 1500 cGy to the tumor bed). Some patients received maintenance chemotherapy and/or boosts to the tumor with brachytherapy. The median survival was 17 months and the overall 4-year actuarial survival was 36% (31). In a retrospective report of the European experience with biliary duct malignancies (6), a subgroup of nine patients received combined chemotherapy (primarily 5-FU) with radiation therapy after palliative drainage and had a remarkable 21-month median survival.

For patients with biliary ductal disease only, without an obvious mass, we administer external beam radiotherapy with radiosensitizing doses of 5-FU and in patients who maintain a good performance status, we add brachytherapy.

Future directions in chemotherapy for biliary malignancies are likely to proceed along two paths: developing more effective agents and abrogating chemotherapy resistance. New agents that have yet to be extensively tested in biliary malignancies include irinotecan (Camptosar), gemcitabine (Gemzar), and the newer oral 5-FU analogs such as capecitabine (Xeloda). The combination of irinotecan and gemcitabine is now in phase I and II studies to determine the response rate in a variety of malignancies. Gemcitabine is also interesting because it is a potent radiosensitizer and is currently being tested in combination with radiation therapy for pancreatic cancer. If the results are promising and the treatment is tolerable, it should be tested in biliary malignancies as well.

Chemotherapy resistance mechanisms, such as expression of the efflux pump P-glycoprotein (PgP), are clearly active in biliary malignancies. In gallbladder carcinoma, the percentage of cases expressing PgP was 69% to 77% by immunohistochemistry, and the percentage of cases expressing MDR1 mRNA measured by polymerase chain reaction was 52%, significantly higher than in normal gallbladder (32). There was a nonsignificant trend for more frequent expression of PgP and MDR1 mRNA at earlier tumor/node/metastasis (TNM) stages than in advanced stages. This suggests that, from the earliest stages, biliary malignancies may be resistant to chemotherapy agents derived from natural sources.

Studies of agents that interfere with PgP activity such as verapamil, cyclosporin A, and PSC833 are being evaluated in other malignancies (33). Once an agent that effectively interferes with MDR activity in vivo with low toxicity to normal tissues is established, it would be reasonable to study it in biliary malignancies. It is also clear that much needs to be learned about the optimal delivery of chemotherapy agents to biliary cancers. In an in vitro study of the 5-FU sensitivity of the gallbladder cancer cell line Mz-ChA-2 and bile duct cancer cell line SK-ChA-1, increasing the duration of exposure to 5-FU decreased the proportion of surviving cells (34). This suggests that the continuous infusion routes of delivery of 5-FU may be more effective in vivo. Also, the Mz-ChA-2 cells were 10 times more sensitive to 5-FU than SK-ChA-1 cells, suggesting gallbladder cancers and cholangiocarcinomas may have different sensitivity to chemotherapy agents.

NOVEL STRATEGIES

The overall modest results with chemotherapy for unresectable biliary malignancies underscores the need to explore other strategies such as immunotherapy, gene therapy, apoptosis induction, and anti-angiogenesis. As these fields are still in their infancy, and the number of patients with biliary neoplasia is small, there are no studies directly evaluating these approaches in biliary cancers. Nonetheless, it is worth speculating on how they might be applied in the future.

Immunotherapy

As observed in other malignancies, patients with more advanced biliary cancer and a poorer prognosis tend to have weaker immune function as well. In one study of patients tested postoperatively after resection for gallbladder cancer, those who subsequently died of their disease were found to have poorer immune responses to delayed-type hypersensitivity skin testing than those who were longer term survivors (35). It is possible that weaker immune function is both a cause and an effect of having more progressive disease and that induction of tumor-specific immunity might result in a clinically relevant effect. Biliary cancers express antigens that have been shown to be targets of immune responses in other malignancies such as mutated k-*ras* (36), carcinoembryonic antigen (CEA) family proteins (37), and c-*erb*B-2 (HER2/neu) (38).

Among the explanations for the failure of the immune system to destroy tumors in patients is the inadequate presentation of the tumor antigens to the effector T cells in a manner that induces T cell activation and proliferation. A number of methods have been proposed for presenting antigen, including immunization with tumor antigens in the form of protein or peptide mixed with an adjuvant (Detox, BCG, GM-CSF); autologous tumors genetically modified to secrete immunostimulatory cytokines; viral vectors (such as vaccinia or fowlpox) containing genes encoding tumor antigens; naked plasmid DNA encoding antigens idiotype possessing the internal image of the tumor antigen; and dendritic cells, the most potent antigen presenting cells, loaded with tumor antigens. These approaches are now being evaluated primarily in patients with melanoma, prostate cancer, breast cancer, and colon cancer. It is also possible to administer antibodies specific for the tumor antigens. A commercially available antibody against HER2/neu (Herceptin) has shown efficacy in breast cancer. Cholangiocarcinomas and gallbladder cancers overexpressing HER2/neu might be amenable to treatment with this agent, but no such trials have been reported. Although the surface epithelium of large bile ducts possesses c-*erb*B-2 protein (39), no significant biliary toxicity has been reported in studies of Herceptin in breast cancer patients.

Gene Therapy

Gene therapy may impact on malignancies by either correcting defects in tumor suppressor genes, interfering with the function of oncogenes, adding genes that increase the susceptibility of tumors to immunologic attack, chemotherapy, or apoptosis, and protecting normal tissue from toxic effects of chemotherapy while leaving tumors susceptible. Mutations and overexpressions of k-*ras* and p53 are detected in 40% to 60% of biliary tract and gallbladder cancer specimens (36).

In one study of cholangiocarcinoma arising in primary sclerosing cholangitis, p53 expression (suggestive of defective p53) was detected in 78.5% of tumor specimens (40). Approaches to targeting p53 defective tumors under development include the injection of adenoviral vectors encoding wild-type p53 and the ONYX-015 virus which lyses p53 deficient cells (41). Suicide gene therapy with the herpes simplex thymidine kinase gene or the cytosine deaminase gene, which when introduced into tumor cells renders them sensitive to gancyclovir and 5-flucytosine, respectively, is being studied in brain, colorectal, mesothelial, melanoma, and ovarian cancer (42). Cholangiocarcinoma cells have been rendered radiation-sensitive in vitro and in vivo by transfection with the cytosine deaminase gene and application of 5-flucytosine which is converted to 5-FU, a potent radiation sensitizer (43). Because of the bystander effect in which untransduced, but neighboring, tumor cells are destroyed along with the gene-expressing cell, introduction of the gene by applying a vector via the biliary tree is a potential approach for disease relatively confined to the bile ducts. Direct administration into the hepatic circulation or directly into the tumor would be necessary for larger masses, but these approaches have not been tested for biliary malignancies.

Another type of gene therapy is the use of antisense oligonucleotides to interfere with the expression of genes that promote oncogenesis. In cholangiocarcinoma cells, antisense specific for bcl-2, an anti-apoptotic molecule, lead to decreased bcl-2 expression and a lowering of the threshold for induction of apoptosis (44).

Anti-angiogenic Therapy

Anti-angiogenic therapy is in its infancy but currently engendering considerable excitement with the approach of clinical trials of angiostatin. Expression of vascular endothelial growth factor (VEGF) by biliary tract and gallbladder cancers has been observed (45) and in some studies has been demonstrated to be a negative prognostic factor (46,47). It is hypothesized that interference with VEGF activity will result in tumor regression or prevent tumor recurrence. Phase I studies using anti-VEGF antibody in patients with metastatic colon cancer are currently ongoing. As further testing is performed and if the results are promising, biliary cancers will be a reasonable setting to apply these agents.

Induction of Apoptosis

Apoptosis is thought to be the final common pathway by which cell death is induced by many therapeutic modalities such as chemotherapy, radiotherapy, and immunotherapy. One mechanism of inducing apoptosis is by activation of the Fas receptor. Early work is now ongoing in identifying pro-apoptotic and anti-apoptotic molecules associated with cholangiocarcinomas. The cholangiocarcinoma cell line SK-ChA-1 heterogeneously expresses Fas receptor. Treatment with an anti-Fas antibody reduced cell viability by 80% in Fas-positive, but not Fas-negative, cells. Furthermore, when injected into mice, only the Fas-negative cells were able to grow tumor nodules (48). Interestingly, tamoxifen, acting through the Fas system and not as an anti-estrogen, was able to induce apoptosis of Fas-positive cells (49).

CONCLUSIONS

Currently available medical approaches to the treatment of biliary malignancy are primarily palliative. Chemotherapy appears to have a palliative benefit compared with best supportive care in advanced gallbladder and bile duct cancers. When used as a radiosensitizer, 5-FU may also give palliative benefit for locally advanced neoplasia. The role of chemotherapy in the adjuvant setting after surgical resection remains to be defined, but we have typically combined it with radiation in patients with positive margins or regional lymph node involvement.

For patients with locally advanced disease who would be surgical candidates if they attained tumor regression, we use systemic chemotherapy as part of a neoadjuvant multimodality approach. As immune, gene, anti-angiogenic, and apoptotic strategies undergo further development, they will likely be applied to biliary cancers.

SUGGESTED READINGS

Glimelius B, Hoffman K, Sjoden P-O, et al. Chemotherapy improves survival and quality of life in advanced pancreatic and biliary cancer. Ann Oncol 1996;7:593–600. This study is one of the few that evaluates quality of life in patients receiving chemotherapy compared with best supportive care in patients with pancreaticobiliary malignancies. It demonstrates that more patients in the chemotherapy group had an improved or prolonged high quality of life compared to those in the best supportive care group.

Oberfield RA, Rossi RL. The role of chemotherapy in the treatment of bile duct cancer. World J Surg 1988;12:105–8. Although a decade old, this paper compiled the published data for intravenous and intra-arterial chemotherapy for biliary malignancies up to 1988 and remains the most comprehensive review of the chemotherapy literature. The only agent with some efficacy evaluated since that time is cisplatin.

Pan G, Vickers SM, Pickens A, et al. Apoptosis and tumorigenesis in human cholangiocarcinoma cells. Involvement of Fas/APO-1 (CD95) and calmodulin. Am J Pathol 1999;155:193–203. A basic research paper that points to potential novel approaches for clinical management of biliary malignancies. In this study, apoptosis could be induced via the Fas receptor in cholangiocarcinoma cells both in vitro and in a murine model.

REFERENCES

1. Kawabata Y, Yano S, Ohishi T, et al. [A case of advanced gallbladder cancer responding to neoadjuvant intra-arterial chemotherapy]. Gan To Kagaku Ryoho 1999;26:365–8.
2. Shikata A, Mori K, Watahiki Y, et al. [A case of unresectable advanced cancer of the gallbladder successfully treated by arterial infusion therapy with cisplatin]. Gan To Kagaku Ryoho 1997;24:1820–4.
3. Amano H, Takada T, Kato H, et al. Five year results of a randomized study of postoperative adjuvant chemotherapy in resected pancreatic-biliary carcinomas. Abstract 1049. Proc Am Soc Clin Oncol 1999;18:273a.
4. Treadwell TA, Hardin WJ. Primary carcinoma of the gallbladder. The role of adjunctive therapy in its treatment. Am J Surg 1976;132:703–6.
5. Urego M, Flickinger JC, Carr BI. Radiotherapy and multimodality management of cholangiocarcinoma. Int J Radiat Oncol Biol Phys 1999;44: 121–6.
6. Gonzalez Gonzalez D, Gerard JP, Maners AW, et al. Results of radiation therapy in carcinoma of the proximal bile duct (Klatskin tumor). Semin Liver Dis 1990;10:131–41.
7. Pitt HA, Nakeeb A, Abrams RA, et al. Perihilar cholangiocarcinoma. Postoperative radiotherapy does not improve survival. Ann Surg 1995;221: 788–98.
8. Schoenthaler R, Phillips TL, Castro J, et al. Carcinoma of the extrahepatic bile ducts. The University of California at San Francisco experience. Ann Surg 1994;219:267–74.
9. Glimelius B, Hoffman K, Sjoden PO, et al. Chemotherapy improves survival and quality of life in advanced pancreatic and biliary cancer. Ann Oncol 1996; 7:593–600.
10. Oberfield RA, Rossi RL. The role of chemotherapy in the treatment of bile duct cancer. World J Surg 1988;12:105–8.
11. Taal BG, Audisio RA, Bleiberg H, et al. Phase II trial of mitomycin C in advanced gallbladder and biliary tree carcinoma. An EORTC-GITCCG study. Ann Oncol 1993;4:607–9.
12. Okada S, Ishii H, Nose H, et al. A phase II study of cisplatin in patients with biliary tract carcinoma. Oncology 1994;51:515–17.
13. Jones DV Jr, Lozano R, Hoque A, et al. Phase II study of paclitaxel therapy for unresectable biliary tree carcinoma. J Clin Oncol 1996;14:2306–10.
14. Falkson G, MacIntyre JM, Moertel CG. Eastern Cooperative Oncology Group experience with chemotherapy for inoperable gallbladder and bile duct cancer. Cancer 1984;54:965–9.
15. Gebbia V, Majello E, Testa A, et al. Treatment of advanced adenocarcinomas of the exocrine pancreas and gallbladder with 5FU, high dose levofolinic acid and oral hydroxyurea on a weekly schedule. Cancer 1996;78:1300–7.
16. Colleoni M, Di Bartolomeo M, Di Leo A, et al. Oral chemotherapy with doxifluridine and folinic acid in biliary tract cancer. Eur J Cancer 1995;31A: 2426–7.
17. Patt Y, Jones D, Hoque A, et al. Phase II trial of intravenous fluorouracil and subcutaneous interferon alpha-2b for biliary tract cancer. J Clin Oncol 1996; 14:2311–15.
18. Rougier P, Fandi A. Ducreux M, et al. Demonstrated efficiency of 5FU continuous infusion and cisplatin in patients with advanced biliary tract carcinoma. Proc Am Soc Clin Oncol 1995;14:205.
19. Polyzos A, Nikou G, Giannopoulos A, et al. Chemotherapy of biliary tract cancer with mitomycin C and 5FU biologically modulated by folinic acid. A phase II study. Ann Oncol 1996;7:644–5.
20. Malzyner A, Caponero R, Donato EM, et al. FALP-M chemotherapy in non-resectable biliary tract adenocarcinoma. Ann Oncol 1992;3(suppl 5):25.
21. Kajanti M, Pyrhonen S. Epirubicin sequential methotrexate 5FU leucovorin treatment in advanced cancer of the extrahepatic biliary system. A phase II study. Am J Clin Oncol 1994;17:223–6.
22. Ellis PA, Norman A, Hill A, et al. Epirubicin, cisplatin, and infusional 5FU (ECF) in hepato-biliary tumours. Eur J Cancer 1995;31A:1594–8.
23. Patt YZ, Hassan MM, Lozano RD, et al. Phase II trial of cisplatin (P), Intron A (I), Adriamycin (A), and 5-fluorouracil (F) (PIAF) for biliary tree cancer (BTC). Abstract 1139. Proc Am Soc Clin Oncol 1999;18:297a.
24. Takada T, Kato H, Matsushiro T, et al. Comparison of 5FU, doxorubicin and mitomycin C with 5FU alone in the treatment of pancreatic-biliary carcinomas. Oncology 1994;51:396–400.
25. Fukuda S, Okuda K, Kinoshita H, et al. [Study of hepatic arterial chemoinfusion with continuous CDDP, 5-FU low dose administration for advanced gallbladder cancer]. Gan To Kagaku Ryoho 1996;23:1610–13.
26. Patt YZ, Hoque A. Multimodality treatment of liver neoplasms. In: Clavien PA, ed. Malignant liver tumors: current and emerging therapies. Malden, MA: Blackwell Science, 1999:208–9.
27. Yokoyama M, Takahashi S, Tateoka H, et al. [A case of recurrent gallbladder cancer with marked response to arterial infusion chemotherapy and transarterial embolization]. Gan To Kagaku Ryoho 1997;24:97–9.
28. Makela JT, Kairaluoma MI. Superselective intra-arterial chemotherapy with mitomycin for gallbladder cancer. Br J Surg 1993;80:912–15.
29. Hsue V, Wong CS, Moore M, et al. A phase I study of combined radiation therapy with 5-fluorouracil and low dose folinic acid in patients with locally advanced pancreatic or biliary carcinoma. Int J Radiat Oncol Biol Phys 1996; 34:445–50.
30. Whittington R, Neuberg D, Tester WJ, et al. Protracted intravenous fluorouracil infusion with radiation therapy in the management of localized pancreaticobiliary carcinoma: a phase I Eastern Cooperative Oncology Group Trial. J Clin Oncol 1995;13:227–32.
31. Minsky BD, Kemeny N, Armstrong JG. Extrahepatic biliary system cancer: an update of a combined modality approach. Am J Clin Oncol 1991;14:433–7.
32. Cao L, Duchrow M, Windhovel U, et al. Expression of MDR1 mRNA and encoding P-glycoprotein in archival formalin-fixed paraffin-embedded gall-bladder cancer tissues. Eur J Cancer 1998;34:1612–17.
33. Sikic BI, Fisher GA, Lum BL, et al. Modulation and prevention of multidrug resistance by inhibitors of P-glycoprotein. Cancer Chemother Pharmacol 1997; 40(suppl):S13–19.
34. Moon Y, Todoroki T, Ohno T, et al. Killing effects of 5-fluorouracil on human biliary tract cancer cell lines. Int J Oncol 1999;14:253–7.
35. Cubillos L, Gonzalez S, Sepulveda C, et al. Immunological evaluation of patients with invasive carcinoma of the gallbladder. J Cancer Res Clin Oncol 1993;119:497–500.
36. Itoi T, Takei K, Shinohara Y, et al. K-*ras* codon 12 and p53 mutations in biopsy specimens and bile from biliary tract cancers. Pathol Int 1999;49:30–7.
37. Hammarstrom S. The carcinoembryonic antigen (CEA) family: structures, suggested functions and expression in normal and malignant tissues. Semin Cancer Biol 1999;9:67–81.
38. Terada T, Ashida K, Endo K, et al. *c-erb*B-2 protein is expressed in hepatolithiasis and cholangiocarcinoma. Histopathology 1998;33:325–31.
39. Chow NH, Huang SM, Chan SH, et al. Significance of *c-erb*B-2 expression in normal and neoplastic epithelium of biliary tract. Anticancer Res 1995;15: 1055–9.
40. Rizzi PM, Ryder SD, Portmann B, et al. p53 protein overexpression in cholangiocarcinoma arising in primary sclerosing cholangitis. Gut 1996;38: 265–8.
41. Bischoff JR, Kirn DH, Williams A, et al. An adenovirus mutant that replicates selectively in p53-deficient human tumor cells. Science 1996;274:373–6.
42. Singhal S, Kaiser LR. Cancer chemotherapy using suicide genes. Surg Oncol Clin N Am 1998;7:505–36.
43. Pederson LC, Buchsbaum DJ, Vickers SM, et al. Molecular chemotherapy combined with radiation therapy enhances killing of cholangiocarcinoma cells in vitro and in vivo. Cancer Res 1997;57:4325–32.
44. Harnois DM, Que FG, Celli A, et al. bcl-2 is overexpressed and alters the threshold for apoptosis in a cholangiocarcinoma cell line. Hepatology 1997;26:884–90.
45. Yamamoto S, Fujii K, Kitadai Y, et al. Expression of vascular endothelial growth factor in human gallbladder lesions. Oncol Rep 1998;5:1065–9.
46. Hida Y, Morita T, Fujita M, et al. Vascular endothelial growth factor expression is an independent negative predictor in extrahepatic biliary tract carcinomas. Anticancer Res 1999;19:2257–60.
47. Okita S, Kondoh S, Shiraishi K, et al. Expression of vascular endothelial growth factor correlates with tumor progression in gallbladder cancer. Int J Oncol 1998;12:1013–18.
48. Pickens A, Pan G, McDonald JM, et al. Fas expression prevents cholangiocarcinoma tumor growth. J Gastrointest Surg 1999;3:374–82.
49. Pan G, Vickers SM, Pickens A, et al. Apoptosis and tumorigenesis in human cholangiocarcinoma cells. Involvement of Fas/APO-1 (CD95) and calmodulin. Am J Pathol 1999;155:193–203.

Section

3

Specific Conditions

Section 3.1

The Gallbladder

Chapter

Natural History and Pathogenesis of Gallstones

KLAUS MERGENER HENNING GERKE

Gallstones are highly prevalent in industrialized countries, affecting 10% to 15% of men and up to 25% of women (1,2). Although the majority of individuals with gallstones remain asymptomatic, symptomatic gallstone disease is considered the most common and costly digestive disease that results in hospitalization in the United States (3). Studies in the 1960s reported cholecystectomy rates of 500,000 per year for the United States (4); with the development of laparoscopic cholecystectomy in the late 1980s, this figure has risen further to an estimated 700,000 operations per year (5). Over the past several decades, there have been major advances in our understanding of gallstone pathogenesis; with the improvements in and wide availability of imaging modalities such as ultrasound and computed tomography, the epidemiology and natural history of cholelithiasis has been studied extensively. In this chapter, we discuss these developments, with special emphasis on their implications for the treatment of gallstone disease.

TYPES OF GALLSTONES

Gallstones are characterized by their chemical composition. They are classified, somewhat arbitrarily, into cholesterol stones (>50% cholesterol content), mixed stones (20% to 50% cholesterol content), and pigment stones (<20% cholesterol content), the latter being composed primarily of calcium bilirubinate. Early epidemiologic studies had suggested that 80% to 90% of all stones in Western countries were of the cholesterol or mixed type and only 10% to 20% were pigment stones (6), but others have found pigment stones in up to 30% of individuals with cholelithiasis (7,8). In Asia, up to 70% of all gallstones are pigment stones (9). Due to the predominance of cholesterol gallstones in the United States, much of the research effort has focused on this type of stone and less is known about the pathogenesis of pigment stones.

Pathogenesis of Gallstone Formation

Components of Normal Bile

The main components of bile are water, electrolytes, and organic solutes, the latter consisting predominantly of bile salts, cholesterol, and phospholipids (10). Bile salts are classified as either primary or secondary. The primary bile acids, cholic and chenodeoxycholic acid, are synthesized in the liver from cholesterol and then conjugated with either glycine or taurine. After excretion with bile fluid into the duodenum, most of the bile acid pool is reabsorbed in the distal small bowel and recirculated via the enterohepatic circulation. A small amount (less than 5%) of bile salts enters the colon, where it undergoes deconjugation by bacteria, resulting in the formation of secondary bile acids (deoxycholic and lithocholic acid) (11,12).

Most of the cholesterol found in bile is synthesized de novo in the liver. Cholesterol is insoluble in water and is therefore dependent on some other vehicle for its solubilization in bile. Understanding the mechanisms responsible for the solubilization of cholesterol has facilitated analysis of the biochemical events occuring during the formation of cholesterol stones (13–15).

Pathogenesis of Cholesterol Stones

The formation of cholesterol gallstones has been separated into three stages: 1) cholesterol solubilization and saturation, 2) nucleation, and 3) stone growth (13,16,17).

Cholesterol is virtually insoluble in bile and therefore requires the interaction with other molecules to be solubilized (13). For many years, it was thought that cholesterol

…maintained in solution almost entirely by the formation of so-called *micelles*, composed of bile acids, phospholipids, and cholesterol. Bile acids are amphipathic compounds, containing both hydrophilic and hydrophobic groups. When the bile acid concentration reaches a certain level (termed *critical micellar level*), individual bile acid molecules aggregate into small clusters with their polar ends oriented outwardly and the hydrophobic portions oriented toward the inside of the cluster. Phospholipids enter this aggregate, leading to swelling of the micelle which in turn facilitates incorporation of cholesterol. Cholesterol molecules are ultimately transported within the matrix of this structure. The concentration of bile acids and phospholipids relative to cholesterol has been thought to be the critical factor in determining cholesterol solubilization, and the relationship between these three substances has commonly been depicted in form of a "cholesterol triangle" (18) (see also Chapter 1, Fig. 1.9) (Fig. 11.1).

The concept of mixed micelle formation and its role in the formation of cholesterol gallstones has recently been challenged by the demonstration that much of the biliary cholesterol exists in a somewhat different structure, termed a *vesicle* (15,19,20). Vesicles are made up of phospholipid bilayers, similar to cell membranes, with interspersed bile acids (21). Cholesterol is solubilized within the hydrophobic portion of the bilayer. The relative importance of micelles and vesicles in cholesterol stone formation remains the subject of intensive research.

The process by which cholesterol monohydrate crystals form and aggregate has been termed *nucleation*. The observation that many normal individuals without gallstones secrete cholesterol-supersaturated bile suggests that factors other than the hepatic secretion of cholesterol-saturated bile are important for the formation of gallstones (22,23). It has been shown that nucleation occurs more rapidly in the gallbladder bile of patients with cholesterol gallstones than in individuals with saturated bile without stones (24). This finding initiated efforts to identify the nature of either pronucleating or antinucleating factors. A heat-labile glycoprotein has been identified in patients with cholesterol gallstones and has been shown to reduce nucleation time significantly (25,26). Increased gallbladder mucus secretion has also been reported to be a potent pronucleating factor (27,28). Mucin secretion is stimulated by prostaglandins. Aspirin, an inhibitor of prostaglandin synthesis, both significantly inhibits mucus secretion and reduces the incidence of experimentally induced cholesterol gallstones in an animal model (29,30). This finding generated considerable enthusiasm as it appeared feasible to prevent gallstone formation through prophylactic usage of prostaglandin inhibitors. However, studies in humans have not found an effect of aspirin usage on gallstone formation (31–34) and this concept has been abandoned. Recently, a bacterial lipopolysaccharide has been shown to induce mucin hypersecretion suggesting that—contrary to the commonly accepted assumption—bacteria may play a role not only in the development of pigment gallstones but also in cholesterol stone formation (35).

In summary, although cholesterol supersaturation is commonly viewed as a prerequisite for cholesterol gallstone for-

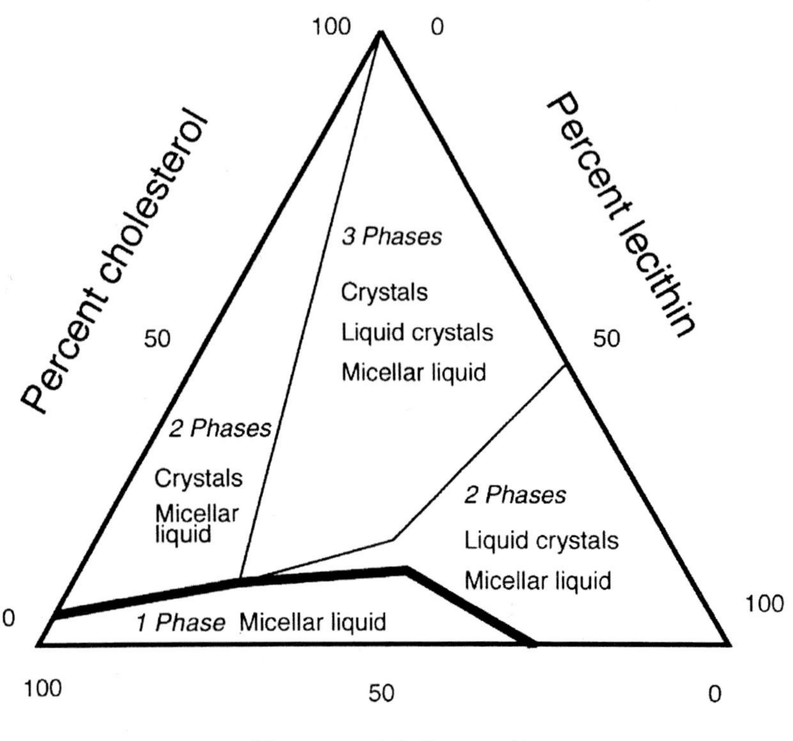

FIGURE 11.1. *Phase-equilibrium diagram of a model bile system consisting of sodium taurocholate, egg yolk lecithin, cholesterol, and water (10 g/dL total lipid concentration, 0.15 mol/L NaCl, pH 7.0, 37°C). (Adapted from Donovan JM, Carey MC. Separation and quantitation of cholesterol "carriers" in bile. Hepatology 1990;12(suppl):S94–104.)*

mation, the impact of pronucleating factors in vivo remains incompletely understood (36). Efforts continue to understand the role of cholesterol supersaturation and the balance between pronucleating and antinucleating factors in the formation of cholesterol stones.

The Role of the Gallbladder

Gallbladder contraction is induced by meals and mediated by the hormone cholecystokinin. When the gallbladder contracts, 70% to 80% of the fasting volume is released into the duodenum (37). Stasis of bile within the gallbladder has been implicated in the increased frequency of gallstone formation in patients after truncal vagotomy and during pregnancy (38–40). Radioisotope and manometric studies have confirmed that gallbladder stasis and decreased gallbladder emptying occur during the early stages of formation of experimentally induced cholesterol gallstones (41,42). High progesterone levels have also been shown to reduce gallbladder contractility in an animal model (43), a mechanism that may contribute to the increased risk for gallstone formation during pregnancy. Further evidence implicating gallbladder stasis as an etiologic factor in cholesterol gallstone formation comes from biliary scintigraphic studies of human patients with gallstones, in whom a decreased motor response to cholecystokinin stimulation has been noted (44). Decreased gallbladder emptying has been demonstrated in patients with cholesterol gallstones (45–47) as well as, in the absence of stones, in individuals with biliary cholesterol crystals (48).

The mechanism by which stasis of bile within the gallbladder promotes cholesterol gallstone formation remains poorly defined. Conceivably, stone growth from cholesterol crystals is a slow process. Even with enough time for microcrystals to nucleate, in subjects with normal gallbladder function these small cholesterol aggregates are likely to be ejected into the duodenum before growing into macroscopic gallstones. Furthermore, gallbladder stasis may be associated with alterations in gallbladder absorptive or secretory function or with sequestration of bile acids in the gallbladder, reducing the amount of bile salts available for cholesterol solubilization (49).

Pathogenesis of Pigment Stones

Pigment stones are characterized by their low cholesterol content and their high concentration of bilirubin, which is usually in excess of 40%. Bilirubin is secreted by the liver into the bile mostly in its diglucuronide form with only small amounts of the monoglucuronide and unconjugated forms. As for cholesterol, bile salts facilitate solubilization of the monoglucuronide and unconjugated forms of bilirubin. The unconjugated form is hydrophobic and may precipitate from solution as calcium salts or bilirubin polymers (50). Pigment stones are speculated to occur when there is supersaturation of bile with unconjugated bilirubin (51). Pigment stones are associated with diverse clinical conditions and can be conveniently divided into "black stone stones."

Black pigment stones occur in patients with chronic hemolysis (52), cirrhosis (53), or compromised ileal function as with Crohn's disease (54–56) or ileal resection (57). In patients with hemolysis, secretion of bilirubin into bile may be increased more than 10-fold, with a shift from diconjugates to monoconjugates. Bilirubin monoconjugates are more liable to hydrolysis by endogenous beta-glucuronidase, leading to accumulation of unconjugated bilirubin which subsequently precipitates with calcium. The pathogenesis of gallstone formation in patients with cirrhosis is less well understood, but mild hemolysis and bile salt hyposecretion leading to reduced solubility of unconjugated bilirubin may play a role. Patients with Crohn´s disease and extensive ileitis have higher levels of bilirubin flux through the liver and higher biliary bilirubin concentrations (55,56). Results from animal experiments suggest that this may be due to bile salt malabsorption in the ileum resulting in high amounts of intracolonic bile salts. This leads to solubilization of intracolonic unconjugated bilirubin, which is then free to be reabsorbed, transported back to the liver, and excreted into the bile, thereby leading to increased concentration of biliary bilirubin (54).

Similar to cholesterol stone formation, a variety of other factors may contribute to pigment stone formation, including secretion by the gallbladder of mucous glycoproteins, biliary stasis, biliary calcium concentration, and bile acidification (49,51,56); the exact contribution of each of these factors remains to be elucidated. The role of bacterial infection in the pathogenesis of *black* pigment stones has long been discussed; there are some indications that bacteria may play a role, but findings have been inconclusive to date (58).

Brown pigment stones can be located throughout the intrahepatic or extrahepatic biliary tract and are the typical type of gallstone associated with bacterial infection and biliary stasis (59). Bacterial enzymes hydrolyse biliary lipids, conjugated bilirubin, and bile salts. The resultant free bile acids, free fatty acids, and unconjugated bilirubin precipitate as such or form insoluble calcium salts. Mucin glycoproteins and bacterial debris may contribute to the growing gallstone.

Common Duct Stones

Gallstones located in parts of the biliary tree other than the gallbladder may be classified as either *primary*, those that formed in the bile duct, or *secondary*, those that formed in the gallbladder and passed through the cystic duct into the common duct or the intrahepatic bile ducts. Epidemiologic evidence suggests that most common duct stones arise in the gallbladder (60,61): most patients with cholesterol stones in the common duct also have gallbladder stones of identical composition. In contrast, patients with pigment stones in the common duct often do not have corresponding stones in the gallbladder. Pigment stones, particularly those of the brown pigment type, are therefore thought to form anywhere in the biliary tree; they probably constitute the majority of primary common duct stones. Although the main factors contributing to the formation of primary common duct stones appear to be biliary bacterial infections and stasis of bile in the common duct, abnormal sphincter of Oddi activity has also been discussed as a contributing factor: Wong and colleagues reported elevated common bile duct pressures at operation in patients with common duct stones (62). However, two other groups could not confirm this finding (63,64). Whether the increased prevalence of gallstones in patients with juxtapapillary duodenal diverticula is due to a motor abnormality of the sphincter of Oddi has also been controversial. It has been suggested that sphincter insufficiency causes higher rates of bacterial contamination of the biliary tree which in turn leads to higher frequencies of brown pigment stone formation (65). Additional studies are needed to clarify the role of motor abnormalities of the sphincter of Oddi in the pathogenesis of primary common duct stones.

Biliary Sludge

Biliary sludge was first described with the advances of abdominal ultrasonography as an echogenic material in the gallbladder that shifts slowly with positioning of the patient (66–68) (Fig. 11.2). Similar pathogenetic mechanisms as in gallstone disease are assumed to apply to the formation of biliary sludge, and the role of biliary sludge as a precursor of cholesterol and pigment gallstones has been proposed by Lee and colleagues (69). Gallbladder sludge, as determined ultrasonographically, has been presumed to be a manifestation of biliary stasis. It has been demonstrated that sludge is composed, in part, of calcium bilirubinate crystals, cholesterol monohydrate crystals, and gallbladder mucus (70). In a study of patients receiving total parenteral nutrition (TPN), sludge could be detected in all patients after 6 weeks of TPN (71). With continuation of TPN, stones developed in almost half of these patients during follow-up. On the other hand, the reinstitution of oral feedings led to disappearance of sludge within 4 weeks.

Risk Factors for Gallstone Formation

A large number of diverse factors predispose individuals to the development of gallstones (Table 11.1). The prevalence of gallstones varies greatly among different ethnic groups suggesting that genetic factors may play an important role. Gallstone prevalence in certain Asian countries is 3% to 5% (72,73), but populations in Europe and North America have an overall prevalence of 10% to 20%; in certain ethnic subgroups such as the North American Pima Indians and Chippewa, gallstones rates reach 60% (74). There is also considerable temporal variation in gallstone prevalence, supporting an influence of dietary factors and lifestyle. It has been argued that the ancient Greeks knew renal colic but did not know gallstone disease, and this has been attributed to their diet and style of living (75). Several studies in more recent times have also shown increases in the prevalence of gallstones over time (76,77).

Gallstones are twice as common in women as in men, and the prevalence increases with age. The family history also seems to be of importance: first-degree relatives of gallstone patients have a 4.5-fold risk of having gallstones compared to matched controls (78). Obesity has long been identified as an important risk factor. One study reported a sixfold increased risk for gallstone formation in very obese women compared to lean women (79). Whether hypertriglyceridemia represents an additional independent risk factor remains controversial.

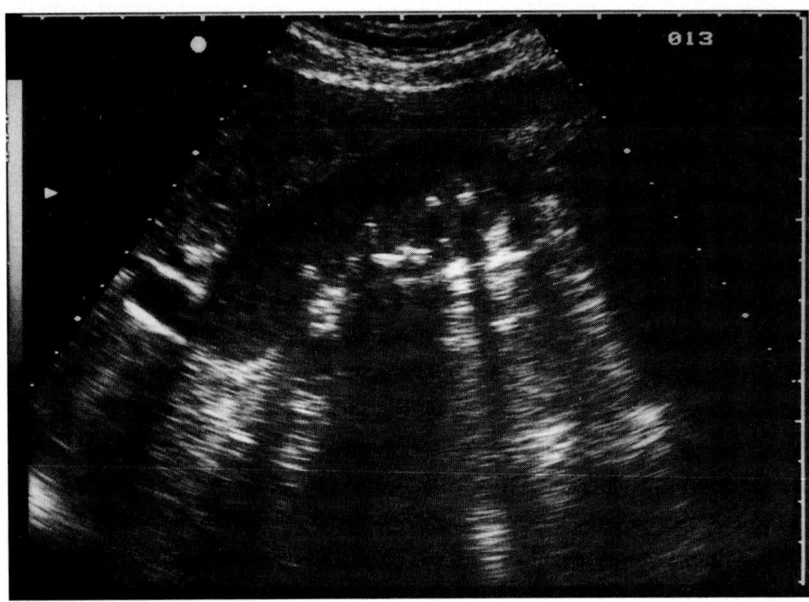

FIGURE 11.2. *Transabdominal ultrasound of a gallbladder containing large amounts of sludge and multiple gallstones generating characteristic acoustic shadowing.*

Table 11.1. Risk factors for gallstone formation

Risk factors
Cholesterol gallstones
American Indians > Hispanics > Whites > Blacks
Western countries
Family history
Female gender
Pregnancy, multiparous
Estrogen supplementation
Obesity
Age
Weight loss
Fasting, total parenteral nutrition
Drugs (Octreotide, Ceftriaxone, Clofibrate, Cholestyramine)
Non-insulin-dependent diabetes mellitus
Black pigment gallstones
Chronic hemolysis
Cirrhosis
Alcoholism
Ileal disease
Age
Brown pigment stones
Rural Asia
Biliary tract infection
Juxtapapillary diverticula

Pregnancy predisposes women to gallstones, probably due to a combination of the effects of estrogens causing an increase in biliary cholesterol saturation and the progesterones causing atony of the gallbladder. In a study by Coelho and colleagues performed in Brazil, 4% of nulliparous women had gallstones compared to 35% of women with six or more pregnancies (80). As mentioned above, biliary sludge commonly develops during pregnancy and may evolve into gallstones or may resolve after the birth.

Medications such as estrogen-containing contraceptives and estrogen given to postmenopausal women raise the risk of gallstones (81–83), as do lipid-lowering agents such as clofibrate and gemfibrozil, which promote biliary cholesterol excretion. Cholestyramine may predispose individuals to gallstone formation by binding to bile acids in the gut and preventing their absorption.

Conditions leading to gallbladder stasis (TPN, diabetes, spinal cord injury, and possibly autonomic dysfunction) are associated with an increased risk of gallstone formation. Some good news for many of us: the consumption of at least 2 cups of coffee per day has recently been reported to be associated with a 40% reduction in the rate of gallstone formation (84)!

Natural History of Gallstones

Gallstones are common and are frequently discovered incidentally in asymptomatic patients. Although their spontaneous disappearance is a rare event—with the exception of stones that formed during pregnancy or weight reduction (85)—gallstones will remain "silent" in more than two-thirds of individuals (86,87). They can, however, cause symptoms and complications, including biliary colic, acute cholecystitis, obstructive jaundice with or without cholangitis, and biliary pancreatitis.

Asymptomatic Gallstones

The management of asymptomatic stones has generated considerable controversy. At one time, cholecystectomy for asymptomatic stones was recommended because prophylactic surgery was assumed to prevent excess morbidity from subsequent symptomatic gallstone disease (88). However, subsequent studies suggested that the cumulative risk for the development of symptoms or complications from asymptomatic gallstones is relatively low, in the range of 1% to 2% per year (89,90). One study found a risk of approximately 10% at 5 years, 15% at 10 years, and 18% at 15 years (89). Patients remaining asymptomatic for 15 years were unlikely to develop symptoms later. Moreover, most patients who did develop complications from their gallstones experienced prior warning symptoms. Decision analysis has suggested that the cumulative risk of death due to asymptomatic gallstone disease while on expectant management is small, and therefore prophylactic cholecystectomy is not warranted for this patient population (85,91).

Some reports have suggested that patients with diabetes mellitus and gallstones may be more susceptible to septic complications (92) and may have an increased risk of perioperative morbidity and mortality (93). This has led some authorities to advise prophylactic cholecystectomy for all diabetic patients with cholelithiasis, irrespective of whether they have developed symptoms. However, when focusing on diabetic patients with *asymptomatic* gallstones, other investigators found that the course of their disease is as benign as it is in nondiabetic patients (94,95). Based on these findings and the decision analysis by Friedman and colleagues (96), prophylactic cholecystectomy in diabetic patients with asymptomatic gallstones does not seem to be warranted.

Gallstones have long been suspected to be a risk factor for the development of carcinoma of the gallbladder. The incidence of gallbladder cancer in patients with cholecystolithiasis is approximately 1 in 10,000, compared to 1 in 30,000 in individuals without gallstones (87). This risk is felt to be too low, however, to justify prophylactic cholecystectomy in every individual with cholelithiasis (80).

Symptomatic Gallstones

Biliary colic is the most common presentation of symptomatic gallstone disease (85,89,97) and is felt to be due to tonic spasm around the cystic duct secondary to temporal obstruction by a gallstone. The resulting intense abdominal pain is typically located in the epigastrium and right upper quadrant and may radiate to the upper back or, less often, the right shoulder. The pain usually begins abruptly, reaches its climax within a few minutes, and remains steady for 30 minutes to several hours. Concomitant symptoms such as nausea, vomiting, and sweating are common.

Because pain in the upper abdomen is a common complaint and may be due to a large variety of diseases in patients who also have (asymptomatic) gallstones, identifying those patients with true symptomatic gallstone disease remains a clinical dilemma. The onset of a biliary colic may be provoked by food (98), but this is a weak discriminator of gallstone disease (99). Intolerance to fried and fatty food is associated with gallstone disease (100), but is very common in general and lacks specificity (101). Dyspeptic symptoms are common in the general population as well as in individuals with gallstones, and a causal relationship remains to be established. In a considerable proportion of patients with gallstones, dyspeptic symptoms are relieved after cholecystectomy (102,103), but these patients cannot be clearly identified preoperatively (102). Identifying patients with symptomatic gallstone disease is important because the annual risk of recurrent pain attacks after an episode of biliary colic ranges from 6% to 40% (99,104). Still, it has been estimated that 30% of patients who experience biliary pain will not have subsequent episodes in the future (85).

Fortunately, serious gallstone-related complications are less common, and occur at an annual rate of 3% to 8% (86,90,91,104). Cholecystitis accounts for the majority of severe gallstone complications occurring in approximately 10% of patients with symptomatic cholelithiasis (90). Obstructive jaundice, cholangitis, and biliary pancreatitis are comparably rare. And 20% to 50% of patients with symptomatic gallstone disease will not have experienced serious complications over the subsequent 20 years (90). Complications are almost always preceded by biliary pain, which may be considered a warning symptom (85). After having experienced a complication, patients have a high risk for recurrence of a symptomatic episode, which occurs in roughly 30% over 3 months in those who do not undergo cholecystectomy (85).

Treatment of Gallstones

Treatment is generally recommended for symptomatic gallstones. In the absence of contraindications to surgery, elective laparoscopic cholecystectomy will be the treatment of choice in most patients. Common duct stones can be removed endoscopically; however, to avoid recurrence of symptomatic gallstone disease, cholecystectomy will still need to be considered in patients with secondary common duct stones and stones remaining in the gallbladder. A sphincterotomy after endoscopic stone extraction will prevent recurrence of biliary pancreatitis (but not cholecystitis) in patients unfit to undergo gallbladder surgery (105).

Oral gallstone dissolution therapy with bile acids may be appropriate in highly selected, mildly symptomatic patients who refuse cholecystectomy or who are felt to be at significant risk for surgery. The treatment is only successful for small stones (less than 0.5 to 1.5 cm) that are noncalcified (as evidenced by plain abdominal x-ray film or abdominal CT scan). Ursodeoxycholic acid (UDCA) is generally considered the agent of choice. A meta-analysis suggests that success rates are higher for UDCA than for chenodeoxycholic acid (CDCA) (106); the latter is associated with considerable dose-related side effects such as elevation of liver enzymes, hypercholesterolemia, and watery diarrhea (107). UDCA therapy given at a dose of 8–12 mg per kg per day for at least 6 months results in complete gallstone dissolution in only 40% of patients (106). The success rate is inversely correlated with gallstone diameter. It approaches 90% in highly selected patients with small (<5 mm) floating stones and is considerably lower for larger stones (106,107). The dissolution rate (if stones dissolve) is generally slow and can be expected to be around 0.5 to 1.0 mm per month. Stones recur after dissolution in about 50% of patients at an annual rate of about 10% during the first 3 to 5 years (14,107).

Extracorporeal shockwave lithotripsy (ESWL) with or without adjuvant UDCA treatment has not generated much enthusiasm in the United States but is available in several countries outside the United States. It is most successful in patients with solitary radiolucent stones with a diameter of less than 2 cm (14).

Topical dissolution therapy of noncalcified stones involves the perfusion of the gallbladder with organic solvents such as methyl tert-butyl ether (MTBE). The solvent is instilled via a catheter introduced into the gallbladder either percutaneously or endoscopically (i.e., via a nasobiliary tube). Gallstones can generally be dissolved within a few hours, regardless of size and number. Unfortunately, stone recurrence is high: 40% for solitary stones and 70% for multiple stones over 5 years (108). Significant complications may occur and are mainly due to the invasive approach. Bile leakage occurs in up to 5% of patients after percutaneous gallbladder puncture. Pancreatitis and cystic duct perforation may complicate endoscopic retrograde cannulation (107). As long as MTBE is contained within the gallbladder, it is well tolerated. Attempts to use MTBE to deal with common bile duct stones, however, have failed due to significant side effects (109–111). MTBE leaking from the bile duct into the duodenum may result in severe duodenitis, and if enough of the ether is absorbed, it causes profound sedation and other systemic effects (e.g., hemolysis or renal insufficiency).

With the advent of minimal invasive surgical techniques such as laparoscopic cholecystectomy and the advances in endoscopic retrograde techniques of stone removal, dissolution therapy and ESWL are rarely needed.

REFERENCES

1. Heaton KW, Braddon FE, Mountford RA, et al. Symptomatic and silent gall stones in the community. Gut 1991;32:316–20.

2. Diehl AK. Epidemiology and natural history of gallstone disease. Gastroenterol Clin North Am 1991;20:1–19.
3. Gallstones and laparoscopic cholecystectomy. NIH Consens Statement 1992; 10:1–28.
4. Ingelfinger FJ. Digestive disease as a national problem. V. Gallstones. Gastroenterology 1968;55:102–4.
5. Lee. Gallstones. In: Yamada T, ed. Textbook of gastroenterology. 3rd ed. Philadelphia: Lippincott Williams & Wilkins, 1999:2258–80.
6. Miyke H, Johnson CG. Gallstones: ethnological studies. Digestion 1968;1: 219–28.
7. Trotman BW, Soloway RD. Pigment vs cholesterol cholelithiasis: clinical and epidemiological aspects. Am J Dig Dis 1975;20:735–40.
8. Trotman BW, Ostrow JD, Soloway RD. Pigment vs cholesterol cholelithiasis: comparison of stone and bile composition. Am J Dig Dis 1974;19:585–90.
9. Soloway RD, Trotman BW, Ostrow JD. Pigment gallstones. Gastroenterology 1977;72:167–82.
10. Busch N, Matern S. Current concepts in cholesterol gallstone pathogenesis. Eur J Clin Invest 1991;21:453–60.
11. Moseley RH. Bile secretion. In: Yamada T, ed. Textbook of gastroenterology. Philadelphia: Lippincott Williams and Wilkins, 1999:380–396.
12. Paumgartner G, Sauerbruch T. Secretion, composition and flow of bile. Clin Gastroenterol 1983;12:3–23.
13. Paumgartner G, Sauerbruch T. Gallstones: pathogenesis. Lancet 1991;338: 1117–21.
14. Portincasa P, van de Meeberg P, van Erpecum KJ, et al. An update on the pathogenesis and treatment of cholesterol gallstones. Scand J Gastroenterol Suppl 1997;223:60–9.
15. Donovan JM, Carey MC. Separation and quantitation of cholesterol "carriers" in bile. Hepatology 1990;12(suppl):S94–104; discussion, S104–5.
16. Carey MC. Pathogenesis of gallstones. Am J Surg 1993;165:410–19.
17. Strasberg SM, Clavien PA, Harvey PR. Pathogenesis of cholesterol gallstones. HPB Surg 1991;3:79–102.
18. Admirand WH, Small DM. The physicochemical basis of cholesterol gallstone formation in man. J Clin Invest 1968;47:1043–52.
19. Somjen GJ, Gilat T. Contribution of vesicular and micellar carriers to cholesterol transport in human bile. J Lipid Res 1985;26:699–704.
20. Lee SP, Park HZ, Madani H, et al. Partial characterization of a nonmicellar system of cholesterol solubilization in bile. Am J Physiol 1987;252:G374–83.
21. Crawford JM, Mockel GM, Crawford AR, et al. Imaging biliary lipid secretion in the rat: ultrastructural evidence for vesiculation of the hepatocyte canalicular membrane. J Lipid Res 1995;36:2147–63.
22. Holzbach RT, Marsh M, Olszewski M, et al. Cholesterol solubility in bile. Evidence that supersaturated bile is frequent in healthy man. J Clin Invest 1973;52:1467–79.
23. Northfield TC, Hofmann AF. Biliary lipid output during three meals and an overnight fast. I. Relationship to bile acid pool size and cholesterol saturation of bile in gallstone and control subjects. Gut 1975;16:1–11.
24. Holan KR, Holzbach RT, Hermann RE, et al. Nucleation time: a key factor in the pathogenesis of cholesterol gallstone disease. Gastroenterology 1979; 77:611–17.
25. Burnstein MJ, Ilson RG, Petrunka CN, et al. Evidence for a potent nucleating factor in the gallbladder bile of patients with cholesterol gallstones. Gastroenterology 1983;85:801–7.
26. Groen AK, Drapers JA, Tytgat GN. Cholesterol nucleation and gallstone formation. J Hepatol 1988;6:383–7.
27. LaMont JT, Smith BF, Moore JR. Role of gallbladder mucin in pathophysiology of gallstones. Hepatology 1984;4(suppl):51S–6S.
28. Smith BF, LaMont JT. The central issue of cholesterol gallstones. Hepatology 1986;6:529–31.
29. Lee SP, Carey MC, LaMont JT. Aspirin prevention of cholesterol gallstone formation in prairie dogs. Science 1981;211:1429–31.
30. MacPherson BR, Pemsingh RS. Ground squirrel model for cholelithiasis: role of epithelial glycoproteins. Microsc Res Tech 1997;39:39–55.
31. Pazzi P, Scagliarini R, Sighinolfi D, et al. Nonsteroidal antiinflammatory drug use and gallstone disease prevalence: a case-control study. Am J Gastroenterol 1998;93:1420–24.
32. Minocha A, Greenbaum DS, Gardiner J. Effect of non-steroidal anti-inflammatory drugs on formation of gallbladder stones. Vet Hum Toxicol 1994;36:514–16.
33. Adamek HE, Buttmann A, Weber J, et al. Can aspirin prevent gallstone recurrence after successful extracorporeal shockwave lithotripsy? Scand J Gastroenterol 1994;29:355–9.
34. Kurata JH, Marks J, Abbey D. One gram of aspirin per day does not reduce risk of hospitalization for gallstone disease. Dig Dis Sci 1991;36:1110–15.
35. Choi J, Klinkspoor JH, Yoshida T, et al. Lipopolysaccharide from Escherichia coli stimulates mucin secretion by cultured dog gallbladder epithelial cells. Hepatology 1999;29:1352–7.
36. Miquel JF, Nunez L, Amigo L, et al. Cholesterol saturation, not proteins or cholecystitis, is critical for crystal formation in human gallbladder bile. Gastroenterology 1998;114:1016–23.
37. Van Erpecum KJ, Van Berge-Henegouwen GP. Gallstones: an intestinal disease? Gut 1999;44:435–8.
38. Pitt HA, Doty JE, DenBesten L. Increased intragallbladder pressure response to cholecystokinin-octapeptide following vagotomy and pyloroplasty. J Surg Res 1983;35:325–31.
39. Glenn F, McSherry CK. Pregnancy, cholesterol metabolism and gallstones. Ann Surg 1969;169:712–23.
40. Pauletzki J, Althaus R, Holl J, et al. Gallbladder emptying and gallstone formation: a prospective study on gallstone recurrence. Gastroenterology 1996; 111:765–71.
41. Gurll NJ, Meyer PD, DenBesten L. Effect of cholesterol crystals on gallbladder function in cholelithiasis. Surg Forum 1977;28:412–13.
42. Roslyn JJ, Pitt HA, Kuchenbecker S, et al. Alterations in biliary tract motility during cholesterol gallstone formation. Surg Forum 1980;31: 205–9.
43. Davis M, Ryan JP. Influence of progesterone on guinea pig gallbladder motility in vitro. Dig Dis Sci 1986;31:513–18.
44. Shaffer EA, McOrmond P, Duggan H. Quantitative cholescintigraphy: assessment of gallbladder filling and emptying and duodenogastric reflux. Gastroenterology 1980;79:899–906.
45. Everson GT. Gallbladder function in gallstone disease. Gastroenterol Clin North Am 1991;20:85–110.
46. Sharma BC, Agarwal DK, Dhiman RK, et al. Bile lithogenicity and gallbladder emptying in patients with microlithiasis: effect of bile acid therapy. Gastroenterology 1998;115:124–28.
47. Jazrawi RP, Pazzi P, Petroni ML, et al. Postprandial gallbladder motor function: refilling and turnover of bile in health and in cholelithiasis. Gastroenterology 1995;109:582–91.
48. Doty JE, Pitt HA, Kuchenbecker SL, et al. Impaired gallbladder emptying before gallstone formation in the prairie dog. Gastroenterology 1983;85: 168–74.
49. Saunders KD, Cates JA, Roslyn JJ. Pathogenesis of gallstones. Surg Clin North Am 1990;70:1197–216.
50. Cahalane MJ, Neubrand MW, Carey MC. Physical-chemical pathogenesis of pigment gallstones. Semin Liver Dis 1988;8:317–28.
51. Trotman BW. Pigment gallstone disease. Gastroenterol Clin North Am 1991; 20:111–26.
52. Bates GL, Brown CH. Incidence of gallbladder disease in chronic hemolytic anemia. Gastroenterology 1952;21:104–9.
53. Davidson JF. Alcohol and cholelithiasis: a necropsy survey of cirrhosis. Am J Med Sci 1962;244:730–6.
54. Brink MA, Slors JF, Keulemans YC, et al. Enterohepatic cycling of bilirubin: a putative mechanism for pigment gallstone formation in ileal Crohn's disease. Gastroenterology 1999;116:1420–7.
55. Shull SD, Wagner CI, Trotman BW, et a!. Factors affecting bilirubin excretion in patients with cholesterol or pigment gallstones. Gastroenterology 1977;72: 625–9.
56. Ko CW, Lee SP. Gallstone formation. Local factors. Gastroenterol Clin North Am 1999;28:99–115.
57. Coyle JJ, Hoyt DB, Sedghat A. Relationship of intestinal bypass operations and cholelithiasis. Surg Forum 1980;31:139–44.
58. Cetta F. The role of bacteria in pigment gallstone disease. Ann Surg 1991;213: 315–26.
59. Kaufman HS, Magnuson TH, Lillemoe KD, et al. The role of bacteria in gallbladder and common duct stone formation. Ann Surg 1989;209:584–91;discussion, 591–82.
60. Saharia PC, Zuidema GD, Cameron JL. Primary common duct stones. Ann Surg 1977;185:598–604.
61. Way LW, Admirand WH. Management of choledocholithiasis. Ann Surg 1973;176:347–51.
62. Wong HN, Frey CF, Gagic NM. Intraoperative common duct pressure and flow measurements. Am J Surg 1985;139:691–6.
63. Toouli J, Geenen JE, Hogan WJ, et al. Sphincter of Oddi motor activity: a comparison between patients with common bile duct stones and controls. Gastroenterology 1982;82:111–17.
64. De Masi E, Corazziari E, Habib FI, et al. Manometric study of the sphincter of Oddi in patients with and without common bile duct stones. Gut 1984;25: 275–8.

65. Lotveit T, Skar V, Osnes M. Juxtapapillary duodenal diverticula. Endoscopy 1988;20(suppl 1):175–8.
66. Conrad MR, Janes JO, Dietchy J. Significance of low level echoes within the gallbladder. AJR Am J Roentgenol 1979;132:967–72.
67. Ko CW, Sekijima JH, Lee SP. Biliary sludge. Ann Intern Med 1999;130:301–11.
68. Lee SP. Pathogenesis of biliary sludge. Hepatology 1990;12(suppl):200S–3S; discussion, 203S–5S.
69. Lee SP, Maher K, Nicholls JF. Origin and fate of biliary sludge. Gastroenterology 1988;94:170–176.
70. Allen B, Bernhoft R, Blanckaert N, et al. Sludge is calcium bilirubinate associated with bile stasis. Am J Surg 1981;141:51–6.
71. Messing B, Bories C, Kunstlinger F, et al. Does total parenteral nutrition induce gallbladder sludge formation and lithiasis? Gastroenterology 1983;84: 1012–19.
72. Huang WS. Cholelithiasis in Singapore. Gut 1970;11:141–6.
73. Stitnimankarn. The necropsy incidence of gallstones in Thailand. Am J Med Sci 1960;240:349–54.
74. Grundy SM, Metzger AL, Alder RD. Mechanisms of lithogenic bile formation in American Indian women with cholesterol gallstones. J Clin Invest 1972;51: 3026–32.
75. Hendry A, O'Leary JP. The history of cholelithiasis. Ann Surg 1998;64:801–2.
76. Kalos A, Delidou A, Kordosis T, et al. The incidence of gallstones in Greece; an autopsy study. Acta Hepatogastroenterol (Stuttg) 1977;24:20–3.
77. Acalovschi M, Dumitrascu D, Caluser I, et al. Comparative prevalence of gallstone disease at 100-year interval in a large Romanian town, a necropsy study. Dig Dis Sci 1987;32:354–7.
78. Sarin SK, Negi VS, Dewan R, et al. High familial prevalence of gallstones in the first-degree relatives of gallstone patients. Hepatology 1995;22:138–41.
79. Maclure KM, Hayes KC, Colditz GA, et al. Weight, diet, and the risk of symptomatic gallstones in middle-aged women. N Engl J Med 1989;321:563–569.
80. Coelho JC, Bonilha R, Pitaki SA, et al. Prevalence of gallstones in a Brazilian population. Int Surg 1999;84:25–8.
81. Strom BL, Tamragouri RN, Morse ML, et al. Oral contraceptives and other risk factors for gallbladder disease. Clin Pharmacol Ther 1986:335–41.
82. Grodstein F, Colditz GA, Hunter DJ, et al. A prospective study of symptomatic gallstones in women: relation with oral contraceptives and other risk factors. Obstet Gynecol 1994;84:207–14.
83. Petitti DB, Sidney S, Perlman JA. Increased risk of cholecystectomy in users of supplemental estrogen. Gastroenterology 1988;94:91–5.
84. Leitzmann MF, Willett WC, Rimm EB, et al. A prospective study of coffee consumption and the risk of symptomatic gallstone disease in men. JAMA 1999;281:2106–112.
85. Ransohoff DF, Gracie WA. Treatment of gallstones. Ann Intern Med 1993;119: 606–19.
86. McSherry CK, Ferstenberg H, Calhoun WF, et al. The natural history of diagnosed gallstone disease in symptomatic and asymptomatic patients. Ann Surg 1985;202:59–63.
87. Angelico F, Del Ben M, Barbato A, et al. Ten-year incidence and natural history of gallstone disease in a rural population of women in central Italy. The Rome Group for the Epidemiology and Prevention of Cholelithiasis (GREPCO). Ital J Gastroenterol Hepatol 1997;29:249–54.
88. Wenckert A, Robertson B. The natural course of gallstone disease: eleven-year review of 781 nonoperated cases. Gastroenterology 1966;50:376–81.
89. Gracie WA, Ransohoff DF. The natural history of silent gallstones: the innocent gallstone is not a myth. N Engl J Med 1982;307:798–800.
90. Friedman GD. Natural history of asymptomatic and symptomatic gallstones. Am J Surg 1993;165:399–404.
91. Ransohoff DF, Gracie WA. Management of patients with symptomatic gallstones: a quantitative analysis. Am J Med 1990;88:154–60.
92. Cucchiaro G, Watters CR, Rossitch JC, et al. Deaths from gallstones. Incidence and associated clinical factors. Ann Surg 1989;209:149–51.
93. Landau O, Deutsch AA, Kott I, et al. The risk of cholecystectomy for acute cholecystitis in diabetic patients. Hepatogastroenterology 1992;39:437–8.
94. Del Favero G, Caroli A, Meggiato T, et al. Natural history of gallstones in non-insulin-dependent diabetes mellitus. A prospective 5-year follow-up. Dig Dis Sci 1994;39:1704–7.
95. Aucott JN, Cooper GS, Bloom AD, et al. Management of gallstones in diabetic patients. Arch Intern Med 1993;153:1053–8.
96. Friedman LS, Roberts MS, Brett AS, et al. Management of asymptomatic gallstones in the diabetic patient. A decision analysis. Ann Intern Med 1988; 109:913–19.
97. Attili AF, De Santis A, Capri R, et al. The natural history of gallstones: the GREPCO experience. The GREPCO Group. Hepatology 1995;21:655–60.
98. Kraagg N, Thijs C, Knipschild P. Dyspepsia—how noisy are gallstones? A meta-analysis of epidemiologic studies of biliary pain, dyspeptic symptoms, and food intolerance. Scand J Gastroenterol 1995;30:411–21.
99. Diehl AK. Symptoms of gallstone disease. Baillieres Clin Gastroenterol 1992;6: 635–57.
100. Festi D, Sottili S, Colecchia A, et al. Clinical manifestations of gallstone disease: evidence from the multicenter Italian study on cholelithiasis (MICOL). Hepatology 1999;30:839–46.
101. Thijs C, Knipschild P. Abdominal symptoms and food intolerance related to gallstones. J Clin Gastroenterol 1998;27:223–31.
102. Bates T, Ebbs SR, Harrison M, et al. Influence of cholecystectomy on symptoms. Br J Surg 1991;78:964–7.
103. Fenster LF, Lonborg R, Thirlby RC, et al. What symptoms does cholecystectomy cure? Insights from an outcomes measurement project and review of the literature. Am J Surg 1995;169:533–8.
104. Thistle JL, Cleary PA, Lachin JM, et al. The natural history of cholelithiasis: the National Cooperative Gallstone Study. Ann Intern Med 1984;101:171–5.
105. Welbourne CRB, Beckley DE, Eyre-Brook IA. Endoscopic sphincterotomy without cholecystectomy for gallstone pancreatitis. Gut 1995;37:119–20.
106. May GR, Sutherland LR, Shaffer EA. Efficacy of bile acid therapy for gallstone dissolution: a meta-analysis of randomized trials. Aliment Pharmacol Ther 1993;7:139–48.
107. Sauerbruch T, Paumgartner G. Gallbladder stones: management. Lancet 1991; 338:1121–4.
108. Hellstern A, Leuschner U, Benjaminov A, et al. Dissolution of gallbladder stones with methyl tert-butyl ether and stone recurrence: a European survey. Dig Dis Sci 1998;43:911–20.
109. Saraya A, Rai RR, Tandon RK. Experience with MTBE as a solvent for common bile duct stones in patients with T-tube in situ. J Gastroenterol Hepatol 1990;5:130–4.
110. Neoptolemos JP, Hall C, Connor HJO, et al. Methyl-tert-butyl-ether for treating bile duct stones: the British experience. Br J Surg 1990;77: 32–5.
111. Ponchon T, Baron J, Pajol B, et al. Renal failure during dissolution of gallstones by methyl-tert-butyl ether. Lancet 1988;30:276–7.

Chapter 12

Acute and Chronic Cholecystitis

LISA A. CLARK THEODORE N. PAPPAS

As far back as 2000 BC, the anatomy of the gallbladder and bile ducts was known, as is proven by clay models found from that period. This knowledge was significant at the time: the Babylonian and Assyrian priests required their patients to breathe into a sheep's mouth, following which the sheep was sacrificed and the liver and gallbladder dissected to determine which area was affected by the patient's breath. Attention was then given to the gallbladder size, color, distension, and any abnormalities were sought and described as a special sign from the gods (1).

The first description of gallstones came in the 5th century by Greek physician Alexander Trallianus, who wrote of calculi within the bile ducts. However, the earliest known human gallstones were discovered in the mummy of a priestess of Amen who lived during the 21st Egyptian Dynasty (1085–945 BC). Abraham Vater discovered the "tubercle" or "diverticulum" at the confluence of the bile and pancreatic ducts, which later became known as the ampulla of Vater (2).

The first known successful cholecystolithotomy was performed by Dr. Joenisius in 1676, when he noted an abdominal wall abscess that had ruptured, with the discharge of pus and bile. By dilating this fistula, he was able to remove the gallstones. Approximately 60 years later Jean Louis Petit used a trocar to aspirate an inflamed gallbladder that had become adherent to the abdominal wall. He then enlarged the incision and removed several calculi. Ninety years later Carre advocated opening the abdomen to affix the gallbladder to the abdominal wall, allowing adhesions to wall off surrounding structures before performing a cholecystostomy (3).

The 19th century brought the development of anesthesia and more detailed knowledge of biliary colic and intermittent fever from obstructive biliary disease, Courvoisier's law (gallbladder dilatation when there is biliary obstruction below the level of the cystic duct), and the performance of the first cholecystostomy, cholecystectomy, and choledochostomy. The first cholecystostomy was performed by John Stough Bobbs in 1867. This particular operation was unplanned, however, as the patient carried a preoperative diagnosis of ovarian cyst. Upon opening the abdomen, inflammation was seen in the gallbladder, and Bobbs removed the fluid and gallstones. The patient subsequently did well (4). The classic description of cholecystostomy and the name for the operation came from James Marion Sims, an early president of the American Medical Association. The operative description for this procedure was included in his "Remarks on Cholecystostomy on Dropsy of the Gall Bladder," which was published in 1878. The patient died 8 days after the operation from a hemorrhage (5). Two years later Kocher performed the first planned cholecystostomy from which the patient recovered (6).

The first cholecystectomy was performed by Carl Johann August Langenbuch, a surgeon from Berlin, who in 1882 remarked,

> The surgery of the gallbladder is still in the infancy of its development, but it does exist and the names of Petit, Thudichum, M. Sims, Kocher, G. Brown, Lawson Tait, Konig and others are in a general way associated with it. Concerned with stone formation, they have until now gone only so far as exposing the gallbladder freely and have been satisfied to widen fistulas and extract stones whenever hydrops or empyema of the gallbladder call for an operation . . . They have busied themselves with the product of the disease, not the disease itself (7).

Langenbuch then developed and performed the first cholecystectomy, which he subsequently described.

The operation proceeded smoothly, through a T incision. The gallbladder was found to be massively full of gall and was emptied by aspiration with a syringe. Two chestnut size cholesterol gallstones were found. When the gallbladder was detached from the liver, a small venous bleeding occurred. This was controlled with a catgut stitch . . . After the operation the patient felt no pain and slept well the following night. Next day his pulse and temperature were normal; he felt no pain and he smoked a cigar. He left his bed on July 27. His old pain had not recurred up to mid-November. He had gained 13 kilograms in weight and he no longer needed morphine (7).

During the first half of the 20th century, the most significant advances in the field pertained primarily to improved diagnosis (ultrasound and cholecystography). The surgical treatment of gallbladder disease remained largely unchanged until the first laparoscopic cholecystectomy was performed by Muhe in 1985. Laparoscopic surgery has added a new dimension to the treatment of cholecystitis by providing a minimally invasive surgical option with decreased patient discomfort and length of hospital stay.

ACUTE CALCULOUS CHOLECYSTITIS

Gallstones are associated with 90% to 95% of episodes of acute cholecystitis. The remaining 5% to 10% are classified as acalculous cholecystitis.

Pathogenesis of Stone Formation

Acute calculous cholecystitis is initiated by cystic duct obstruction by gallstones. Gallstones, which represent the failure to maintain biliary solutes (cholesterol, calcium salts, etc.) in solution, are fully described in Chapters 1 and 11.

Biliary sludge is defined as the mixture of bile and precipitated bile solutes. The clinical course varies and can include complete resolution, waxing and waning, and the production of gallstones. Situations that are associated with biliary sludge include rapid weight loss, pregnancy, ceftriaxone or other medications, octreotide therapy, and bone marrow or solid organ transplantation (8).

Pathophysiology of Calculous Cholecystitis

Generally, an episode of cholecystitis begins when a stone becomes impacted in the infundibulum or cystic duct. This leads to pain as the gallbladder contracts against a fixed obstruction and dilates. Stone-induced damage to the mucosa and mucosal edema lead to lymphatic and venous obstruction, and possibly localized areas of ischemia. Bile salts become concentrated in the gallbladder and cause further mucosal injury. This injury can further progress to frank abscess or perforation. Bacteria are found in 50% to 70% of cases of acute cholecystitis. It is unclear if this bacteria is the cause of inflammation or translocates to the gallbladder in the presence of inflammation.

Presentation

Acute cholecystitis is more common in the middle-aged and the elderly. It affects women more than men, and occurs 3:1 in patients under age 50 and 1.5:1.0 in those over 50. In fact, the most common patient to present with gallbladder pathology carries the five "F"s: forties, female, fair, fat, and fertile. Of affected patients, 60% to 80% have had previous biliary tract symptoms, the remainder presenting with acute cholecystitis as the first indication of biliary tract disease. The episode is often preceded by a large, heavy meal; as the fat reaches the duodenum, it stimulates cholecystokinin release and subsequent gallbladder contraction. The presentation is generally that of epigastric and right upper quadrant pain, which may radiate to the back. The right upper quadrant tenderness is best elicited by Murphy's sign, an examination originally described by biliary surgeon Dr. John B. Murphy in 1912. Murphy's sign entails percussion of the right midsubcostal region with the bent middle finger of the left hand, using the right hand to strike the dorsum of the left hand with hammer-like blows. This causes acute pain and inspiratory arrest in those with cholecystitis (9).

Nausea and vomiting are often described in acute cholecystitis. Classic teaching and texts indicate that fever and leukocytosis are generally present, but there is no supportive data for these signs, and recent studies have found them to be inconsistent. A 1996 retrospective study of patients with acute, nongangrenous cholecystitis found only 29% to be febrile (temperature greater than 100°F) and 68% to have leukocytosis (white blood cell count greater than 11,000 mm^3), with 28% of patients lacking either sign (10). Electrolyte abnormalities are based upon degree of sepsis and/or dehydration. The associated complications of common bile duct obstruction (choledocholithiasis) or gallstone-induced pancreatitis will lead to elevations in liver enzymes (transaminases, bilirubin, and alkaline phosphatase) or pancreatic enzymes (amylase and lipase), respectively.

Imaging Studies

Ultrasound

The first diagnostic test obtained is generally a right upper quadrant ultrasound (see Chapter 3). This study can demonstrate gallstones, gallbladder wall thickening, pericholecystic fluid, biliary ductal dilatation, and a sonographic Murphy's sign (maximal pain with probe pressure directly over the gallbladder). Gallstones are defined as echogenic foci that have an acoustic shadow and seek gravitational dependence (Fig. 12.1). The procedure is without risk to the patient and relatively inexpensive. It carries a relatively high specificity of 95%, with a sensitivity that is impossible to quantitate,

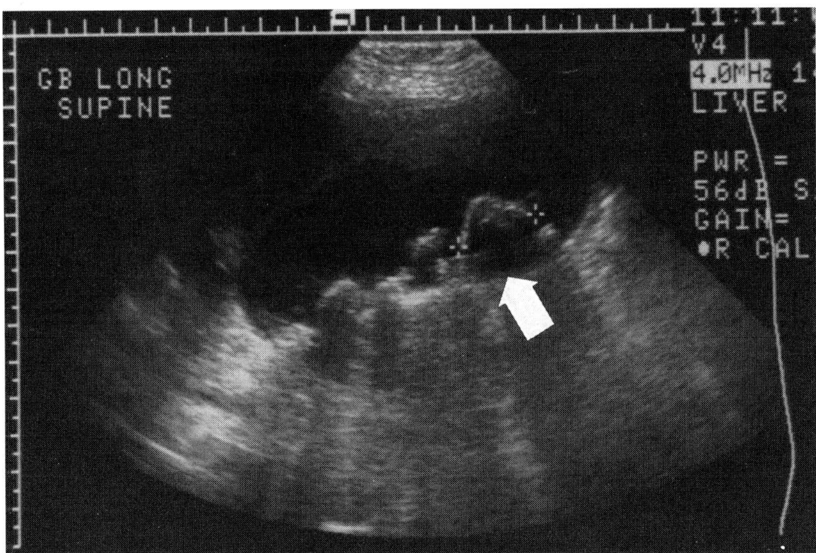

FIGURE 12.1. *Ultrasound of cholelithiasis; arrow indicates gallstones.*

as those with a negative ultrasound do not undergo routine surgical intervention (11).

Oral Cholecystogram

The oral cholecystogram has been used since 1924 to detect stones and assess gallbladder function. Oral contrast agents are given and are absorbed from the gastrointestinal tract. These contain a triiodinated benzene ring which becomes conjugated to glucuronide in the liver for excretion in the bile. The tablets are given with a fat-containing meal and the patient subsequently fasts overnight before imaging the following morning. Visualization of the gallbladder is expected in a normal study. If the gallbladder fails to visualize, a second dose is given and the patient is reexamined the following day. This test is rarely used today because it is comparable to ultrasound in specificity and sensitivity yet ultrasound is less expensive and requires less time to perform.

Radioisotope Cholescintigraphy

Radioisotope cholescintigraphy, often called an HIDA (hepatobiliary iminodiacetic acid) scan, is a nuclear imaging study used to diagnose cystic duct obstruction. A radioactive technetium-labeled iminodiacetic acid derivative (99m technetium iminodiacetic analogue) is injected intravenously and will normally be taken up by the liver and then the gallbladder. Uptake by the liver and excretion into the duodenum without filling of the gallbladder is indicative of acute cholecystitis (Fig. 12.2). This test has a sensitivity of greater than 95% and specificity of 90% in the correct clinical setting. False-positive results can be reduced by the injection of morphine, which increases common bile duct pressure and aids in visualization of the gallbladder. A "rim" of increased pericholecystic activity is seen in the presence of gangrene. The spillage of isotope into the free peritoneal cavity indicates gallbladder perforation. HIDA works poorly in cholestasis, when the serum bilirubin exceeds 10 mg/dL, and its benefit in evaluating common bile duct patency has not been proven (11).

Plain X-ray

X-ray studies are of limited usefulness in acute cholecystitis, as only 15% to 20% of gallstones are seen on plain radiographs. Emphysematous cholecystitis can sometimes be visualized as an air bubble in the right upper quadrant (Fig. 12.3).

Computed Tomography

In patients with presumed acute cholecystitis, ultrasonography and cholescintigraphy are considered the first-choice imaging techniques. However, prior to imaging, patient symptomatology may lead the clinician to consider intra-abdominal abscess or other abdominal findings and order a computed tomography (CT) as the first test. This is a common step with the critically ill patient who has leukocytosis or vague abdominal complaints. Common CT findings in acute cholecystitis have been reviewed by Fidler et al. (12) from Duke University and include gallbladder wall thickening, pericholecystic stranding and fluid, gallbladder distension, subserosal edema, high-attenuation bile, and sloughed membranes (Fig. 12.4). Unfortunately, although many studies have investigated the findings of CT scans, there have been no large prospective studies to define its sensitivity and specificity.

Magnetic Resonance Imaging/Magnetic Resonance Cholangiopancreatography

In the evaluation of acute cholecystitis, ultrasound is superior to magnetic resonance (MR) studies in the evaluation of gallbladder wall thickening; however, MR is superior in the depiction of cystic duct and gallbladder

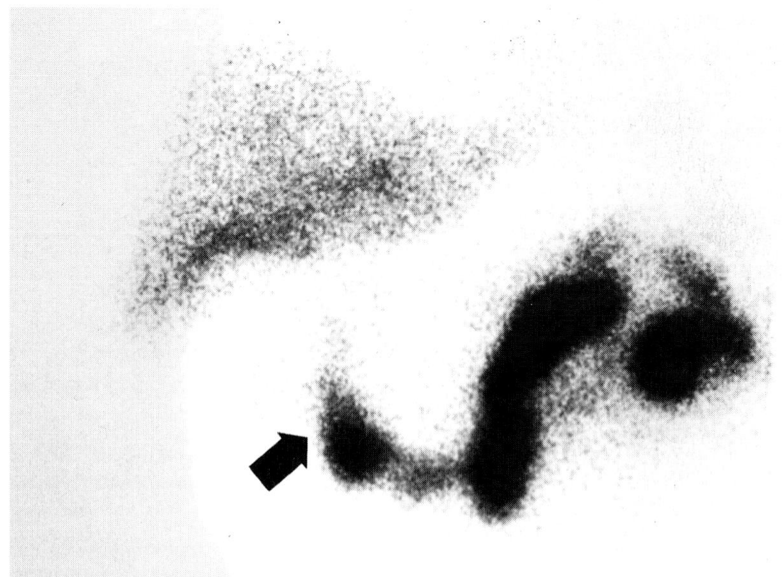

FIGURE 12.2. *HIDA showing uptake of tracer by the liver and excretion into the small bowel without visualization of the gallbladder. Arrow indicates the small bowel.*

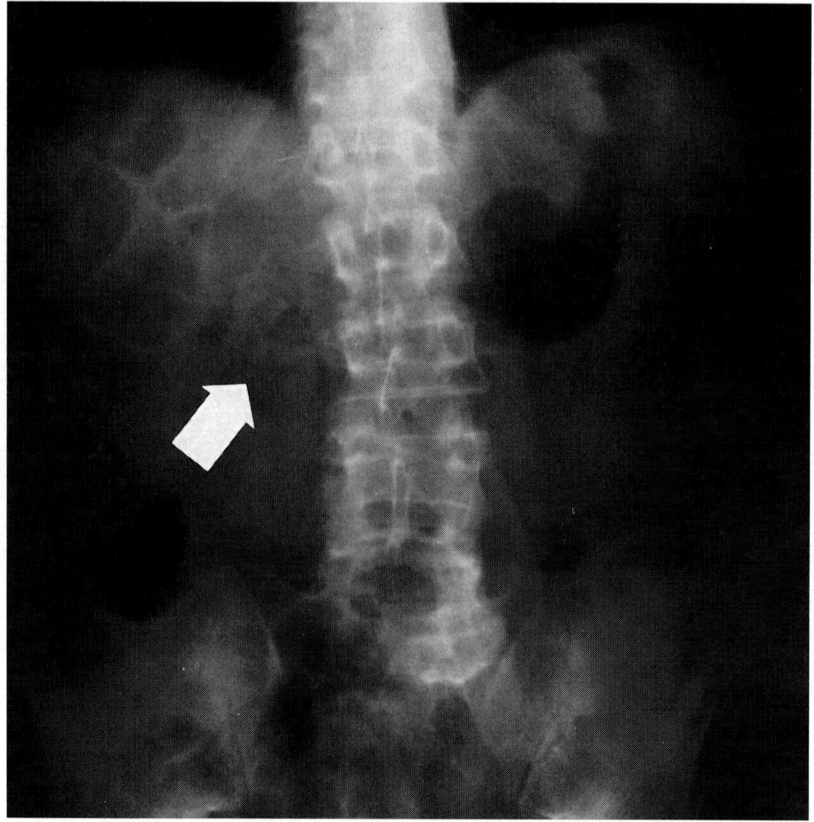

FIGURE 12.3. *Gas in the gallbladder on plain film; arrow indicates gallbladder.*

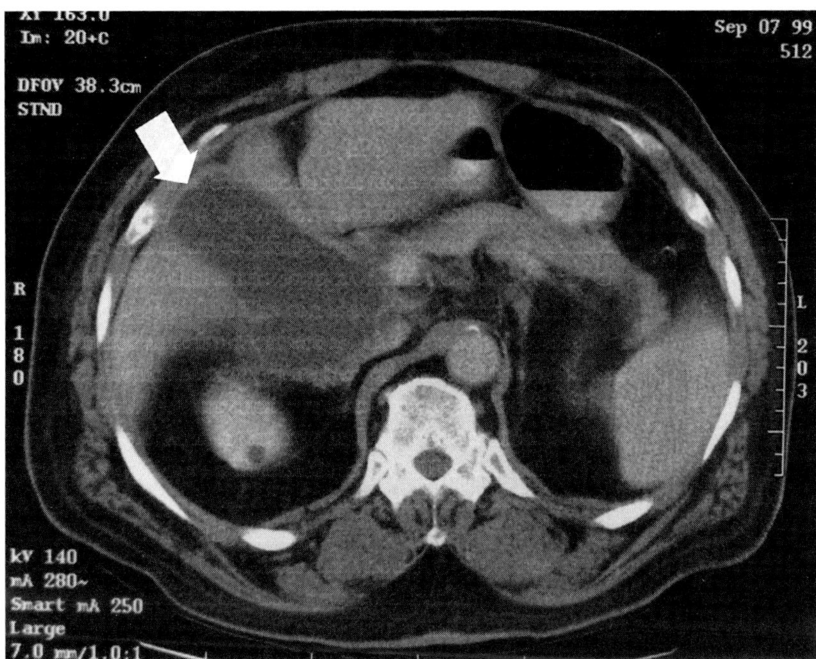

FIGURE 12.4. *CT scan of acute cholecystitis; arrow indicates gallbladder.*

neck calculi obstructions (13). Magnetic resonance imaging/magnetic resonance cholangiopancreatography (MRI/MRCP) is being used with increasing frequency to detect common bile duct stones in a noninvasive manner. Although this test is diagnostic and not therapeutic, its use may limit the number of endoscopic cholangiograms performed for stones suspected prior to or following cholecystectomy (14).

Endoscopic Retrograde Cholangiopancreatography

Endoscopic retrograde cholangiopancreatography (ERCP) can be helpful in differentiating acute cholecystitis from cholangitis and/or in the diagnosis of common bile duct stones. In this case, the common bile duct is evaluated for stones or other causes of obstruction and is cleared, if possible. In addition, ERCP can be used in cases of Mirizzi's syndrome for decompression of the obstructed bile duct.

Bacteriology

Positive bile cultures are found in 40% to 60% of patients and include common enteric organisms. These are gram-positive and gram-negative aerobes and anaerobes: *Escherichia coli*, *Klebsiella*, *Streptococcus faecalis*, *Clostridium welchii*, *Proteus*, *Enterobacter*, and anaerobic streptococci. In a study undertaken to define the bacteriology of gallstone disease, control subjects without symptomatic gallstone disease were found to have no bacteria, whereas 22% of patients with symptomatic gallstones and 46% of patients with acute cholecystitis were found to have positive cultures. The bacteria most frequently isolated were *E. coli*, *Streptococcus* D, *Klebsiella*, and *Enterobacter* (15).

Therapy

The ultimate goal of therapy is to decrease pain, remove the diseased gallbladder and calculi, relieve obstruction, and control infection.

Pain Control

Traditional opiate therapy has included meperidine (Demerol). As morphine has been cited as increasing sphincter of Oddi pressure, it is therefore considered less helpful in biliary tract disease. However, a careful review of the literature reveals minimal data to support this theory. It would seem reasonable to treat the patient with whichever narcotic is well tolerated and provides symptomatic relief (16).

Antibiotics

Antibiotics are chosen that broadly cover routine enteric organisms (such as a second-generation cephalosporin) and can be changed with the results of bile/blood cultures or failure of clinical improvement. Dosage alterations should be considered when obstructive jaundice is present, as this will greatly decrease the excretion of antibiotics into bile.

Surgical Treatment

The definitive therapy for acute cholecystitis clearly involves the surgical drainage or removal of the gallbladder. The key controversies have been *how* and *when* to perform the procedure. The question of cholecystectomy immediately upon diagnosis of cholecystitis versus delayed surgery after antibiotic therapy has been widely debated. Several studies are now available that confirm that surgery performed within 72 hours of symptom onset is both safe and effective, including a prospective, randomized study performed in China and published in 1998 (17). In this study, 99 patients with acute cholecystitis were randomized to receive immediate versus delayed laparoscopic cholecystectomy. The immediate group received surgery within 72 hours of onset of symptoms. The alternate group received medical therapy, which consisted of hospital admission and intravenous antibiotics until clinical improvement was demonstrated, followed by planned laparoscopic cholecystectomy 8 to 12 weeks later. Eight of 41 patients randomized into the delayed group required urgent operation due to clinical deterioration. The delayed group had a significantly higher rate of complications, with no significant difference in rate of conversion to open procedure, which was approximately 15%.

Questions have also been raised as to the risks and benefits of laparoscopic surgery in the setting of acute cholecystitis. Initially, it was thought that the acute inflammation would increase the number of complications. However, as experience has increased with the laparoscopic technique, acute disease is no longer a contraindication to this approach. A study from Spain has confirmed this (18). In this trial, patients were selected for laparoscopic surgery based on the surgeon's experience. Conversion from laparoscopic to open procedure was required in 15% of patients. The operative time was shorter in the open group (mean time of 77 minutes vs. 88 minutes in the laparoscopic group); the number of complications was similar in both groups, and the length of stay significantly shorter in the laparoscopic group (3.3 days vs. 8.1 days for the open group). An additional study performed in Finland was reported in 1998 (19). This prospective study randomized 63 patients to open versus laparoscopic cholecystectomy. Conversion to an open procedure was required in 16% of patients, in most cases due to severe inflammation. The rate of postoperative complications was significantly higher in the open group, and the length of stay and medical sick leave were significantly shorter in the laparoscopic group. Complications in the open group included pneumonia, femoral artery embolism, serious wound infection, incisional hernia, adhesive intestinal obstruction, and retained stone in the common bile duct.

Partial Cholecystectomy

In cases of acute infection with severe inflammation or fibrosis in which it is not possible to clearly identify tissue planes, the risk of injury to vital structures is increased, and it may be safest to perform a partial cholecystectomy. This was described in 1985 by Bornman (20). This is accomplished by the careful dissection of the free wall of the gallbladder, with identification and ligation of the cystic duct whenever possible and adequate drainage of the gallbladder bed, particularly if the cystic duct cannot be ligated. Increasing experience with laparoscopic techniques has made possible laparoscopic subtotal cholecystectomy. A report of this technique and case examples by Michalowski et al. (21) in 1998 revealed similar complications and mortality with the open technique.

Cholecystostomy Tube

Although cholecystectomy is the standard of care for the majority of patients with acute cholecystitis, the morbidity and mortality are substantially increased in those patients with a serious underlying illness; the documented average mortality is none to 0.8% in the average population, versus 14% to 30% in severely debilitated patients (22). Percutaneous cholecystostomy involves the placement of a small drainage catheter directly into the gallbladder, either in the operating room through a small incision, or, more commonly, in the radiology suite, with ultrasound guidance, under local anesthesia (Fig. 12.5). This can provide an immediate, minimally invasive approach for the interim management of acute cholecystitis in the patient not fit enough for surgery. Additionally, it can provide diagnostic information on an ill patient for whom studies are equivocal and the source of infection is being sought. A review of patients who had undergone this procedure at Duke University Medical Center by England et al. (23) revealed the following factors predictive of cholecystostomy tube success: patients with

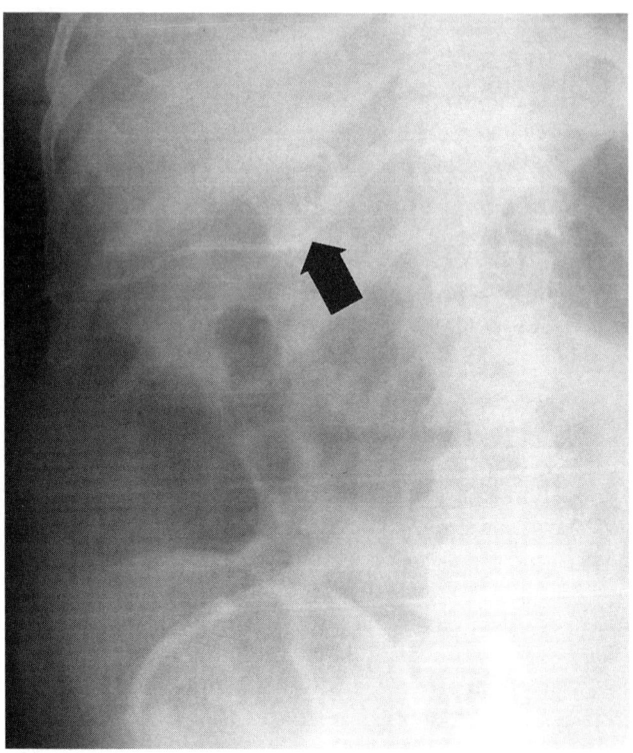

FIGURE 12.5. *Plain film of cholecystostomy tube; arrow indicates tube.*

gallstones and symptoms and signs localized to the right upper quadrant of the abdomen, and gallbladder wall thickening, distension, and pericholecystic fluid. Their mortality rate was 2%, complication rate was 10%, and response rate by clinical improvement after tube placement was 73%. Complications included bleeding, exacerbation of infection, injury to intra-abdominal structures, and failure to improve the clinical status (23). Elective cholecystectomy is performed once the patient's clinical status has improved and the acute inflammation has been resolved. In the severely debilitated patient with a short lifespan, the cholecystostomy tube may be left in indefinitely.

Approach to Common Bile Duct Stones

Common bile duct (CBD) stones are present in 10% to 20% of patients with acute calculous cholecystitis. The presence of CBD stones is indicated by elevation in liver function tests (particularly γ-glutamyltransferase and bilirubin) or by dilation of the CBD on ultrasound. The identification and treatment of CBD stones has changed since the introduction of laparoscopic cholecystectomy. Although laparoscopic CBD exploration is possible, it is seldom performed because of the difficulty of the procedure and high success of ERCP in stone identification and retrieval.

A reasonable algorithm involves the stratification of patients into high, medium, and low risk categories for CBD stones by the assessment of duct size and elevation in transaminases. Those in the high risk category receive preoperative ERCP. Those in the medium category undergo intraoperative cholangiography (Fig. 12.6). Intraoperative cholangiography is appropriate if stones are found and the surgeon is skilled with laparoscopic common duct exploration; otherwise, a decision can be made as to the relative possibility of postoperative ERCP/stone extraction or an open CBD exploration. Those in the low-risk category are observed for symptoms only (24).

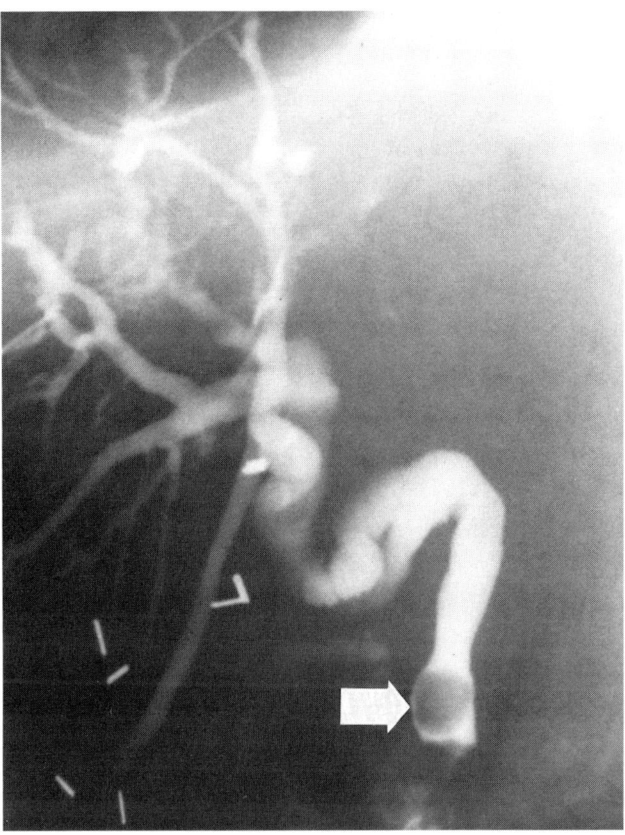

FIGURE 12.6. *Intraoperative cholangiogram revealing choledocholithiasis; arrow indicates stone in the common bile duct.*

ACUTE ACALCULOUS CHOLECYSTITIS

Approximately 5% to 10% of cases of acute cholecystitis are not associated with gallstones. This process is therefore termed *acalculous cholecystitis*. The first known case was reported in 1844 by Duncan (25). In contrast to calculous cholecystitis, males predominate in acute acalculous cholecystitis by a ratio of 1.5 to 1.0. Frequently, acalculous cholecystitis occurs in the setting of other conditions, such as trauma, sepsis, major surgery, infections, or autoimmune diseases, although it can occur spontaneously, especially in diabetics. The incidence of gangrene and the mortality rate are higher than in acute calculous cholecystitis. It is unclear whether the disease process is more severe or the increase is due to comorbidities and overall patient status causing a delay in diagnosis.

There is no clear cause for acalculous cholecystitis, although there appear to be a number of physiologic insults that can lead to the final common pathway of gallbladder mucosal hypoxia and inflammation. This can be attributed to systemic hypotension with gallbladder mucosa hypoperfusion and ischemia, systemic capillary leak syndrome (such as sepsis), and gallbladder wall inflammation and edema, or infection with migration of microorganisms to the gallbladder. Once the mucosa is injured, the gallbladder wall is directly exposed to the concentrated bile, causing further injury.

Histologic features include intensive wall injury with necrosis of blood vessels in the muscularis and serosa of the gallbladder wall (26).

Presentation of Acalculous Cholecystitis

Acalculous cholecystitis patients present in a similar fashion to acute calculous cholecystitis patients, with the exception of a higher incidence of comorbid processes.

Imaging

The imaging procedures are the same as for calculous cholecystitis. Ultrasound can be nonspecific, but may demonstrate a contracted, empty gallbladder or one filled with sludge, and there may be a sonographic Murphy's sign. Initial reports on ultrasound studies found it to be very good for acute acalculous cholecystitis. However, recent studies have revealed a high false-negative rate with significant underestimation of the severity of disease (27,28). CT may be unrevealing, or may demonstrate stranding or pericholecystic fluid. Diagnosis may best be made by HIDA scan, which shows nonfilling of the gallbladder and is 95% to 98% sensitive but less specific (60% to 88%) because of patient factors such as total parenteral nutrition, fasting, or hepatic dysfunction. The use of morphine may increase specificity.

Therapy

Pain control and broad spectrum antibiotics are given. Patient fitness for surgery is assessed. In those patients unable to tolerate a general anesthetic, percutaneous cholecystostomy can alleviate the symptoms at a decreased risk. The remaining patients undergo laparoscopic cholecystectomy, with open cholecystectomy required if this is unsuccessful. An operative cholangiogram should be performed to rule out bile duct stones, if clinically indicated.

Outcome

A recent review of the outcome of acute acalculous cholecystitis by Kalliafas et al. (29) revealed an incidence of 0.19% in the ICU population, accounting for 14% of all cases of acute cholecystitis. They found morphine cholescintigraphy to have the highest sensitivity in diagnosis. These patients had a 63% incidence of gangrene, 15% perforation, and 4% abscess, with a mortality rate of 41%. They concluded that acute acalculous cholecystitis is a rare but severe disease, and that it requires a high index of suspicion to avoid any delay in diagnosis.

CHRONIC CALCULOUS CHOLECYSTITIS

Chronic calculous cholecystitis, or symptomatic cholelithiasis, occurs in the setting of low-grade inflammation from the presence of stones within the gallbladder. Symptomatology is that of intermittent, subacute right upper quadrant pain which may radiate to the back. This results from transient obstruction of the cystic duct by stones. The pain lasts minutes to hours and is often preceded by a fatty meal, which precipitates gallbladder contraction against the stones. No fever or other signs of inflammation are present, although nausea and vomiting are common. Between attacks, patients are asymptomatic.

These patients undergo standard imaging, as for acute cholecystitis, and often require only ultrasound for diagnosis of stones if the symptoms are classic. Elective cholecystectomy is performed in those patients fit enough for surgery, and medical management such as Actigall stone dissolution is used for patients too ill for surgery. This therapy is most useful when the stones are pure or predominantly cholesterol.

CHRONIC ACALCULOUS CHOLECYSTITIS

Chronic acalculous cholecystitis, also known as gallbladder dyskinesia, is defined as biliary colic symptoms (primarily pain) in the absence of identifiable stones on imaging studies. The clinical presentation is that of nonspecific symptoms, including right upper quadrant/epigastric pain, nausea, bloating, and/or altered bowel habits. The physical exam, laboratory studies, and ultrasound are often unrevealing. In some patients, ultrasound reveals a thickened gallbladder wall (3 to 5 mm) and/or sludge. The oral cholecystogram may show nonvisualization of the gallbladder. Radioisotope cholescintigraphy is generally the most useful study, showing decreased tracer uptake. This classically reveals decreased ejection fraction of isotope and reproduces biliary colic pain when gallbladder contraction is stimulated with cholecystokinin (CCK-HIDA scan).

An ejection fraction less than 35% is considered abnormal and surgical removal of the gallbladder is performed on an elective basis. Of the gallbladders removed for this diagnosis, 90% reveal chronic inflammation (Fig. 12.7). However, autopsy series and histologic studies of gallbladders removed incidentally at surgery show a 75% to 90% incidence of similar pathologic changes (30).

Outcome

The application of the CCK-HIDA and the advent of laparoscopy—providing cholecystectomy with less pain and a shorter length of stay—has given rise to an increased use of cholecystectomy in the treatment of chronic acalculous cholecystitis. The demographics of these patients include a greater number of white women and a younger age range than those with calculous cholecystitis. In a study by Jones-Monahan and Gruenberg from Michigan, a 78% incidence of symptom resolution was reported for laparoscopic cholecystectomy for acute acalculous cholecystitis (32). An additional study by Khosla et al. (33) from Missouri evaluated laparoscopic cholecystectomy for the treatment of gallbladder dyskinesia in those patients with a documented decrease in ejection fraction. They found that 67% had resolution of pain, 27% had partial improvement, and 7% had no change. This was significantly different than those patients with decreased ejection fraction who did not undergo cholecystectomy. They concluded that cholecystectomy is indicated for patients with acute acalculous cholecystitis associated with a reduced gallbladder ejection fraction.

Special Situations

Emphysematous Cholecystitis

Emphysematous cholecystitis is a severe form of cholecystitis in which there is gas in the gallbladder lumen, wall, or

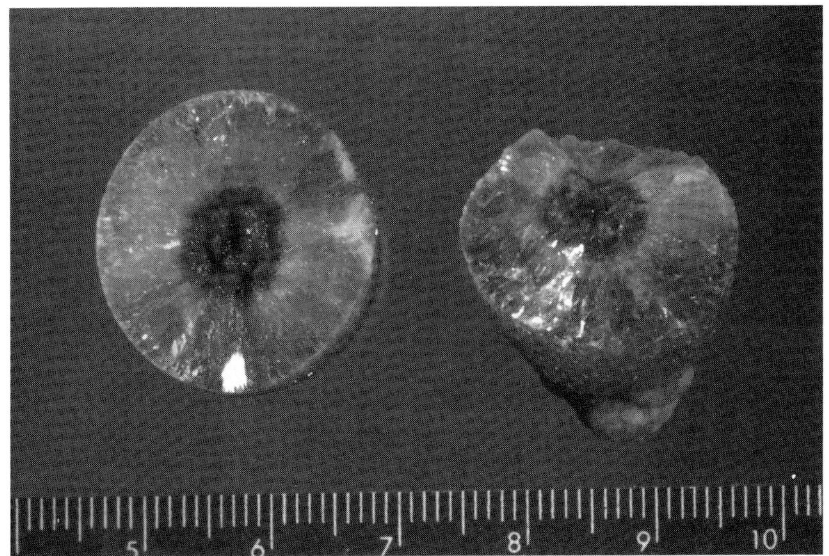

FIGURE 12.7. *Gallbladder specimen with marked chronic acalculous cholecystitis.*

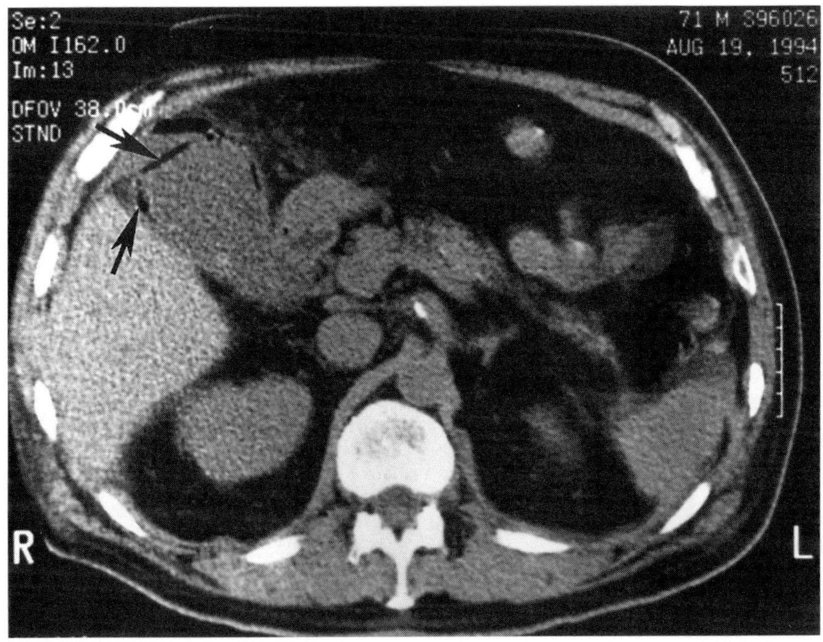

FIGURE 12.8. *CT scan of emphysematous cholecystitis; arrows indicate gas in the wall of the gallbladder.*

pericholecystic tissues in the absence of an abnormal communication between the biliary system and the gastrointestinal tract (Fig. 12.8). This occurs in 1% of patients with acute cholecystitis when acute inflammation is complicated by a secondary infection with gas-forming bacilli. It is more common in men than women and has a more rapid, acute onset with a more severe course, and a higher incidence of gangrene and perforation. Gallstones are found in 40% of cases and many patients are diabetic.

Gas is seen in the gallbladder wall by plain film or ultrasound. Treatment includes high-dose antibiotics to cover clostridia and other gas-forming organisms and an urgent cholecystectomy, with cholecystostomy tube placement in those patients not fit for surgery. A laparoscopic procedure can be attempted, but carries a higher conversion rate (30% to 50%) than usual.

Cholecystitis in Pregnancy

Cholecystitis during pregnancy presents special challenges. Fortunately, ultrasound can be safely performed for diagnosis during pregnancy. In addition, a recent study reviewing open and laparoscopic cholecystectomies performed during pregnancy revealed that laparoscopic surgery is equally safe as open, with similar occurrences of premature labor and fetal mortality (34). As in all procedures in the pregnant patient, cholecystectomy should be delayed until the second trimester whenever possible as there is an increased rate of miscarriage during the first trimester.

SUGGESTED READINGS

Karam J, Roslyn J. Cholelithiasis and cholecystectomy. In: Zinner MJ, Schwartz SI, Ellis H, eds. Maingot's abdominal operations. 10th ed. Stamford, CT: Appleton & Lange, 1997:1717–38.

Nahrwold DL. Acute cholecystitis. In: Sabiston DC, Kim LH, eds. Textbook of surgery: the biological basis of modern surgical practice. 15th ed. Philadelphia: WB Saunders, 1997:1126–32.

Peterson BT, Thistle JL. Medical-surgical management of cholelithiasis. In: Kaplowitz N, ed. Liver and biliary diseases. 2nd ed. Baltimore: Williams & Wilkins, 1996:693–705.

REFERENCES

1. Bettman OL. Pictorial history of medicine. Springfield, IL: Charles C Thomas, 1956.
2. Vater A. Dissertatio anatomica, qua novum bilis diverticulum ut et valvulosum colli vesicae felleae constructionem, etc. In: Haller's disputationum anatomicarium selectarium, Gottinger, 1970;3:259.
3. Glenn F. Historical considerations. In: Atlas of biliary tract surgery. New York: Macmillan, 1963.
4. Bobbs JS. Case of lithotomy of gallbladder. Tr State Med Soc Indiana 1868;18:68–73.
5. Sims JM. Remarks on cholecystostomy in dropsy of gallbladder. BMJ 1878;1:811–15.
6. Kocher T. Mannskopfgrossesmyem der gallenblase: Heilung durch incision. Cor. B. F. schweiz. Basel: Aerzte, 1880;8:577–83.
7. Langenbuch CJA. Ein fall von exstirpation der gallenblase wegen chronisher cholelithiasis; Heilung Berl Klin Wchnschr 1982;19:725–7.
8. Ko CW, Sekijima JH, Lee SP. Biliary sludge. Ann Intern Med 1999;130:301–11.
9. Schmitz RL, Oh TT, eds. The remarkable practice of John Benjamin Murphy. Urbana-Champaign: University of Illinois Press, 1993:29.
10. Gruber PJ, Silverman RA, Gottesfeld S, Flaster E. Presence of fever and leukocytosis in acute cholecystitis. Ann Emerg Med 1996;28:273–7.
11. Zeman RK, Garra BS. Gallbladder imaging—the state of the art. Gastroenterol Clin North Am 1991;2:127–56.
12. Fidler J, Paulson EK, Layfield L. CT evaluation of acute cholecystitis: finding and usefulness in diagnosis. AJR Am J Radiol 1996;166:1085–8.
13. Park MS, Yu JS, Kim YH, et al. Acute cholecystitis: comparison of MR cholangiography and US. Radiology 1998;209:781–5.
14. Liu TH, Consorti ET, Kawashima A, et al. The efficacy of magnetic resonance cholangiography for the evaluation of patients with suspected choledocholithiasis before laparoscopic cholecystectomy. Am J Surg 1999;178:480–4.
15. Csendes A, Burdiles P, Maluenda F, et al. Simultaneous bacteriologic assessment of bile from gallbladder and common bile duct in control subjects and patients with gallstones and common bile duct stones. Arch Surg 1996;131:389–94.
16. Lee F, Cundiff D. Meperidine vs. morphine in pancreatitis and cholecystitis. Arch Intern Med 1998;158:2399.
17. Lo CM, Liu CL, Fan ST, et al. Prospective randomized study of early versus delayed laparoscopic cholecystectomy for acute cholecystitis. Ann Surg 1998;227:461–7.
18. Lujan JA, Parilla P, Robles R, et al. Laparoscopic cholecystectomy vs. open cholecystectomy in the treatment of acute cholecystitis. Arch Surg 1998;133:173–5.
19. Kiviluoto T, Siren J, Luukkonen P, Kivilaakso E. Randomized trial of laparoscopic versus open cholecystectomy for acute and gangrenous cholecystitis. Lancet 1998;351:321–5.
20. Bornman PC, Terblanche J. Subtotal cholecystectomy for the difficult gallbladder in portal hypertension and cholecystitis. Surgery 1985;98:1–6.
21. Michalowski PC, Bornman PC, Krige JEJ, et al. Laparoscopic subtotal cholecystectomy in patients with complicated acute cholecystitis or fibrosis. Br J Surg 1998;85:904–6.
22. Hamy A, Visset J, Likholanikov D, et al. Percutaneous cholecystostomy for acute cholecystitis in critically ill patients. Surgery 1997;121:398–401.
23. England RE, McDermott VG, Smith TP, et al. Percutaneous cholecystostomy: who responds? AJR Am J Roentgenol 1997;168:1247–51.
24. Hammarstrom L, Ranstam J. Factors predictive of bile duct stones in patients with acute calculous cholecystitis. Dig Surg 1998;15:323–7.
25. Frazee RC, Nagorney DM, Much P Jr. Acute acalculous cholecystitis. Mayo Clin Proc 1989;64:163–7.
26. Glenn F, Becker CG. Acute acalculous cholecystitis: an increasing entity. Ann Surg 1982;195:131–6.
27. Blankenberg F, Wirth R, Jeffrey RB Jr, et al. Computed tomography as an adjunct to ultrasound in the diagnosis of acute acalculous cholecystitis. Gastrointest Radiol 1991;16:149–53.
28. Shuman WP, Rogers JV, Rudd TG, et al. Low sensitivity of sonography and cholescintigraphy in acalculous cholecystitis. AJR Am J Roentgenol 1984;142:531–4.
29. Kalliafas S, Siegler DW, Flancbaum L, Choban PS. Acute acalculous cholecystitis; incidence, risk factors, diagnosis, and outcome. Ann Surg 1998;64:471–5.
30. Yap L, Wycherly AG, Morphett AD, Toouli J, Acalculous biliary pain: cholecystectomy alleviates symptoms in patients with abnormal cholescintigraphy. Gastroenterology 1991;101:786–93.
31. Fink-Bennett D, DeRiddler P, Kolozsi WZ, et al. Cholecystokinin cholescintigraphy: detection of abnormal gallbladder motor function in patients with chronic acalculous gallbladder disease. J Nucl Med 1991;32:1695–9.
32. Jones-Monahan K, Gruenberg JC. Chronic acalculous cholecystitis: changes in patient demographics and evaluation since the advent of laparoscopy. J Soc Laparoendosc Surg 1999;90:1087–90.
33. Khosla R, Singh A, Jiedema BW, Marshall JB. Cholecystectomy alleviates acalculous biliary pain in patients with a reduced gallbladder ejection fraction. South Med J 1997;90:1087–90.
34. Barone JE, Bears S, Chen S, et al. Outcome study of cholecystectomy during pregnancy. Am J Surg 1999;177:232–6.

Chapter

13

Biliary Fistula, Gallstone Ileus, and Mirizzi's Syndrome

Hannes A. Rüdiger Pierre-Alain Clavien

In this chapter, we first discuss biliary fistulas with a focus on gallstone ileus, its major complication. Then, Mirizzi's syndrome will be covered in a separate section.

A biliary fistula is an abnormal passage or communication from the biliary system to another location. *Internal fistulas* are abnormal communications between the biliary tract and any other thoracal and abdominal organs or cavities. *External fistulas* are connections between the biliary tract and the skin. *Gallstone ileus* is a complication of a bilioenteric fistula in which bowel obstruction is caused by impaction of one or more gallstones within the enteric system.

Biliary fistulas and gallstone ileus were first mentioned by Bartholini in 1654 (1). Thilesus described the first external biliary fistula in 1670 (2). A thorough analysis of biliary fistula was first presented by Courvoisier in 1890, reporting a large series of about 500 cases, including 131 patients with gallstone ileus and 169 patients with spontaneous external biliary fistula (3).

Biliary fistulas are usually the result of acute suppurative cholecystitis associated with cholelithiasis (4). The suppurative process leads to necrosis and perforation. The site of spontaneous perforation and subsequent fistula is in the gastroenteric system, the thoracic cavity, or more rarely through the abdominal wall.

INTERNAL BILIARY FISTULAS

Ninety percent of the internal biliary fistulas are related to complicated gallstone disease (5). The common sites are between the gallbladder and duodenum, stomach, colon, and more rarely the jejunum. Other routes include between the common bile duct and duodenum or between hepatic duct and duodenum. Multiple biliary fistulas, such as cholecystoduodenocolic, are very rare. As the symptomatology varies, the diagnosis is difficult and often delayed until operation. Biliobiliary fistulas and Mirizzi's syndrome are discussed in a separate section below.

Biliary-enteric Fistulas

Biliary-enteric fistulas represent the most common forms of biliary fistulas. The localization of spontaneous biliary-enteric fistulas is detailed in Table 13.1. The most frequent type is the *cholecystoduodenal fistula* representing about three-quarters of all biliary-enteric fistulas (6). In a series of 300 laparoscopic cholecystectomies, Sharma et al. (7) found a cholecystoduodenal fistula in 1.7% of the cases. Cholecystitis with associated cholelithiasis is the main etiology, as in almost all fistulas involving the gallbladder. Most of them are asymptomatic or result in unspecific digestive complaints. Gallstones may occasionally pass the fistula tract and cause gallstone ileus. A preoperative diagnosis of an uncomplicated cholecystoduodenal fistula is exceptionally made (Fig. 13.1). Surgery is unnecessary in asymptomatic or high-risk patients (6). If a cholecystoduodenal fistula is discovered incidentally during abdominal surgery, a cholecystectomy and closure of the duodenal defect is sufficient in low-risk patients.

Cholecystocolic fistulas represent the second largest group, with 15.5% of cases of biliary-enteric fistulas. The spontaneous development of cholecystocolic fistulas is characterized by the sudden change of mild biliary symptoms to those of an acute disease due to the influx of bacteria into the biliary tract. Fever, chills, and abdominal pain are usually present. Because the ileum, as the main site of bile resorption, is bypassed, a choleric enteropathy may develop as sign of bile acid loss. The patients present with nausea, weight loss, and steatorrhea. Radiologic diagnosis can be difficult. The plain abdominal film reveals air in the gallbladder only in half of the cases. Barium enema may significantly increase the sen-

Table 13.1. Localization of biliary-enteric fistulas in a series of 109 cases

Type of Fistula	Percent
Cholecystoduodenal	76
Cholecystocolic	16
Cholecystogastric	2
Choledochoduodenal	1
Other types	5

Source: Morrissey K, McSherry C. Internal biliary fistula and gallstone ileus. In: Surgery of the liver and biliary tract. Philadelphia: Churchill-Livingstone, 1994:909–22.

sitivity of this examination by demonstrating the fistula (8). Immediate surgical treatment is indicated, including cholecystectomy and closure of the fistulous communication (9). A laparoscopic approach has been recently described (9). Segmental resection of the colon can be necessary (10).

Spontaneous *choledochoduodenal fistulas* are rare. They occur in more than 80% of cases (11) as a complication of duodenal peptic ulcer disease, and are usually not associated with cholelithiasis as are most other types of biliary fistulas. Hepatobiliary neoplasms are also known to occasionally cause choledochoduodenal fistula (12), and have been described almost exclusively in men. The interval between the onset of peptic ulcer symptoms and formation of the fistula is usually long, ranging in one series between 7 to 11 years (11). These fistulas are usually diagnosed incidentally, because they are rarely associated with biliary symptoms. In rare instances, cholangitis, jaundice, and abnormal liver function tests may occur as indicators of a concomitant biliary tract infection and obstruction (11). An upper gastrointestinal series, endoscopy, or endoscopic retrograde cholangiopancreatography can be sensitive tools to confirm the diagnosis. Treatment of the uncomplicated choledochoduodenal fistula is usually not indicated (11,13,14). Most authors agree that the therapy is dictated by the symptoms of the underlying peptic ulcer and not by presence of the fistula (11,15,16). Closure of the fistula may be achieved by conservative management of the ulcer disease. Surgical treatment of the fistula may be necessary in presence of severe ulcer disease with perforation, bleeding, or obstruction, or upon the onset of acute cholangitis. The latter has been observed in 11% of patients with cholecystoduodenal fistula and 60% with cholecystocolonic fistula (17–19). Another long-term complication of biliary-enteric fistula is gallbladder cancer (17–19). The risk of cancer can be avoided by removing the gallbladder in a one-stage procedure.

Parapapillary fistulas are a subgroup of choledochoduodenal fistulas, which have recently received increased attention due to the development of endoscopic retrograde cholangiopancreatography. They usually represent a complication of choledocholithiasis (20), but may also develop in presence of carcinoma of the papilla (13,21) or as an iatrogenic complication following papillotomy. The latter can be avoided by performing the papillotomy through the papillary opening (13,22). The treatment consists usually of endoscopic papillotomy with removal of the calculus (22).

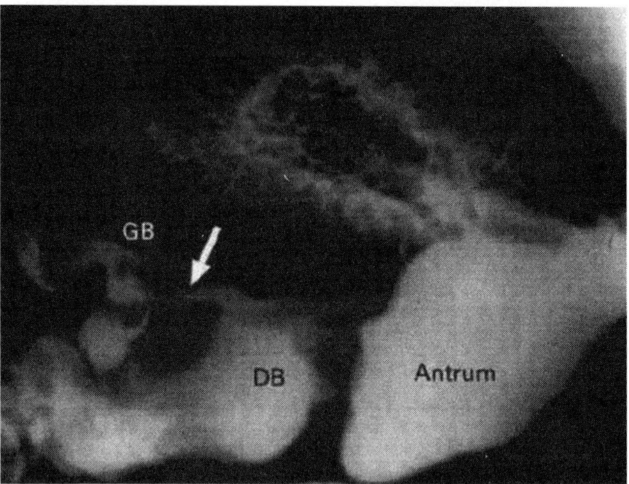

(A)

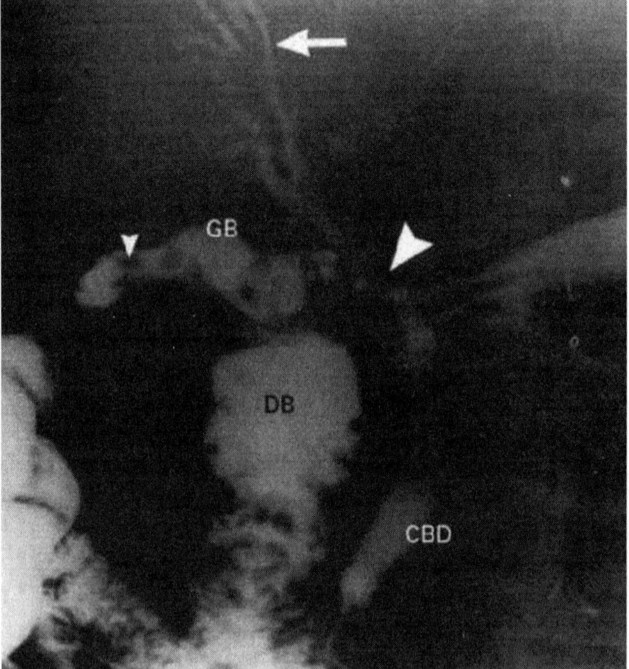

(B)

FIGURE 13.1. *Cholecystoduodenal fistula. **(A)** An upper gastrointestinal series reveals a fistula (arrow) between the duodenal bulb (DB) and the gallbladder (GB). **(B)** The biliary tree is visible as a result of the retrograde flow of contrast material from the duodenal bulb into the gallbladder and cystic duct (larger arrowhead) and then into the intrahepatic ducts (arrow) and common bile duct (CBD). The semilunar lucencies within the gallbladder are gallstones (small arrowhead). (Reprinted by permission of the New England Journal of Medicine, from Singh N, Stempel K. Images in clinical medicine. Cholecystoduodenal fistula. N Engl J Med 1997; 336:266.)*

Thoracobiliary and Bronchobiliary Fistulas

Thoracobiliary and bronchobiliary fistulas are rare disorders, defined as the opening of a passage between the bronchial tree and the biliary tract. They are usually associated with significant morbidity. The causes are manifold, and include thoracoabdominal trauma, malignancies, liver abscess, parasitic liver disease (i.e., mainly echinococcosis or amebic disease), choledocholithiasis, postoperative biliary stenosis, or rare congenital disorders. In Western countries, the most common cause of bronchobiliary fistulas is bile duct obstruction, usually secondary to postoperative bile duct stenosis (23). Echinococcal cysts and amebic liver abscesses are probably the most common causes in developing countries. Pathogenesis of bronchobiliary fistulas caused by bile duct obstruction involves local inflammatory processes (cholangitis), followed by abscess and rupture toward the pleural space, and progression of the inflammation with erosion of the bronchial tree. Thoracobiliary fistulas have also been described as a rare complication of percutaneous biliary drainage.

The hallmark of a bronchobiliary fistula is the presence of bile pigments in the sputum (biliptysis). Biliptysis is suggested by bitter taste and a cough that produces yellow sputum (24). Bronchiolitis is usually present. Other symptoms include right upper abdominal and pleuritic chest pain. Fever, chills, or leukocytosis is noted in only half the cases. A right pleural effusion is almost always present, whereas massive biliothorax and gallstone migration are rarities (25). Jaundice is usually not present.

Surgery remains the mainstay of treatment in congenital bronchobiliary fistulas (26). Excision of the fistula through a right thoracotomy is usually performed (27). Interventional radiology and endoscopic techniques, including stenting to reduce distal biliary obstruction, may provide a safe treatment of acquired fistulas (24,26,28). Currently, operative approaches should only be considered if percutaneous or endoscopic interventions have failed (26).

A communication between the biliary tree and a blood vessel is usually associated with hemobilia, that is, the blood flow into the biliary tree (29). In contrast, bilhemia with bile flow through a *biliary-vascular fistula* into the venous system is exceptionally diagnosed, and remains a widely unknown entity. It was first described in 1952 by Brown, who reported a case of fatal bile embolism after liver biopsy (30). Bilhemia is usually preceded by a blunt abdominal trauma with central rupture of the liver veins and bile ducts or by a needle biopsy. Bilhemia is also a well-described complication of transhepatic portocaval shunts (TIPS) (31–33). However, the prevalence of biliary-vascular fistulas after placement of TIPS is unknown. The few reported cases were often associated with 1) fever, 2) bacteremia due to subsequent contamination of the venous circulation with enteric flora, and 3) recurrent thrombosis of the stent due to the procoagulant properties of bile (mucine and anionic bile salts) (31–34). Accumulating evidence supports the theory that communication with the biliary system is an important etiologic factor of early stenosis or occlusion of the transhepatic stent (35). Bilhemia has also been proposed as a major stimulus of pseudointimal hyperplasia and metaplastic biliary epithelial cell proliferation within the TIPS (34–36).

Biliary obstruction increases the risk of massive bile flow in the venous system. The low pressure in the caval vein may lead to flow of bile into the blood circulation. An alternative pathogenesis is the creation of a flap of tissue acting as a one-way valve between a bile duct and a vein (29). Bile dissolves into the bloodstream and rapidly leads to an extreme increase of direct bilirubin (37). However, liver enzymes are only moderately elevated. The constellation of excessive direct hyperbilirubinemia and low liver enzyme levels should raise the suspicion of bilhemia (37). Bilhemia can be diagnosed by endoscopic retrograde cholangiopancreatography. High-pressure injection of contrast material into the TIPS using a diagnostic catheter or by manual injection through a balloon occlusion catheter represents sensitive alternative (31).

Treatment of the biliary tract stenosis, when present, is usually sufficient for closure of the fistula (29). In cases of distal bile duct obstruction, a nasobiliary drainage may lead to spontaneous closure of the fistula. In cases of blunt abdominal trauma or if the endoscopic approaches have failed, surgery is usually advised (37). Several surgical options have been proposed: 1) hepatic resection, 2) liver transplantation, 3) T-tube suction drainage of the common bile duct, and 4) drainage and tamponade of the rupture or necrotic cavity to create a percutaneous bile fistula, which may eventually resolve (29,37). Bilhemia as a complication of TIPS placement has been successfully treated by sealing the TIPS with stents covered with polytetrafluoroethylene (PTFE) (31). Sphincterotomy and biliary stenting to decrease pressure in the biliary tree, and broad-spectrum antibiotics, may improve the outcome in a number of cases (33).

EXTERNAL BILIARY FISTULAS

Spontaneous external biliary fistulas were reported in several series prior to 1900. This type of fistulas was first described by Thilesus in 1670 (2). In Courvoisier's report on 500 cases of gallbladder perforation in 1890, one-third of the cases were external fistulas (3). However, spontaneous external biliary fistulas are now extremely rare due to better diagnosis, and the wide availability of surgical therapy for stone-related biliary disease (38,39). Less than 100 cases were reported in the 20th century.

Spontaneous external biliary fistulas are usually a complication of acute cholecystitis with underlying cholelithiasis (40). They are diagnosed more often in women than men, especially between the fifth and seventh decades (39). Virtually all spontaneous external biliary fistulae are single, with the fistulous opening usually in the right upper quadrant or, via the falciform ligament, in the umbilicus (40). Diagnosis of biliary fistula and identification of the fistulous tract is best done by a sinogram with injection of contrast into the external opening or, if this fails, by performing an endoscopic retrograde cholangiopancreatography (41). Definitive treatment requires removal of the gallbladder and excision of the fistulous tract. Alternatively, the fistula may be curetted and left to heal spontaneously (25,39,40).

An *iatrogenic external biliary fistula* is a serious and difficult complication of biliary surgery that often results in unexpected prolongation of hospitalization. Iatrogenic injury at operation more often results in an external rather than an internal fistula. It complicates about 4% of cases of hydatoid cysts (42). Obstruction of bile flow in the distal common bile duct by stones or strictures may add to bile leakage due to the high pressure in the biliary system (43). Both fistulography (sinogram) and cholangiography performed endoscopically or by the percutaneous approach can delineate the fistula tract (41). Delayed surgical repair with a biliodigestive anastomosis after resolution of the inflammation is often preferable. However, this type of surgery is associated with a high morbidity (43). When the fistula is well contained and the patient does not present with any signs of sepsis or bile peritonitis, a nonsurgical treatment can be advised. A conservative treatment with endoscopic sphincterotomy, stenting, or placing of a nasobiliary catheter to reduce intraductal pressure can facilitate spontaneous healing (44).

GALLSTONE ILEUS

Gallstone ileus is a mechanical bowel obstruction that is caused by impaction of one or more gallstones within the lumen of the enteric system. It represents a complication of biliary-enteric fistulas. In 1890, Courvoisier reported a 44% mortality after surgery in a series of 131 patients. Over the past century the mortality rate has declined to 5% to 24% (45–49).

Incidence

As an infrequent complication of cholelithiasis, gallstone ileus is often misdiagnosed. About 0.4% to 1.5% of patients with cholelithiasis develop gallstone ileus (50). Virtually all cases of gallstone ileus are associated with a cholecystenteric fistula and significant surrounding inflammation (8,50). It accounts for 1% to 3% of all cases of nonstrangulated small bowel obstruction (51). Gallstone ileus is a geriatric emergency; most studies report an average age between 65 and 78 years (45,46,52). In patients over the age of 65, gallstone ileus accounts for 25% of nonstrangulated bowel obstruction. Increasing longevity in Western countries has increased the incidence of gallstone ileus, which is estimated to approach 1 case per 117,000 people per year (46). However, the youngest patient in the literature was 13 years of age (47). Concomitant geriatric diseases are present in as many as 80% to 90% of cases. Reisner reported in a review of 1001 cases a ratio of female to male of 3.5 : 1 (46).

A minimal stone size of 2.0 to 2.5 cm in diameter is required to cause intestinal obstruction (47,53). Multiple stones are found in up to 40% of cases and are often the cause for early recurrence. Once a stone enters the gastrointestinal tract, it may be vomited, passed spontaneously, or become impacted (45). It is likely that more than 80% of stones entering the gut through a biliary-enteric fistula will be uneventfully excreted (54). However, once a stone is obstructed, spontaneous passage is exceptional (45). The most common sites of stone impactions are detailed in Table 13.2. The ileocecal valve as the narrowest part of the bowel is the most frequent site of stone impaction. Duodenal obstruction by gallstones is also known as gastric outlet obstruction or Bouveret's syndrome (55). In these cases, early vomiting is a common sign. Colonic stone impaction is rare but can occur with cholecystocolonic fistulas (45). Colonic gallstone ileus is usually found in association with an underlying pathological narrowing of the colon, such as postdiverticulitis stenosis or carcinoma. It may exceptionally be found without colonic abnormality in cases of cholecystocolonic fistula and very large stones (10).

Table 13.2. Site of stone impaction in cases of gallstone ileus

Site	%
Stomach	14%
Duodenum	4%
Jejunum	17%
Ileum	61%
Colon	4%

Clinical Signs

The clinical presentation of gallstone ileus is rarely specific, and as many as half of the patients have no history of biliary symptoms (45,56,57). The symptoms do not differ from bowel obstruction of any other etiologies. The patient is usually acutely ill and dehydrated and typically complains about vomiting, abdominal pain, and distention with bowel sound of obstructive quality (58). The mean duration of these symptoms before admission was reported to be 3.9 days (57). Signs of local peritonitis in the right upper quadrant may indicate acute cholecystitis.

Diagnosis

The diagnosis is made before the operation in less than half of the patients (46). Delay in surgical treatment may lead to serious complications, such as electrolyte imbalance, ischemic lesions, ulcerations of the small bowel, abscess formation, and occasionally free perforation and peritonitis (59,60).

Plain Abdominal Films

Plain abdominal films are widely used as a screening in patients with acute abdomen. Rigler (61) described four radiologic signs of gallstone ileus on plain abdominal film:

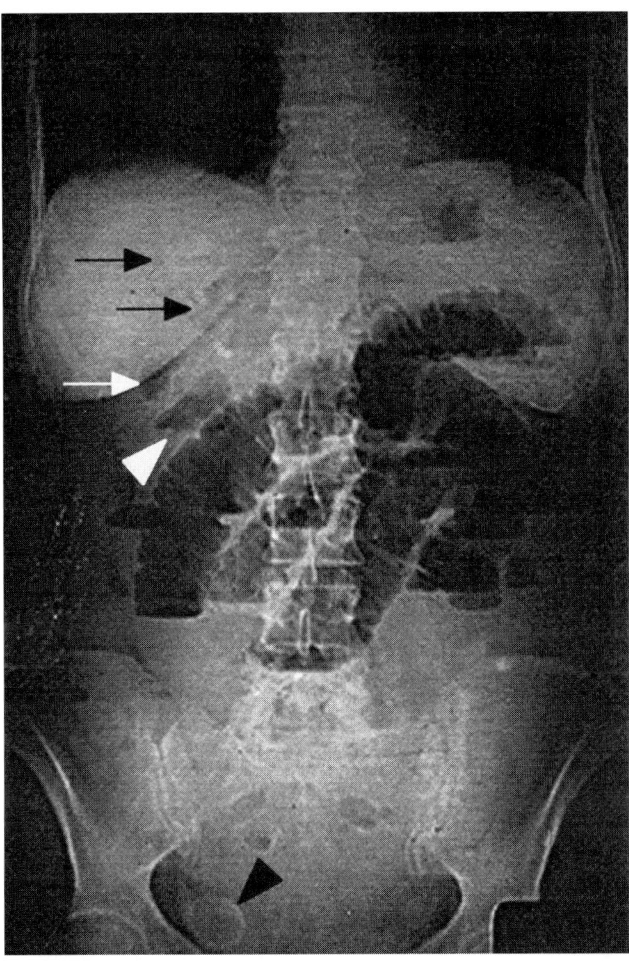

FIGURE 13.2. *Typical presentation of gallstone ileus on plain abdominal radiograph with mechanical ileus, pneumobilia (black arrows), and aberrantly located gallstone (black arrowhead). Balthazar's sign consists of air in the gallbladder (white arrow) and in the duodenal bulb (white arrowhead).*

1) air in the biliary tree (pneumobilia), 2) bowel obstruction, 3) visualized stone, and 4) migration of a previously observed stone (Fig. 13.2). The presence of two of the first three signs has been considered pathognomonic of gallstone ileus (45). However, these characteristic signs are rarely completely present (59,60). Plain x-ray examination is diagnostic in only 35% of the cases (41,62).

Pneumobilia is the most important radiographic sign of Rigler's tetrade. However, it is observed in only 30% to 50% of cases with fistulas (63). Concomitant occlusion of the cystic duct prevents the development of pneumobilia. The latter is not pathognomonic of biliary-enteric fistula because it is also seen in presence of insufficient sphincter of Oddi following sphincteroplasty or endoscopic sphincterotomy. Emphysematous cholecystitis may also cause pneumobilia.

Balthazar (8) reported a small series of patients with gallstone ileus, in which air in the gallbladder is visible on plain films in most cases. In contrast, air in the duodenal bulb or biliary radicles is more rarely detected. The combination of air in the gallbladder and air in the duodenum (double air bubble in the right upper quadrant) was observed in 7 out of 11 patients and is also known as Balthazar's sign (see Fig. 13.2) (59,60).

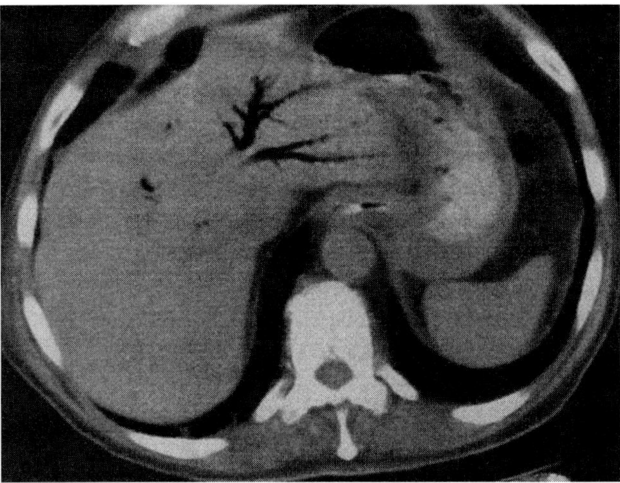

FIGURE 13.3. *Pneumobilia is demonstrated on abdominal computed tomography. (Lobo DN, Jobling JC, Balfour TW. Gallstone ileus: diagnostic pitfalls and therapeutic successes. J Clin Gastroenterol 2000;30:72–6.)*

A significant higher diagnostic accuracy (80% to 90%) may be achieved using contrast examinations (59,60). The demonstration of a diverticulum-like structure or a fistulous tract adjacent to the first duodenal segment associated with an intestinal obstruction on the delayed films suggests the correct diagnosis (59,60).

Ultrasonography

Ultrasonography may be more sensitive than plain films in patients with gallstone ileus due to the small volume of intestinal air associated with ileal of higher obstruction. The most characteristic ultrasonographic findings include 1) location of a gallstone in a fluid filled intestine, 2) a severely diseased gallbladder, and 3) pneumobilia (64). In some cases, ultrasonography may provide definitive diagnosis of gallstone ileus, and obviate the need for any further tests.

CT Scan

Computed tomography (CT) is increasingly used as a screening modality in patients with an acute abdomen. CT is often used in the elderly population, in whom signs and symptoms of abdominal pathologies are particularly vague and unspecific (63). Rigler's criteria for gallstone ileus are also frequent findings in the CT scan (Figs. 13.3 and 13.4).

Treatment

Long-standing controversies surround the treatment of patients with gallstone ileus, and several therapeutic approaches have been proposed. Most authors agree that the immediate relief of the intestinal obstruction remains the cornerstone of management.

Two main surgical strategies were proposed: first, enterotomy with removal of the impacted stone and fistula repair including cholecystectomy in a *one-stage* operation; second, a *two-stage* operation with surgical removal of the obstructing stone from the gut without biliary surgery. Biliary surgery and closure of the fistula are then eventually performed in a second operation (47).

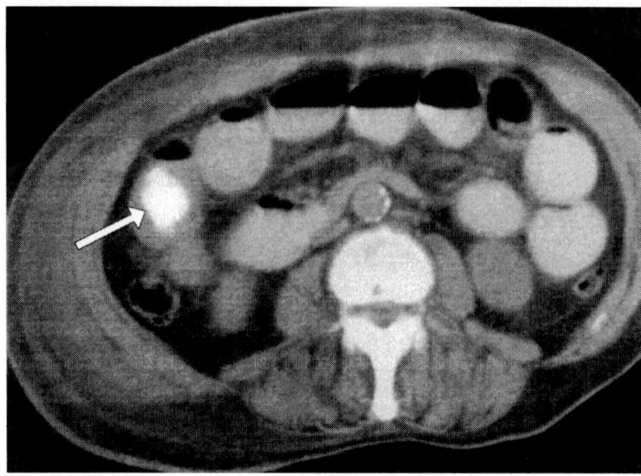

FIGURE 13.4. *Gallstone ileus. Abdominal computed tomography after oral contrast shows a calcified stone (arrow) obstructing the small bowel. (Lobo DN, Jobling JC, Balfour TW. Gallstone ileus: diagnostic pitfalls and therapeutic successes. J Clin Gastroenterol 2000;30:72–6.)*

Most investigators favor enterolithotomy alone in the initial surgical treatment of gallstone ileus due to the lower operative mortality (48,50). Some have pointed out that a number of fistulae spontaneously close once the stone has passed, particularly when the cystic duct is patent, and when there are no residual stones left in the gallbladder. In addition, cholecystectomy is often technically difficult because of the underlying chronic cholecystitis with concomitant adhesions. However, complications arising from the untreated fistula in the two-stage procedure may contribute to a higher morbidity. For example, untreated fistulas may lead to recurrent gallstone ileus (50). A large review of 1001 cases has reported a similar mortality of the one-stage operation compared with the two-stage approach, or enterolithotomy alone (Table 13.3) (46). Therefore, the one-stage operation has recently become more popular (45,65), and is recommended whenever local and general conditions permit.

It is important to search for additional stones in the bowel, which often lead to recurrence of gallstone ileus. Manual propulsion of the smallest stones to the enterotomy of the larger stones may be used successfully, but caution is

Table 13.3. Largest series of gallstone ileus reported since 1980 in the English literature

Authors	Year	Location	Period	No. of Patients	One Stage			Two Stage/ Enterolithotomy Alone			Overall Operative Mortality
					No.	%[c]	Mortality	No.	%[c]	Mortality	
Lobo et al. (49)	2000	United Kingdom	1992–97	15	1	6	0	14	93	7	7
Rodriguez-Sanjuan et al. (48)	1997	Spain	1975–94	25	9	36	33[d]	16	64	19	24
Zuegel et al. (65)	1997	Germany	1986–94	16	14	88	7	2	13	0	6
Reisner et al. (46)[a]	1994	USA	1953–93	1001	113	12	17[d]	801	88	12	18
Schutte et al. (72)	1992	Chile	1975–87	74	1	1	N/A	73	99	N/A[e]	14
Clavien et al. (45)	1990	Switzerland	1976–87	37	8	22	25[d]	29	78	17	19
Moss et al. (95)	1987	USA	1965–84	20	1	5	0	18	95	11	11
Illuminati et al. (96)	1987	Italy	1975–85	23	0	0	—	23	100	17	17
Deitz et al. (97)	1986	USA	1953–84	24	4	17	N/A	19	21	N/A	13
Kurtz et al. (98)	1985	USA	1938–82	45	3	8	N/A	36	92	N/A	23
Hesselfeldt et al. (52)	1982	Denmark	1960–76	39	2	6	0	34	94	15	14
Glenn et al. (19)	1981	USA	1932–78	22	2	9	0	20	91	5	5
Svartholm et al. (57)	1982	USA	1960–79	83	3	4	0.0	73	96	23	22
Heuman et al. (54)	1980	Sweden	1968–79	20	—	—	—	20	100	5	5
Kasahara et al. (47)[b]	1980	Japan	1903–78	112	16	16	19	85	84	7	9

[a] Meta-analysis from all reported cases in the world literature from 1953 to 1993.
[b] Meta-analysis from all reported cases in the Japanese literature from 1903 to 1978.
[c] Percent of operatively treated patients.
[d] Not significantly different from the mortality rate in the two-stage group.
[e] 16 patients underwent secondary repair of the fistula, no death occurred among these patients.

recommended because of the risk of injury of the intestinal mucosa (45). Attempts to crush impacted stones manually without enterolithotomy should be avoided for the same reason. Multiple enterotomies are safer than aggressive attempts at extracting all stones through one incision.

Laparoscopic treatment of gallstone ileus has been described but is often difficult as extensive adhesions occur in the area of the gallbladder (66). A two-stage operation is therefore usually advised. Laparoscopy may be useful to establish the diagnosis and offers a minimally invasive treatment of the ileus. This approach may possibly reduce mortality and morbidity in elderly and high-risk patients (66). Laparoscopy also reduces the risk of wound infection, which still represents the most common postoperative complication following treatment of gallstone ileus (46,67). In any case, the laparoscopic approach should only be performed by experienced surgeons.

Alternative nonsurgical modalities have been proposed, including endoscopic removal of the gallstone, endoscopic sphincterotomy in cases of concurrent choledocholithiasis, and extracorporeal shockwave lithotripsy (68–71). These methods may avoid emergency laparotomy, but they should be considered only in high-risk patients. In addition, they do not definitively manage the biliary disease (67).

Morbidity and Mortality

The morbidity and mortality are mostly determined by the presence of comorbid diseases of the patient and the duration of the ileus (50). In large series, it varies between 4.5% and 24% (see Table 13.3). These figures are 5 to 10 times higher than in patients with intestinal obstructions from other causes. The most important factors influencing the risk of mortality include advanced age, comorbidities, delayed consultation, misdiagnosis, delayed surgery, and postoperative complications (72). The most common postoperative complications include wound infection (27%), pulmonary infection (26%), and peritonitis (15%) (72). Postoperative antibiotic treatment has failed to lower the rate of wound infection and is therefore not routinely indicated. Severe postoperative bleeding has also been described, generally arising from the erosion of a blood vessel during the passage of the gallstones (73–75).

MIRIZZI'S SYNDROME

In 1905, Kehr first reported on external compression of the bile duct following stone impaction in the cystic duct (76). However, the syndrome was named after Pablo Mirizzi, who described in 1948 a hepatic duct obstruction due to cholelithiasis and cholecystitis (77). Mirizzi's syndrome is caused by an impacted gallstone in the cystic duct or the neck of the gallbladder that compresses the adjacent bile duct and results in complete or partial obstruction of the common hepatic bile duct.

Cholecystobiliary fistulas are a rare entity, representing a later stage of Mirizzi's syndrome. In 1942, Pestow first described a case of spontaneous internal biliary fistula (78). Initially, a stone is impacted in the neck of the gallbladder, compressing the common hepatic duct and causing jaundice and repeated attacks of cholecystitis. Eventually, the stone erodes its way into the common hepatic duct creating a cholecystocholedochal fistula.

Classification

McSherry et al. (79) initially classified this syndrome into two types. Type I involves the external compression of the common hepatic duct due to a stone impacted in the neck of the gallbladder or the cystic duct. Type II refers to cholecystocholedochal fistula and stone migration into the common hepatic duct. A further modification of this classification was suggested by Csendes et al. (80), in which type II is an obstruction that involves less than one-third of the bile duct, type III is an obstruction involving up to two-thirds of the duct, and type IV is complete obstruction of the bile duct. The classification used in this chapter differentiates three types and is detailed in Fig. 13.5.

Incidence

In the largest series, including 17,000 patients undergoing surgery for gallstone disease, 219 patients (1.3%) had

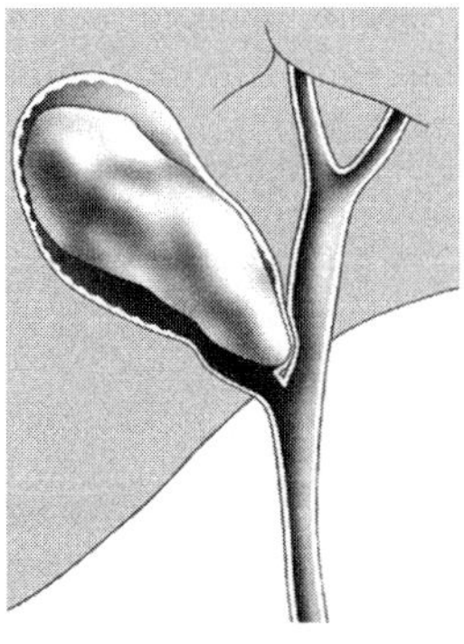

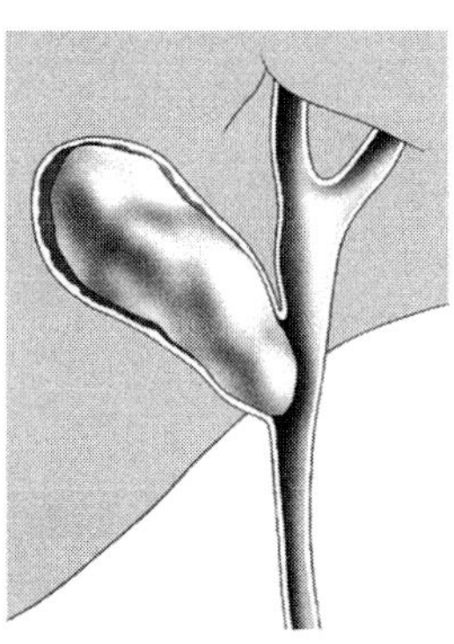

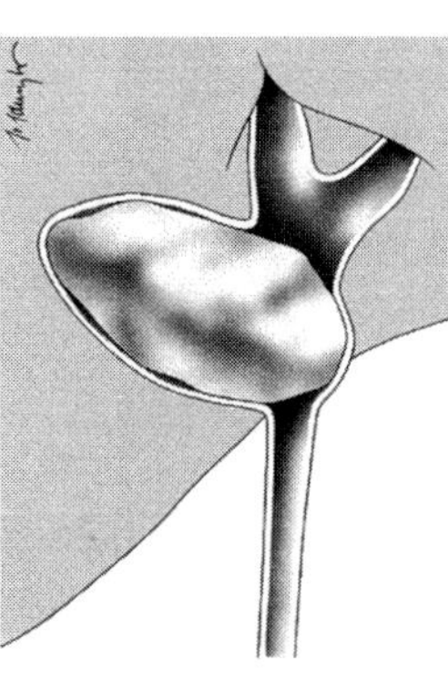

FIGURE 13.5. *Mirizzi's syndrome. Three types are differentiated. Type A is characterized by external compression of the hepatic duct without fistula. In type B, a cholecystobiliary fistula is present with partial obstruction of the bile duct. Complete obstruction is present in type C.*

Mirizzi's syndrome and/or cholecystobiliary fistula (80). This figure may rise up to 2.7% in high-risk populations such as native American Indians (81). Approximately 50% to 77% of all patients reported are women, probably reflecting the increased frequency of the gallstone disease in this group. A correlation was also noted between the stage of the disease and the mean age of patients (80). In patients with type A disease the mean age was 44 years; the mean age was 62 years in patients with type C lesions.

Pathophysiology

Mirizzi's syndrome may be caused by either a single large stone or multiple small stones impacted in the Hartmann's pouch of the gallbladder or in the cystic duct. Anatomically, a long cystic duct parallel to the bile duct predisposes to the development of this syndrome (82–84). Recurrent cystic duct obstruction may lead to repeated attacks of cholecystitis and may cause gallbladder dilatation, thickening, and inflammation. If the inflamed gallbladder is in close proximity to the bile duct, inflammation and adhesions may further contribute to the obstruction of the bile duct. Over time, the stone causes pressure necrosis and erodes into the common hepatic duct producing a cholecystobiliary fistula. This hypothesis is supported by the observation that in most cases the cholecystocholedochal fistula is occupied by a large impacted gallstone in the fistula tract (85).

Clinical Signs

Mirizzi's syndrome is typically seen in the setting of long-standing biliary symptoms. Obstructive jaundice is the key feature of Mirizzi's syndrome and is frequently accompanied with pain and fever. This presentation often suggests acute cholangitis. Rarely, patients may be anicteric at presentation. Patients can also present with cholecystitis or pancreatitis. Laboratory data are not specific, with hyperbilirubinemia as the most encountered laboratory abnormality. Elevated alkaline phosphatase and transaminases levels are also common. Leukocytosis is a frequent presence in concomitant acute cholecystitis, pancreatitis, or cholangitis.

Diagnosis

An early diagnosis is important to prevent major complications. However, in clinical practice, the diagnosis is rarely made preoperatively.

Endoscopic retrograde cholangiopancreatography (ERCP) is the procedure of choice to establish the diagnosis and to classify the lesion. Mirizzi type A presents as an extrinsic compression of the common hepatic duct by a distended gallbladder with dilatation of the intrahepatic biliary tree. ERCP is also essential in determining the presence of a fistula preoperatively. Percutaneous transhepatic cholangiography (PTC) can provide similar information. However, ERCP can identify a low-lying cystic duct that may be missed by PTC. In addition, PTC may not visualize the distal common bile duct because of the obstruction in the hepatic duct. Finally, as discussed below, ERCP offers the opportunity to exercise a variety of therapeutic options including stone retrieval and stenting (86,87).

On ultrasonography, a solitary stone or multiple impacted stones in the cystic duct and gallbladder may be seen. A dilated intrahepatic biliary tree and common bile duct suggest the diagnosis of Mirizzi's syndrome (88).

The literature regarding the use of CT scans for the diagnosis of Mirizzi's syndrome is controversial. Some authors feel that CT does not provide any additional information beyond what can be obtained with ultrasonography (89,90); also, the presence of periductal inflammation can be misinterpreted as carcinoma of the gallbladder. Overall, CT may be helpful in excluding malignancies in the pancreas, the porta hepatis area, or the liver.

The differential diagnosis includes other causes of obstructive jaundice such as malignancies (e.g., cholangiocarcinoma, carcinoma of the gallbladder, or pancreatic cancer) and sclerosing cholangitis (81).

Treatment

Surgery remains the treatment of choice for Mirizzi's syndrome (80,83). The choice of surgery is determined by whether a fistula into the bile duct is present. The common surgical approach is usually an incision in the gallbladder fundus and removal of the impacted stone. A gush of bile indicates a fistula, because the cystic duct is usually occluded. In cases with intact common bile duct (type A) and no inflammatory processes, cholecystectomy is advised. If the viability of the common duct is questionable or an advanced stage is present (types B and C), a T-tube (91) or a choledochoduodenostomy or a hepaticojejunostomy (Roux-en-Y) is to be preferred. In any case, excellent drainage should be achieved. An intraoperative frozen section of the gallbladder wall should be sampled—in particular in the presence of markedly elevated CA19-9 levels—to exclude carcinoma (92).

A serious complication of the surgical approach is the ligation of the hepatic duct because a normal caliber hepatic duct may be mistaken for a dilated cystic duct that runs parallel to it. The laparoscopic approach appears to carry a considerable risk for this serious complication (86) and should be used exclusively for type A disease. For types B and C, an open approach is advised.

Recently, investigators have become increasingly interested in endoscopic treatment not only for the evaluation, but also for the treatment of Mirizzi's syndrome. Whether it is used as primary therapy or as an adjunct to surgical treatment, ERCP is an attractive alternative and may be the only option for high-risk patients (93). In general, endoscopic management includes both biliary drainage and stone removal. Endoscopic sphincterotomy is generally recommended for stone extraction. Standard stone removal techniques are usually used and include baskets, balloons, and mechanical and electrohydraulic lithotripsy. The latter may be a valuable modality as standard techniques have failed. However, multiple treatment sessions may be required and leakage of contrast material from the cystic duct into the peritoneal cavity has been described after the fragmentation of large stones (94). Further advances in the design of retrograde cholangioscopes may make this option more attractive in the future.

Mortality and Morbidity

In the largest series, Csendes (80) reported no operative mortality (within 30 days of operation) in patients with type A disease, 2% to 12% with type B, and 11% with type C disease. Late mortality due to biliary disease was below 5% with any stages of the disease (80).

Postoperative morbidity includes mainly the development of external biliary fistula, bile peritonitis, and subphrenic abscess. The incidence of benign strictures of the bile duct occurs in 4% to 11% of patients (80).

SUGGESTED READINGS

Clavien PA, Richon J, Burgan S, Rohner A. Gallstone ileus. Br J Surg 1990;77:737–42. This article is a review of the literature and a report of a single institution experience from a region with a high incidence of gallstone ileus. Clinical presentations, risk factors, and radiological and operative findings are thoroughly analyzed. Indications for the one and two-stage operations are discussed.

Csendes A, Carlos Diaz J, Burdiles P, Maluenda F, Nava O. Mirizzi syndrome and choecystobiliary fistula: a unifying classification. Br J Surg 1989;76:1139–43. This is the largest series of patients with Mirizzi syndrome. This article represents a detailed description of the syndrome including careful analysis of various surgical treatments according to the staging of the disease.

Reisner RM, Cohen JR. Gallstone ileus: a review of 1001 reported cases. Am Surg 1994;60:441–6. This is the largest meta-analysis on gallstone ileus. Preoperative findings and outcome of surgical and non-operative treatments are carefully and critically evaluated.

REFERENCES

1. Martin F. Intestinal obstruction due to gallstones. Ann Surg 1912;55:725.
2. Peacock T. Case in which a hydatid cyst of the liver communicates with the lungs. Edinburgh Med J 1850;74:33–46.
3. Courvoisier L. Beiträge zur Pathologie und Chirurgie der Gallenwege. Leipzig, FCW Vogel, 58, 1890.
4. Yang HK, Fondacaro PF. Enterolith ileus: a rare complication of duodenal diverticula. Am J Gastrol 1992;87:1846–8.
5. Rosato F. Gallstone ileus and fistula. In Sabiston D, ed. Textbook of surgery. Philadelphia: WB Saunders, 1991:1017.
6. Morrissey K, McSherry C. Internal biliary fistula and gallstone ileus. In: Surgery of the liver and biliary tract. Philadelphia: Churchill-Livingstone, 1994:909–22.
7. Sharma A, Sullivan M, English H, Foley R. Laparoscopic repair of cholecystoduodenal fistulae. Surg Laparosc Endosc Percutan Tech 1994;4:433–5.
8. Balthazar EJ, Schechter LS. Air in gallbladder: a frequent finding in gallstone ileus. AJR Am J Roentgenol 1978;131:219–22.
9. Gentileschi P, Forlini A, Rossi P, et al. Laparoscopic approach to cholecystocolic fistula: report of a case. J Laparoendosc Surg 1995;5:413–7.
10. Phillips DE, Doran J. Obstruction of the colon by a giant gallstone. Br J Hosp Med 1986;36:444.
11. Wagner GR, Passaro E Jr. Choledochoduodenal fistula secondary to duodenal ulcer. Arch Surg 1971;103:21–4.
12. Walker G, Large A. Choledochoduodenal fistula: its surgical management. Ann Surg 1954;139:510.
13. Tanaka M, Ikeda S. Parapapillary choledochoduodenal fistula: an analysis of 83 consecutive patients diagnosed at ERCP. Gastrointest Endosc 1983;29:89–93.
14. Naga M, Mogawer MS. Choledochoduodenal fistula: a rare sequel of duodenal ulcer. Endoscopy 1991;23:307–8.
15. Topal U, Savci G, Sadikoglu MY, Tuncel E. Choledochoduodenal fistula secondary to duodenal peptic ulcer. A case report. Acta Radiologica 1997;38:1007–9.
16. Iso Y, Yoh R, Okita K, et al. Choledochoduodenal fistula: a complication of a penetrated duodenal ulcer. Hepatogastroenterology 1996;43:489–91.
17. Safaie-Shirazi S, Zike WL, Printen KJ. Spontaneous enterobiliary fistulas. Surg Gynecol Obstet 1973;137:769–72.
18. Cooperman AM, Dickson ER, ReMine WH. Changing concepts in the surgical treatment of gallstone ileus: a review of 15 cases with emphasis on diagnosis and treatment. Ann Surg 1968;167:377–83.
19. Glenn F, Reed C, Grafe WR. Biliary enteric fistula. Surg Gynecol Obstet 1981;153:527–31.
20. Hunt DR, Blumgart LH. Iatrogenic choledochoduodenal fistula: an unsuspected cause of post-cholecystectomy symptoms. Br J Surg 1980;67:10–3.
21. Imaeda K, Katagiri K, Ando T, et al. Multiple parapapillary choledochoduodenal fistulas with ampullary carcinoma. Hepatogastroenterology 1998;45:2097–100.
22. Jorge A, Diaz M, Lorenzo J, Jorge O. Choledochoduodenal fistulas. Endoscopy 1991;23:76–8.
23. Rose DM, Rose AT, Chapman WC, et al. Management of bronchobiliary fistula as a late complication of hepatic resection. Am Surg 1998;64:873–6.
24. Brem H, Gibbons GD, Cobb G, et al. The use of endoscopy to treat bronchobiliary fistula caused by choledocholithiasis. Gastroenterology 1990;98:490–2.
25. Delco F, Domenighetti G, Kauzlaric D, et al. Spontaneous biliothorax (thoracobilia) following cholecystopleural fistula presenting as an acute respiratory insufficiency. Successful removal of gallstones from the pleural space. Chest 1994;106:961–3.
26. Poullis M, Poullis A. Biliptysis caused by a bronchobiliary fistula. J Thorac Cardiovasc Surg 1999;118:971–2.
27. Yamaguchi M, Kanamori K, Fujimura M, et al. Congenital bronchobiliary fistula in adults. South Med J 1990;83:851–2.
28. Moreira VF, Arocena C, Cruz F, et al. Bronchobiliary fistula secondary to biliary lithiasis. Treatment by endoscopic sphincterotomy. Dig Dis Sci 1994;39:1994–9.
29. Verhille MS, Munoz SJ. Acute biliary-vascular fistula following needle aspiration of the liver. Gastroenterology 1991;101:1731–3.
30. Brown C, Walsh G. Fatal bile embolism following liver biopsy. Ann Intern Med 1952;36:1529–33.
31. Sze DY, Vestring T, Liddell RP, et al. Recurrent TIPS failure associated with biliary fistulae: treatment with PTFE-covered stents. Cardiovasc Intervent Radiol 1999;22:298–304.
32. Boyvat F, Cekirge S, Balkanci F, Besim A. Treatment of a TIPS-biliary fistula by stent-graft in a 9-year-old boy. Cardiovasc Intervent Radiol 1999;22:67–8.
33. Mallery S, Freeman ML, Peine CJ, et al. Biliary-shunt fistula following transjugular intrahepatic portosystemic shunt placement. Gastroenterology 1996;111:1353–7.
34. Saxon RR, Mendel-Hartvig J, Corless CL, et al. Bile duct injury as a major cause of stenosis and occlusion in transjugular intrahepatic portosystemic shunts: comparative histopathologic analysis in humans and swine. J Vasc Intervent Radiol 1996;7:487–97.
35. Ducoin H, El-Khoury J, Rousseau H, et al. Histopathologic analysis of transjugular intrahepatic portosystemic shunts. Hepatology 1997;25:1064–9.
36. LaBerge JM, Ferrell LD, Ring EJ, Gordon RL. Histopathologic study of stenotic and occluded transjugular intrahepatic portosystemic shunts. J Vasc Intervent Radiol 1993;4:779–86.
37. Glaser K, Wetscher G, Pointner R, et al. Traumatic bilhemia. Surgery 1994;116:24–7.
38. Smith AC, Schapiro RH, Kelsey PB, Warshaw AL. Successful treatment of nonhealing biliary-cutaneous fistulas with biliary stents. Gastroenterology 1986;90:764–9.
39. Ruderman RL, Laird W, Reingold MM, Rosen IB. External biliary fistula. CMAJ 1975;113:875–8.
40. Reed MW, Tweedie JH. Spontaneous simultaneous internal and external biliary fistulae. Br J Surg 1985;72:538.
41. Oikarinen H, Paivansalo M, Tikkakoski T, Saarela A. Radiological findings in biliary fistula and gallstone ileus. Acta Radiol 1996;37:917–22.

42. Barros JL. Hydatid disease of the liver. Am J Surg 1978;135:597–600.
43. Vagianos C, Polydorou A, Karatzas T, et al. Successful treatment of postoperative external biliary fistula by selective nasobiliary drainage. HPB Surg 1992;6:115–20.
44. Sauerbruch T, Weinzierl M, Holl J, Pratschke E. Treatment of postoperative bile fistulas by internal endoscopic biliary drainage. Gastroenterology 1986;90:1998–2003.
45. Clavien PA, Richon J, Burgan S, Rohner A. Gallstone ileus. Br J Surg 1990;77:737–42.
46. Reisner RM, Cohen JR. Gallstone ileus: a review of 1001 reported cases. Am Surg 1994;60:441–6.
47. Kasahara Y, Umemura H, Shiraha S, et al. Gallstone ileus. Review of 112 patients in the Japanese literature. Am J Surg 1980;140:437–40.
48. Rodriguez-Sanjuan JC, Casado F, Fernandez MJ, et al. Cholecystectomy and fistula closure versus enterolithotomy alone in gallstone ileus. Br J Surg 1997;84:634–7.
49. Lobo DN, Jobling JC, Balfour TW. Gallstone ileus: diagnostic pitfalls and therapeutic successes. J Clin Gastroenterol 2000;30:72–6.
50. Doogue MP, Choong CK, Frizelle FA. Recurrent gallstone ileus: underestimated. Austral N Z J Surg 1998;68:755–6.
51. Fevang B, Fevang J, Stangeland L, et al. Complications and detach after surgical treatment of small bowel obstruction: a 35-year institutional experience. Ann Surg 2000;231:529–37.
52. Hesselfeldt P, Jess P. Gallstone ileus. A review of 39 cases with emphasis on surgical treatment. Acta Chir Scand 1982;148:431–3.
53. Wills VL, Smith RC. Gallstone ileus: post cholecystectomy. Aust N Z J Surg 1994;64:650–2.
54. Heuman R, Sjodahl R, Wetterfors J. Gallstone ileus: an analysis of 20 patients. World J Surg 1980;4:595–8.
55. Bouveret L. Rev de Med 1896;16:1–16.
56. van Hillo M, van der Vliet JA, Wiggers T, et al. Gallstone obstruction of the intestine: an analysis of ten patients and a review of the literature. Surgery 1987;101:273–6.
57. Svartholm E, Andren-Sandberg A, Evander A, et al. Diagnosis and treatment of gallstone ileus. Report of 83 cases. Acta Chir Scand 1982;148:435–8.
58. Sobolewski VJ. Gallstone ileus: criteria for preoperative diagnosis. J Am Osteopath Assoc 1987;87:484–7.
59. Balthazar EJ, Schechter LS. Air in gallbladder: a frequent finding in gallstone ileus. AJR Am J Roentgenol 1978;131:219–22.
60. Balthazar EJ, Schechter LS. Gallstone ileus. The importance of contrast examinations in the roentgenographic diagnosis. AJR Am J Roentgenol 1975;125:374–9.
61. Rigler L, Borman C, Noble J. Gallstone obstruction: pathogenesis and roentgen manifestations. JAMA 1941;117:1753–9.
62. Kirkland K, Croce E. Gallstone intestinal obstruction: review of the literature and presentation of 12 cases, including 3 recurrences. JAMA 1961;176:494–7.
63. Swift SE, Spencer JA. Gallstone ileus: CT findings. Clin Radiol 1998;53:451–4.
64. Lasson A, Loren I, Nilsson A, et al. Ultrasonography in gallstone ileus: a diagnostic challenge. Eur J Surg 1995;161:259–63.
65. Zuegel N, Hehl A, Lindemann F, Witte J. Advantages of one-stage repair in case of gallstone ileus. Hepatogastroenterology 1997;44:59–62.
66. Montgomery A. Laparoscope-guided enterolithotomy for gallstone ileus. Surg Laparosc Endosc Percutan Tech 1993;3:310–4.
67. Franklin ME Jr, Dorman JP, Schuessler WW. Laparoscopic treatment of gallstone ileus: a case report and review of the literature. J Laparoendosc Surg 1994;4:265–72.
68. Sauerbruch T, Delius M, Paumgartner G, et al. Fragmentation of gallstones by extracorporeal shock waves. N Engl J Med 1986;314:818–22.
69. Meyenberger C, Michel C, Metzger U, Koelz HR. Gallstone ileus treated by extracorporeal shockwave lithotripsy. Gastrointest Endosc 1996;43:508–11.
70. Elewaut A, Crape A, Afschrift M, et al. Results of extracorporeal shock wave lithotripsy of gall bladder stones in 693 patients: a plea for restriction to solitary radiolucent stones. Gut 1993;34:274–8.
71. Elewaut A, Afschrift M, Barbier F. Gallstone ileus treated with extracorporeal shock wave lithotripsy. J Clin Ultrasound 1993;21:343–5.
72. Schutte H, Bastias J, Csendes A, et al. Gallstone ileus. Hepatogastroenterology 1992;39:562–5.
73. Buetow G, Blaubitz J, Crampton R. Recurrent gallstone ileus. Surgery 1963;54:716–24.
74. Oakland DJ, Denn PG. Endoscopic diagnosis of gallstone ileus of the duodenum. Dig Dis Sci 1986;31:98–9.
75. Kaplan BJ. Massive lower gastrointestinal hemorrhage from cholecystocolic fistula. Dis Colon Rectum 1967;10:191–6.
76. Starling J, Matallana R. Benign mechanical obstruction of the common hepatic duct (Mirizzi's syndrome). Surgery 1980;88:737–40.
77. Mirizzi P. Sindrome del conducto hepatico. J Int Chir 1948;8:731–77.
78. Pestow C. Spontaneous internal biliary fistula. Am Surg 1942;115:1043–54.
79. McSherry C, Ferstenberg H, Virshup M. The Mirizzi syndrome: suggested classification and surgical therapy. Surg Gastroenterol 1982;1:219–25.
80. Csendes A, Carlos Diaz J, Burdiles P, et al. Mirizzi syndrome and cholecystobiliary fistula: a unifying classification. Br J Surg 1989;76:1136–43.
81. Curet M, Rosendale D, Congilosi S. Mirizzi syndrome in a native American population. Am J Surg 1994;168:616–21.
82. Lubbers E. Mirizzi's syndrome. World J Surg 1983;7:780–5.
83. Pemberton M, Wells A. The Mirizzi syndrome. Postgrad Med J 1997;73:487–90.
84. Suchy F. Anatomy, anomalies, and pediatric disorders of the biliary tract. In: Fortran SA, ed. Textbook of gastrointestinal and liver disease. Philadelphia: WB Saunders, 1998:905–23.
85. Yip A, Chow W, Chan J. Mirizzi syndrome with cholecystocholedochal fistula: preoperative diagnosis and management. Surgery 1992;111:335–8.
86. Cozart C, Aliperti G. Endoscopic management of Mirizzi's syndrome. Gastrointest Endosc 1997;46:290–2.
87. Toscano R, Taylor P, Peters J. Mirizzi syndrome. Am Surg 1994;60:889–91.
88. Toursarkissian B, Holley D, Kearney P. Mirizzi's syndrome. Southern Med J 1994;87:471–5.
89. Becker C, Hassler H, Terrier F. Preoperative diagnosis of the Mirizzi syndrome: limitation of sonography and computed tomography. AJR Am J Roentgenol 1984;142:591–6.
90. Berland L, Lawson T, Stanley R. CT appearance of Mirizzi syndrome. J Comput Assist Tomogr 1984;8:165–6.
91. Baer H, Matthews J, Schweizer W. Management of the Mirizzi syndrome and the surgical implications of the cholecystocholedochal fistula. Br J Surg 1990;77:743–5.
92. Redaelli C, Buchler M, Schilling M, et al. High coincidence of Mirizzi syndrome and gallbladder carcinoma. Surgery 1997;121:58–63.
93. Delcenserie R, Joly J, Dupas J. Endoscopic diagnostic and treatment of Mirizzi's syndrome. J Clin Gastroenterol 1992;15:343–6.
94. Binmoeller K, Thonke F, Soehendra N. Endoscopic treatment of Mirizzi's syndrome. Gastrointest Endoscop 1993;39:532–6.
95. Moss JF, Bloom AD, Mesleh GF, et al. Gallstone ileus. Am Surg 1987;53:424–8.
96. Illuminati G, Bartolucci R, Leo G, Bandini A Jr. Gallstone ileus: report of 23 cases with emphasis on factors affecting survival. Ital J Surg Sci 1987;17:319–25.
97. Deitz DM, Standage BA, Pinson CW, et al. Improving the outcome in gallstone ileus. Am J Surg 1986;151:572–6.
98. Kurtz RJ, Heimann TM, Beck AR, Kurtz AB. Patterns of treatment of gallstone ileus over a 45-year period. Am J Gastroenterol 1985;80:95–8.

Chapter

14

Benign and Malignant Gallbladder Tumors

Malcolm M. Bilimoria Christopher H. Crane Jean-Nicolas Vauthey

Carcinoma of the gallbladder is a rare disease affecting less than 4000 patients each year in the United States (1). Despite this it remains the most common biliary tract cancer and accounts for 5% of all cancers found at autopsy (2). Likewise, benign tumors of the gallbladder are also quite rare and often detected incidentally during ultrasound examination or by the pathologist after cholecystectomy. This chapter highlights the diagnosis and treatment of benign and malignant gallbladder tumors.

POLYPS AND BENIGN TUMORS

There are numerous types of polyps that can arise within the gallbladder, the most common of which are cholesterol polyps. Cholesterol polyps do not represent a neoplastic process but rather are the result of excess lipid and foamy macrophage deposits within the gallbladder epithelium. A single cholesterol polyp can occur, but more often there are numerous small cholesterol polyps within the gallbladder when they occur. Adenomyomas of the gallbladder are also not a true neoplastic process in that it is a form of adenomyomatosis forming projections of the gallbladder mucosa that resemble a polyp. These polyps usually are found in the fundus of the gallbladder (3). Inflammatory polyps of the gallbladder are small sessile polyps that are composed of granulation tissue, fibrous tissue, lymphocytes, and plasmocytes. These polyps are usually discovered after cholecystectomy is performed for cholecystitis.

There are little data regarding whether adenomas represent premalignant lesions. Some authors have recommended follow-up ultrasounds every 6 months for asymptomatic gallbladder polyps less than 10 mm in size (4). Moriguchi et al. (5) prospectively followed the natural history of polypoid gallbladder lesions in 109 asymptomatic patients. After examining these patients by ultrasonography once or twice a year for 5 years, only one gallbladder carcinoma was identified, and its location was distinct from that of the preexisting polyp. In addition, 88% of the polyps were unchanged in size over the study period. The authors concluded that most of the gallbladder polyps that are identified incidentally are benign.

Despite the paucity of compelling evidence supporting a polyp-to-cancer sequence, other studies have clearly shown that larger polyps (>10 metastasis) are frequently malignant (6,7). Boulton and Adams (8) reviewed this issue and presented an algorithm for managing gallbladder polyps (Fig. 14.1). We concur with their strategy.

GALLBLADDER CARCINOMA

Clinical Presentation

Gallbladder carcinoma is diagnosed in 2.5 out of every 100,000 people in the United States each year (9). Gallbladder carcinoma is primarily a disease of older women with an average age of onset of 72 years. Women develop the disease more commonly than men do by a ratio of 3:1. The disease also has a predominance in certain ethnic groups that mirrors the incidence of cholelithiasis in these groups. Alaskan and American Indian natives have a frequency of gallbladder cancer that is six times the frequency of the rest of the country (10).

The association between gallbladder carcinoma and gallstones has been well established. Patients with gallbladder carcinoma have a 70% to 90% incidence of concurrent cholelithiasis. Correspondingly, approximately 1% of all patients undergoing cholecystectomy for cholecystitis will have carcinoma found at pathologic examination (11). Other pathologic conditions have also been associated with gallbladder carcinoma. There is a 15% incidence of gallbladder

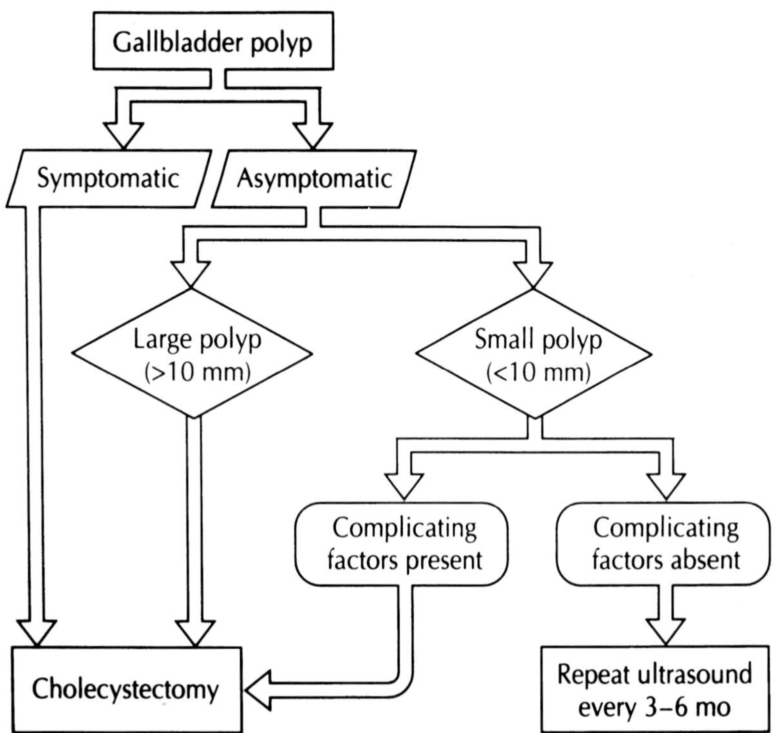

FIGURE 14.1. *Strategies for the management of gallbladder polyps. "Complicating factors" include age greater than 50 years and cholelithiasis. (Adapted by permission from Boulton RA, Adams DH. Gallbladder polyps: when to wait and when to act. Lancet 1997;349:817–21.)*

cancer in patients who have or have had a cholecystenteric fistula (12). Likewise, patients with a calcified or porcelain gallbladder have a 20% to 60% incidence of gallbladder cancer. A porcelain gallbladder likely results from years of chronic cholecystitis and therefore represents a gallbladder that is at high risk for subsequent malignancy. Identification of a porcelain gallbladder, even in the absence of symptoms, is therefore an indication for cholecystectomy.

Redaelli et al. (13) reviewed 18 cases of Mirizzi's syndrome, a syndrome associated with advanced pericystic inflammation resulting in common duct obstruction. Five of the 18 patients were found to have carcinoma, likely resulting from years of advanced inflammatory disease. Finally, the risk of developing gallbladder carcinoma in patients who are typhoid carriers, a chronic inflammatory condition of the gallbladder, is six times that of the general population (14).

Symptoms of gallbladder cancer often mimic symptoms of benign gallbladder disease. Common symptoms include right upper quadrant abdominal pain, nausea, fatty food intolerance, fever, chills, anorexia, and weight loss. Unfortunately, most patients have advanced disease at the time of diagnosis. If a gallbladder cancer is suspected preoperatively, usually as a result of an abnormally thickened gallbladder wall on ultrasound, then further investigation with contrast enhanced computerized tomography scan or magnetic resonance imaging is warranted (Fig. 14.2).

Surgical Therapy

A cure for gallbladder carcinoma can only be achieved by a complete surgical resection. The extent of surgery, however, for many stages of gallbladder carcinoma remains controversial (15). Current recommendations regarding surgical therapy are based on the primary tumor (T) as defined by the American Joint Committee on Cancer (Table 14.1) (see also Table 2.10).

Table 14.1. Primary tumor (T)

TX	Primary tumor cannot be assessed
T0	No evidence of primary tumor
Tis	Carcinoma in situ
T1	Tumor invades lamina propria or muscle layer
	T1a Tumor invades lamina propria
	T1b Tumor invades muscle layer
T2	Tumor invades perimuscular connective tissue; no extension beyond serosa or into liver
T3	Tumor perforates the serosa (visceral peritoneum) or directly invades one adjacent organ, or both (extension 2 cm or less into liver)
T4	Tumor extends more than 2 cm into liver, and/or into two or more adjacent organs (stomach, duodenum, colon, pancreas, omentum, extrahepatic bile ducts, any involvement of liver)

Shirai et al. (16) addressed the issue of the inapparent carcinoma of the gallbladder. In this scenario, an unsuspected gallbladder cancer is removed during simple cholecystectomy, and it is learned only from the final pathology that the specimen contained a carcinoma. These authors reviewed 98 cases and concluded that cholecystectomy alone was appropriate for patients with pT1 cancer, conferring a 100% 5-year survival rate. However, survival following cholecystectomy alone yielded a 40% survival rate for pT2

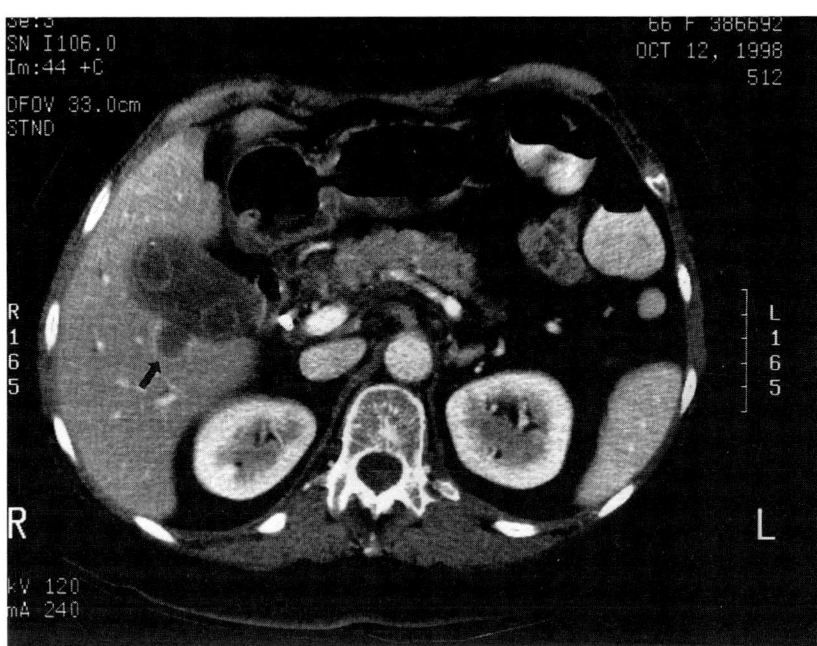

FIGURE 14.2. *A 66-year-old woman with cholelithiasis and a contrast enhanced mass arising from the gallbladder wall (arrow). In the absence of other signs of cholecystitis (diffusely thickened gallbladder wall or pericholecystic effusion), the diagnosis of gallbladder carcinoma should be made preoperatively. In this patient a preoperative percutaneous fine-needle aspiration confirmed adenocarcinoma.*

and no survival for pT3 lesions. Performance of a radical second operation (in most patients, wedge resection of the gallbladder bed, resection of the supraduodenal segment of the extrahepatic bile duct, and en bloc dissection of the regional lymph nodes) improved the pT2 5-year survival to 90% ($P < 0.05$). Because of the small number of patients, there was no definitive conclusion regarding improvement in survival after radical surgery for pT3 or pT4 patients.

Yamaguchi et al. (17) reviewed 2616 laparoscopic cholecystectomies performed over 4 years and found 24 gallbladder carcinomas. In situ carcinomas and T1 tumors (confined to the mucosa) accounted for eight of the patients, all of whom were alive and without evidence of disease at a follow-up examination of 2 to 19 months. The remaining 16 patients had T2 (tumor invades perimuscular connective tissue) or T3 (tumor perforates serosa or invades one adjacent organ or invades ≤2 cm into liver) tumors, with five cancer-related deaths 5 to 18 months after the operation. Trocar site metastases were reported in 19% of patients with T2 or T3 tumors. The authors concluded that Tis and T1 tumors of the gallbladder could be safely removed by laparoscopic cholecystectomy but that suspicious T2 or T3 tumors should prompt further surgery. Ricardo et al. (18), however, dispute the increased association between laparoscopic procedures and subsequent wound recurrences. They found no difference in wound implants in patients undergoing laparoscopic versus open procedures for gallbladder carcinoma. The authors concluded that wound implants were determined more by the biology of the disease than the type of surgery performed. Wibbenmeyer et al. (11) reviewed 928 laparoscopic cholecystectomies and found nine gallbladder carcinomas. They also concluded that T2 and T3 lesions warrant open cholecystectomy with a hepatoduodenal lymphadenectomy, wedge resection of the liver, and wide local excision of all trocar sites. The authors also reported peritoneal seeding after intra-operative gallbladder rupture in the presence of an in situ cancer.

In another study patient outcome with respect to tumor stage and extent of surgery were analyzed (19). Of the 70 patients with gallbladder carcinoma all 12 with T1 lesions were alive 4 to 82 months after cholecystectomy or extended cholecystectomy. Of the 30 patients with T2 tumors, the 3-year survival was 28% for those undergoing cholecystectomy versus 91% for those undergoing extended cholecystectomy. Likewise, for T3 and T4 tumors the survival appeared to improve with more radical resections. Of the 28 patients with advanced disease (T3 and T4 tumors) the 2-year survival was 10% for those undergoing cholecystectomy versus 17% and 23% for those undergoing extended cholecystectomy and hepatectomy, respectively (17). Many surgeons have used these data to support a surgical resection that is commensurate with the T stage of the tumor. Clearly, in situ and T1 tumors can be treated with cholecystectomy alone whereas tumors staged T2 and greater require segment IVB and V liver resection or formal hepatic lobectomy in combination with regional lymph node dissection.

To evaluate the effectiveness of radical reoperation in patients with advanced gallbladder cancer Bartlett et al. (20) reviewed the results of 149 patients with advanced gallbladder cancer. Only 58 of the patients underwent exploration with 35 found to be unresectable at the time of laparotomy. Twenty-three patients underwent resection for cure. The median survival for the unresectable patients was 5 months; the 5-year survival for those undergoing complete resection was 58%.

Table 14.2. Survival following resection for gallbladder carcinoma

Study	Patients (n)	Morbidity (%)	Mortality (%)	Survival (%)		
				1 Year	3 Year	5 Year
Donohue et al. (26)	40	13	5	—	—	33
Ogura et al. (24)	984	23	5	87	66	51
Shirai et al. (27)	40	—	0	—	—	65
Ouchi et al. (28)	25	—	0	95	70	61
Chijiiwa and Tanaka (29)	17	—	—	—	—	53
Bartlett et al. (20)	23	26	0	81	66	58

Clearly, the extent of resection for gallbladder carcinoma continues to be an issue of great debate. As previously noted, most surgeons agree that Tis and T1 lesions are adequately treated with cholecystectomy. As T2 and T3 tumors have a 62% and 81% incidence of portal lymph node metastases, respectively, it is not sufficient to treat these tumors with cholecystectomy alone (21). These patients are best treated with a portal lymph node dissection in conjunction with segment IVB and V liver resection. Other surgeons advocate more radical procedures as they feel that all posterior pancreaticoduodenal lymph nodes must be removed. Hepatopancreatoduodenectomies have been used to achieve this goal; however, the procedure has been associated with a mean hospital stay of as much as 58 days and an 85% complication rate (22,23). The short median survival of 12 months has made it difficult to justify these radical procedures. Despite this, some surgeons continue to advocate these procedures, noting that 30% of advanced gallbladder cancer patients will have disease that is encompassed by this extensive procedure (24).

In addition to advanced stage disease, other poor prognostic indicators have also been identified. Henson et al. (25) reviewed the SEER survival data for 3038 patients with gallbladder carcinoma and found that patients with papillary adenocarcinoma had a 5-year survival of 32% compared to 10% for all other types of gallbladder cancer. They also noted that the presence of vascular invasion led to a 13% 5-year survival compared to 31% for those patients without vascular invasion noted in their cancer.

Table 14.2 displays the various survival rates for patients undergoing surgical resection for gallbladder carcinoma (20,24,26–29). Although the studies reflect a heterogeneous group of patients treated with various types of resections, making a comparison between studies difficult, the individual reports support increased survival after operative resection in selected patients with gallbladder carcinoma.

Adjuvant Therapy

Unfortunately, adjuvant chemotherapy has not proved overly useful in patients with gallbladder carcinoma. Most studies evaluating systemic therapy for this disease are limited by the number of patients in the study and the frequent inclusion of cholangiocarcinoma patients in the study. The most studied chemotherapeutic in gallbladder cancer remains 5-fluorouracil (5-FU). Despite its inclusion in multiple regimens and its varied modes of delivery, 5-FU has been associated with response rates of only 10% to 24% (30–32). Phase II trials of mitomycin-C or *cis*-platinum used in single agent regimens proved no better than 5-FU with partial responses noted in less than 10% of patients (33,34). In a multidrug regimen of 5-FU, leucovorin, methotrexate, and epirubicin (a phase II study) no responses were seen in the 21 patients enrolled in the study (35). Thus, to date there are no multidrug regimens that have proven better than 5-FU alone.

Given the dismal responses noted with systemic chemotherapy, regional infusion of chemotherapy by hepatic artery infusion has been studied. Oberfield and Rossi (36) noted a partial response in 15 of 38 patients treated with hepatic artery infusion, but failed to show any difference in survival.

The argument for the addition of postoperative chemoradiation is based on the pattern of failure. After complete resection, relapse is common in the tumor bed as well as the regional nodes (37,38). Due to the rarity of gallbladder cancer, postoperative adjuvant chemoradiation has not been adequately evaluated. However, a suggestion of improved locoregional control has been suggested by single arm studies. Improved median survival has been reported with the use of radiation alone (39). The European Organization for Research on Treatment of Cancer (EORTC) has also reported improvement in median survival with the use of postoperative radiation in patients with positive margins in other biliary tract cancers (40). Although these data are not controlled, it is likely that there is a selection bias against the treated group in both studies because patients are usually only referred for postoperative therapy if they are considered high risk. The addition of radiosensitizing protracted venous infusion 5-FU has not been evaluated, but is reasonable based on the results of randomized trials showing improvement in survival with the combination of radiation and chemotherapy in other gastrointestinal sites (41). Phase III studies are needed to establish a role for postoperative therapy, but are probably only feasible with the participation of multiple cooperative groups.

Significant palliation of the symptoms of unresectable disease is frequent with the use of palliative radiotherapy, but long-term local control is unlikely with conventional treatment techniques. Conformal radiotherapy, novel sensitizers, or novel radioprotectors may improve the therapeutic index and the possibility of long-term disease control in patients with unresectable disease, and should be evaluated prospectively.

SUGGESTED READINGS

Bartlett DL, Fong Y, Fortner JG, et al. Long-term results after resection for gallbladder cancer: implications for staging and management. Ann Surg 1996;224:639–46. This study evaluates the effectiveness of radical reoperation for patients with gallbladder cancer. Only 23 of the 58 patients undergoing laparotomy actually had a resection for potential cure. Median survival for the unresectable patients was five months compared to a 58% five-year survival for those undergoing complete resection.

Moriguchi H, Tazawa J, Hayashi Y, et al. Natural history of polypoid lesions in the gallbladder. Gut 1996;39:860–2. This study reviews the natural history of benign gallbladder polyps incidentally identified and concludes that asymptomatic gallbladder polyps can be safely followed by ultrasound.

Yamaguchi K, Chijiiwa K, Saiki S, et al. Retrospective analysis of 70 operations for gallbladder cancer. Br J Surg 1997;84:200–4. This study confirms that survival for gallbladder cancer patients is closely correlated with their T stage. Patients with T2 lesions had an increase in three-year survival when liver resection was added to cholecystectomy for treatment of their cancer.

REFERENCES

1. Cancer facts and figures. Atlanta: American Cancer Society, 1998.
2. Arminski TC. Primary carcinoma of the gallbladder: a collective review with the addition of twenty-five cases from the Grace Hospital. Cancer 1949;2:379.
3. Joseph M, Vauthey JN. Biliary tract cancer. Curr Opinion Gastroenterol 1998;14:402–7.
4. Aldridge MC, Bismuth H. Gallbladder cancer: the polyp-cancer sequence. Br J Surg 1990;77:363–4.
5. Moriguchi H, Tazawa J, Hayashi Y, et al. Natural history of polypoid lesions in the gallbladder. Gut 1996;39:860–2.
6. Koga A, Watanabe K, Fukuyama T, et al. Diagnosis and operative indications for polypoid lesions of the gallbladder. Arch Surg 1988,123:26–9.
7. Yang HL, Sun YG, Wang Z, et al. Polypoid lesions of the gallbladder: diagnosis and indications for surgery. Br J Surg 1992,79:227–9.
8. Boulton RA, Adams DH. Gallbladder polyps: when to wait and when to act. Lancet 1997;349:817–21.
9. Breda MA, Hoffman AL, Sher L, et al. Hepatobiliary tumors. In: Harvey JC, Beattie EJ, eds. Cancer surgery. Philadelphia: WB Saunders, 1996:88–119.
10. Diehl AK. Epidemiology of gallbladder cancer: a synthesis of recent data. J Natl Cancer Inst 1980;65:1209–12.
11. Wibbenmeyer LA, Wade TP, Chen RC, et al. Laparoscopic cholecystectomy can disseminate in situ carcinoma of the gallbladder. J Am Coll Surg 1995;181:504–10.
12. Berliner SD, Burson LC. One-stage repair of cholecystoduodenal fistula and gallstone ileus. Arch Surg 1965;90:313–16.
13. Redaelli CA, Buchler MW, Schilling MK, et al. High coincidence of Mirizzi syndrome and gallbladder carcinoma. Surgery 1997;121:58–63.
14. Wanebo HJ. Treatment of gallbladder cancer. In: Wanebo HJ, ed. Surgery for gastrointestinal cancer. Philadelphia: Raven-Lippincott, 1997:577–88.
15. Corsetti RL, Wanebo HJ. Gallbladder cancer. In: Cameron JL, ed. Current surgical therapy. St. Louis: Mosby, 1998:462–8.
16. Shirai Y, Yoshida K, Tsukada K, Muto T. Inapparent carcinoma of the gallbladder. Ann Surg 1992;215:326–31.
17. Yamaguchi K, Chijiiwa K, Ichimiya H, et al. Gallbladder carcinoma in the era of laparoscopic cholecystectomy. Arch Surg 1996;131:981–4.
18. Ricardo AE, Feig BW, Ellis LM, et al. Gallbladder cancer and trocar site recurrences. Am J Surg 1997;174:619–23.
19. Yamaguchi K, Chijiiwa K, Saiki S, et al. Retrospective analysis of 70 operations for gallbladder cancer. Br J Surg 1997;84:200–4.
20. Bartlett DL, Fong Y, Fortner JG, et al. Long-term results after resection for gallbladder cancer: implications for staging and management. Ann Surg 1996;224:639–46.
21. Shimada H, Endo I, Togo S, et al. The role of lymph node dissection in the treatment of gallbladder carcinoma. Cancer 1997;79:892–9.
22. Tsukada K, Yoshida K, Anono T, et al. Major hepatectomy and pancreaticoduodenectomy for advanced carcinoma of the biliary tract. Br J Surg 1994;81:108–10.
23. Nakamura S, Nishiyama R, Yokoi Y, et al. Hepatopancreaticoduodenectomy for advanced gallbladder carcinoma. Arch Surg 1994;129:625–9.
24. Ogura Y, Mizumoto R, Isaji S, et al. Radical operations for carcinoma of the gallbladder: present status in Japan. World J Surg 1991;15:337–41.
25. Henson DE, Albores-Saavedra J, Corle D. Carcinoma of the gallbladder: histologic types, stage of disease, grade and survival rates. Cancer 1992;70:1493–7.
26. Donohue JH, Nagorney DM, Grant CS, et al. Carcinoma of the gallbladder: does radical resection improve outcome? Arch Surg 1990;125:237–41.
27. Shirai Y, Yoshida K, Tsukada K, et al. Radical surgery for gallbladder carcinoma: long-term results. Ann Surg 1992;216:565–8.
28. Ouchi K, Suzuki M, Saijo S, et al. Do recent advances in diagnosis and operative management improve the outcome of gallbladder carcinoma? Surgery 1993;113:324–9.
29. Chijiiwa K, Tanaka M. Carcinoma of the gallbladder: an appraisal of surgical resection. Surgery 1994;115:751–6.
30. Falkson G, Macinityre JM, Moertel CG. Eastern Cooperative Oncology Group experience with chemotherapy for inoperable gallbladder and bile duct cancer. Cancer 1984;54:965–70.
31. Harvey JH, Smith FP, Sehien PS. 5-fluorouracil, mitomycin, and doxorubicin (FAM) in carcinoma of the biliary tract. J Clin Oncol 1984;2:1245–9.
32. Takada F, Kuttot S, Matsushiro T, et al. Comparison of 5-fluorouracil, doxorubicin, and mitomycin with 5-fluorouracil alone in the treatment of pancreatic-biliary carcinoma. Oncology 1994;51:396–402.
33. Taal BG, Audisio RA, Bleiberg H, et al. Phase II trial of mitomycin C in advanced gallbladder and biliary tract carcinoma. An EORTC Gastrointestinal Tract Cooperative Group Study. Ann Oncol 1993;4:407–12.
34. Okada S, Ishii F, Nose H, et al. A phase II study of cisplatinum in patients with biliary tract carcinoma. Oncology 1994;51:515–19.
35. Kajanti M, Pyrhonen S. Epirubicin-sequentila methotrexate, 5-fluorouracil, leucovorin treatment of advanced cancer of the extrahepatic biliary system: a phase III trial. Am J Clin Oncol 1994;17:223–39.
36. Oberfield RA, Rossi RL. The role of chemotherapy in the treatment of bile duct cancer. World J Surg 1988;12:105–12.
37. Kopelson G, Galdabini J, Warshaw AL, Gunderson LL. Patterns of failure after curative surgery for extra-hepatic biliary tract carcinoma: implications for adjuvant therapy. Int J Radiat Oncol Biol Phys 1981;7:413–17.
38. Kopelson G, Gunderson LL. Primary and adjuvant radiation therapy in gallbladder and extrahepatic biliary tract carcinoma. J Clin Gastroenterol 1983;5:43–50.
39. Vaittinen E. Carcinoma of the gall-bladder. A study of 390 cases diagnosed in Finland 1953–1967. Ann Chir Gynaecol Fenn Suppl 1970;168:1–81.
40. Gonzalez Gonzalez D, Gerard JP, Maners AW, et al. Results of radiation therapy in carcinoma of the proximal bile duct (Klatskin tumor). Semin Liver Dis 1990;10:131–41.
41. O'Connell M, Martenson JA, Wieand HS, et al. Improving adjuvant therapy for rectal cancer by combining protracted-infusion fluorouracil with radiation therapy after curative surgery. N Engl J Med 1994;331:502–7.

Section

3.2

The Intrahepatic and Extrahepatic Bile Ducts

Chapter 15

Acute Cholangitis

ANDY S. YU JOSEPH W. LEUNG

Acute cholangitis is a common cause for emergency hospital admissions. It develops as a result of bacterial colonization and overgrowth within a stagnant or obstructed biliary system. Historically, emergency surgery was necessary for urgent biliary decompression. With the advances in therapeutic biliary endoscopy and interventional radiology over the last two decades, most cases can now be managed acutely without surgery and in a minimally invasive manner with significant improvement in the clinical outcome. The cornerstone of acute management includes empiric broad-spectrum antibiotic coverage and, if necessary, prompt biliary decompression. Eighty percent of patients respond to conservative management, but 20% will require urgent drainage because of suppurative cholangitis associated with complete bile duct obstruction.

ETIOLOGY

Obstruction of the common bile duct by stones is the most common cause of acute cholangitis, accounting for 80% of cases seen in the Western world (1). Such stones often originate from the gallbladder and, hence, are termed secondary common bile duct (CBD) stones. On the other hand, in East Asian countries, patients may develop primary pigment stones in the CBD that are typically associated with recurrent pyogenic cholangitis or Oriental cholangiohepatitis (2). The role of biliary parasites in cholangitis remains controversial (3,4). It is possible that *Ascaris lumbricoides* (5,6) and *Clonorchis sinensis* (7) may cause biliary obstruction and serve as a nidus for intrahepatic ductal stone formation or hepatolithiasis. This is supported by the presence of remains of adult worms and ova in the center of pigment stones (8–10).

Other causes of cholangitis include benign strictures, neoplasms, papillary stenosis, chronic pancreatitis, and sclerosing cholangitis. Foreign bodies, such as biliary endoprosthesis and surgical sutures, may also lead to acute cholangitis. Of 99 patients who presented from 1966 to 1976, two-thirds of their obstructions were caused by stones or benign strictures (11). Acute cholangitis may also be a complication from direct cholangiography due to failed drainage procedures in patients with malignant obstructive jaundice. Mirizzi's syndrome, an external compression on the common hepatic duct by a stone impacted in the cystic duct or neck of the gallbladder, can precipitate concomitant acute cholecystitis and cholangitis (12).

PATHOGENESIS

The three major pathogenic factors involved in the development of acute cholangitis are 1) bacteriobilia, 2) bile stasis, and 3) local propagation of bacteria (13). The normal biliary system is sterile (14) except for transient bacteriobilia. The biliary defense mechanisms against bacterial invasion include 1) the sphincter of Oddi guarding bacterial entry from the duodenum or ascending infection, 2) constant unidirectional bile flow, 3) bacteriostatic bile salts, 4) immunoglobulin (IgA) secretion from cholangiocytes, 5) phagocytic activity of the Kupffer cells, and 6) mucinous coating and tight intercellular junctions of the bile duct epithelium (15–17). The last two play a role in preventing descending infection from the portal circulation.

It has been shown in a feline model that bacteria could gain entry to the biliary tree via the portal venous system (15). Bacteriobilia can occur without bacteremia if there is no obstruction, as seen after sphincterotomy or biliary drain placement with a patent endoprosthesis (18). Chronic obstruction renders the biliary system more susceptible to cholangitis (19) by causing bile stasis and a raised intrabiliary pressure within the bile duct. The nutrient-rich bile serves as a good culture medium for bacteria to multiply.

The raised biliary pressure causes reflux of bacteria into the lymphatics and hepatic sinusoids, leading to endotoxemia and septicemia. This is classically known as cholangiovenous reflux (20).

The normal biliary pressure ranges from 8 to 16 cm H_2O. What is known as cholangiovenous reflux was demonstrated in a canine model when the intrabiliary pressure exceeded 25 cm H_2O (21). In human studies, cholangitis presents when the biliary pressure exceeds 20 cm H_2O. Bile secretion stops completely when biliary pressure exceeds 30 cm H_2O (22,23). A continued elevation of bile duct pressure eventually overwhelms the integrity of the biliary epithelium, leading to bacterial reflux into the systemic circulation. The clinical severity and mortality of acute cholangitis correlate well with the intraductal pressure (24). In fact, forceful injection of contrast during direct cholangiography was shown to cause bacteremia (25).

Endotoxin, which is released during the breakdown of the cell wall of gram-negative bacteria, is usually metabolized by the liver and excreted in bile. It may also be refluxed into the sinusoidal spaces under high biliary pressure in the face of acute cholangitis. Relief of biliary obstruction allows endotoxin excretion to be resumed. This is demonstrated by a study on 40 patients with calculous cholangitis. A significant association was demonstrated between the clinical features of acute cholangitis and the serum and bile levels of endotoxin. Furthermore, significant reductions in both bile and serum endotoxin levels were achieved within 24 hours after successful endoscopic drainage (26). In a separate study, biliary decompression is shown to promote the excretion of antibiotics into bile and resumption of IgA secretion (27). Hence, biliary decompression plays a crucial role in the management of acute cholangitis.

Table 15.1. Frequency (%) of polymicrobial infections in bile and blood

Number of Species	Bile (n = 579)	Blood (n = 121)
1	29	94
2	33	6
3	29	0
4	8	0
5	1	0

Reproduced by permission from Leung JW, Ling TK, Chan RC, et al. Antibiotics, biliary sepsis, and bile duct stones. Gastrointest Endosc 1994;40:716–21.

Table 15.2. Species of bacteria isolated from bile, stones, and blood in patients with bacterobilia-cholangitis

Organisms Isolated	Bile[a] (%)	Stone[b] (%)	Blood[c] (%)
E. coli	27	22	71
Klebsiella spp	17	18	14
Enterobacter spp	8	8	5
P. aeruginosa	7	9	4
Citrobacter spp	3	1	2
Proteus spp	3	3	0
Acinetobacter spp	1	3	0
Bacteroides spp	1	1	1
Enterococcus spp	17	12	0
Streptococcus spp	8	9	0
Staphylococcus spp	2	6	3
Clostridium spp	2	1	0
Candida spp	4	1	0
Others	0	8	0

[a] Isolated from 579 patients (1236 species).
[b] Isolated from 70 patients (152 species).
[c] Isolated from 121 patients with septicemia (128 species).

Reproduced by permission from Leung JW, Ling TK, Chan RC, et al. Antibiotics, biliary sepsis, and bile duct stones. Gastrointest Endosc 1994;40:716–21.

BACTERIOLOGICAL FINDINGS

There have been many bacteriological studies of bile cultures in patients with acute cholangitis (28–31). Some of these studies have also compared blood and bile bacterial isolates in cases complicated by septicemia. A more recent study conducted in Hong Kong analyzed the bile, the biliary stones, and the blood cultures in 579 patients who presented over a 7-year period (32). The blood cultures were positive in 121 patients (21%), and almost always yielded a single organism (Table 15.1), predominantly *Escherichia coli*. In contrast, over two-thirds of the bile cultures showed mixed infection of two or more organisms; and culture of bile duct stones always showed mixed flora. Two-thirds of the patients with bacteremia had similar organisms isolated from blood and bile. Analysis of bile and stone cultures showed that *E. coli*, *Klebsiella* spp, *Enterobacter* spp, *Enterococcus* spp, and *Streptococcus* spp were the most commonly isolated bacteria (Table 15.2).

Anaerobic organisms, most commonly *Bacteroides* spp, can be found in elderly patients and in patients who have suffered cholangitis in iatrogenic settings. *Pseudomonas* infections were linked to biliary sepsis outbreaks following biliary endoscopies (33,34). Gram-positive organisms are isolated more often following percutaneous drainage of the biliary system (35). *Candida albicans* is the most common fungal cause of cholangitis, but is usually associated with an immunocompromised state. As previously mentioned, *Ascaris lumbricoides* and *Clonorchis sinensis* may serve as the nidus for intrahepatic stone formation and contribute to recurrent pyogenic cholangitis.

CLINICAL FEATURES

Most cases of acute cholangitis arise de novo, although patients with recurrent pyogenic cholangitis may have a history of previous attacks. Also, 50% to 70% of the patients may present with Charcot's triad, which includes right upper quadrant abdominal pain, spiking fever, and increasing jaundice (36). Fever is consistently the most common presentation, which occurs in over 90% of the cases. Abdominal pain ranges from mild to severe, but may not be localized to the right upper quadrant. Jaundice may be absent in the early stages. However, profound jaundice suggests a malignant etiology (37). Rigor, which is a profound chill associated with piloerection and severe shivering, reflects intermittent bacteremia (38). Elderly patients may present solely with mental confusion and a deterioration of their general condition. The combination of confusion, hypotension, and Charcot's triad constitutes the Reynolds' pentad (38a), which is invariably fatal without urgent decompression of the biliary system. The term "toxic cholangitis" is also used to describe this severe condition (39).

Recurrent pyogenic cholangitis presents as bouts of Charcot's triad. A typical attack may last for several hours or days before subsiding spontaneously. Chronic biliary obstruction may give rise to multiple liver abscesses, liver atrophy, and eventually secondary biliary cirrhosis (40). The clinical course is characterized by recurrent attacks of pain and cholangitis that require multiple operative interventions. The incidence of residual stones is 77% and the incidence of recurrent stones is 15% after surgery (4). Silent cholangiocarcinoma may develop even after the complete removal of intrahepatic stones because bile stasis, the culprit for carcinogens, is not corrected (41).

Organ failures and sepsis may develop in severe forms of acute cholangitis. Uncontrolled infections can also give rise to liver abscesses, sclerosing cholangitis, and strictures. The spread of infection or inflammation into the portal circulation can lead to pyelophlebitis and portal vein thrombosis. Cholecystitis and/or pancreatitis may be complicated by cholangitis or caused by the same underlying process (Table 15.3). Rupture of a terminal bile ductule under elevated intrabiliary pressure leads to bile peritonitis.

Although acute cholangitis is a very serious illness, its mortality rate can be kept below 10% with appropriate treatment. In a multivariate analysis (42), seven risk factors were identified to predict the mortality in acute cholangitis: 1) age over 50 years, 2) female gender, 3) associated liver abscess, 4) associated cirrhosis, 5) cholangitis due to a high-grade malignant stricture, 6) cholangitis after percutaneous transhepatic choledochography, and 7) acute renal failure. In a separate analysis of the risk factors responsible for therapeutic failure in acute cholangitis, the following comorbid parameters were identified: 1) malignancy, 2) bacteremia, 3) two or more species of organisms or a pan-resistant species recovered from the bile, and 4) a serum bilirubin of 2.2 mg/dL or higher.

LABORATORY FINDINGS

Leukocytosis with a left shift is the most common laboratory finding. Depending on the degree and duration of biliary obstruction, elevations in serum liver enzymes may present in either a cholestatic or a hepatocellular fashion. With acute gallstone obstruction of the CBD and sudden biliary pressure increase, the level of serum aminotransferases may reach the thousands within 24 to 48 hours, then rapidly decline to lower values (43). Elevated serum alkaline phosphatase and direct hyperbilirubinemia levels are seen in over 80% of all acute cholangitis cases (13), but they may lag behind the clinical picture by more than one day.

Concurrent pancreatitis, which may be due to an ampullary stone, can lead to high serum amylase and lipase levels. However, mild hyperamylasemia can be found in 40% of cholangitis patients without concomitant pancreatitis. The levels of serum CA 19-9, which is a rather nonspecific and nonsensitive tumor marker for both cholangiocarcinoma and pancreatic adenocarcinoma, can be elevated in obstructive jaundice and acute cholangitis (44). It is not used routinely for the diagnosis and acute management of cholangitis.

Table 15.3. Common complications of cholangitis

Local
Liver abscess (solitary or multiple)
Secondary sclerosing cholangitis
Secondary strictures
Cholangiocarcinoma
Portal vein thrombosis/pylephlebitis
Cholecystitis
Pancreatitis
Systemic
Disseminated intravascular coagulopathy
Acute renal failure
Respiratory failure
Sepsis/septic shock
Mental obtundation

Reproduced by permission from Köksal R, Lo SK. Pyogenic cholangitis. In: Brandt L, ed. Clinical practice of gastroenterology. Philadelphia: Saunders, 1999:1079–88.

RADIOLOGIC INVESTIGATIONS

Plain x-ray is generally unhelpful, as most gallstones are radio-opaque. However, a clinical picture of an acute abdomen certainly would require one. There may be an incidental finding of an ileus. Pneumobilia, or air in the biliary tree, may suggest a spontaneous biliary-enteric fistula, a previous biliary-enteric bypass, or a sphincterotomy.

A combination of abdominal ultrasound, computed tomography (CT), and direct cholangiography complements the radiologic investigation of acute cholangitis. Abdominal ultrasound is fast, inexpensive, and noninvasive. It demonstrates the presence of stones and dilated ducts, plus the level of obstruction. Stones appear in the form of acoustic shadows. Furthermore, ultrasound may possibly reveal a tumor, an abscess, cholecystitis, or acute pancreatitis.

Ultrasound, however, is operator dependent. Any overlying bowel gas, abdominal scars from prior surgeries, and pneumobilia can obscure the images. Besides, ultrasound is nonsensitive in the detection of choledocholithiasis, especially stones impacted in the distal duct. However, in the presence of a dilated biliary tree together with the typical clinical signs and symptoms, a presumptive diagnosis of acute cholangitis can be made. Ultrasound is more sensitive in detecting stones in the dilated intrahepatic system. It should be considered the initial method of choice for investigating patients with suspected biliary sepsis.

CT is only slightly more sensitive than ultrasound in the diagnosis of choledocholithiasis, but is less sensitive for the detection of intrahepatic stones. Analogous to ultrasound, an unremarkable CT scan does not exclude the possibility of cholangitis. However, it is superior to ultrasound in the evaluation of the extent of liver damage associated with intrahepatic stones, such as ductal dilation, abscess formation, and relative atrophy and hypertrophy of different liver lobes. It provides a good preoperative assessment of the disease and localizes obstructed segmental ducts not filled or visualized by direct cholangiography. It is useful to detect associated cholangiocarcinoma or metastatic cancer. For staging purposes, it reveals splenomegaly as associated with portal hypertension from biliary cirrhosis (45).

Direct cholangiography to delineate the exact ductal pathology is often necessary before deciding the appropriate management. It is the gold standard for diagnosing acute cholangitis. The choice between endoscopic retrograde cholangiopancreatography (ERCP) and percutaneous transhepatic cholangiography (PTC) depends on the availability of an operator with expertise and the nature and level of biliary obstruction. They both serve to define the extent of ductal involvement. ERCP is less invasive, but the obstructed ducts may not be visualized unless an occlusion cholangiogram is performed with contrast injected under pressure to fill the segments proximal to the obstruction. As previously mentioned, the increase in intrahepatic pressure can iatrogenically aggravate bacteremia and worsen the preexisting cholangitis. ERCP has also the advantage of offering therapeutic measures, including stone extraction and biliary drainage, immediately at the same setting.

PTC is used to define the ductal anatomy and the extent of disease, especially when ERCP has already failed or in patients who have the anatomy of a bilioenteric anastomosis. Where ERCP did not opacify a ductal segment, PTC can confirm the presence of dilated ducts with complete obstruction. Once percutaneous access to the biliary system is established, transhepatic biliary drainage and placement of a stent can be undertaken to decompress the obstructed segment. Nevertheless, PTC is more invasive than ERCP and can produce complications including hemobilia, hepatic arteriovenous shunting, and bile peritonitis.

Magnetic resonance cholangiopancreatography (MRCP) serves as a good diagnostic tool in the setting of failed ERCP, incomplete delineation of the biliary anatomy, or biliary-enteric anastomosis. It produces high-quality images without the injection of contrast agents (Fig. 15.1). Its sensitivity in defining stones and strictures is similar to that of conventional direct cholangiography (46–48). Furthermore, it is less operator dependent and its images are easily reproducible. It provides additional information on adjacent soft tissue that cannot be obtained from ERCP or PTC (49). Its major limitation is that it cannot offer therapeutic options.

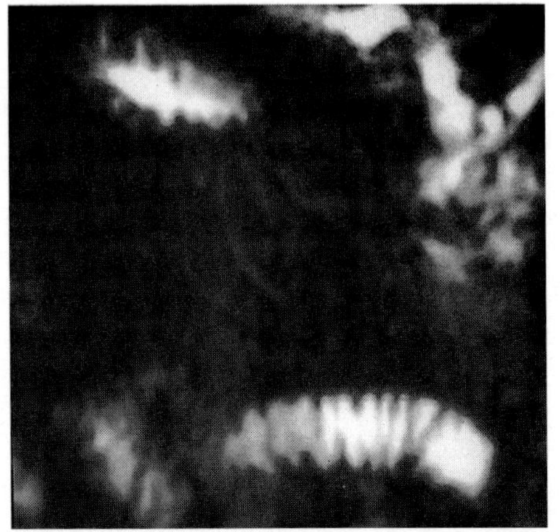
(A)

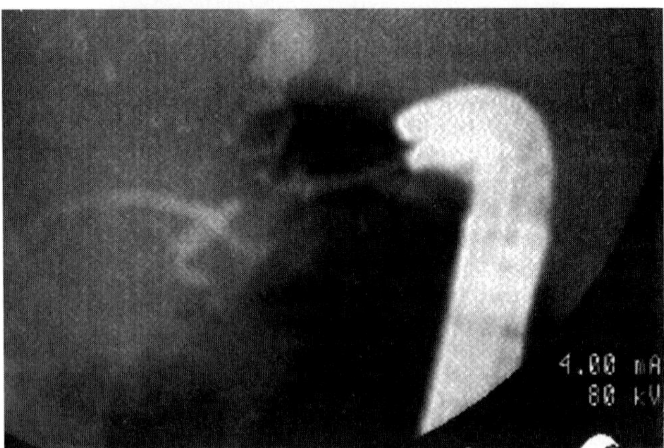

(B)

FIGURE 15.1. ***(A)*** *Magnetic resonance cholangiopancreatography (MRCP) showing an 8-mm common duct stone above a distal common bile duct stricture.* ***(B)*** *Endoscopic retrograde cholangiopancreatography (ERCP) showing the 8-mm stone above a distal common bile duct stricture.*

MANAGEMENT

General Principles of Management

Untreated acute cholangitis is uniformly fatal. Management begins with early recognition of the condition. Empiric broad-spectrum antibiotics and prompt biliary decompression are the mainstay of therapy. Approximately 80% of patients will improve with conservative management, which includes broad-spectrum antibiotic coverage (50). However, medical therapy only temporarily stabilizes the patient and controls the infection. Further cholangiographic investigations and definitive treatment on a more elective basis are required to correct the offending lesion.

For the remaining 20% of patients who continue to deteriorate despite conservative management, an urgent biliary decompression is necessary. These are patients who present with swinging fever despite antibiotic treatment over a period of 48 hours, or those who develop mental confusion, hemodynamic instability, or multisystemic involvement. Progressive tachycardia, declining blood pressure, and oliguria are warning signs of impending sepsis. The prime objective of management is focused on reducing the biliary pressure effectively by a safe and expeditious method, rather than on eliminating the underlying obstruction.

There are three major therapeutic options for urgent biliary decompression. Until recently surgery was the only choice available. The advances and successes in therapeutic endoscopy and interventional radiology over the last 20 years have made urgent surgical drainage mainly the last resort. The choice between endoscopic decompression and percutaneous transhepatic biliary drainage (PTBD) is determined by the anatomy of the disease and the availability of local expertise. In the following sections, we will examine the different modalities of management.

Conservative Management

Medical management must be initiated immediately once a presumptive diagnosis of acute cholangitis is made. Therapy consists of close monitoring to detect any clinical deterioration, intravenous fluid to maintain adequate perfusion of vital organs, and broad-spectrum antibiotics right after blood cultures have been obtained. All oral intakes should be stopped. The patient must be followed closely for mental condition, pulse, blood pressure, and urinary output. The underlying coagulopathy needs to be corrected with vitamin K and perhaps with fresh frozen plasma. For patients who are frail, elderly, or seriously ill, monitoring in the intensive care unit is necessary. Circulatory support and artificial ventilation may be required in cases of septicemia and shock.

An ideal antibiotic regimen should cover gram-negative coliforms such as *E. coli*, *Klebsiella*, *Streptococcus* spp, and anaerobes. A frequently used combination includes a third-generation cephalosporin to cover gram-negative bacilli, ampicillin to cover gram-positive cocci (including streptococcal organisms), and metronidazole to cover anaerobes. An alternative choice is ureidopenicillins, which can be in the form of azlocillin, mezlocillin, or piperacillin (51–53). This monotherapy provides similar antimicrobial coverage.

In addition, an ideal antibiotic should achieve high levels in the bile. Unfortunately many antibiotics that are normally excreted in bile no longer enter the biliary tree when the system is completely obstructed (54). It has been demonstrated that biliary obstruction impairs both active and passive excretions of antibiotics into bile. After relief of biliary obstruction, it takes some time for an actively excreted drug to build up its bile concentration. This is due to the delayed recovery of hepatocytes' active secretory processes. Although an antibiotic may be effective for treating septicemia in cholangitis, it may not achieve sufficient concentration in bile for the effective treatment of biliary infection.

Ciprofloxacin alone has been demonstrated to be an adequate therapy for patients with acute cholangitis. Among a group of patients with bile duct obstruction (32,55), the biliary excretion profile of five different antibiotics were studied. These antibiotics included ceftazidime, cefoperazone, imipenem, netilmicin, and ciprofloxacin. With the sole exception of ciprofloxacin, the bile obtained from over 90% of the patients immediately after endoscopic drainage contained no detectable level of antibiotic. The bile concentration of ciprofloxacin was only 20% of the mean peak serum concentration, but it was still higher than the necessary minimum inhibitory concentration for gram-negative bacteria.

In a prospective randomized clinical trial of 100 patients with acute cholangitis, ciprofloxacin monotherapy was compared with the triple combination of ampicillin, ceftazidime, and metronidazole (56). Eighty-five percent of patients in the monotherapy group and 77% of those in the triple-regimen group responded to therapy. The mean durations of fever, septicemic shock, and hospitalization were similar in the two treatment groups. Similar proportions of patients in the two treatment groups required urgent endoscopy or surgery for uncontrolled infection. The mortality rates were 4% in the ciprofloxacin group and 2% in the triple-therapy group (Table 15.4).

Antibiotics should be continued for 1 to 2 weeks, depending on the patient's response. They may be switched to oral antibiotics once clinical stability has been achieved. It should also be noted that aminoglycosides are nephrotoxic and should be used with caution in patients with obstructive jaundice (57). Acute renal failure can be easily precipitated, especially in the setting of sepsis and dehydration. Also, aminoglycosides have a poor bile–serum ratio.

Endoscopic Drainage

If an experienced endoscopist is available, endoscopic drainage should be considered the treatment of choice for acute cholangitis when biliary sepsis progresses despite an adequate trial of antibiotics. Unstable patients should undergo the procedure immediately in the intensive care unit, because any delay will only worsen the clinical status. Intravenous sedation should be kept to a minimum, and vital signs (including oxygen saturation) should be closely monitored throughout the entire procedure.

During ERCP cannulation should be performed as quickly as possible without being reckless. Bile ducts should be deeply cannulated and the purulent bile should be aspi-

Table 15.4. Clinical responses of evaluable patients in the two treatment groups

	Treatment Group	
	Cipro (n = 46)	Triple (n = 44)
No. (%) of patients who responded to therapy	39 (85)	34 (77)
No. (%) of patients who failed therapy	7 (15)	10 (23)
Mean (± SD) duration of fever (days)	1.7 ± 1.4	2.4 ± 2.0
Duration of shock (number of patients)		
<1 day	4	4
>1 day	2	3
Mean (± SD) hospital stay (days)	6.6 ± 4.3	7.7 ± 5.2
Need for emergency endoscopy/surgery [no. (%) of patients]	6 (13)	7 (16)
Fever recurrence during hospitalization [no. (%) of patients]	1 (2)	3 (7)
Mortality attributable to infection [no. (%) of patients]	1 (2)	1 (2)

Reproduced by permission from Sung JY, Lyon DJ, Suen R, et al. Intravenous ciprofloxacin as treatment for patients with acute suppurative cholangitis: a randomized, controlled clinical trial. J Antimicrob Chemother 1995;35:855–64.

rated to decompress the bile ducts before obtaining a cholangiogram. The amount of contrast injection should be minimized to avoid increasing the intrahepatic pressure and cholangiovenous reflux. Occlusion cholangiography with balloon catheters should also be avoided. Once the ductal pathology is delineated, the endoscopist has to decide on the best mode of drainage based on the obstructing factor and the patient's condition. The prime objective of an urgent endoscopy is to reduce the biliary pressure effectively by a safe and expeditious method, rather than to eliminate the underlying obstructive lesion.

Sphincterotomy with stone removal is reserved for stable patients with single or small stones. It requires skilled assistance and extensive instrumentation of the biliary system. Although immediate extraction of all ductal calculi was once widely practiced, such an aggressive approach carried an increased morbidity of 28% even in experienced hands. Complications such as bleeding and retroduodenal perforations, which require emergency exploration, are highly undesirable especially at the time of a severe cholangitic attack (39). Prolonged biliary manipulation delays effective drainage until ductal clearance is achieved, thus lengthening the exposure to sepsis and increasing the risks of conscious sedation, including hemodynamic and respiratory compromise.

Insertion of a nasobiliary drain provides urgent biliary decompression while allowing more definitive procedures to be performed on an elective basis (Figs. 15.2 and 15.3). It can be performed without a prior sphincterotomy. This mode of drainage is preferable for unstable patients or

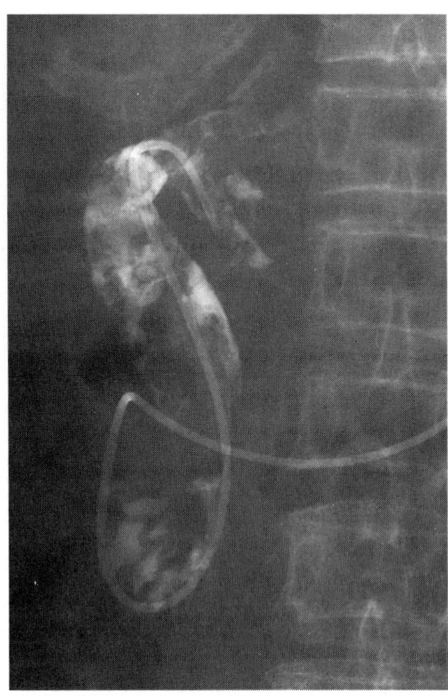

FIGURE 15.2. *Nasobiliary catheter drainage for acute cholangitis. The cholangiogram shows a nasobiliary drain and multiple large common bile duct stones.*

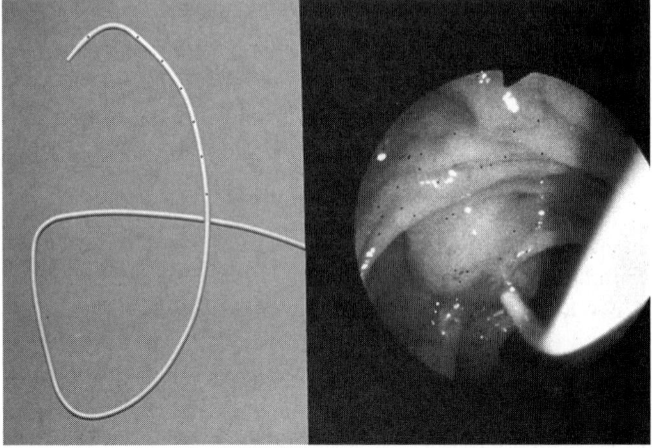

FIGURE 15.3. *An example of a nasobiliary catheter (Leung-6.5–7.0, Wilson Cook Medical) on left and insertion of nasobiliary catheter without a sphincterotomy on right.*

patients with technically difficult or large stones. In a study of 105 patients with acute cholangitis who underwent emergency endoscopy, biliary drainage was successful in 102 patients and clinical improvement was achieved in 99 of them. Defervescence within 3 days was observed in 90% of patients. Even though 40% of these patients were in septic shock prior to the endoscopic procedure, the overall 30-day mortality was only 4.7% and was limited to those who had

Table 15.5. Outcomes of nasobiliary drainage

Outcome	ES Group (n = 73)	Non-ES Group (n = 93)
Timing of drainage[a]		
Urgent	47 (64%)	65 (70%)
Early	26 (36%)	28 (30%)
Successful placement	69 (95%)	89 (96%)
Effective drainage	67 (92%)	87 (94%)
Complications	8 (11%)	2 (2%)[b]
Acute pancreatitis	1 (1%)	1 (1%)
Hemorrhage	3 (4%)	0[b]
Acute cholecystitis	3 (4%)	0[b]
Withdrawal of catheter	1 (1%)	1 (1%)
Perforation	0	0
Death	0	0

[a] Urgent drainage, performed within 72 hours of the onset of cholangitis; early drainage, performed between 72 hours and 7 days.
[b] $P < 0.05$ vs ES group.

Reproduced by permission from Sugiyama M, Yutaka A. The benefits of endoscopic nasobiliary drainage without sphincterotomy for acute cholangitis. Am J Gastroenterol 1998;93:2065–8.

presented initially with shock. Besides the 13% of patients who underwent stone extraction with or without sphincterotomy, 64% of patients had sphincterotomy followed by nasobiliary drain placement, and the remaining 23% of patients had nasobiliary drain placement without sphincterotomy (58).

As seen in the previous study, nasobiliary drainage with sphincterotomy is a simple, safe, and effective treatment for acute cholangitis. The bile duct can be directly cannulated using the nasobiliary tube without going through the tedious exchange process. The small yet significant risk of post-sphincterotomy bleeding can be completely prevented. This procedure is especially useful for patients who are critically ill or severely coagulopathic. This idea was further examined in a retrospective nonrandomized study involving a total of 166 patients suffering from acute cholangitis: 120 with choledocholithiasis, 10 with benign strictures, and 36 with malignancy (59). Although not randomized, the 93 patients in the nonsphincterotomy group were comparable in the major demographic and clinical variables to the 73 patients in the sphincterotomy group. Effective drainage was established in 94% of the nonsphincterotomy group and 92% of the sphincterotomy group. Procedure-related complications occurred in two nonsphincterotomy patients and eight sphincterotomy patients. No mortality was observed (Table 15.5).

The nasobiliary drain carries several advantages and disadvantages. It provides a continuous external access to the biliary system, allowing for 1) follow-up bile fluid collection, 2) intermittent irrigation, 3) further cholangiographic imaging, and 4) instillation of solvent for stone dissolution. However, it causes irritation in the patient's nose and throat.

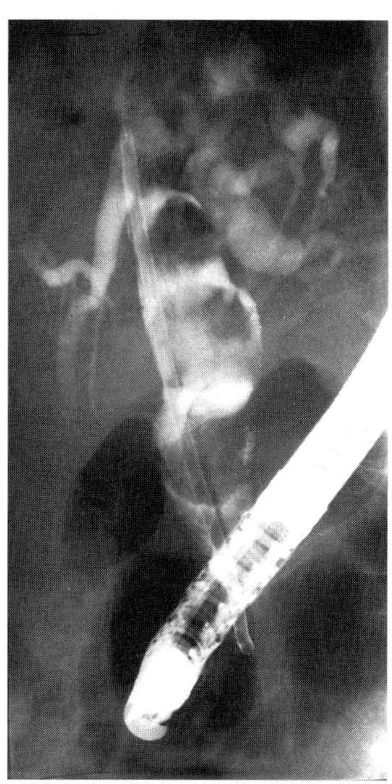

FIGURE 15.4. *Endoscopic stenting for acute cholangitis. The cholangiogram shows a biliary stent and multiple large common bile duct stones.*

It also can be cosmetically unappealing, as the proximal end of the catheter is taped onto the face, and the external collection bag is physically cumbersome. The small-caliber catheter may kink or occlude. The risk of dislodging this life-saving device—either accidentally or intentionally by a confused or uncooperative patient—is a major concern (60).

Insertion of an indwelling biliary stent (61) serves as a valuable medium-term temporizing measure for unstable patients or patients with large common duct stones that cannot be cleared in one single session (Fig. 15.4). An indwelling stent cannot be dislodged manually by the patient, so in a confused or combative patient, it is definitely preferred to nasobiliary tube placement. Among 27 patients who presented with acute cholangitis (62), 7 French biliary endoprosthesis placement was achieved in all cases without sphincterotomy. Complications included one case of early stent occlusion and another case of Dormia basket entrapment during stone extraction. No mortality was observed. Biliary endoprosthesis placement is easy and safe to perform. Its relative disadvantages include 1) a tendency to be blocked by viscous pus in the absence of access for irrigation and 2) the need for a follow-up endoscopy session to remove the stent. It can be removed at the time of subsequent stone extraction.

There are three additional comments that deserve mentioning on nasobiliary tubes and indwelling stents. During endoscopic deployment of the stent, its proximal tip should be placed proximal to the level of obstruction, as confirmed

Table 15.6. Clinical course after surgery or endoscopic biliary drainage in 82 patients with severe acute cholangitis[a]

Variable	Surgical Group (n = 41)	Endoscopic Group (n = 41)
Time to normalization of temperature	38 (22–54) hours	26 (15–36) hours
Time to stabilization of blood pressure	10 (5–15) hours	10 (6–13) hours
Duration of ventilatory support	80 (27–134) hours	47 (19–75)[b] hours
Duration of fasting	80 (55–106) hours	51 (40–63)[b] hours

[a] Values are means, with 95% confidence intervals in parentheses.
[b] $P < 0.05$, for the comparison with the surgery group.

Reprinted by permission of the New England Journal of Medicine, from Lai EC, Mok FP, Tan ES, et al. Endoscopic biliary drainage for severe acute cholangitis. N Engl J Med 1992;326:1582–6.

fluoroscopically and/or endoscopically by effective drainage of purulent bile. When a sphincterotomy is not performed, iatrogenic pancreatitis from occlusion of the pancreatic orifice by stent placement rarely occurs (63). In a large retrospective study of 444 patients with large or difficult choledocholithiasis who underwent endoscopic stenting, a small and yet statistically significant reduction in stone size was observed over a median follow-up period of 63 days (64). This change in stone size was thought to be secondary to 1) mechanical grinding of the stone continuously against the stent, and 2) changes in the bile biochemistry during stenting, thus facilitating stone dissolution.

In the scenario of a difficult cannulation, the endoscopist is confronted with the dilemma of whether to persist or to resort to other means of biliary decompression, including PTBD and surgical sphincteroplasty or exploration of the CBD. In a study of needle-knife precut sphincterotomy for calculous cholangitis due to ampullary stone impaction, cannulation was achieved in 95% of the 20 cases. The last patient who failed ERCP underwent surgery. However, four patients developed mild post-sphincterotomy bleeding, which was immediately controlled by an epinephrine injection. In three of the four patients who bled, stone extraction was not feasible at the time and a nasobiliary catheter was placed for temporary drainage. No perforation, clinical pancreatitis, or iatrogenic cholangitis occurred. Eventually stone extraction and ductal clearance were accomplished in all but one patient. A word of caution is that, since precut sphincterotomy is performed with a free wire, control over the wire is more difficult compared to a standard sphincterotome (65). Previous literature did report significant morbidity and mortality (66–68).

The result of successful endoscopic biliary drainage is dramatic and gratifying. The patient may feel an almost immediate amelioration of pain when the intrabiliary pressure is reduced (69). Over the next 24 to 48 hours, defervescence occurs with appropriate antibiotic therapy, along with resolution of delirium and bile clearance. The patient becomes ambulant a few hours after the procedure and can resume an oral diet very soon thereafter. Several papers demonstrate that the outcome following endoscopic drainage is far superior to that of surgery. A retrospective study on acute cholangitis comparing endoscopic sphincterotomy with surgical or medical treatment showed a 30-day mortality of 4.7%, 21.4%, and 36.4%, respectively. This was a significant difference, considering that the patients in the endoscopic group were comparatively much older and sicker.

The superiority of endoscopic drainage was subsequently confirmed in a prospective, randomized, controlled trial of 82 patients with severe acute cholangitis secondary to choledocholithiasis (70). These patients were randomized to undergo either 1) sphincterotomy and nasobiliary drainage under conscious sedation or 2) urgent diagnostic ERCP followed by exploratory laparotomy under general anesthesia. Half of them presented initially with shock and positive blood cultures. Both groups stabilized and defervesced one day after the procedure. However, more patients in the surgical group required ventilatory support for a longer duration. The hospital mortality rates were 10% and 32%, respectively (Table 15.6). A more recent study, retrospectively done on 27 patients with acute cholangitis secondary to choledocholithiasis, demonstrated similar mortality rates of 5% and 33%, respectively (71).

After acute cholangitis is stabilized, further definitive therapy can be planned according to the general condition of the patient and the underlying obstructing pathologies. This follow-up treatment should not take place until after a full week of antibiotics. In a relatively young patient with suitable anatomy, curative therapy might entail endoscopic sphincterotomy, lithotripsy, and stone extraction. For high-risk, debilitated patients who failed stone extraction during the initial urgent endoscopy session, long-term indwelling stent placement may be the only feasible option (72,73). For patients who suffer from recurrent pyogenic cholangitis, the definitive management is a multidisciplinary approach and may encompass endoscopic balloon dilatation of a biliary stricture, biliary stenting, and stone extraction (69); percutaneous transhepatic cholangioscopy (74); surgical choledochoscopy (75), and postsurgical T-tube tract cholangioscopy (76); various forms of mechanical, extracorporeal shockwave

(77,78), and laser lithotripsy (79,80); hepatic resection (81); and creation of a cutaneous hepaticojejunostomy (81a). The interested reader is referred to more comprehensive reviews on the subject of hepatolithiasis (45).

On the other hand, for patients who do not respond promptly to the initial endoscopic drainage, the following possibilities should be entertained and excluded: 1) the presence of undrained hepatic segments, especially in cases of malignant hilar obstruction or recurrent pyogenic cholangitis, 2) coexisting acute cholecystitis, and 3) cholangitic abscesses (37). In these scenarios, it is necessary to resort to PTBD and/or surgical drainage.

Percutaneous Transhepatic Biliary Drainage

The percutaneous transhepatic access to the biliary tract is performed under local anesthesia by using a Chiba fine needle. Under ultrasound or fluoroscopic guidance, multiple passes are made until a dilated bile duct is entered. A guidewire is then introduced. After dilating up the percutaneous tract, a biliary catheter is then advanced over the guidewire for external drainage. Success rates of PTBD range from 80% to 100% (82–84). Similar to endoscopic decompression, PTBD only offers temporary relief for the acute cholangitis. When the patient becomes stabilized, more definitive therapy is necessary to correct the underlying obstructive lesion.

PTBD is associated with multiple adverse events, including hemobilia, intra-abdominal bleeding, bile leak, biliary-vascular fistula, and catheter-related sepsis. Septic bile peritonitis may occur as a result of puncturing an infected and distended bile duct segment. Patients with underlying cirrhosis, coagulopathy, and ascites are particularly susceptible to complications. With the use of fine needles, the mortality rate of PTBD is reduced to below 5% (85).

Surgical Drainage

Surgical drainage for acute cholangitis is indicated when ERCP and PTBD are unsuccessful or unavailable. The procedure consists of CBD exploration and placement of a large-caliber T-tube. Other surgical options include surgical sphincteroplasty, bile duct resection, or bypass with a bilioenteric anastomosis. Biliary decompression is the major concern. Any attempt to achieve ductal clearance at the expense of prolonged instrumentation should be prohibited. A follow-up choledochoscopy in the postoperative period can be performed to remove any residual stone.

Historically, surgical drainage was the classic method for biliary decompression. However, it does carry formidable postoperative morbidity and mortality rates. Among 86 patients with acute cholangitis who underwent emergent surgery, five risk factors were identified (86):

1. concomitant medical problems
2. arterial blood pH <7.4
3. total serum bilirubin level >90 μmol/L
4. platelet count <150 × 10^9/L
5. serum albumin concentration <30 g/L

In the presence of three or more risk factors, postoperative morbidity and mortality rates were 91% and 55%, respectively. In contrast, the corresponding rates were 34% and 6%, respectively, in those patients with two or fewer risk factors. Endoscopic drainage came out as a superior alternative in the acute setting, with a significantly reduced morbidity and mortality (70,71). PTBD, however, has not been carefully studied to compare its efficacy against surgery. Some institutions still prefer a surgical approach to PTBD once therapeutic endoscopy has failed (87).

CONCLUSION

The management of acute cholangitis begins with early recognition of the condition, followed by aggressive antibiotic coverage. Approximately 80% of patients will improve with conservative management. For the remaining 20% of patients who continue to deteriorate despite antibiotics, urgent biliary drainage is required. Emphasis is placed on reducing the biliary pressure effectively by a safe and expeditious method, rather than on eliminating the underlying obstructive pathology. With its significant reductions in morbidity and mortality in clinical trials, therapeutic endoscopy stands out as the method of choice for biliary decompression. When endoscopic drainage is unavailable or unsuccessful, then PTBD and surgery should be contemplated. Immediate surgical drainage, with its formidable mortality and morbidity rates, is now considered the last resort. PTBD has yet to be carefully studied to compare its efficacy against surgery. Once acute cholangitis is stabilized, a detailed treatment plan can be carried out electively to remove the underlying obstruction.

REFERENCES

1. Schonfield LJ, Carey MC, Marks JW, et al. Gallstone: an update. Am J Gastroenterol 1989;84:999–1007.
2. Stock FE, Fung JH. Oriental cholangiohepatitis. Arch Surg 1962;84:409–12.
3. Ker CG, Huang TJ, Sheen PC. Intrahepatic stones: etiological study. Taiwan I Hseuh Hui Chih 1981;80:698–711.
4. Cheung KL, Lai EC. The management of intrahepatic stones. Adv Surg 1996;29:111–29.
5. Fung J. Liver fluke infestation and cholangiohepatitis. Br J Surg 1961;48:404–15.
6. Ong GB. A study of recurrent pyogenic cholangitis. Arch Surg 1962;84:199–225.
7. Teoh TB. A study of gallstones and worms in recurrent pyogenic cholangitis. J Pathol Bacteriol 1963;86:123–9.
8. Maki T. Cholelithiasis in the Japanese. Arch Surg 1961;82:599–612.
9. Maki T. Pathogenesis of calcium bilirubinate gallstones: role of E. coli, β-glucuronidase and coagulation by inorganic ions, polyelectrolytes and agitation. Ann Surg 1966;164:90–100.
10. Seel DJ, Park YK. Oriental infestational cholangitis. Am J Surg 1983;146:366–70.
11. Boey JH, Way LW. Acute cholangitis. Ann Surg 1980;191:264–70.
12. Csendes A, Diaz JC, Burdiles P, et al. Mirizzi syndrome and cholecystobiliary fistula: a unifying classification. Br J Surg 1989;76:1139–43.

13. Hanau LH, Steigbigel NH. Cholangitis: pathogenesis, diagnosis and treatment. Curr Clin Top Infect Dis 1995;15:153–78.
14. Csendes A, Fernandez M, Uribe P. Bacteriology of the gallbladder bile in normal subjects. Am J Surg 1975;129:629–31.
15. Sung JY, Leung JW, Olson ME, et al. Demonstration of transient bacteriobilia by foreign body implantation in the feline biliary tract. Dig Dis Sci 1991;36:943–8.
16. Sung JY, Shaffer EA, Olson ME, et al. Bacterial invasion of the biliary system by way of the portal-venous system. Hepatology 1991;142:313–17.
17. Sung JY, Costerton JW, Shaffer EA. Defense system in the biliary tract against bacterial infection. Dig Dis Sci 1992;37:689–96.
18. Sung JY, Leung JW, Shaffer EA, et al. Ascending infection of the biliary tract after surgical sphincterotomy and biliary stenting. J Gastroenterol Hepatol 1992;7:240–5.
19. Yu JL, Ljungh A. Infections associated with biliary drains. Scand J Gastroenterol 1996;31:625–30.
20. Raper SE, Barker ME, Jones AL, et al. Anatomic correlates of bacterial cholangiovenous reflux. Surgery 1989;105:352–9.
21. Huang T, Bass JA, Williams RD. The significance of biliary pressure in cholangitis. Arch Surg 1969;98:629–32.
22. Csendes A, Sepulveda A, Burdiles P, et al. Common bile duct pressure in patients with common bile duct stones with or without acute suppurative cholangitis. Arch Surg 1988;123:697–9.
23. Ohshio G, Manabe T, Tamura K, et al. Effects of percutaneous transhepatic biliary drainage in blood-bile permeability and selective IgA transport in patients with biliary obstruction. Ann Surg 1990;211:428–32.
24. Lygadakis NJ, Brummelkamp WH. The significance of intrabiliary pressure in acute cholangitis. Surg Gynecol Obstet 1985;161:465–9.
25. Yoshimoto H, Ikeda S, Tanaka M, Matsumoto S. Relationship of biliary pressure to cholangiovenous reflux during endoscopic retrograde balloon catheter cholangiography. Dig Dis Sci 1989;34:16–20.
26. Lau JY, Ip SM, Chung SC, et al. Endoscopic drainage aborts endotoxemia in acute cholangitis. Br J Surg 1996;83:181–4.
27. Sung JY, Leung JC, Tsui CP, et al. Biliary IgA secretion in obstructive jaundice: the effects of endoscopic drainage. Gastrointest Endosc 1995;42:439–44.
28. Muller EL, Pitt HA, Thompson JE, et al. Antibiotics in infections of the biliary tract. Surg Gynecol Obstet 1987;1654:285–92.
29. Leung JW, Sung JY, Costerton JW. Bacteriological and electron microscopy examination of brown pigment stones. J Clin Microbiol 1989;27:915–21.
30. Brook I. Aerobic and anaerobic microbiology of biliary tract disease. J Clin Microbiol 1989;27:2373–5.
31. Thompson JE, Pitt HA, Doty JE, et al. Broad-spectrum penicillin as an adequate therapy for acute cholangitis. Surg Gynecol Obstet 1990;171:275–82.
32. Leung JW, Ling TK, Chan RC, et al. Antibiotics, biliary sepsis, and bile duct stones. Gastrointest Endosc 1994;40:716–21.
33. Allen JI, Allen MO, Olson MM, et al. *Pseudomonas* infection of the biliary system resulting from use of a contaminated endoscope. Gastroenterology 1987;92:759–63.
34. Classen DC, Jacobson JA, Burke JP, et al. Serious *Pseudomonas* infections associated with endoscopic retrograde cholangiopancreatography. Am J Med 1988;84:590–6.
35. Levine GJ, Botet J, Kurtz RC. Microbiological analysis of sepsis complicating non-surgical biliary drainage in malignant obstruction. Gastrointest Endosc 1990;36:364–8.
36. Charcot JM. Leçons sur les maladies du foie, des voies biliaires et des reins. Paris: Faculté de Médecine de Paris, 1877.
37. Lee DW, Chung SC. Biliary infection. Bailliere's Clin Gastroentrol 1997;11:707–24.
38. Sinanan MN. Acute cholangitis. Infect Dis Clin North Am 1992;6:571–99.
38a. Reynolds BM, Dargan EL. Acute obstructive cholangitis: a distinct clinical syndrome. Ann Surg 1959;150:299–303.
39. Lai EC, Chu KM, Ngan H. Acute cholangitis. In: Pitt HA, Carr-Locke DL, Ferrucci JT, eds. Hepatobiliary and pancreatic disease: the team approach to management. Boston: Little, Brown, 1995:229–38.
40. Chou ST, Chan CW. Recurrent pyogenic cholangitis: a necropsy study. Pathology 1980;12:415–28.
41. Chijiiwa K, Ichimiya H, Kuroki S, et al. Late development of cholangiocarcinoma after the treatment of hepatolithiasis. Surg Gynecol Obstet 1993;177:279–82.
42. Gigot JF, Leese T, Dereme T, et al. Acute cholangitis. Multivariate analysis of risk factors. Ann Surg 1988;209:435–8.
43. Abbruzzese A, Jeffrey RL. Marked elevations of serum glutamic oxaloacetic transaminase and lactic dehydrogenase activity in chronic extrahepatic biliary disease. Am J Dig Dis 1969;14:332–8.
44. Leung JW, Yu AS. Update on cholangiocarcinoma. In: Syllabus book: American Society for Gastrointestinal Endoscopy 14th Interim Postgraduate Course 73–78, 1998.
45. Leung JW, Yu AS. Hepatolithiasis and biliary parasites. Bailliere's Clin Gastroentrol 1997;11:681–706.
46. Liessi G, Cesari S, Dell'Antonio C, et al. Cholangiopancreatography with magnetic resonance. Clinical use of a new "inversion-recovery" sequence. Radiol Med 1996;92:252–6.
47. Pavone P, Laghi A, Catalano C, et al. Biliary-enteric anastomosis: role of cholangiography with magnetic resonance. Radiol Med 1996;92:247–51.
48. Chan YL, Chan AC, Lam WW, et al. Choledocholithiasis: comparison of MR cholangiography and endoscopic retrograde cholangiography. Radiology 1996;200:85–9.
49. Barish MA, Soto JA, Yucel EK. Magnetic resonance cholangiopancreatography of the biliary ducts: techniques, clinical applications, and limitations. Top Magn Reson Imaging 1996;8:302–11.
50. Leung JW, Venezuela RR. Cholangiosepsis: endoscopic drainage and antibiotic therapy. Endoscopy 1991;23:220–3.
51. Wise R, Gillet AP, Andrews JM, et al. Activity of azlocillin and mezlocillin against gram-positive organisms: comparison with other penicillins. J Antimicrob Chemother 1982;9(suppl A):1–9.
52. Gerecht WB, Henry NK, Hoffman WW, et al. Prospective randomized comparison of mezlocillin therapy alone and combined ampicillin and gentamicin therapy for patients with cholangitis. Arch Intern Med 1989;149:1279–84.
53. Giron A, Meyers BR, Hirschmann SZ. Biliary concentrations of piperacillin in patients undergoing cholecystectomy. Antimicrob Agents Chemother 1981;19:309–11.
54. Leung JW, Chan RC, Cheung SW, et al. The effect of obstruction on the biliary excretion of cefoperazone and ceftazidime. J Antimicrob Chemother 1990;25:399–406.
55. Leung JW, Chan CY, Lai CW, et al. Effect of biliary obstruction on the hepatic excretion of imipenem-cilastatin. Antimicrob Agents Chemother 1992;36:2057–60.
56. Sung JY, Lyon DJ, Suen R, et al. Intravenous ciprofloxacin as treatment for patients with acute suppurative cholangitis: a randomized, controlled clinical trial. J Antimicrob Chemother 1995;35:855–64.
57. Desai TK, Tsang TK. Aminoglycosides nephrotoxicity in obstructive jaundice. Am J Med 1988;85:47–50.
58. Leung JW, Chung SC, Sung JY, et al. Urgent endoscopic drainage for acute suppurative cholangitis. Lancet 1989;1:1037–9.
59. Sugiyama M, Yutaka A. The benefits of endoscopic nasobiliary drainage without sphincterotomy for acute cholangitis. Am J Gastroenterol 1998;93:2065–8.
60. Leung JW, Cotton PB. Endoscopic nasobiliary catheter drainage in biliary and pancreatic disease. Am J Gastroenterol 1991;86:389–94.
61. Soehendra N, Reynders-Frederix V. Palliative bile duct drainage—a new endoscopic method of introducing a transpapillary drain. Endoscopy 1980;12:8–11.
62. Misra SP, Dwivedi M. Biliary endoprosthesis as an alternative to endoscopic nasobiliary drainage in patients with acute cholangitis. Endoscopy 1996;28:746–9.
63. Huibregtse K, Tytgat GNJ. Palliative treatment of obstructive jaundice by transpapillary introduction of large bore bile duct endoprosthesis. Gut 1982;23:371–5.
64. Chan AC, Ng EK, Chung SC, et al. Common bile duct stones become smaller after endoscopic biliary stenting. Endoscopy 1989;30:356–9.
65. Leung JW, Banez VP, Chung SC. Precut (needle knife) papillotomy for impacted common bile duct stone at the ampulla. Am J Gastroenterol 1990;85:991–3.
66. Sloof M, Baker R, Lavelle MI, et al. What is involved in endoscopic sphincterotomy for gallstones? Br J Surg 1980;67:18–21.
67. Passi RB, Raval B. Endoscopic papillotomy. Surgery 1982;92:581–8.
68. Booth F, Doerr R, Khalafi F, et al. Surgical management of complications of endoscopic sphincterotomy with precut papillotomy. Am J Surg 1990;159:132–5.
69. Leung JW, Venezuela RR, Banez VP, et al. Endoscopic management of intrahepatic stones. Gastrointest Endosc 1991;35:226–31.
70. Lai EC, Mok FP, Tan ES, et al. Endoscopic biliary drainage for severe acute cholangitis. N Engl J Med 1992;326:1582–6.
71. Chijiiwa K, Kozaki N, Naito T, et al. Treatment of choice for choledocholithiasis in patients with acute obstructive suppurative cholangitis and liver cirrhosis. Am J Surg 1995;170:356–60.
72. Cotton PB, Forbes A, Leung WC, et al. Endoscopic stenting for long-term treatment of large bile duct stones: 2- to 5-year follow-up. Gastrointest Endosc 1987;33:411–13.

73. Chen JH, Yang KC, Liu YH, et al. Clinical experience with endoscopic stents for treatment of common bile duct stones. J Formos Med Assoc 1999;98:128–32.
74. Yeh YH, Huang MH, Yang JC, et al. Percutaneous transhepatic cholangioscopy and lithotripsy in the treatment of intrahepatic stones: a study with 5 year follow-up. Gastrointest Endosc 1995;42:13–18.
75. Choi S, Choi TK, Wong J. Intraoperative flexible choledochoscopy for intrahepatic and extrahepatic biliary calculi. Surgery 1987;101:571–6.
76. Fan ST, Choi TK, Lo CM. Treatment of hepatolithiasis: improvement of result by a systemic approach. Surgery 1991;109:474–80.
77. Binmoeller KF, Bruckner M, Thonke F, et al. Treatment of difficult bile duct stones using mechanical, electrohydraulic and extracorporeal shock wave lithotripsy. Endoscopy 1993;25:201–6.
78. Dagenais M, Lapointe R, Dery R, et al. Role of extracorporeal shock wave lithotripsy in the treatment of common bile duct and intrahepatic calculi. Ann Chir 1995;49:659–63.
79. Jakobs R, Maier M, Kohler B, et al. Peroral laser lithotripsy of difficult intrahepatic and extrahepatic bile duct stones: laser effectiveness using an automatic stone-tissue discriminator system. Am J Gastroenterol 1996;91:468–73.
80. Brambs HJ, Duda SH, Rieber A, et al. Treatment of bile duct stones: value of laser lithotripsy delivered via percutaneous endoscopy. Eur Radiol 1996;6:734–40.
81. Chijiiwa K, Kameoka N, Komura M, et al. Hepatic resection for hepatolithiasis and long-term results. J Am Coll Surg 1995;180:43–8.
81a. Stain SC, Incarbone R, Guthrie CR, et al. Surgical treatment of recurrent pyogenic cholangitis. Arch Surg 1995;130:527–32.
82. Chen MF, Jan YY, Lee TY. Percutaneous transhepatic biliary drainage for acute cholangitis. Int Surg 1987;72:131–3.
83. Pessa ME, Hawkins IF, Vogel SB. The treatment of acute cholangitis. Percutaneous transhepatic biliary drainage before definitive therapy. Ann Surg 1987;205:389–92.
84. Sirinek KR, Levine BA. Percutaneous transhepatic cholangiography and biliary decompression. Invasive, diagnostic, and therapeutic procedures with too high a price? Arch Surg 1989;124:885–8.
85. Mueller PR, van Sonnenberg E, Simeone JF. Fine-needle transhepatic cholangiography. Indications and usefulness. Ann Intern Med 1982;97:567–72.
86. Lai EC, Tam PC, Paterson IA, et al. Emergency surgery for severe acute cholangitis: the high-risk patients. Ann Surg 1990;211:55–9.
87. Köksal R, Lo SK. Pyogenic cholangitis. In: Brandt L, ed. Clinical practice of gastroenterology. Philadelphia: Saunders, 1999:1079–88.

Chapter

16

Cystic Diseases of the Biliary System

ROBERT J. PORTE PIERRE-ALAIN CLAVIEN

Cystic lesions of the bile ducts and liver can result from a variety of pathologic processes. They occur as solitary or multiple. Cystic abnormalities occurring within the liver parenchyma that are not in continuity with the biliary tree are referred to as liver cysts. Cystic lesions that are in direct continuity with the bile ducts are considered as biliary duct cysts. The aim of this chapter is primarily to focus on cystic lesions of the bile duct, which are characterized by an epithelial lining. However, because of the assumed common pathogenesis of these biliary duct lesions and the noncommunicating liver cysts, the latter will be discussed in this chapter as well. Cystic lesions of the liver with an infectious origin (e.g., echinococcus or hydatid cysts, liver abscesses) and pseudocysts are outside the scope of this chapter and are not discussed.

Cysts of the liver and bile ducts can occur as single entities, but are frequently found in various combinations of intrahepatic or extrahepatic cystic abnormalities. The heterogenicity of these lesions has led to problems in classification and nomenclature in the past. More recently, the majority of the cystic lesions of the liver or intrahepatic bile ducts are considered as part of one family of congenital disorders, characterized by persistence or lack of remodeling of the embryonic ductal plate (1). The ductal plate is a layer of cells surrounding the portal vein branches that develops during the first weeks of gestation. After subsequent remodeling and partial involution, the biliary ducts are formed out of the ductal plate. The various intrahepatic cystic disorders most likely reflect abnormalities at different levels of the ductal plate. Although cystic abnormalities of the extrahepatic bile ducts are historically classified as acquired entities, more recent evidence raised the possibility of a common congenital origin involving embryologic malformation (2,3). Furthermore, combinations of cystic abnormalities of both intrahepatic and extrahepatic bile ducts may occur in one patient, which supports the theory of a common pathogenesis (2,4).

In general, true or epithelialized liver and biliary cysts can be divided into two groups: a neoplastic and a non-neoplastic group. The neoplastic group primarily comprises biliary cystadenoma and cystadenocarcinoma, which are discussed in the second part of this chapter. The non-neoplastic group can be subdivided in sporadic cysts and cysts associated with embryonic ductal plate abnormalities, also known as fibropolycystic diseases (Table 16.1).

SPORADIC HEPATIC CYSTS

Simple Cysts

Simple hepatic cysts are also known as benign, nonparasitic, or solitary cysts; the latter is a poor name, as these are multiple in 50% of the cases. These cysts are usually considered as rare lesions, although they have been found after careful examination in 1% to 2% of autopsy studies (5). The exact pathogenesis of simple hepatic cysts is unknown, but it has been suggested that they develop from biliary microhamartoma or aberrant bile ducts that have lost contact with other parts of the biliary system during the early embryological stages (6). Although simple hepatic cysts are usually not classified as part of the ductal plate malformations or fibropolycystic diseases, one could argue that they represent isolated manifestations of embryonic remnants of the ductal plate. This hypothesis, as well as the differential diagnosis with other types of hepatic and biliary cystic disorders, justifies a discussion of simple hepatic cysts in this chapter, despite their lack of direct continuity with the biliary tree.

Simple cysts can be found at all ages, although the prevalence increases with increasing age and women are more often affected than men. Most cysts have a round or oval shape and size can vary from a few millimeters to more than 30 cm (6). They are usually asymptomatic and coincidentally found during ultrasound examination of the abdomen for unrelated symptoms or conditions. Occasionally large cysts can cause vague upper abdominal complaints and/or compression of the gastrointestinal tract with (partial) obstruction. Large cysts in the hepatic hilum can cause compression of the hepatic duct or portal vein, causing obstructive jaundice or portal hypertension (7–9). Acute abdominal pain can result from rupture or bleeding into the cyst. Depending on the size and localization within the liver, cysts can sometimes be found at physical examination. Serum values of the hepatic enzymes may be increased, but are usually within the normal range (6).

Table 16.1. Classification of hepatic and biliary cysts

Non-neoplastic
Sporadic
Simple cysts
Periductal hilar cysts
Fibropolycystic Diseases
Autosomal recessive polycystic disease/congenital hepatic fibrosis
Autosomal dominant polycystic disease
Caroli's disease
Choledochal cysts
Neoplastic
Biliary cystadenoma
Biliary cystadenocarcinoma

Histologically, the inner cystic lining is formed by a single layer of cuboidal or columnar epithelium that resembles biliary epithelium (6). The cystic fluid is usually clear yellow and serous, but may appear bloody or purulent under some circumstances. The presence of numerous microhamartomas in the surrounding liver or the combination of multiple cysts should raise the possibility of autosomal dominant polycystic disease (1). Malignant degeneration, either to squamous cell carcinoma, adenocarcinoma, or a mixed type, is a very rare but serious complication (10–12).

The diagnosis of simple cysts is usually made by ultrasonography or computer tomography (5). Differentiation from abscesses, hematomas, and solid tumors is not difficult when using these radiological techniques (Fig. 16.1). The differentiation between simple cysts and echinococcal (hydatid) cysts can be somewhat more difficult, although simple cysts are always unilocular and never have calcifications, whereas echinococcal cysts usually are septated and frequently have calcifications in the wall (13). Serological studies will be helpful in this situation. Cysts with irregularities of the cystic wall or papillary projections into the cystic cavity should raise a very high suspicion for cystadenoma or cystadenocarcinoma. In these cases, CA 19-9 serum concentrations are usually elevated, which is not the case for simple cysts (14). Occasionally, metastasis from other tumors can present as cystic lesions due to central necrosis and cavity formation (5).

Treatment is not indicated in case of asymptomatic simple cysts. For symptomatic cysts different approaches have been described. Simple percutaneous puncture and aspiration of the cystic content is not effective, as it is immedi-

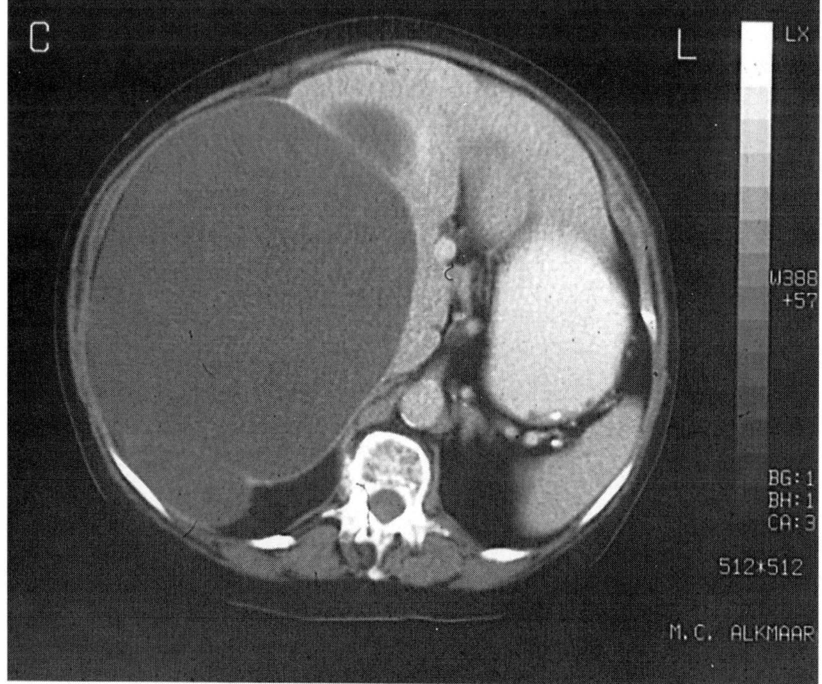

FIGURE 16.1. *Computer tomography of the upper abdomen showing a simple cyst in an otherwise normal liver.*

ately followed by refilling of the cysts (15). Percutaneous aspiration of the cyst followed by the injection of a sclerosing agent (95% alcohol or minocycline) has a higher success rate of up to 70% (16,17). However, for a long-term success, repeated procedures are usually required, which carry the risk of infection or sclerosing cholangitis (18). The use of alcohol can be complicated by pain, fever, or alcoholic intoxication. Laparoscopic unroofing of the external part of the cyst, followed by transposition of an omental flap into the remaining cyst cavity, is currently considered to be the treatment of choice for symptomatic cysts (8,19). However, experience with this technique is still limited and long-term follow-up data are not available yet. Open surgery is indicated when cysts cannot be approached laparoscopically (e.g., the posterior segments VI and VII, and segment IVa), or when a potentially malignant disease cannot be excluded (8). If aspiration of the cystic contents, with precautions to avoid contamination of the abdominal cavity, provides evidence for a malignancy, a partial liver resection is indicated (20).

Multiple Periductal Cysts

Small cystic lesions of 1 to 2 mm are incidentally found within Glisson's capsule along the large intrahepatic or extrahepatic bile ducts. These rare cystic lesions have been referred to as mucinous hamartoma or periductal cysts (21,22). They usually occur in chronically diseased livers, but isolated presentations in otherwise normal livers have been reported as well (23). Occasionally they are found in transplanted livers and are a cause of obstructive jaundice after liver transplantation (24). The cysts contain watery or mucoid material and have been considered as retention cysts, resulting from obstructed periductal glands. The inner lining is constituted of a mucinous epithelial lining and cysts are surrounded by a mild chronic inflammatory reaction. Although they are most frequently found in patients with severe chronic liver disease and portal hypertension, periductal cysts are usually asymptomatic and are an incidental finding at autopsy (21). When they occur in an otherwise normal liver and cause biliary obstruction, differentiation from a malignancy can be difficult and resection of the affected part of the liver can be indicated (23).

FIBROPOLYCYSTIC DISEASES OF THE LIVER

The group of fibropolycystic diseases is considered to be part of the larger family of ductal plate malformations, and includes various disorders characterized by malformation and dilatation of the bile ducts and a variable degree of fibrosis (1). The level at which malformations in the ductal plate develop is believed to determine the clinical disorder and symptoms: congenital liver fibrosis and autosomal recessive polycystic disease (small intrahepatic bile ducts), autosomal dominant polycystic disease (intermediate intrahepatic bile ducts), Caroli's syndrome (large intrahepatic bile ducts), and choledochal cyst (extrahepatic bile duct) (1,25). In case of the latter, the association with ductal plate malformations is less clear and other mechanisms have been proposed as well (see below). In addition to this, bile duct microhamartomas or von Meyenburg complexes are considered to be part of this group of ductal plate malformation disorders (1). These small and often multiple lesions can be incidentally found in otherwise normal livers or in association with polycystic disease or congenital hepatic fibrosis. Isolated bile duct microhamartomas are mostly asymptomatic and of no clinical relevance.

Autosomal Recessive Polycystic Disease/Congenital Hepatic Fibrosis

Autosomal recessive polycystic disease (also known as infantile polycystic disease) and congenital hepatic fibrosis are often seen in combination. It has been debated whether these entities are two distinct disorders or are a different expression of the same underlying developmental disorder at the level of the intermediate or small intrahepatic bile ducts (1,26). Both conditions are frequently associated not only with other liver malformations, such as Caroli's disease and von Meyenburg complexes, but also with renal dysgenesis such as polycystic renal disease, renal dysplasia, or nephronophthisis (27,28). Liver abnormalities are very similar in both clinical entities and are characterized by fibrous enlargements of the portal tracts containing numerous abnormally shaped and ectatic bile ducts. Macroscopically visible cysts are usually not present in the liver (1).

Which term is used in an individual patient mostly depends on the amount of renal involvement. The term *autosomal recessive polycystic disease* is preserved for those cases with renal involvement as the most prominent feature. Because cystic dilatations are not the main feature of these conditions, a further discussion would be outside the scope of this chapter. A more detailed discussion is found in Chapter 21.

Autosomal Dominant Polycystic Disease

Autosomal dominant polycystic liver disease, also known as adult-type polycystic disease, is characterized by the development of multiple liver cysts during life. Although there is a close association with polycystic renal disease, polycystic liver disease is far less common than its renal counterpart (29–31). The prevalence at autopsy studies is about 0.13% (32). Hepatic cysts are more frequently found with increasing age and in women, especially after multiple pregnancies or the use of drugs containing sex hormones (33). In addition to liver and kidney cysts, patients with this disorder may also develop cysts in different organs such as the pancreas, spleen, ovaries, uterus, testes, thyroid, and mesenterium. Other associated disorders are colon diverticula, vascular aneurysms, and inguinal hernias (33). Polycystic liver disease is considered to result from progressive dilatation of the abnormal ducts in microhamartomas or von Meyenburg complexes, as part of a ductal plate malformation at the level of the small intrahepatic bile ducts (1). These small bile ducts have lost continuity with the remaining bile ducts, which explains the noncommunicating nature of the cysts in polycystic liver disease. On histologic examination the cysts are very similar to simple hepatic cysts. The inner wall is formed by a single layer of more or less cuboidal epithelium that resembles biliary epithelium, and they are surrounded by a thin fibrous wall (34,35).

Polycystic liver disease is usually asymptomatic and an incidental finding. Symptoms occur in 10% to 20% of the patients and usually not before the third decade (29,31). Most symptoms center around the massive hepatomegaly and include upper abdominal pain and discomfort, abdominal distention, and dyspnea. Hepatic function is well preserved in most cases and serum levels of liver enzymes are either normal or only slightly elevated (36). In symptomatic patients the liver can usually be felt on physical examination and may extend downward into the pelvis. Complications may occur from infection, compression, bleeding, or rupture of the cysts. Infection of hepatic cysts occurs in up to 3% of patients with autosomal dominant polycystic disease who have end-stage renal failure, but in less than 1% of such patients before end-stage renal failure (37). Compression of the bile ducts may result in icterus. Isolated cases of compression of the inferior caval vein or portal vein that resulted in an inferior caval syndrome or portal hypertension have been reported (31,38). Malignant degeneration is extremely rare and has been described in a few case reports (39).

Modern radiologic studies, like ultrasonography, computer tomography, or magnetic resonance imaging (MRI) can be helpful in making the diagnosis or defining the cause of complications. Diagnostic puncture and aspiration of the cyst contents will facilitate making the diagnosis when a cyst infection is suspected.

Most patients with polycystic liver disease do not require treatment. When kidney disorders are present, these abnormalities and kidney function (rather than that of the liver) define the long-term prognosis of these patients (29). Treatment of liver cysts is indicated in cases with serious complaints of compression or pain and/or infection (31,40). In similarity with simple liver cysts, decompressing puncture alone does not provide long-term relief of symptoms. Chemical ablation is only indicated when one or two dominant cysts can be held responsible for the symptoms. The indication for surgical interventions is less evident than for simple cysts. Possible options are laparoscopic or open fenestration, partial liver resection, and liver transplantation (41–44). Relief of symptoms is often transient and the long-term effect of most surgical interventions is disappointing. In general, the indication for surgical interventions in polycystic liver disease is limited and it should always be viewed in relationship with the risk of postoperative complications such as infection or massive ascites production. In selected cases with diffuse bilobar polycystic disease and massive hepatomegaly, liver transplantation with or without combined kidney transplantation should be considered (41,45).

Caroli's Disease and Caroli's Syndrome

Caroli's disease is a developmental anomaly characterized by segmental dilatations of the large intrahepatic ducts without an obstructive cause (46,47). Typical for this disease are localized and saccular dilatations of the large bile ducts, resembling a picture of multiple cyst-like structures of varying size. Although this disorder has been historically described as a separate entity, it is now generally considered as part of the ductal plate malformations (1). Two types have been described: a type with bile duct abnormalities alone, and a type with bile duct abnormalities in combination with periportal fibrosis, similar to congenital hepatic fibrosis (1). Based on the combinations of lesions, it has been suggested that in the latter type the developmental malformations have occurred simultaneously at different levels of the ductal plate and the intrahepatic biliary tree. This combined type is also known as Caroli's syndrome and has been reported more frequently than the pure type, or Caroli's disease.

In Caroli's disease, saccular dilatations of the large bile ducts are more frequently seen on the left side of the liver (Fig. 16.2). In 30% to 40% of the cases, abnormalities are confined to one segment or sector of one side of the liver (48). Bilateral abnormalities are more frequently seen in the second type, Caroli's syndrome (49). The abnormal bile ducts are in continuity with the remaining normal bile tree and, therefore, contain bile. Biliary stasis, leading to stone formation, is commonly seen in the dilated ducts and predisposes the patient to the development of recurrent cholangitis and septicemia (47). Other complications include amyloidosis and cholangiocarcinoma, the latter of which is found in 7% to 10% of the patients (48,50).

Caroli's syndrome is associated with renal disorders (i.e., nephrospongiosis and renal cysts) in 30% to 40% of patients (51). Patients with Caroli's disease do not have a higher incidence of renal disorders. Choledochal cysts, however, have been described in combination with both types (3).

The disorder usually becomes symptomatic during childhood or early adult life, although initial symptoms may also be delayed until later ages (49). Males are slightly more affected than females. Typically, the clinical features are related to cholangitis and/or portal hypertension (in case of Caroli's syndrome), and may include recurrent episodes of abdominal pain, chills, and fever (52). Icterus may develop secondary to obstruction of the extrahepatic bile ducts by stones migrated from the intrahepatic ducts. In combination with congenital hepatic fibrosis (Caroli's syndrome), symptoms from portal hypertension such as hematemesis from bleeding esophageal varices usually occur at an earlier age than cholangitis (49). In this situation hepatomegaly and splenomegaly can be found during physical examination,

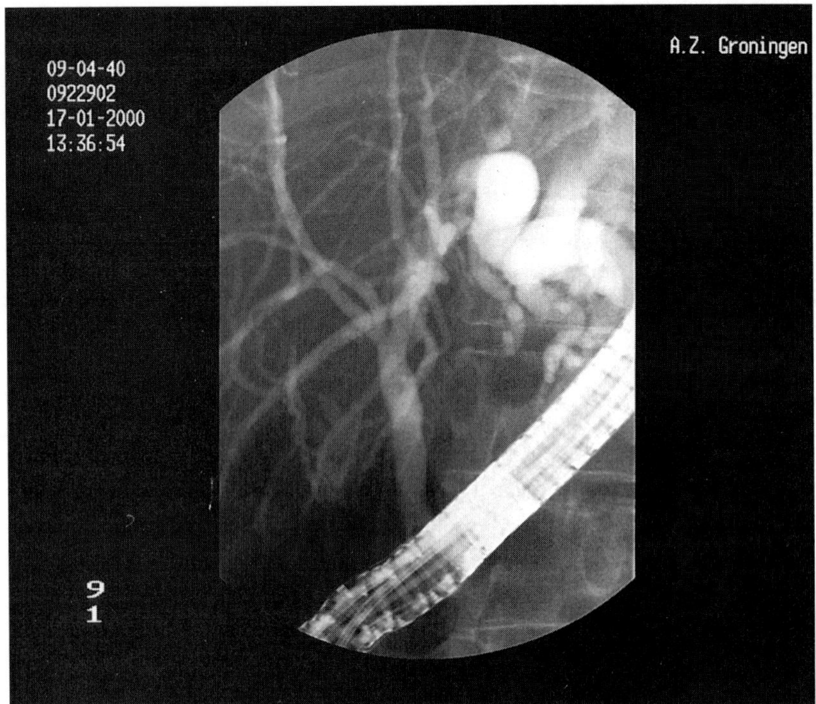

FIGURE 16.2. *Endoscopic retrograde cholangiopancreatography in a patient with cystic dilatations of the left-sided intrahepatic bile ducts (Caroli's disease).*

whereas usually no abnormalities are found on physical examination in patients with Caroli's disease. Abnormal laboratory studies of liver function are usually not found, but will be compatible with obstructive cholestasis in patients with stones in the extrahepatic bile ducts.

The diagnosis is usually made by radiologic studies such as ultrasonography or computer tomography, or by cholangiography during endoscopic retrograde cholangiopancreatography (ERCP) (49,53). Typical findings are saccular or cystically dilated intrahepatic ducts up to 5 cm in diameter, filled with stone material or sludge (see Fig. 16.2). Differential diagnoses include primary sclerosing cholangitis, dilatations secondary to obstruction, and Oriental cholangitis. Primary sclerosing cholangitis can usually be differentiated by the concomitant multiple strictures of the intrahepatic and extrahepatic bile ducts in this disorder (see also Chapter 19) (54). In biliary obstruction due to a malignant tumor along the bile duct, the entire biliary tree proximal to the mass is dilated, including the small peripheral intrahepatic ducts. In Asian populations, differential diagnosis with recurrent pyogenic cholangitis or Oriental cholangitis can be difficult (55). Oriental cholangitis usually occurs at a older age and is associated with a straightening and rigidity of the dilated large ducts, with acute peripheral tapering (see also Chapter 15).

In uncomplicated cases, without signs of cholangitis or obstruction, conservative therapy with observation is indicated. Medical treatment of complicated cases should focus on drainage of the obstructed infected ducts and treatment of the bacterial cholangitis (52). In these cases surgical interventions are usually required to reduce the risk of recurrent cholangitis and formation of secondary biliary cirrhosis or cholangiocarcinoma. Surgical procedures may vary from drainage of the hepatic bifurcation via a hepaticojejunostomy, to a partial liver resection with or without hepaticojejunostomy (48,56). Liver transplantation should be considered in selected patients with generalized disease or with concomitant liver fibrosis and portal hypertension (Caroli's syndrome).

Choledochal Cysts

Choledochal cysts are relatively rare disorders characterized by cystic dilatation of main bile ducts. The first classification, as proposed by Alonso Lej and colleagues in 1959, included three types located in the extrahepatic bile duct (57). This classification was modified by Todani et al. (58) in 1977, who identified two more types and included intrahepatic cystic dilatations of the large bile ducts as found in Caroli's disease (Fig. 16.3). Type 1, a segmental or diffuse dilatation of the common bile duct, is most frequently found, and accounts for 75% to 95% of all cases. Type 2 represents a diverticulum of the common bile duct, whereas type 3 has been identified as a choledochocele of the distal end of the common bile duct, protruding into the duodenum. Type 4 has been recognized as a combination of cysts, either extrahepatic alone (type 4B) or as combination of extrahepatic and intrahepatic (Caroli-like) cysts (type 4A). Multiple cysts of the large intrahepatic ducts (Caroli's disease) were identified as type 5. The cyst wall is thickened and fibrotic, and the mucosa severely inflamed or even absent and replaced by granulation tissue.

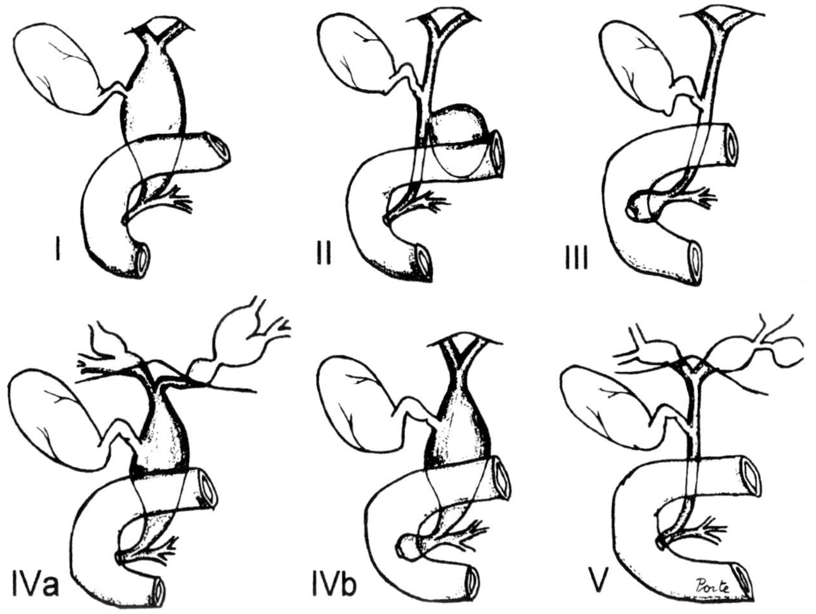

FIGURE 16.3. *Todani's modification of Alonso Lej's classification of choledochal cysts. Types I and II are extrahepatic choledochal cysts; type II is a diverticulum of the common bile duct. Type III is choledochocele of the distal end of the common bile duct. Type IVa is a combination of intrahepatic and extrahepatic cysts, and type IVb is a combination of extrahepatic cysts. Type V represents multiple cysts of the large intrahepatic bile ducts (Caroli's disease).*

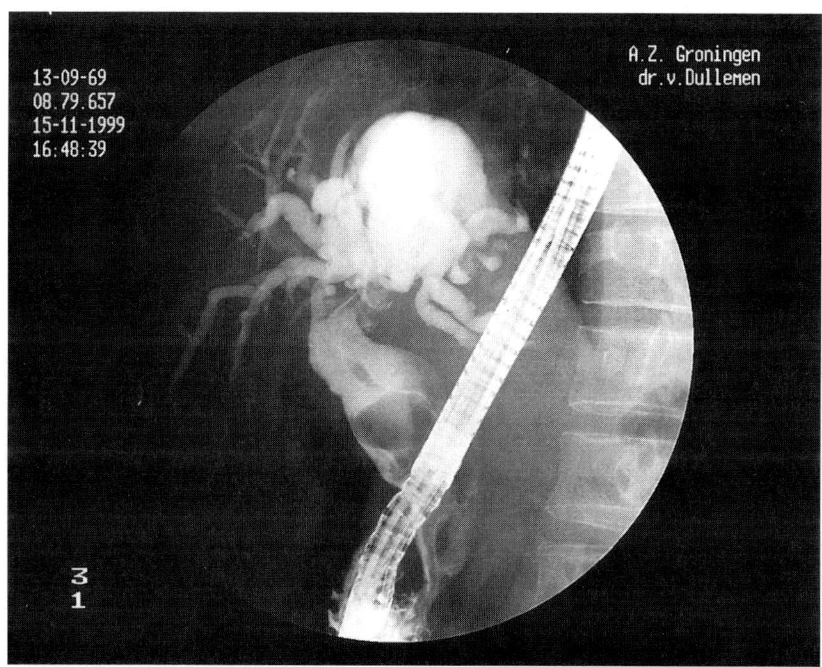

FIGURE 16.4. *Endoscopic retrograde cholangiopancreatography in a patient with cystic dilatation of the common bile duct in combination with left-sided (Caroli-like) cystic dilatations of the intrahepatic bile ducts (type 4A). Sludge and concrements can be seen in the common bile duct.*

About 75% of the choledochal cysts occur in women, and lesions are far more common in the Far East than in Western countries (58,59). The prevalence in the United States is estimated to be about 1 per 13,000 live births (60). The cause of choledochal cysts is unknown, but two different theories have been suggested. In the first theory, choledochal cysts are seen as part of the congenital fibropolycystic diseases, or ductal plate malformations (1,25). This theory is supported by the occasional finding of combinations of intrahepatic and extrahepatic bile disorders, with or without concomitant liver fibrosis (25) (Fig. 16.4). The second theory is based on an anomalous pancreaticobiliary junction, which is seen in up to 85% of the patients with a choledochal cyst (61,62). In this anomaly, which is also known as the "long common channel," the common duct enters the duct of Wirsung abnormally proximal to the ampulla of Vater. It has been suggested that this "long common channel" contributes to reflux of pancreaticobiliary juices into the common bile duct, leading to damage of the wall and subsequent dilatation. Probably both congenital and acquired mechanisms can be involved.

Most choledochal cysts become symptomatic during

childhood (63,64). However, symptoms can be nonspecific, and the diagnosis can be missed until adolescence. The classic clinical triad of symptoms includes intermittent upper abdominal pain, jaundice, and a palpable mass in the right upper quadrant of the abdomen (65). Occasionally, patients remain asymptomatic and the choledochal cyst is incidentally found during ERCP, computer tomography, or magnetic resonance cholangiopancreatography (MRCP) performed for unrelated symptoms. Secondary biliary cirrhosis is a rare complication in untreated patients in whom the diagnosis has been missed for several years (66). In infants, the disorder has to be differentiated from other diagnoses that belong to the group of infantile obstructive cholangiopathies (see Chapter 23). In adults, differentiation with symptomatic bile stone disease usually cannot be made on the clinical symptoms alone (67). The definite diagnosis is usually made by radiologic imaging studies, similar to what was previously discussed for Caroli's disease (59,66).

To treat or prevent complications such as recurrent cholangitis and secondary cirrhosis, surgical treatment is generally indicated (59,68). Another argument for surgical intervention is the risk of malignant degeneration, which has been reported in 2.5% to 30.0% of the patients in different series (68–70). The current treatment of choice is a complete resection of the cyst and a hepaticojejunostomy, with a meticulous mucosa-to-mucosa anastomosis (Fig. 16.5) (63,68,71). Endoscopic unroofing and sphincterotomy of the common bile duct has been successfully performed in patients with symptomatic small choledochoceles (type 3 choledochal cyst) (72). The endoscopist, however, must be aware that an ampullary carcinoma may develop in a choledochocele, and complete surgical excision remains the treatment of choice in cases with large or abnormal looking

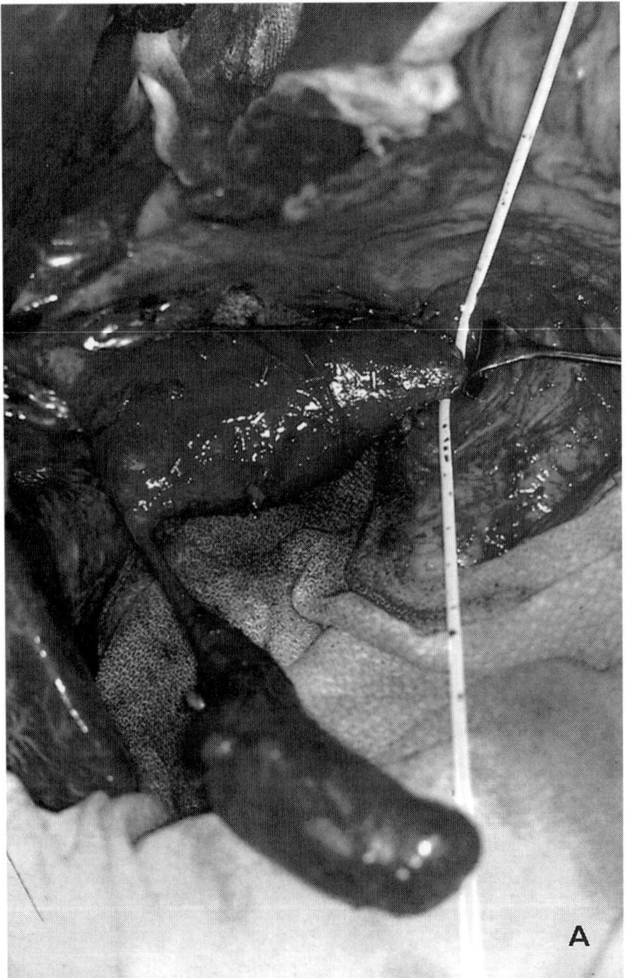

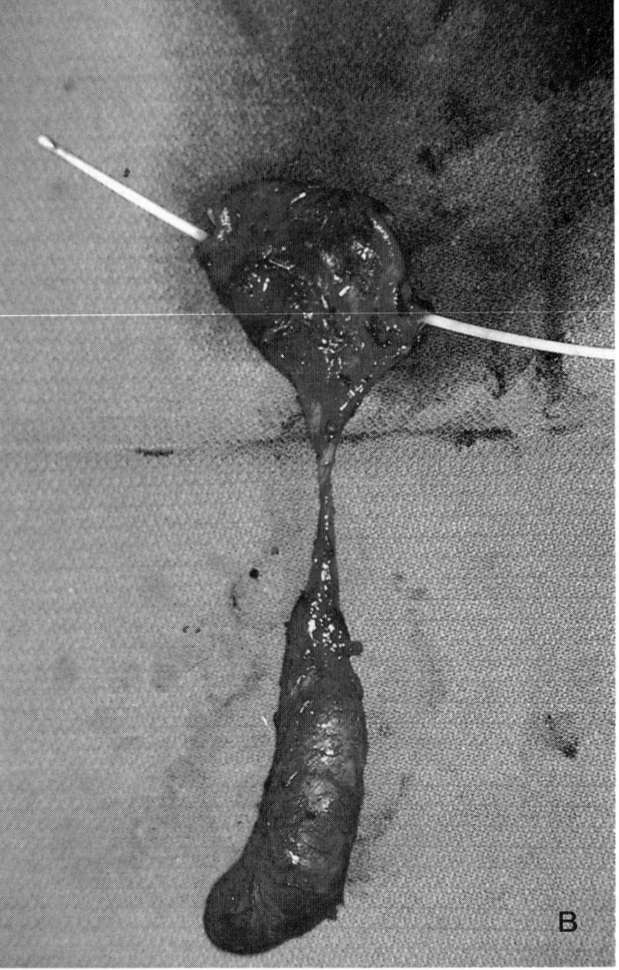

FIGURE 16.5. *Intraoperative views of a choledochal cyst (type 1) with the dissected gallbladder still attached. The cystic duct enters the common bile duct at the level of the cyst.* ***(A)*** *In situ presentation with a yellow vessel loop encircling the common bile duct just cranial from the pancreas.* ***(B)*** *The excised choledochal cyst of the common bile duct in continuity with the cystic duct and gallbladder. A white probe is passed through the lumen of the cyst. (Photographs courtesy P.M.J.G. Peeters, MD, University Hospital Groningen, The Netherlands.)*

choledochoceles (73). A partial liver resection may be indicated in patients with cysts of type 4A and type 5 (Caroli's disease). Liver transplantation should be considered in the rarer patients with concomitant diffuse intrahepatic abnormalities such as congenital liver fibrosis or secondary biliary cirrhosis.

Simple drainage of the cyst alone by a cystenterostomy is generally regarded as an obsolete procedure because of the high risk of late complications (anastomotic stricture formation, malignant degeneration). Especially in adults, however, the cyst wall is sometimes so adherent to the portal vein or the hepatic artery that a plane of dissection cannot be identified. In these cases, the cyst must be entered, and the entire mucosal lining excised, leaving the external wall attached to the adjacent structures (74). Mucosal lining of a choledochal cyst is currently considered as a precancerous condition, warranting complete excision (69). Although some investigators have found an increased risk for neoplasia developing anywhere in the biliary tract, gallbladder, or pancreas in patients after resection of a choledochal cyst (69), others could not find malignant changes in the remnant proximal hepatic duct or terminal bile duct after a mean follow-up of 9.1 years (75). The prognosis for patients who have developed a cancer in the cyst is very poor, even after surgery (68,76).

BILIARY CYSTADENOMA AND CYSTADENOCARCINOMA

Biliary cystadenomas are rare tumors, constituting about 2% to 5% of all intrahepatic tumors of biliary origin. Malignant degeneration into a cystadenocarcinoma is even less frequently seen. The size of biliary cystadenomas varies between 0.5 and 30 cm, with an average diameter of 10 cm (77). Usually they have a multilocular and multilobular aspect, with papillary foldings. The tumors arise from the intrahepatic (and rarely from the extrahepatic) bile ducts or gallbladder. Cystadenomas are most frequently found in middle-aged females, but a nearly equal sex distribution has been found for cystadenocarcinomas (78). The inner lining of the cysts is formed by columnar epithelium with or without a densely cellular ("ovarian-like") stroma. Cystadenocarcinomas surrounded by an ovarian-like stroma are exclusively found in females, whereas the ones without a distinctive cellular stroma are seen in males. The presence of a true epithelial lining distinguishes these cysts from infectious lesions and pseudocysts. Another distinguishing feature is the mucinous content of these cysts compared to the more serous fluid content of simple cysts (77,78).

The etiology of biliary cystadenomas is largely unknown. It has been suggested that they develop from ectopic remnants of primitive foregut sequestered within the liver. According to this theory cystadenoma is a congenital rather than an acquired disorder (79). Cystadenocarcinomas are considered to result from malignant degeneration of cystadenomas. A transition zone between benign and malignant parts is often encountered on histologic examination of cystadenocarcinomas, which supports this theory (77,78).

The clinical presentation and symptoms are usually mild and atypical (80). Cystadenomas are slowly growing tumors that usually remain asymptomatic until the second or third decade of life. In more than 80% of the patients, the presenting symptoms include upper abdominal pain or discomfort, nausea, jaundice, and a palpable mass (78,80). Less than 20% are discovered coincidentally. Complications are also seen in about 20% and include cholangitis or sepsis secondary to compression of bile ducts, portal hypertension due to portal vein compression, bleeding, and rupture (77). Laboratory studies usually reveal normal liver function tests and normal serum levels of alpha-fetoprotein and CEA. CA 19-9 levels, however, are elevated in most cases and measurement can be helpful in making the diagnosis (14,81,82).

On ultrasonography and computer tomography, cystadenomas are usually recognized as multilobular cysts with internal septation and/or small polyps (83–85). Cystadenomas need to be differentiated from simple cysts, with or without malignant degeneration, hydatid cysts, metastatic cystadenocarcinomas, primary or metastatic neoplasms with central necrosis, and post-traumatic cysts (84).

Cystadenocarcinomas should be highly suspected when large papillary or solid parts are found inside the cyst during imaging studies. Preoperative differentiation between a congenital cyst with malignant degeneration and a cystadenocarcinoma can be very difficult, if not impossible. Percutaneous aspiration of the cystic fluid and needle biopsy have been propagated to facilitate the diagnosis. However, these techniques may cause seeding metastasis of the needle track, so this procedure should be avoided (86).

The treatment of choice is a radical excision of the mass (77,86). This can be done either as a typical lobectomy or as an extra-anatomical excision with a wide margin of normal liver tissue, depending on the size and localization of the tumor. Partial excision of cystadenomas is associated with a recurrence rate of 90% (87). Even after radical excision, recurrences are seen in 5% of the patients, so they should receive extensive follow-up reexaminations. In general, however, the prognosis is good in patients with cystadenoma if the tumor can be completely resected with free margins of normal liver tissue. Patients with cystadenocarcinomas accompanied by an ovarian-like stroma who have been treated with radical excision also have a relatively good prognosis (80). However, cystadenocarcinomas lacking a distinctive (ovarian-like) surrounding stroma usually follow a more aggressive course and are more likely to result in the patient's death. In one series, the median survival for male patients with cystadenocarcinomas was 3 years, whereas no deaths were seen during 30 patient years of follow-up in women with cystadenocarcinomas that were surrounded by a mesenchymal stroma (80). Distal metastases are rarely seen, but can occur in the liver, lungs, and bones (88).

SUGGESTED READINGS

Fibropolycystic Hepatobiliary Diseases

Desmet VJ. Congenital diseases of intrahepatic bile ducts: variations on the theme "ductal plate malformations." Hepatology 1992;16:1069–83. A review of current evidence for the theory of ductal plate malformation as the common underlying cause of cystic and fibropolycystic hepatobiliary diseases.

Bile Duct Cysts

Lenriot JP, Gigot JF, Segol P, et al. Bile duct cysts in adults. A multi-institutional retrospective study. Ann Surg 1998;228:159–66. A recent large analysis of the French Associations for Surgical Research of clinical presentation, radiologic presurgical evaluation, and current surgical treatment for bile duct cysts in 17 institutions.

Todani T, Watanabe Y, Narusue M, et al. Congenital bile duct cysts. Classification, operative procedures, and review of the thirty-seven cases including cancer arising from choledochal cyst. Am J Surg 1977;134:263–9. The currently used classification for choledochal cysts.

Cystadenoma and Cystadenocarcinoma

Devaney K, Goodman ZD, Ishak KG. Hepatobiliary cystadenoma and cystadenocarcinoma. A light microscopic and immunohistochemical study of 70 patients. Am J Surg Pathol 1994;18:1078–91. A series of 70 patients with cystadenoma or cystadenocarcinoma in which light microscopic features of the tumors were correlated with immunohistochemical and follow-up data.

REFERENCES

1. Desmet VJ. Congenital diseases of intrahepatic bile ducts: variations on the theme "ductal plate malformation." Hepatology 1992;16:1069–83.
2. O'Neill J Jr. Choledochal cyst. Curr Probl Surg 1992;29:361–410.
3. Landing BH. Considerations of the pathogenesis of neonatal hepatitis, biliary atresia and choledochal cyst—the concept of infantile obstructive cholangiopathy. Prog Pediatr Surg 1974;6:113–39.
4. Cheney M, Rustad DG, Lilly JR. Choledochal cyst. World J Surg 1985;9:244–9.
5. Gaines PA, Sampson MA. The prevalence and characterization of simple hepatic cysts by ultrasound examination. Br J Radiol 1989;62:335–7.
6. Sanfelippo PM, Beahrs OH, Weiland LH. Cystic disease of the liver. Ann Surg 1974;179:922–5.
7. Martin IJ, McKinley AJ, Currie EJ, et al. Tailoring the management of nonparasitic liver cysts. Ann Surg 1998;228:167–72.
8. Krahenbuhl L, Baer HU, Renzulli P, et al. Laparoscopic management of nonparasitic symptom-producing solitary hepatic cysts. J Am Coll Surg 1996;183:493–8.
9. Cappell MS. Obstructive jaundice from benign, nonparasitic hepatic cysts: identification of risk factors and percutaneous aspiration for diagnosis and treatment. Am J Gastroenterol 1988;83:93–6.
10. Bloustein PA, Silverberg SG. Squamous cell carcinoma originating in an hepatic cyst. Case report with a review of the hepatic cyst-carcinoma association. Cancer 1976;38:2002–5.
11. Pliskin A, Cualing H, Stenger RJ. Primary squamous cell carcinoma originating in congenital cysts of the liver. Report of a case and review of the literature. Arch Pathol Lab Med 1992;116:105–7.
12. Theise ND, Miller F, Worman HJ, et al. Biliary cystadenocarcinoma arising in a liver with fibropolycystic disease. Arch Pathol Lab Med 1993;117:163–5.
13. Roemer CE, Ferrucci JT Jr, Mueller PR, et al. Hepatic cysts: diagnosis and therapy by sonographic needle aspiration. AJR Am J Roentgenol 1981;136:1065–70.
14. Horsmans Y, Laka A, Gigot JF, Geubel AP. Serum and cystic fluid CA 19-9 determinations as a diagnostic help in liver cysts of uncertain nature. Liver 1996;16:255–7.
15. Saini S, Mueller PR, Ferrucci JT Jr, et al. Percutaneous aspiration of hepatic cysts does not provide definitive therapy. AJR Am J Roentgenol 1983;141:559–60.
16. Kairaluoma MI, Leinonen A, Stahlberg M, et al. Percutaneous aspiration and alcohol sclerotherapy for symptomatic hepatic cysts. An alternative to surgical intervention. Ann Surg 1989;210:208–15.
17. Cellier C, Cuenod CA, Deslandes P, et al. Symptomatic hepatic cysts: treatment with single-shot injection of minocycline hydrochloride. Radiology 1998;206:205–9.
18. Castellano G, Moreno Sanchez D, Gutierrez J, et al. Caustic sclerosing cholangitis. Report of four cases and a cumulative review of the literature. Hepatogastroenterology 1994;41:458–70.
19. Klingler PJ, Gadenstatter M, Schmid T, et al. Treatment of hepatic cysts in the era of laparoscopic surgery. Br J Surg 1997;84:438–44.
20. Iwatsuki S, Todo S, Starzl TE. Excisional therapy for benign hepatic lesions. Surg Gynecol Obstet 1990;171:240–6.
21. Nakanuma Y, Kurumaya H, Ohta G. Multiple cysts in the hepatic hilum and their pathogenesis. A suggestion of periductal gland origin. Virchows Arch A Pathol Anat Histopathol 1984;404:341–50.
22. Fujioka Y, Kawamura N, Tanaka S, et al. Multiple hilar cysts of the liver in patients with alcoholic cirrhosis: report of three cases. J Gastroenterol Hepatol 1997;12:137–43.
23. Yuasa N, Nimura Y, Hayakawa N, et al. Multiple hepatic cysts along the intrahepatic bile duct—case report. Hepatogastroenterology 1997;44:1262–6.
24. Colina F, Castellano VM, Gonzalez Pinto I, et al. Hilar biliary cysts in hepatic transplantation. Report of three symptomatic cases and occurrence in resected liver grafts. Transpl Int 1998;11:110–6.
25. Summerfield JA, Nagafuchi Y, Sherlock S, et al. Hepatobiliary fibropolycystic diseases. A clinical and histological review of 51 patients. J Hepatol 1986;2:141–56.
26. Murray Lyon IM, Ockenden BG, Williams R. Congenital hepatic fibrosis—is it a single clinical entity? Gastroenterology 1973;64:653–6.
27. Hildebrandt F, Waldherr R, Kutt R, Brandis M. The nephronophthisis complex: clinical and genetic aspects. Clin Investig 1992;70:802–8.
28. Pahl MV, Vaziri ND, Dure Smith B, et al. Hepatobiliary pathology in hemodialysis patients: an autopsy study of 78 cases. Am J Gastroenterol 1986;81:783–7.
29. Gabow PA, Johnson AM, Kaehny WD, et al. Risk factors for the development of hepatic cysts in autosomal dominant polycystic kidney disease. Hepatology 1990;11:1033–7.
30. Pirson Y, Lannoy N, Peters D, et al. Isolated polycystic liver disease as a distinct genetic disease, unlinked to polycystic kidney disease 1 and polycystic kidney disease 2. Hepatology 1996;23:249–52.
31. Vauthey JN, Maddern GJ, Kolbinger P, et al. Clinical experience with adult polycystic liver disease. Br J Surg 1992;79:562–5.
32. Kwok MK, Lewin KJ. Massive hepatomegaly in adult polycystic liver disease. Am J Surg Pathol 1988;12:321–4.
33. Sherstha R, McKinley C, Russ P, et al. Postmenopausal estrogen therapy selectively stimulates hepatic enlargement in women with autosomal dominant polycystic kidney disease. Hepatology 1997;26:1282–6.
34. Everson GT, Emmett M, Brown WR, et al. Functional similarities of hepatic cystic and biliary epithelium: studies of fluid constituents and in vivo secretion in response to secretin. Hepatology 1990;11:557–65.
35. Balli M, Zhao M, Zimmermann A. Polycystic liver disease: immunohisto-chemical characterization of cyst epithelia and extracellular matrix. Contrib Nephrol 1995;115:127–33.
36. Everson GT, Scherzinger A, Berger Leff N, et al. Polycystic liver disease: quantitation of parenchymal and cyst volumes from computed tomography images and clinical correlates of hepatic cysts. Hepatology 1988;8:1627–34.
37. Grunfeld JP, Albouze G, Jungers P, et al. Liver changes and complications in adult polycystic kidney disease. Adv Nephrol Necker Hosp 1985;14:1–20.
38. Uddin W, Ramage JK, Portmann B, et al. Hepatic venous outflow obstruction in patients with polycystic liver disease: pathogenesis and treatment. Gut 1995;36:142–5.
39. Bloustein PA. Association of carcinoma with congenital cystic conditions of the liver and bile ducts. Am J Gastroenterol 1977;67:40–6.
40. Telenti A, Torres VE, Gross JB Jr, et al. Hepatic cyst infection in autosomal dominant polycystic kidney disease. Mayo Clin Proc 1990;65:933–42.
41. Washburn WK, Johnson LB, Lewis WD, Jenkins RL. Liver transplantation for adult polycystic liver disease. Liver Transpl Surg 1996;2:17–22.
42. Kabbej M, Sauvanet A, Chauveau D, et al. Laparoscopic fenestration in polycystic liver disease. Br J Surg 1996;83:1697–701.
43. Henne Bruns D, Klomp HJ, Kremer B. Non-parasitic liver cysts and polycystic liver disease: results of surgical treatment. Hepatogastroenterology 1993;40:1–5.
44. Newman KD, Torres VE, Rakela J, Nagorney DM. Treatment of highly symptomatic polycystic liver disease. Preliminary experience with a combined hepatic resection-fenestration procedure. Ann Surg 1990;212:30–7.
45. Starzl TE, Reyes J, Tzakis A, et al. Liver transplantation for polycystic liver disease. Arch Surg 1990;125:575–7.

46. Caroli J, Soupault R, Kossakowski J, et al. La dilatation congenitale des voies biliaires intrahepatiques. Semin Hop Paris 1958;34:488–95.
47. Caroli J. Diseases of the intrahepatic biliary tree. Clin Gastroenterol 1973;2:147–61.
48. Dagli U, Atalay F, Sasmaz N, et al. Caroli's disease: 1977–1995 experiences. Eur J Gastroenterol Hepatol 1998;10:109–12.
49. Taylor AC, Palmer KR. Caroli's disease. Eur J Gastroenterol Hepatol 1998;10:105–8.
50. Fozard JB, Wyatt JI, Hall RI. Epithelial dysplasia in Caroli's disease. Gut 1989;30:1150–3.
51. Terada T, Nakanuma Y. Congenital biliary dilatation in autosomal dominant adult polycystic disease of the liver and kidneys. Arch Pathol Lab Med 1988;112:1113–6.
52. Caroli Bosc FX, Demarquay JF, Conio M, et al. The role of therapeutic endoscopy associated with extracorporeal shock-wave lithotripsy and bile acid treatment in the management of Caroli's disease. Endoscopy 1998;30:559–63.
53. Mujahed Z, Glenn F, Evans JA. Communicating cavernous ectasia of the intrahepatic ducts (Caroli's disease). Am J Roentgenol Radium Ther Nucl Med 1971;113:21–6.
54. Geneve J, Dubuc N, Mathieu D, et al. Cystic dilatation of intrahepatic bile ducts in primary sclerosing cholangitis. J Hepatol 1990;11:196–9.
55. Lim JH. Oriental cholangiohepatitis: pathologic, clinical, and radiologic features. AJR Am J Roentgenol 1991;157:1–8.
56. Mercadier M, Chigot JP, Clot JP, et al. Caroli's disease. World J Surg 1984;8:22–9.
57. Alonso Lej F, Revor WB, Passagno DJ. Congenital choledochal cyst, with a report of 2, and an analysis of 94 cases. Surg Gynecol Obstet 1959;108:1–30.
58. Todani T, Watanabe Y, Narusue M, et al. Congenital bile duct cysts: classification, operative procedures, and review of thirty-seven cases including cancer arising from choledochal cyst. Am J Surg 1977;134:263–9.
59. Lenriot JP, Gigot JF, Segol P, et al. Bile duct cysts in adults: a multi-institutional retrospective study. French Associations for Surgical Research. Ann Surg 1998;228:159–66.
60. Ryckman FC, Noseworthy J. Neonatal cholestatic conditions requiring surgical reconstruction. Semin Liver Dis 1987;7:134–54.
61. Ono J, Sakoda K, Akita H. Surgical aspect of cystic dilatation of the bile duct. An anomalous junction of the pancreaticobiliary tract in adults. Ann Surg 1982;195:203–8.
62. Todani T, Watanabe Y, Fujii T, Uemura S. Anomalous arrangement of the pancreaticobiliary ductal system in patients with a choledochal cyst. Am J Surg 1984;147:672–6.
63. Chaudhary A, Dhar P, Sachdev A, et al. Choledochal cysts—differences in children and adults. Br J Surg 1996;83:186–8.
64. Vanderpool D, Lane BW, Winter JW, Ettinger J. Choledochal cysts. Surg Gynecol Obstet 1988;167:447–51.
65. Tan KC, Howard ER. Choledochal cyst: a 14-year surgical experience with 36 patients. Br J Surg 1988;75:892–5.
66. Shian WJ, Wang YJ, Chi CS. Choledochal cysts: a nine-year review. Acta Paediatr 1993;82:383–6.
67. Lipsett PA, Pitt HA, Colombani PM, et al. Choledochal cyst disease. A changing pattern of presentation. Ann Surg 1994;220:644–52.
68. Stain SC, Guthrie CR, Yellin AE, Donovan AJ. Choledochal cyst in the adult. Ann Surg 1995;222:128–33.
69. Fieber SS, Nance FC. Choledochal cyst and neoplasm: a comprehensive review of 106 cases and presentation of two original cases. Am Surg 1997;63:982–7.
70. Kagawa Y, Kashihara S, Kuramoto S, Maetani S. Carcinoma arising in a congenitally dilated biliary tract. Report of a case and review of the literature. Gastroenterology 1978;74:1286–94.
71. Chen HM, Jan YY, Chen MF, et al. Surgical treatment of choledochal cyst in adults: results and long-term follow-up. Hepatogastroenterology 1996;43:1492–9.
72. Martin RF, Biber BP, Bosco JJ, Howell DA. Symptomatic choledochoceles in adults. Endoscopic retrograde cholangiopancreatography recognition and management. Arch Surg 1992;127:536–8.
73. Ladas SD, Katsogridakis I, Tassios P, et al. Choledochocele, an overlooked diagnosis: report of 15 cases and review of 56 published reports from 1984 to 1992. Endoscopy 1995;27:233–9.
74. Lilly JR. Total excision of choledochal cyst. Surg Gynecol Obstet 1978;146:254–6.
75. Ishibashi T, Kasahara K, Yasuda Y, et al. Malignant change in the biliary tract after excision of choledochal cyst. Br J Surg 1997;84:1687–91.
76. Nagorney DM, McIlrath DC, Adson MA. Choledochal cysts in adults: clinical management. Surgery 1984;96:656–63.
77. Ishak KG, Willis GW, Cummins SD, Bullock AA. Biliary cystadenoma and cystadenocarcinoma: report of 14 cases and review of the literature. Cancer 1977;39:322–38.
78. Devaney K, Goodman ZD, Ishak KG. Hepatobiliary cystadenoma and cystadenocarcinoma. A light microscopic and immunohistochemical study of 70 patients. Am J Surg Pathol 1994;18:1078–91.
79. Subramony C, Herrera GA, Turbat Herrera EA. Hepatobiliary cystadenoma. A study of five cases with reference to histogenesis. Arch Pathol Lab Med 1993;117:1036–42.
80. Tsiftsis D, Christodoulakis M, de Bree E, Sanidas E. Primary intrahepatic biliary cystadenomatous tumors. J Surg Oncol 1997;64:341–6.
81. Lee JH, Chen DR, Pang SC, Lai YS. Mucinous biliary cystadenoma with mesenchymal stroma: expressions of CA 19-9 and carcinoembryonic antigen in serum and cystic fluid. J Gastroenterol 1996;31:732–6.
82. Thomas JA, Scriven MW, Puntis MC, et al. Elevated serum CA 19–9 levels in hepatobiliary cystadenoma with mesenchymal stroma. Two case reports with immunohistochemical confirmation. Cancer 1992;70:1841–6.
83. Federle MP, Filly RA, Moss AA. Cystic hepatic neoplasms: complementary roles of CT and sonography. AJR Am J Roentgenol 1981;136:345–8.
84. Itai Y, Araki T, Furui S, et al. Computed tomography of primary intrahepatic biliary malignancy. Radiology 1983;147:485–90.
85. Buetow PC, Buck JL, Pantongrag Brown L, et al. Biliary cystadenoma and cystadenocarcinoma: clinical-imaging-pathologic correlations with emphasis on the importance of ovarian stroma. Radiology 1995;196:805–10.
86. Nakajima T, Sugano I, Matsuzaki O, et al. Biliary cystadenocarcinoma of the liver. A clinicopathologic and histochemical evaluation of nine cases. Cancer 1992;69:2426–32.
87. Lewis WD, Jenkins RL, Rossi RL, et al. Surgical treatment of biliary cystadenoma. A report of 15 cases. Arch Surg 1988;123:563–8.
88. Davies W, Chow M, Nagorney D. Extrahepatic biliary cystadenomas and cystadenocarcinoma. Report of seven cases and review of the literature. Ann Surg 1995;222:619–25.

Chapter

17

Laparoscopic Biliary Injuries

STEVEN M. STRASBERG

Biliary injury is the most severe common complication of cholecystectomy. It is always morbid, is occasionally fatal, increases cost (1–3), and often results in litigation (4,5). Bile duct injury has always been a risk of cholecystectomy but its incidence increased sharply when laparoscopic surgery for cholecystolithiasis was introduced. Not only has laparoscopic cholecystectomy led to more injuries, but certain types of injury such as ductal lacerations, bile leaks, and aberrant duct injuries are more common than they were previously. The causes of injury are becoming better understood, and improved methods for preventing injury are available. When injury occurs, a high rate of permanent cure is possible in specialized centers using advanced techniques of reconstruction.

CLASSIFICATION OF BILIARY INJURIES

Bismuth's classification was the standard classification of biliary injuries in the era of open cholecystectomy. It divides biliary injuries into five types mainly based on the upper level of injury. This classification became somewhat less useful as the injury pattern altered due to laparoscopic cholecystectomy (6–14). In 1995 we introduced a new classification that retained the essence of the Bismuth classification for major injuries but allowed inclusion of other injuries that were being seen with increasing frequency (15); this new classification has found considerable acceptance (16–18). Other classification schemes have been proposed by McMahon et al. (19), Stewart and Way (20), Schol et al. (21).

Our classification is based on anatomical location and on severity of the injury (Fig. 17.1).

Type A

A type A injury is a bile leak from a minor duct. Continuity with the common bile duct is retained. These leaks are usually caused by a failure to adequately secure closure of the cystic duct or by an injury of a small bile duct in the liver bed (Fig. 17.2). Occasionally, a 1- to 2-mm bile duct lies immediately under the gallbladder plate and is readily injured if the dissection is carried into the plane of liver tissue. Type A biliary injuries are the least serious, because major ducts are not involved and there is little chance of progression to a more serious form of injury. However, even these injuries can be quite morbid. They are usually lateral injuries to the biliary tract, so decreasing intrabiliary pressure by endoscopic sphincterotomy results in healing without loss of continuity of any part of the biliary tract. In terms of severity grade (22), type A injuries are rarely more than grade 2b complications.

Types B and C

The type B and C injuries involve creation of a discontinuity of part of the biliary tree with occlusion (type B) or intraperitoneal leak (type C). These are end injuries that isolate a part of the biliary tree. They usually result from an injury to an aberrant right hepatic duct, although rarely an aberrant left duct or a normally situated duct may be involved. For instance, a completely occluded or transected but normally located right hepatic duct would be classified here. About 2% of patients have an aberrant low-lying right duct that most commonly drains one or two segments of the right hemiliver (23). A key anatomical feature contributing to the likelihood of injury is that in many cases the cystic duct joins the aberrant duct, which then continues to join the main ductal system. The appearance of the junction of the aberrant duct with the hepatic duct is like that of the junction of the cystic duct with the hepatic duct and as a result there is great potential for injury.

When the injury is a ductal occlusion, it is designated

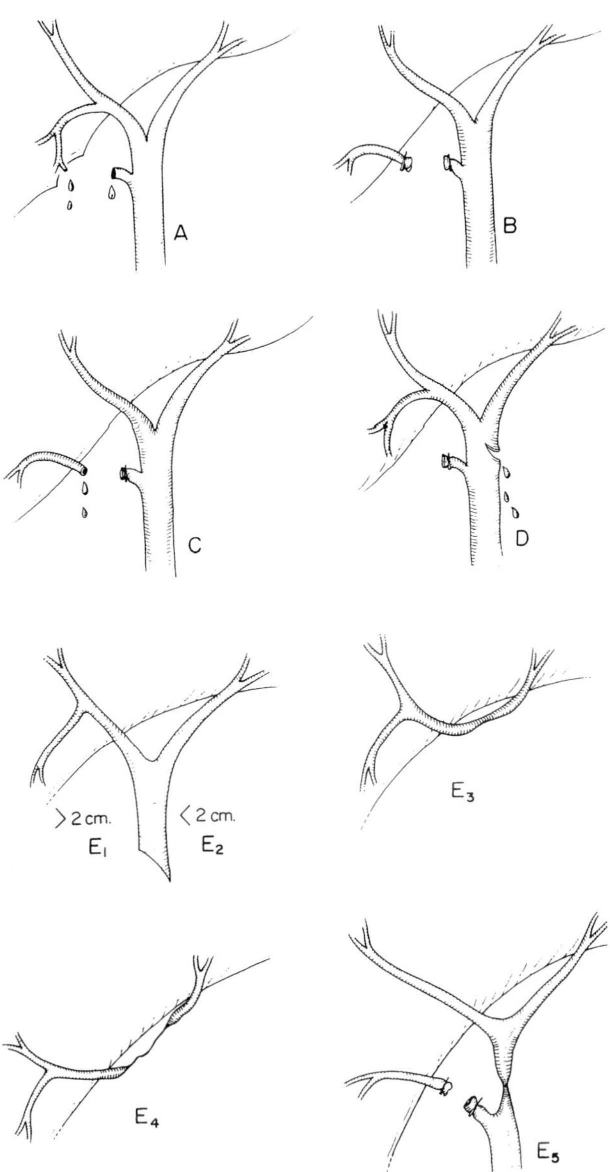

FIGURE 17.1. *Classification of laparoscopic injuries to the biliary tract. Injury types A to E are illustrated. Type E injuries are subdivided according to the Bismuth classification. Type A injuries are cystic duct leaks or leaks from small ducts in the liver bed. Type B and C injuries almost always involve aberrant right hepatic ducts. Type D injuries are lateral injuries to major bile ducts. The notations >2 cm and <2 cm in type E1 and type E2 indicate the length of common hepatic duct remaining. (Reproduced by permission of the Journal of the American College of Surgeons from Strasberg SM, Hertl M, Soper NJ. An analysis of the problem of biliary injury during laparoscopic cholecystectomy. J Am Coll Surg 1995;180:101–25.)*

type B (see Fig. 17.1). When it is a transection without occlusion it is termed type C (see Fig. 17.1). The reason for the difference in classification is that the presentation, management, and often prognosis are very different. Generally, occlusions (type B) are injuries of lesser severity. They are often asymptomatic (Fig. 17.3A), or if symptomatic may not cause symptoms such as cholangitis for months (Fig. 17.3B) or years. The liver behind a type B injury atrophies and the remaining liver undergoes compensatory hyperplasia. Transections without occlusion (type C) result in local intraperitoneal bile collections or bilious ascites and peritonitis. Type C injuries usually present in the early postoperative period and almost always require treatment (Fig. 17.4). These and subsequent types of injury should probably be considered level 3 surgical complications (22) because there is actual or life-long potential for loss of functional liver.

In the Bismuth classification these B and C injuries are considered to be level 5 injuries along with a more serious injury in which an aberrant duct injury is combined with a common hepatic duct injury. Because isolated aberrant duct injuries are so much more common in the laparoscopic era they were separated out in our classification.

Type D

Type D is a lateral injury to a major bile duct. These are partial disruptions, usually lacerations of the common bile duct or common hepatic duct. Like the type A variant, they are lateral injuries and will often resolve after decompression by postoperative endoscopic sphincterotomy. If they are discovered at the time of surgery they may be repaired with sutures and the placement of a T-tube. Unlike type A injuries, type D injuries have the potential to be much more serious injuries, particularly if they are thermal in origin or associated with devascularization of the bile duct; in these cases they may progress to complete obstruction, which is a type E injury. Type D injuries may occur to other major ducts. Right hepatic duct injuries similar to that shown in Figure 17.5 have been reported (11,13). Type C and type D injuries involving the right bile duct are very similar, but there are major therapeutic implications to complete transection (type C) versus lateral injury (type D).

Inadvertent incision of the common bile duct instead of the cystic duct when attempting to delineate ductal anatomy by operative cholangiography might be considered to be a type D injury. Provided the only consequence is that a T-tube is placed in the common bile duct without later consequences such as bile duct stricture or leakage, we do not consider this to be a biliary injury. Cannulation of the bile duct to protect it during abdominal surgery is an accepted procedure and is not in itself considered a complication.

Type E

Type E injuries are circumferential injuries of major bile ducts (Bismuth class 1 to 5). These are circumferential injuries of major bile ducts, as described by Bismuth. Subclassification into types E1 to E4 is based on the level of injury (Figs. 17.6 and 17.7), whereas the E5 is a combination of common hepatic duct and aberrant right duct injury (Fig. 17.8). Type E injuries separate the hepatic parenchyma from the lower biliary tract as a result of stenosis, simple

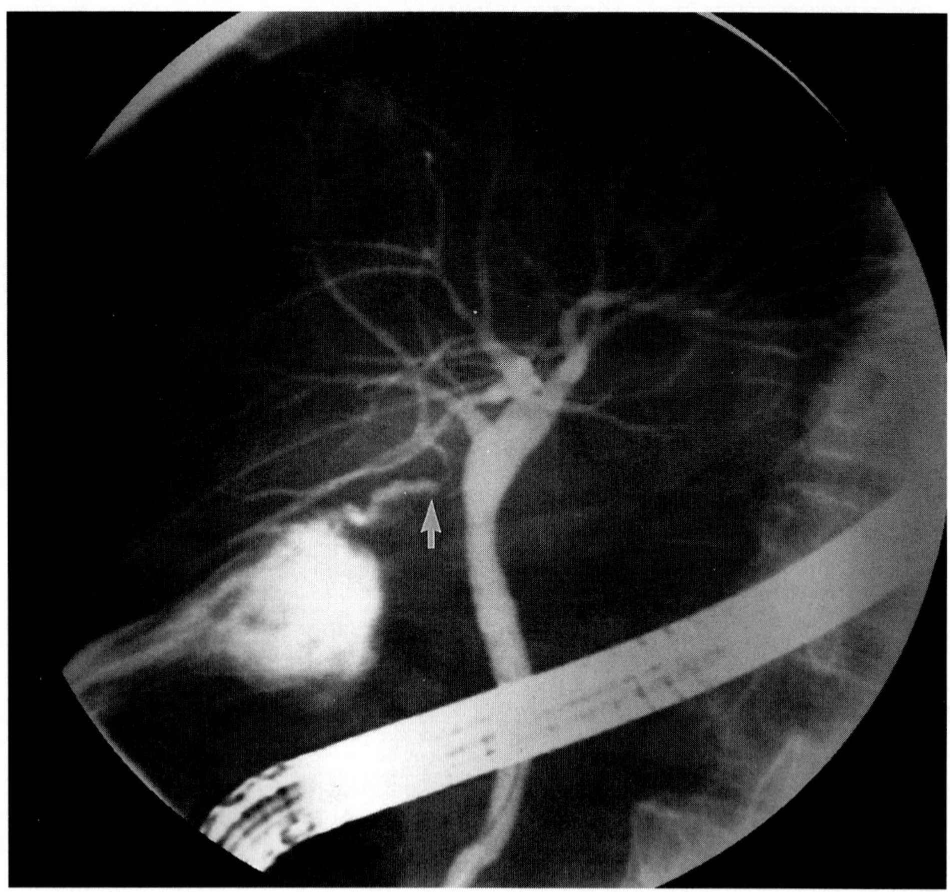

FIGURE 17.2. *ERCP for a patient with a type A injury. Note that the injury is to a small branch of a hepatic duct. The arrow points to the contrast leak from the duct. Sphincterotomy resolved the problem. (Reproduced by permission of the Journal of the American College of Surgeons from Strasberg SM, Hertl M, Soper NJ. An analysis of the problem of biliary injury during laparoscopic cholecystectomy. J Am Coll Surg 1995;180:101–25.)*

occlusion or transection, or occlusion or transection accompanied by resection of bile ducts. To classify the injury properly it must be stated which of these is present and if bile duct resection has occurred, the length of excised duct should be noted: e.g., "E2, simple, complete occlusion," or "E3, 3-cm duct length excised, transection without proximal occlusion, distal occlusion present." For purposes of the repair, the upper limit of injury is the key variable and this is given in the E type itself.

THE INCIDENCE OF LAPAROSCOPIC BILIARY INJURY

An increase in biliary injuries was an unpredicted accompaniment of laparoscopic cholecystectomy. The first indication of the problem was a sudden surge of referrals of biliary injuries to specialized hepatopancreaticobiliary units. To determine the true incidence of injury, large, accurate, representative studies were needed. Institutional or multi-institutional studies, studies of fewer than several thousand cases, and studies with less than 100% reporting, including mail surveys, fail to satisfy these conditions.

Several excellent reports exist, including statewide evaluations from New York (24) and Connecticut (25), a report from the armed services (26), and several from Europe (16,27,28). In all, a significant increase in the injury rate has been noted. Although injury rates remain elevated, it is encouraging that two studies have found that the injury rate has been decreasing toward normal (25,28). One may conservatively estimate that 1500 to 2500 laparoscopic biliary injuries are now occurring annually in the United States.

RISK FACTORS FOR BILIARY INJURY

Training and Experience

Early reports suggested that the high rate of injury was due mainly to inexperience in the procedure; this is referred to as the "learning curve" effect (29,30). It seems unquestionable that inexperience did initially contribute to the high incidence of injury, but other factors are responsible for the still elevated rates of injury today.

Local Operative Risk Factors

As during open cholecystectomy, biliary injuries seem more likely to occur during difficult laparoscopic cholecystectomies (21,25,31). Based on a very large series of patients in a state of Connecticut registry, Russell et al. (25) reported that the incidence of injury when laparoscopic cholecystec-

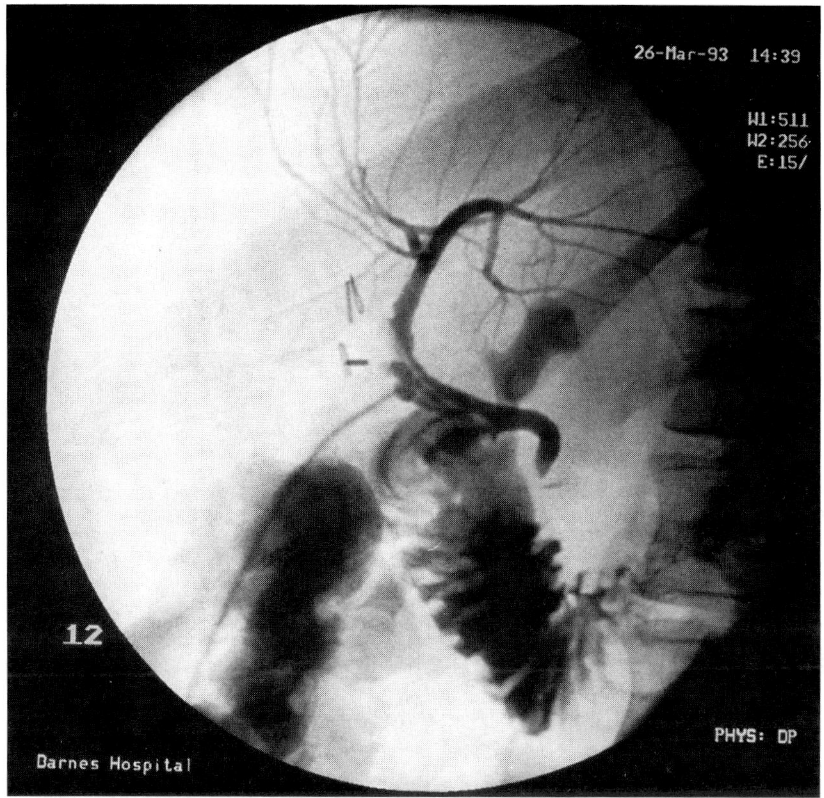

(A)

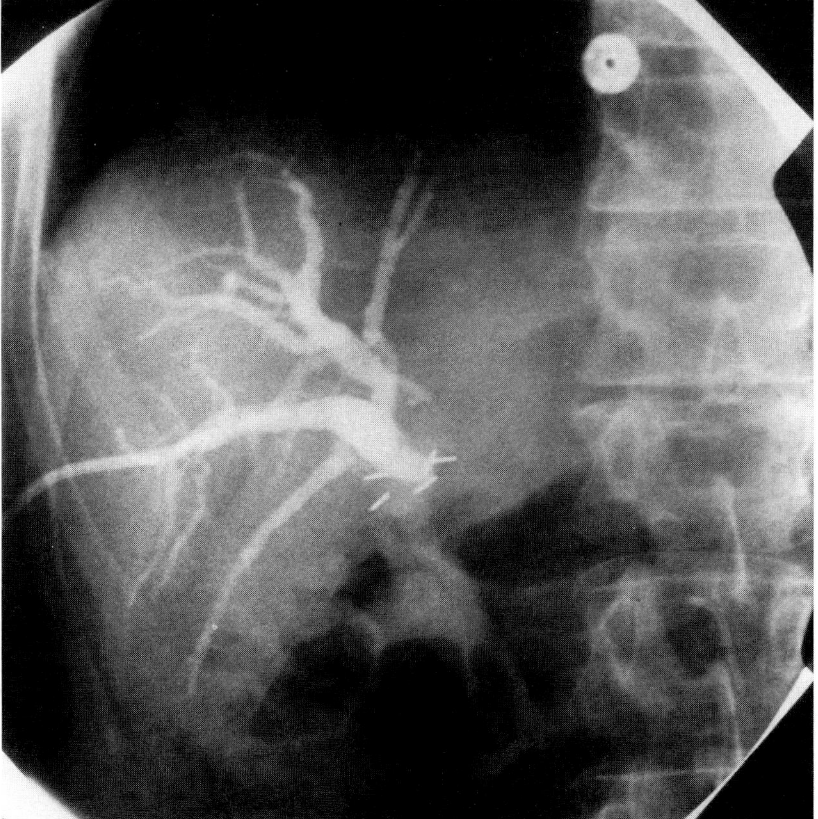

(B)

FIGURE 17.3. ***(A)*** *A postoperative ERCP demonstrating a type B injury. Note absence of right posterior sectional ducts (ducts to segments VI and VII). This patient has been asymptomatic for many years.* ***(B)*** *Another type B injury involving the whole right side of the liver. This patient complained of heaviness in the right upper quadrant beginning several months after cholecystectomy and required reconstruction. (Reproduced by permission of the Journal of the American College of Surgeons from Strasberg SM, Hertl M, Soper NJ. An analysis of the problem of biliary injury during laparoscopic cholecystectomy. J Am Coll Surg 1995;180:101–25.)*

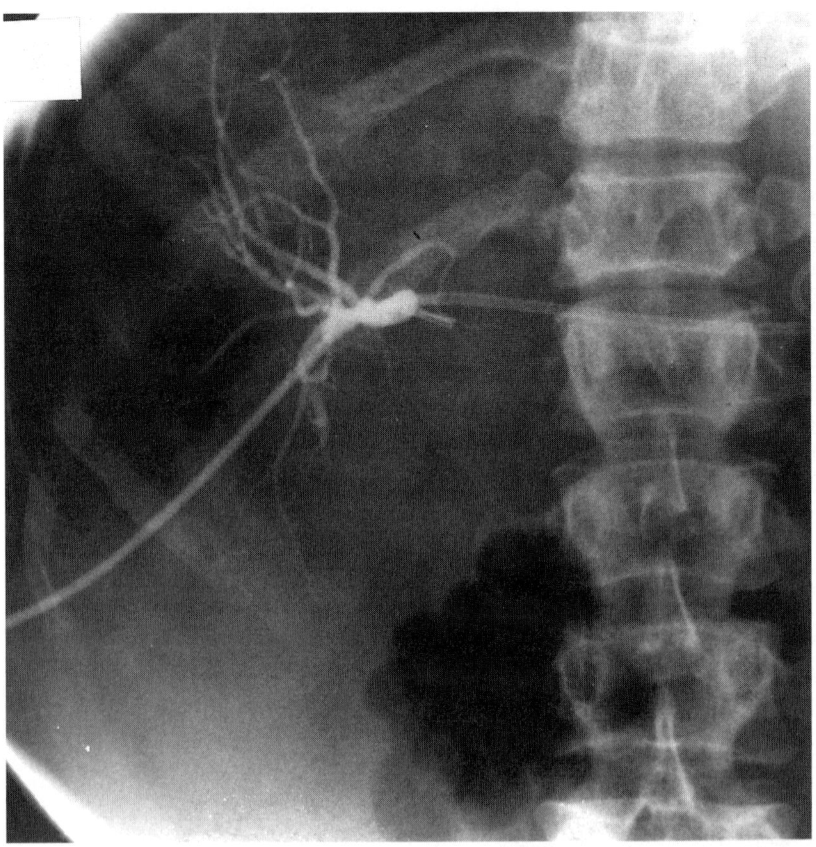

FIGURE 17.4. *A percutaneous cholangiogram in a patient with a type C injury. A segment of the right posterior sectional duct had been excised and a postoperative biloma resulted. Note the percutaneous stent used to drain biloma and guide surgical repair. (Reproduced by permission of the Journal of the American College of Surgeons from Strasberg SM, Hertl M, Soper NJ. An analysis of the problem of biliary injury during laparoscopic cholecystectomy. J Am Coll Surg 1995;180:101–25.)*

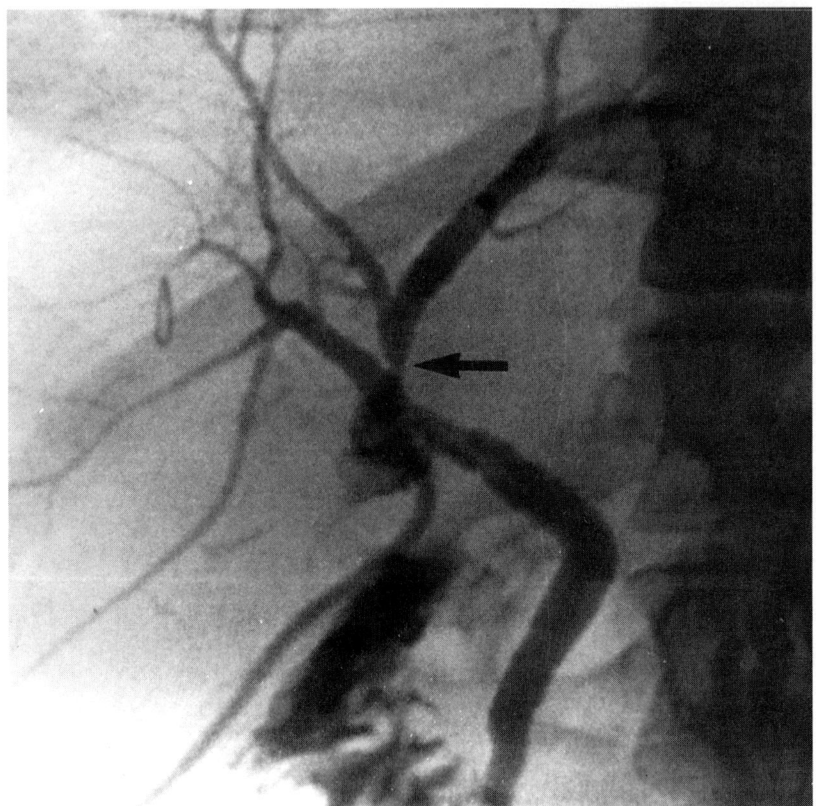

FIGURE 17.5. *Type D injury to the right hepatic duct/common hepatic duct junction. A T-tube is in place. Note the dye extravasation. (Reproduced by permission of the Journal of the American College of Surgeons from Strasberg SM, Hertl M, Soper NJ. An analysis of the problem of biliary injury during laparoscopic cholecystectomy. J Am Coll Surg 1995;180:101–25.)*

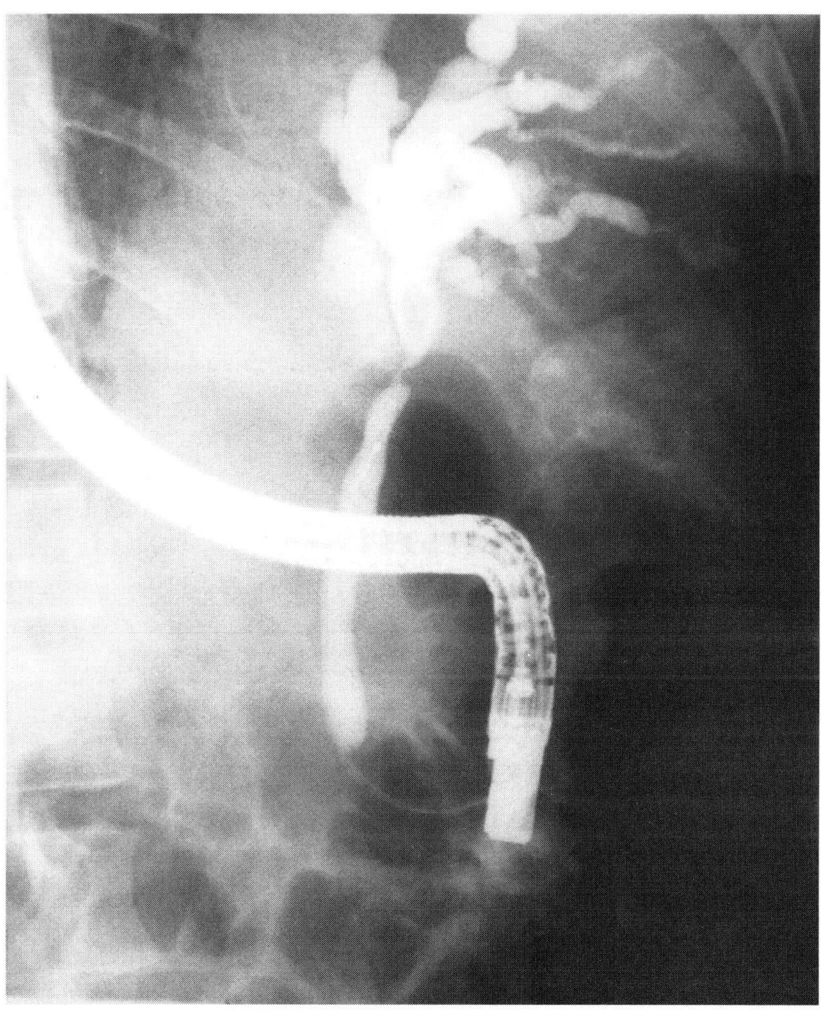

FIGURE 17.6. *Type E2 injury with a stenosis just below the bifurcation of the hepatic ducts.*

tomy was performed for acute cholecystitis (0.51%) was three times higher than that for elective laparoscopic cholecystectomy and twice as high as open cholecystectomy for acute cholecystitis. Thousands of patients are required to see this difference (21,25) and one should be wary of concluding that the procedure is as safe as elective cholecystectomy based on reports of a few hundred patients. Chronic inflammation with dense scarring (16), operative bleeding obscuring the field, or fat in the portal area were cited as contributing factors in 15% to 35% of injuries (5,7,8,13). Blood in the field hampers dissection much more often in laparoscopic than in open cholecystectomy, and gentle dissection is required, especially when inflammation is present, to avoid bleeding that then obscures vision (5,32,33). The role of obesity is difficult to evaluate, as it is so often present in patients with cholelithiasis.

Aberrant Anatomy

Aberrant anatomy is a well-described danger in biliary surgery. The aberrant right hepatic duct anomaly referred to in the discussion of type B and type C injuries is the most common problem. There are several reports of injury to aberrant right hepatic ducts during laparoscopic cholecystectomy (5,7,11,13,34,35). These injuries are probably underreported because type B injuries may be asymptomatic (36). Isolated injuries to aberrant right ducts did occur before the advent of laparoscopic cholecystectomy, but such ducts appear to be particularly prone to injury during laparoscopic cholecystectomy (15).

Equipment

Laparoscopic equipment must be well maintained. Thermal injuries to bile ducts or surrounding structures (37) may occur due to focal loss of insulation on the instruments used for cauterization.

DIRECT CAUSES OF LAPAROSCOPIC BILIARY INJURY

Biliary injury is caused either by anatomical misidentification of the cystic duct or by technical problems, especially the misuse of cautery.

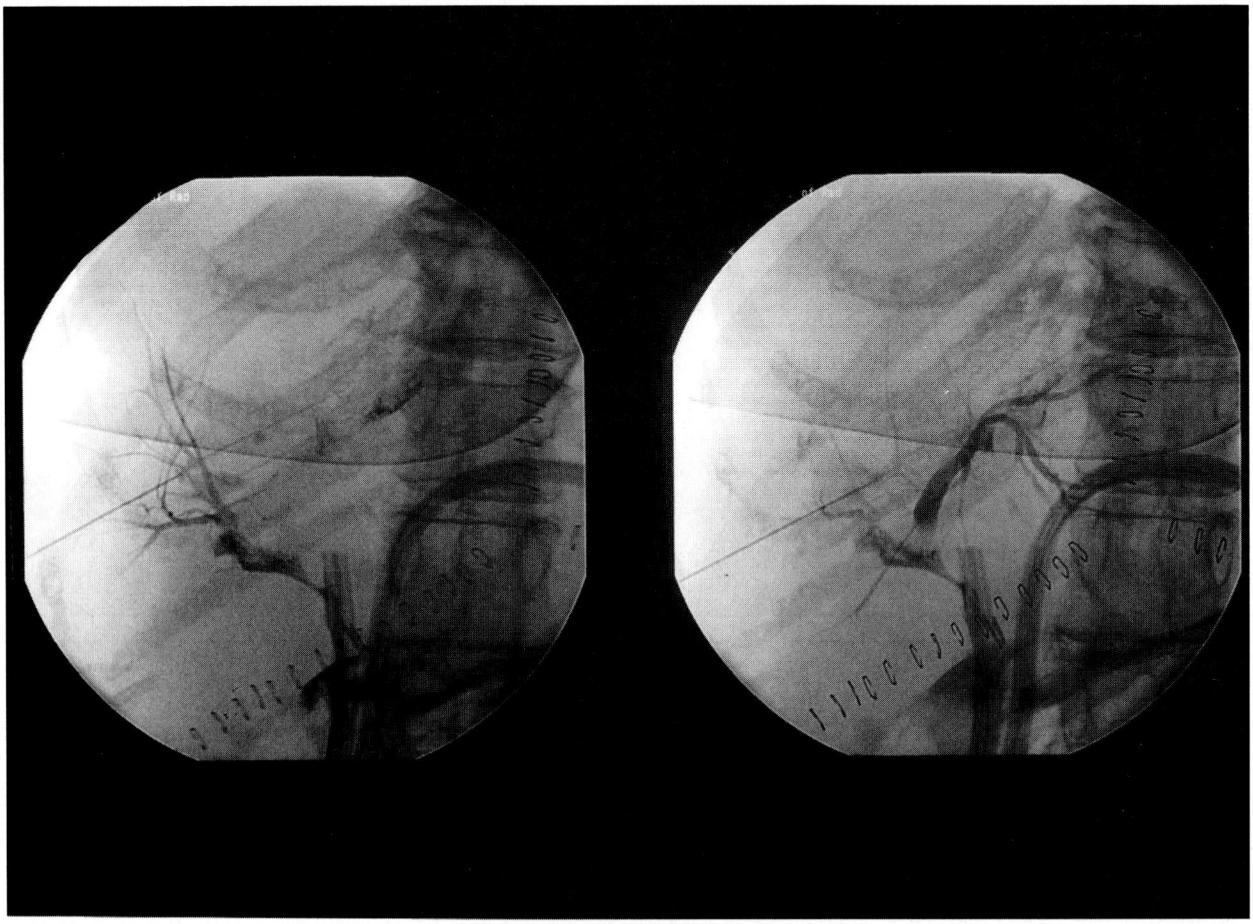

FIGURE 17.7. *An E4 injury in which the right hepatic duct (left panel) and the left hepatic duct (right panel) have been isolated by resection of the bifurcation of the hepatic ducts. This percutaneous cholangiogram preceded the placement of stents immediately prior to surgery.*

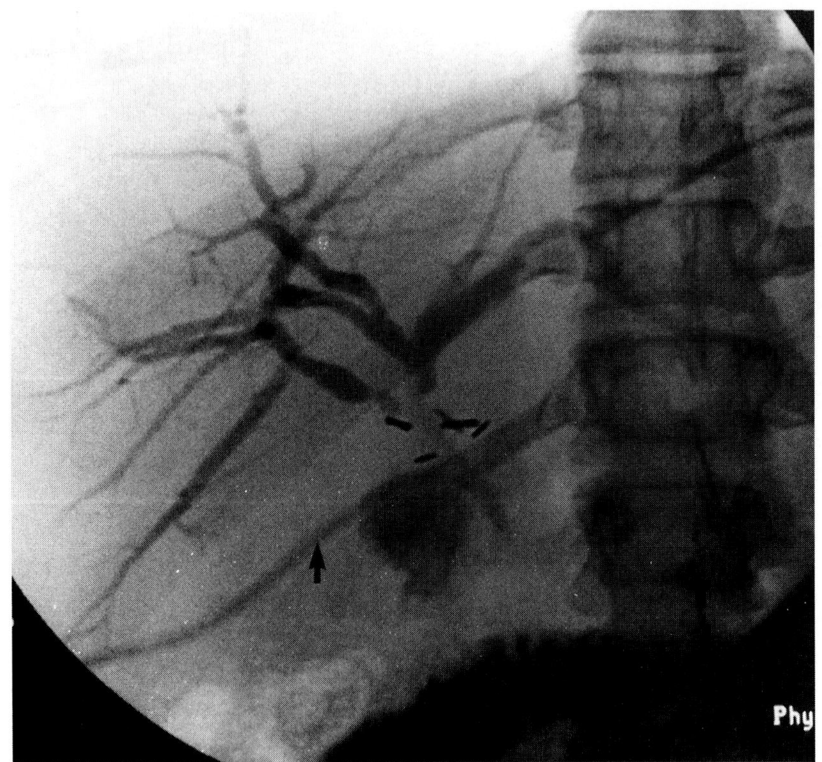

FIGURE 17.8. *E5 injury initially treated by a double-barreled choledochocholedochostomy and splinted with a T-tube (arrow) divided at the upper limb to go up both the hepatic duct and the aberrant right duct. These anastomoses strictured. (Reproduced by permission of the Journal of the American College of Surgeons from Strasberg SM, Hertl M, Soper NJ. An analysis of the problem of biliary injury during laparoscopic cholecystectomy. J Am Coll Surg 1995;180:101–25.)*

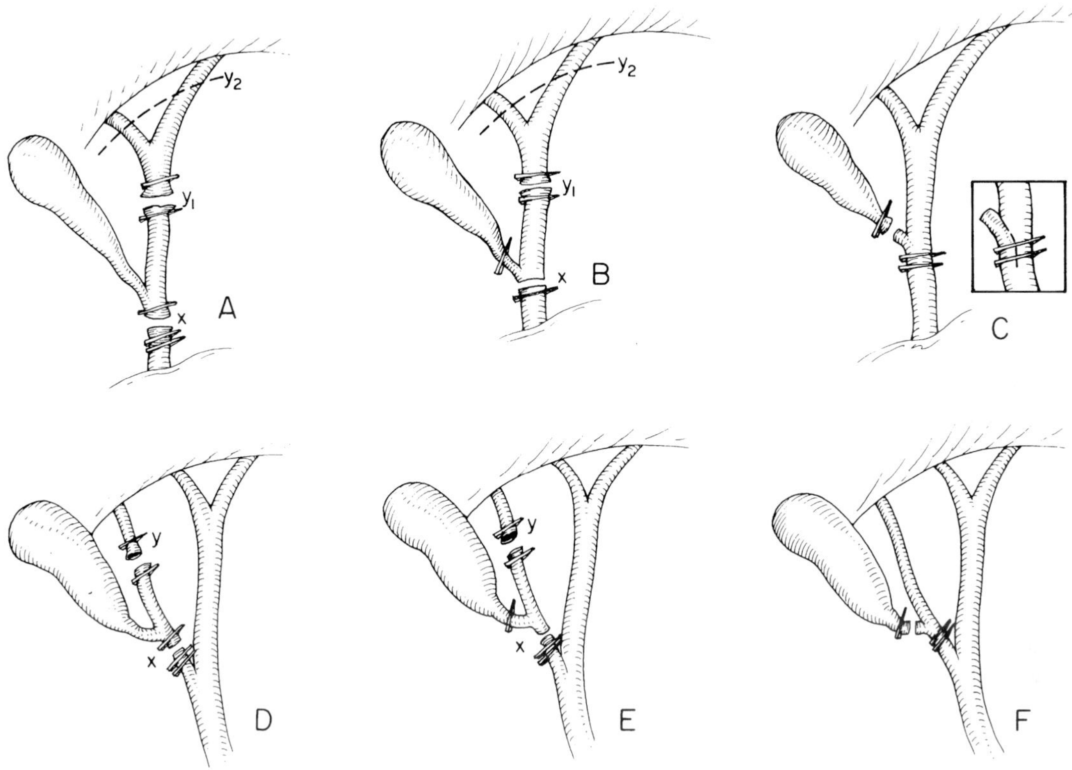

FIGURE 17.9. *Patterns of biliary injury due to misidentification.* ***(A)*** *The classic type E injury in which the common duct is divided between clips at point x. The ductal system is later divided again to remove the gallbladder either at point y_1, producing E1 or E2 injuries, or at point y_2, producing E3 or E4 injuries.* ***(B)*** *Variant of type E injury that leads to bile leakage into the operative field and thereby an increased chance of recognition before the entire injury evolves.* ***(C)*** *Variant of type E injury leading to clipping but not excision of the duct. This injury also causes intraoperative bile leakage, except when cystic and common bile ducts are both occluded, as shown in the inset.* ***(D—F)*** *Variants of injury to aberrant right hepatic duct, producing type B or type C injuries. The injuries shown in D, E, and F correspond to the injuries shown in A, B, and C but affect the aberrant right duct. (Reproduced by permission of the Journal of the American College of Surgeons from Strasberg SM, Hertl M, Soper NJ. An analysis of the problem of biliary injury during laparoscopic cholecystectomy. J Am Coll Surg 1995;180:101–25.)*

Misidentification is the most common cause of serious injuries. There are two scenarios. In the first, the common duct is mistaken for the cystic duct and is clipped and divided (Fig. 17.9A, point x). To complete the excision of the gallbladder the bile ducts must be divided again. The type of injury produced varies from E1 to E4 and depends on the level of this second division (see Fig. 17.9A, points y_1 and y_2). Frequently, a "second cystic duct" or "accessory duct" that is actually the common bile duct or even more proximal ducts is reported in the operative notes of these procedures, but just as often the second transection is not noted. High transections are probably due to traction on the gallbladder, which actually pulls the hepatic ducts down during transection of the biliary tree. Hepatic ducts may either be clipped or divided, resulting in either obstruction or bile leak. This injury is often associated with an injury to the right hepatic artery, with brisk bleeding that leads to conversion and diagnosis of biliary injury or simply to occlusion and division of the right hepatic artery. Either may aggravate the biliary injury due to ischemia of the remaining bile duct. (30). At the time of reconstruction there is often evidence of dissection on the left side of the common duct, even to the point of exposure of the portal vein (11).

Sometimes one clip is placed on the cystic duct (see Fig. 17.9B) and the point of division is either the common duct (see Fig. 17.9B) or cystic duct (see Fig. 17.9C). If the common duct is transected, bile drains from the cut end, sometimes leading to recognition of injury. However, equally often this gets attributed to a second cystic duct, and the full-blown injury shown in Figure 17.9C evolves. The least harmful type of misidentification occurs when the cystic duct is divided (Fig. 17.9C), because if the injury is recognized by observation of bile in the field, the clip on the common bile duct may simply be removed. Bile leak will not occur if cystic and common ducts run in a common sheath and the clip is placed across both (Fig. 17.9C, inset). Clip removal (29), balloon dilatation (14), or stenting (38) of the clipped duct may occasionally resolve the injury even when the injury is recognized postoperatively; in other patients late stricture occurs after clip removal (11).

The misidentification scenario leads to injury to an aberrant right hepatic duct, which is present in 2% of cases. The

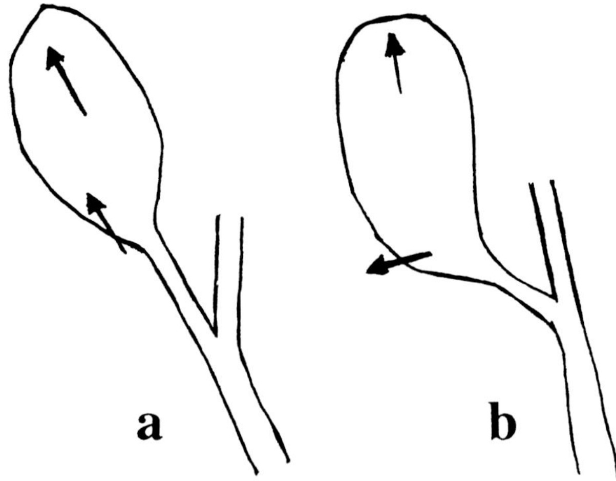

FIGURE 17.10. *Effect of the direction of traction on the appearance of the bile ducts at surgery.* ***(a)*** *Both graspers pulling superiorly bring the common and cystic ducts into alignment, producing the appearance of a single duct.* ***(b)*** *When the grasper on the pouch of Hartmann is pulling laterally to the right, the cystic and common ducts appear as separate structures and the common bile duct is less likely to be mistaken for the cystic duct and injured.*

segment of the aberrant right hepatic duct between where the cystic duct enters it and the point at which it joins the common hepatic is thought to be the cystic duct. The misidentified segment is clipped and usually cut (Fig. 17.9D). To remove the gallbladder, the aberrant duct must be cut again at a higher level. Variations of this injury are shown in Figure 17.9E and F.

It is widely appreciated that the direction of traction of the gallbladder may contribute to the appearance that the common bile duct is the cystic duct, leading to the misidentification injury. When the pouch of Hartmann is pulled superiorly rather than laterally, the common bile duct and the cystic bile duct align and appear to be a single structure (Fig. 17.10). Although incorrect traction has undoubtedly contributed to some injuries—especially early in the learning curve—it is our opinion that it is the reliance on the appearance of the lower end of the gallbladder for identification of the cystic duct that is responsible for many misidentification injuries. In this method the surgeon follows the putative cystic duct up to the gallbladder where it can be seen flaring out to become the infundibulum, thus identifying it as the actual cystic duct. However, when the common bile duct is surrounded and followed upward it may "flare" at the point where the cystic and common hepatic ducts connect to it. This false infundibulum is most likely to appear when there is a short cystic duct, a large stone in the pouch of Hartmann, and severe acute and chronic inflammation, all of which make retraction and display of the real cystic duct difficult. The end stage of this pathology is Mirizzi's syndrome, in which stones efface the cystic duct so that the gallbladder communicates directly with the common bile duct.

Misidentification is also more common when adhesive bands tether the gallbladder to the common bile duct (39). Misidentification may lead to injury of the bile duct without division or clipping, as extensive dissection may cause devascularization (11) especially if ductal arteries, thought to be the cystic artery, are divided (29). This type of injury may present later as a stricture (40).

The chief technical causes of laparoscopic ductal injury are failure to occlude the cystic duct securely, too deep a plane of dissection when taking the gallbladder off the liver bed, tenting injuries, and thermal injuries to the bile duct. The cystic duct is routinely occluded with clips that are less reliable than ligatures or suture ligatures, the standard methods of securing the cystic duct during open cholecystectomy. Retained stones in the bile duct may contribute to clip failure by raising biliary tract pressures (41), but the main cause is the inappropriate use of clips rather than another occlusion device on a thick rigid cystic duct. Clips may also "scissor" during application, resulting in faulty closure; or they may be loosened by subsequent dissection close to the clip. Injury to ducts in the liver bed is due to dissection in too deep a plane when excising the gallbladder. It usually occurs when the dissection is difficult (as when acute or severe chronic inflammation is present) or when the gallbladder is intrahepatic.

Tenting injury was well described in the open cholecystectomy era. There are few reports of this injury during laparoscopic cholecystectomy, and it actually may be less common during laparoscopic cholecystectomy due to the excellent visualization of properly identified cystic ducts. In the tenting injury, the junction of the common bile duct and hepatic bile ducts is occluded when a clip is placed at the bottom end of the cystic duct while forcefully pulling up on the gallbladder.

Cautery-induced injuries are more likely to occur in the presence of severe inflammation, which may lead to the use of excessively high cautery settings to control hemorrhage. Misuse of cautery has led to some very serious bile duct injuries, characteristically type E injuries with loss of ductal tissue due to thermal necrosis.

PREVENTION OF BILIARY INJURIES

General

Laparoscopic cholecystectomy should be performed only by surgeons who have been trained and proctored in the operation. Experience should be graded and difficult procedures should not be attempted until experience has been gained. Laparoscopic cholecystectomy is more difficult in the presence of acute inflammation, and biliary injury is more likely under these circumstances (25). It is also more difficult when the patients are males, elderly, or when there have been repeated attacks of pain (42)—these factors are additive. A previous attack of acute cholecystitis also is a significant contributing factor to operative difficulty (42). Inexperienced surgeons should be aware of these predictive factors and take appropriate steps to ensure adequate assistance in the operating room. For credentialing purposes, laparoscopic cholecystectomy during an attack of acute cholecystitis should be considered to be an advanced laparoscopic technique.

Avoidance of Misidentification of Ducts

Misidentification results when there has been a failure to identify the cystic structures conclusively. The cystic duct and artery are the only structures that require division during a cholecystectomy, so the objective of dissection is to identify these structures conclusively (15). Furthermore, only these structures need to be identified.

The key phrase is "conclusive identification." Such a method was available during open cholecystectomy. It consisted of tentative identification of the cystic structures by dissection in the triangle of Calot followed by dissection of the gallbladder off the liver bed. After complete detachment of the gallbladder, the conclusive identification of the cystic structures as the only two structures entering the gallbladder could be made.

In 1995 we introduced a technique for conclusive identification of the cystic structures at laparoscopic cholecystectomy based on a "critical view of safety" (Fig. 17.11). In this technique the triangle of Calot is cleared of all fat and fibrous tissue. After this is done only two structures remain connected to the lower end of the gallbladder, and the lowest part of the gallbladder attachment to the liver bed has been exposed. The latter is an important step that is equivalent in the open technique to taking the gallbladder off the liver bed. It is not necessary to see the common duct. Once the critical view is attained, the cystic structures may be occluded, as they have been conclusively identified. Failure to achieve the critical view is an absolute indication for conversion or possibly cholangiography to define ductal anatomy. As discussed previously, we believe that there is considerable danger on relying simply on the appearance of the "cystic duct" to gallbladder junction because this may be deceiving, especially in the presence of severe inflammation.

Some useful technical suggestions to aid clearing the triangle of Calot are to dissect the triangle of Calot from both its dorsal and ventral aspects by the use of a combination of pulling techniques, gentle spreading with forceps, hook cautery, and blunt dissection with a nonactivated spatula cautery tip or anchored pledgets (5,7,15,43). The pouch of Hartmann should be pulled laterally and interiorly to open the anterior-left side of Calot's triangle and create an angle between the cystic duct and common bile duct (see Fig. 17.10) (7). The plane of dissection should always be maintained on the gallbladder or cystic duct. To do so, the gallbladder should be followed down to the presumed point of the infundibulum to the cystic duct junction, and dissection started there. "Dome-down" cholecystectomy is not a substitute for conclusive identification by the critical view technique, although it is a useful way to take the gallbladder off the liver bed once identification is achieved.

Whether anatomical identification by routine operative cholangiography (RIOC) prevents biliary injury is hotly debated. A recent population study in Australia found that RIOC reduced the incidence of injury (44). This is an

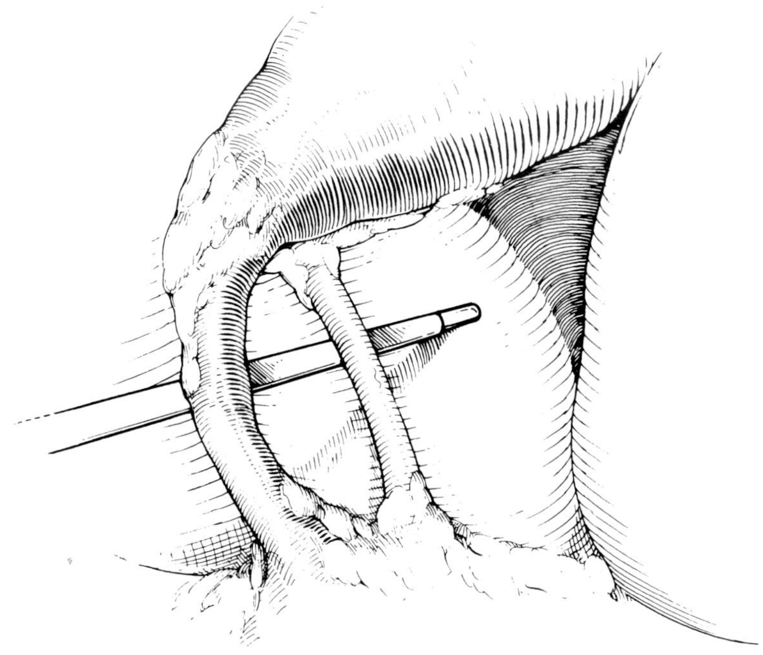

FIGURE 17.11. *The critical view of safety. The triangle of Calot is dissected free of all tissue except for cystic duct and artery and the base of the liver bed is exposed. When this view is achieved, the two structures entering the gallbladder can only be the cystic duct and artery. It is not necessary to see the common bile duct. (By permission of the Journal of the American College of Surgeons.)*

important study because it adjusted for confounding variables such as age, gender, hospital type, and severity of disease. Other studies suggest that the severity but not the incidence of biliary injury is reduced by RIOC (45–47). Operative cholangiography is best at detecting a misidentification of the common bile duct as the cystic duct and will prevent excisional injuries of bile ducts, provided that the cholangiogram is interpreted properly. However, operative cholangiograms have been misinterpreted frequently in the presence of injury (5,29,48,49). The most common misinterpretation is the failure to recognize that the bile duct rather than the cystic duct has been incised and cannulated when only the lower part of the biliary tree is seen. Such an incisional injury of the common bile duct made to perform RIOC may not be innocuous. At the least, it requires conversion and repair over a T-tube, and at worst requires biliary reconstruction. Furthermore, RIOC is very poor at detecting aberrant right ducts that unite with the cystic duct before joining the common duct (Figs. 17.12 and 17.13). The aberrant duct appears to be the cystic duct

(A)

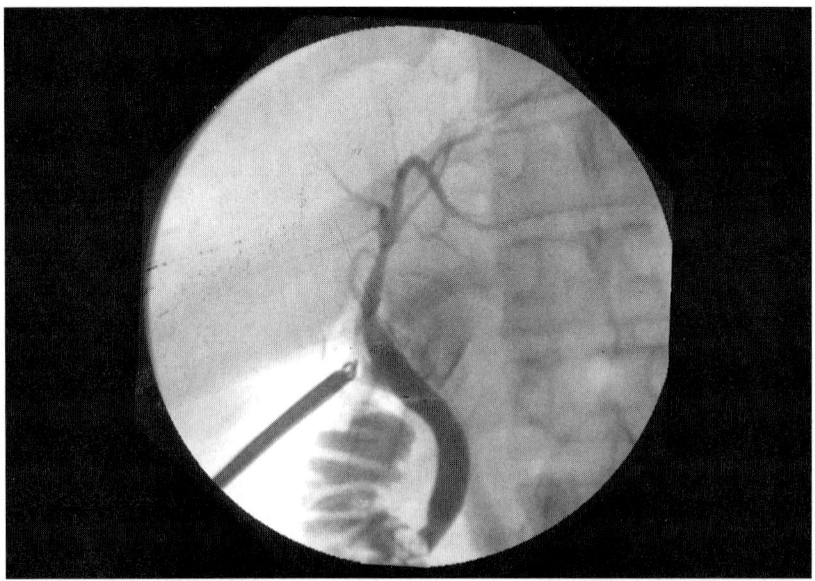

(B)

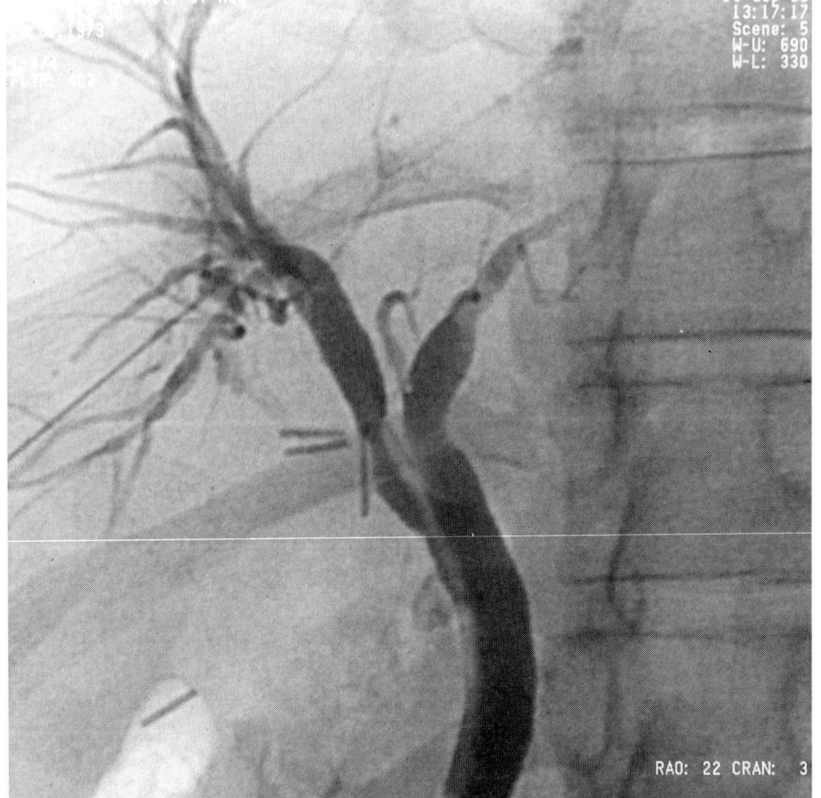

FIGURE 17.12. ***(A)*** *"Normal" cystic duct cholangiogram obtained at laparoscopic cholecystectomy. Failure to completely fill the right-sided ducts was interpreted as being a result of rapid emptying from below into the duodenum.* ***(B)*** *Percutaneous cholangiogram performed several days after surgery demonstrating that a large part of the right side of the liver is drained by an aberrant duct that was joined by the cystic duct. This demonstrates the limitation of cystic duct cholangiography in identifying aberrant ducts.*

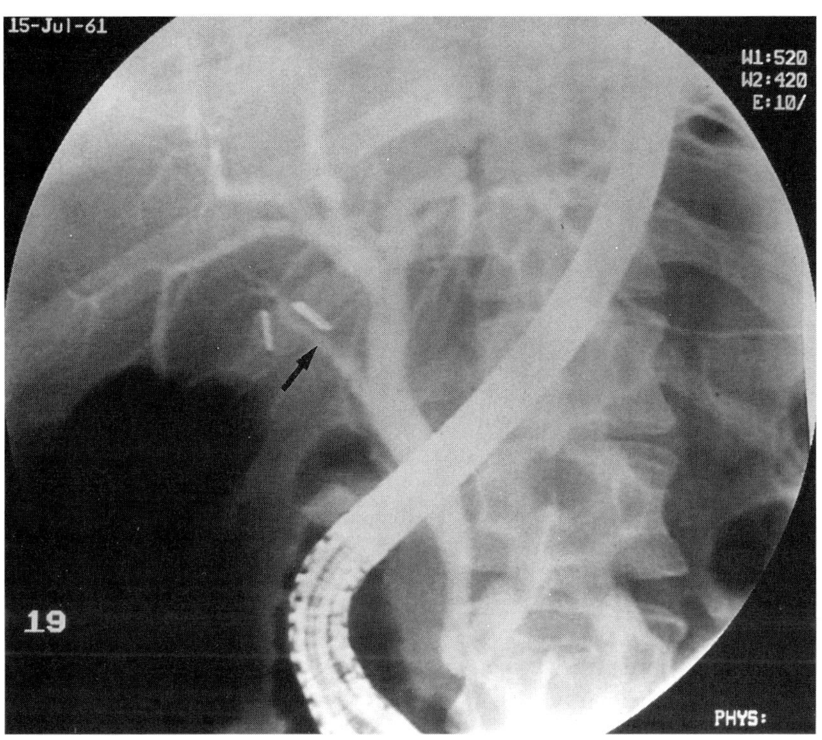

FIGURE 17.13. *Postoperative ERCP in a patient with an aberrant right hepatic duct (arrow). Clips indicate the position of cystic duct and artery. Note how the point of union of the aberrant duct with the common hepatic duct looks like a cystic duct/common duct junction. Mistakenly doing a cholangiogram through the aberrant duct rather than identifying it by dissection would have led to a ductal injury that would have been difficult to repair because of the small size of the aberrant duct. Also, a cholangiogram done through the aberrant duct would probably have been read as normal because it only supplied a part of the right hemiliver. (Reproduced by permission of the Journal of the American College of Surgeons from Strasberg SM, Hertl M, Soper NJ. An analysis of the problem of biliary injury during laparoscopic cholecystectomy. J Am Coll Surg 1995;180:101–25.)*

visually and on x-ray because other right-sided ducts fill. As a result, many argue that meticulous dissection of the triangle of Calot, as was done during the open era, is the correct means of anatomical identification (15,50,51). Our view is that conclusive identification of the anatomy by the "critical view" technique is the method of choice for identification of biliary anatomy during laparoscopic cholecystectomy. If this method is not used, and cystic duct identification is performed by the infundibular technique, then RIOC should always be used to confirm the procedure.

Avoidance of Technical Errors

Clips should be placed so that the tips can be seen projecting beyond the duct, free of extraneous material. Clips should not be manipulated in the subsequent dissection. Clips should not be used when the cystic duct is thick—rather, two preformed ligature loops should be applied and tightened to occlude the cystic duct. Applying extra clips is not the answer and may lead to tenting injury. Tenting injury can also be avoided by not pulling up on the gallbladder forcefully when applying clips, and by ensuring, via direct observation, that a piece of cystic duct remains below the clip applied closest to the common bile duct end of the cystic duct.

Avoidance of ductal injury in the liver bed depends upon staying in the correct plane of dissection. Use of the spatula dissector combined with irrigation to keep the field clear of blood is often helpful. The cautery scissors are also useful, but there is no substitute for meticulous technique and experience in this dissection.

Cautery should not be used or must be used only with great care in the triangle of Calot. Great care means low cautery settings and coagulation of small pieces of tissue at one time; that tissue must be lifted off and be free of any adjacent tissue. Low cautery settings are mandatory as higher settings may lead to arcing of the current to the ducts. Cautery should never be used to divide the cystic duct because this may lead to thermal necrosis of the cystic duct stump or adjacent bile duct (52).

Bleeding should never be controlled by blind application of clamps, clips, or cautery. Brisk bleeding is an indication for conversion. Lesser degrees of hemorrhage may appear more serious than they really are, because of the magnification of laparoscopy. The operating surgeon must use good judgment in such cases, as the bleeding often stops spontaneously or with direct pressure.

PRESENTATION AND INVESTIGATION

About 10% of type A injuries are identified intraoperatively; most of the rest are diagnosed in the first postoperative week (15). Type B injuries are infrequently diagnosed intraoperatively; usually they present months or years later with right-sided abdominal pain or jaundice (36). Type C and D injuries, which produce bilomas like type A injuries, tend to be diagnosed in the early postoperative period. The type of injury most likely to be identified during the procedure is type E. Of type E injuries, 25% to 40% are diagnosed intraoperatively according to most literature reports (15). Most of the remaining type E injuries are identified in the first 30 days after surgery (15), with the remaining presenting months to years after the laparoscopic cholecystectomy (15). The preceding comments refer to the first presentation of injury. In large series, 30% to 40% of repairs are performed on patients who have had a prior repair at the institution where the injury occurred (20).

Intraoperative identification of injury may occur by recognition of bile in the field, indicating a cut bile duct; by cholangiography; or rarely by direct observation of a divided duct. At other times, the actual diagnosis of biliary injury is made after conversion for bleeding or inability to proceed in a difficult dissection.

Postoperative presentations are influenced by the type of injury and whether a drain has been left. Pathologic processes leading to symptoms are biloma, fistula, or bile ascites; partial or complete biliary obstructions; and superinfection. These may occur in various combinations. The most common presentations are pain with sepsis with or without jaundice, and jaundice without other symptoms. Biliary fistula is also a common presentation. Some patients present only with distention and malaise. The latter is a particularly insidious presentation and is usually due to bile ascites. Many times vague complaints of this type have been passed over by overly optimistic surgeons only to evolve into much more ominous complaints—the lesson is that patients should feel well after laparoscopic cholecystectomy and that such complaints should be heeded. Delay in diagnosis of this type of injury has been a key factor in litigation (4). There have been many papers written on the subject of investigation of symptoms developing after laparoscopic cholecystectomy, but there are no comparative trials of different algorithms. The least invasive and most economical approach seems to be one based on the type of presentation.

Pain and Sepsis

Pain and sepsis usually occur in injuries leading to bilomas: injury types A, C, and D. Most patients with type A injury present with the pain/sepsis symptom complex; jaundice is very uncommon but hyperbilirubinemia (2–3 mg/dL) is often found (9), as is elevation of alkaline phosphatase level (12). Few of the more serious type E injuries present only with pain and sepsis.

The purpose of investigation in the pain/sepsis group is to determine whether there is a biloma or bile ascites, whether there is continuing bile leakage, and whether the site of the leakage is from the biliary tree. A computed tomography (CT) scan is performed first to localize the fluid collections, which may then be aspirated to determine if they are bilious. In most cases a drain is placed in the biloma and an endoscopic retrograde cholangiopancreatography (ERCP) follows. Magnetic resonance imaging (MRI) with magnetic resonance cholangiography (MRC) has the potential to replace these investigations with a single one (53), but MRC does not see collapsed ducts well and is more likely to be useful when there is obstruction of the biliary tree than perforation with free drainage of bile into the peritoneal cavity.

Because most patients presenting with pain/sepsis have type A or D injuries, definitive treatment is possible at the time of endoscopy. Very stable patients with bile ascites may be treated in the same manner, but laparotomy and drainage is advisable for other patients with generalized bile ascites. Another more circuitous approach when a collection is found is to perform a hepatobiliary iminodiacetic acid (HIDA) scan if bile is aspirated and proceed to drain placement and ERCP only if continuing leakage is demonstrated. The latter may be suitable for the minimally symptomatic patient.

Jaundice

The presence of jaundice strongly suggests that the patient has sustained a type E injury. Type E injuries present with jaundice in about 70% of cases. Occlusions usually present with jaundice as the sole symptom, but transections are often accompanied by pain and sepsis due to accumulation of bile in the peritoneal cavity (15). ERCP is the first-line investigation today, although it may be supplanted by MRC in the future. The duct may be found to be completely occluded—often clips are seen at the point at which the dye column stops (Fig. 17.14); or the duct may be transected, with loss of continuity to the upper biliary tract. Next, percutaneous transhepatic cholangiography (PTC) is performed to delineate the proximal ducts and to provide external drainage of bile. If partially occluded stenotic rather than totally occluded ducts are found, the entire extent of injury may be diagnosed by ERCP. The presence of bile collections may require percutaneous drainage as well.

Bile Fistula

About one-third of patients with type A patients present with bile fistula, but any injury in which there is a bile leak may do so. Because as bile has egress, local collections or obstruction to bile flow is unlikely and sepsis and jaundice are usually absent. The first-line investigation is a fistulogram. Subsequent management depends upon anatomical findings.

Vague Symptoms

A few patients present only with vague symptoms such as distention, malaise, anorexia, complaints of discomfort, or requirements for more than the usual amount of analgesia. Such complaints are all too easy to dismiss, but they might be the only manifestations of a serious biliary injury. Hepatic bile is dilute and could cause little irritation until an infection occurs. The suggested line of investigation is the same as for pain/sepsis.

Hemobilia is a rare presentation of biliary injury and is due to pseudoaneurysm formation (54–56) at the site of an associated arterial injury with subsequent erosion into the biliary tree (54,55).

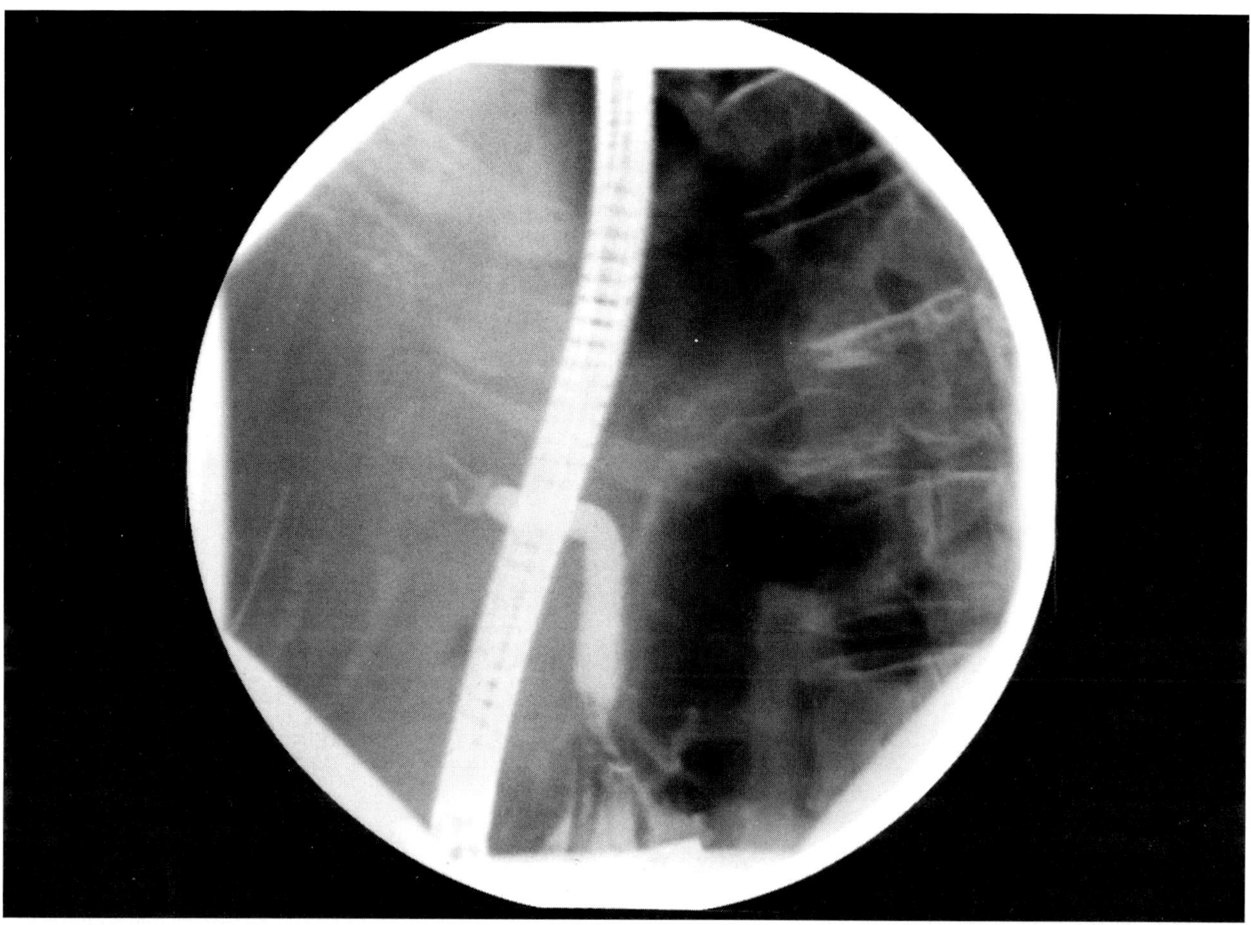

FIGURE 17.14. *Postoperative ERCP for a patient who was noted to have bile in the operative field at the time of surgery. The surgeon placed a drain in the right upper quadrant and referred the patient for further management. Note the complete occlusion of the bile duct and the position of clips at the top of the column of dye.*

MANAGEMENT OF BILIARY INJURIES

Management of Injuries Recognized at the Initial Operation

There is little written about the conduct of a laparoscopic cholecystectomy once a biliary injury is suspected. The following is based on our experience with referred biliary injuries. It is also predicated on highly suggestive evidence that the repair of difficult biliary injuries frequently fails when it is performed by surgical teams that are infrequently engaged in upper biliary tree surgery such as liver resections and bile duct resections (4,15,20,57).

Intraoperative recognition of biliary injury is usually an indication for conversion (but not always, as will be discussed later). The following two guidelines are suggested when laparotomy is undertaken for suspected injury:

1. A repair should be attempted only if the techniques of dissection or reconstruction required for the repair are commonly used by the operating team.
2. The injury should not be worsened by attempting a dissection for the purpose of making an exact diagnosis.

Repair of type A, type D, and type E1 injuries normally requires techniques that are commonly practiced by most general surgeons. Type B, C, and E2 to E5 injuries require operative techniques that are more likely to be available only at specialized hepatobiliary units. When such techniques are not available at the time of injury, closed suction drains should be placed in the right upper quadrant and the patient should be referred. Simple drainage of the right upper quadrant seems to be safe (see Fig. 17.13), and there have been no reports of problems arising as a result of this strategy (15). If an injury is recognized during the laparoscopic cholecystectomy and is of a type that the operating surgeon would normally refer for repair, then laparotomy is not indicated unless it is needed to control blood loss. Laparoscopic drainage and referral without laparotomy is preferable.

Type A injuries, recognized at the time of surgery, are repaired by suture of the cystic duct and drainage. Type D injuries are repaired by closure of the defect using fine absorbable sutures over a T-tube and placement of a closed suction drain in the vicinity of the repair. Nonabsorbable sutures are contraindicated because they form a nidus for stone formation. The T-tube should be brought out through a separate incision in the duct, if possible. Avulsion of the cystic duct, a variant of type D injury, may be managed in the same manner. Complete transection should be repaired with a Roux-en-Y hepaticojejunostomy, applying the principles of anastomosis given below. Other reconstructive techniques such as choledochocholedochostomy or choledochoduodenostomy should not be used, because of considerations of blood supply and tension.

Management of Biliary Injuries Diagnosed Postoperatively

Management depends on the type of injury, the type of initial management and its result, and the time elapsed since the initial operation or repair.

Type A Injuries

Intraperitoneal bile collections are drained percutaneously. If bile leakage is continuing, intrabiliary pressure is reduced by endoscopic sphincterotomy with placement of a stent or a nasobiliary catheter (see Fig. 17.2). Most investigators recommend placement of a stent or a nasobiliary catheter (58) in addition to sphincterotomy and there is experimental evidence supporting this policy (59). Infrequently, balloon dilatation and stenting rather than sphincterotomy and stenting have also been used. The stent should not occlude the lumen; the bile should be able to flow around as well as through the stent. If ERCP fails, percutaneous transhepatic cholangiography may also be used to decompress the duct. There is little indication for reoperation as the first line of management of this type of injury except when the patient has generalized bile ascites or peritonitis.

Type B Injuries

Type B injuries may remain asymptomatic or present years later with right upper quadrant discomfort or pain. Type B injuries may also present with cholangitis (36). They are sometimes diagnosed in asymptomatic patients on the basis of abnormal liver function tests found on routine screening. Symptomatic patients require hepaticojejunostomy or hepatic resection if biliary-enteric anastomosis is not possible. In asymptomatic patients, treatment is not recommended when the section of liver affected is small or if the injury was remote and the isolated portion has atrophied. When the injury is recent and the section of liver is large (e.g., the whole right hemiliver) repair is empirically recommended (see Fig. 17.14).

Type C Injuries

Type C injuries require drainage of the bile collections and biliary-enteric anastomosis or ligation of the transected duct. If the duct is very small (i.e., <2 mm), biliary-enteric anastomosis is unlikely to be successful and ligation is preferable. Insertion of a transhepatic catheter prior to duct reconstruction is a useful aid to locating the duct at operation. It also may be used to control bile drainage and to drain the subhepatic bile collection preoperatively (see Fig. 17.4). Liver resection may occasionally be required when other techniques fail.

Type D Injuries

For type D injuries, ERCP and stenting (60) are the treatment of choice in the postoperative period (see Fig. 17.5). Failure of ERCP to control biliary drainage is an indication for operative repair. These patients should be followed closely because their injury may evolve into a type E injury, especially when the cause was a thermal injury or when there has been concomitant vascular injury. When an operation is required, the technique of repair is the same as when the problem is discovered at time of initial surgery.

Type E Injuries

Many studies have emphasized that the best chance for lasting repair is the first chance (15,20,61). Strictures and sometimes clip occlusions (14,29,38) may be treated by dilatation and stents placed either by ERCP or percutaneously through the liver. One series suggested that the results are equivalent to an operation (60); however, in this study the mean interval between cholecystectomy and presentation was several years and the mean bilirubin level was 4.3 mg/dL. Therefore, the study population had mild and late appearing stenoses, not the early severe stenoses that seem to be much more common after laparoscopic surgery. Other papers have reported frequent successes, although long-term follow-up is not commonly available (62–64) and there seems to be declining enthusiasm for this approach except in selected circumstances.

In our experience, nonsurgical therapy is most likely to be successful when the strictures are mild, appear months to years after surgery, or are of short length. Lillemoe et al. (65) reported a 64% success rate with interventional techniques. The failures tended to be E3 or E4 lesions with prior hepaticojejunostomy that presented early after that procedure with a re-stenosis. An operation is required for failure of stent therapy and when there is ductal discontinuity.

Timing of Surgery

With fresh injuries there is a choice between immediate or delayed repair. Factors favoring immediate repair are early referral, lack of right upper quadrant bile collections, simpler injuries that can be rapidly diagnosed and are unlikely to involve vascular injury, and a stable patient. Many patients are referred 1 to 6 weeks after the primary operation, a time when local inflammation may be expected to be great. In these patients percutaneous tubes are placed to relieve obstruction from affected segments, to drain subhepatic col-

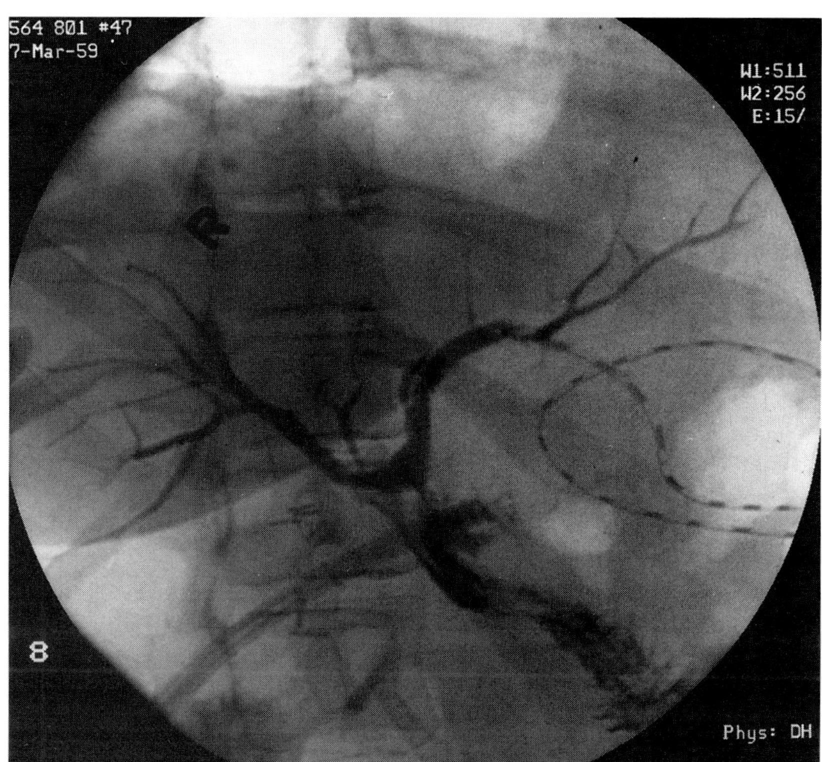

FIGURE 17.15. *Postoperative cholangiogram showing the typical appearance of a repair performed by the Hepp-Couinaud approach. Dye is draining through a side-to-side anastomosis between the left hepatic duct and the jejunum. The injury (E3) was at the bifurcation. The tube was removed after cholangiography. (Reproduced by permission of the Journal of the American College of Surgeons from Strasberg SM, Hertl M, Soper NJ. An analysis of the problem of biliary injury during laparoscopic cholecystectomy. J Am Coll Surg 1995;180:101–25.)*

lections, and to control sepsis. Sometimes subhepatic drains alone are sufficient to provide egress of bile from all parts of the liver, and percutaneous transhepatic stents are inserted only on the day prior to repair to guide the dissection. Repair is performed when the inflammation has settled, usually about 3 months after the last operation.

This delayed approach is sometimes used even when the patient is referred within the first week, especially for complex injuries (E4, E5) and those in which either a thermal etiology or concomitant ischemic injury is suspected. This permits the injury to evolve to a stable state in which the upper extent of ischemic damage is clear. In a recent small series in which immediate repair of fresh injuries was the standard policy regardless of the preceding considerations, the re-stricture rate at just over 1 year was 25% (66). Immediate repair may also be undertaken when the injury is diagnosed months after surgery, such as when stenting of a stenosis has failed or a biliary-enteric anastomosis has had a late failure.

Preoperative Preparation

It is essential to completely diagnose the injury prior to an operation (6,15,20,61). Failure to do so may result in exclusion of bile ducts from the repair (6). The percutaneous transhepatic tubes placed to ensure biliary drainage from all liver segments also serve as guides to the position of the injured ducts at surgery (8,48) (see Fig. 17.7). Our policy is to perform a conciliation between CT and PTC studies to be sure that all ducts in the liver are accounted for. All isolated sections of the biliary tree are intubated preoperatively.

Other principles of repair are that the anastomosis be tension free with a good blood supply, be mucosa to mucosa, and be of adequate caliber (61). Hepaticojejunostomy is used in preference to either choledochocholedochostomy or choledochoduodenostomy, because a tension-free anastomosis is always possible with hepaticojejunostomy. Choledochocholedochostomy has the additional disadvantage that blood supply to the anastomosis may be poor. Whenever possible, an anterior longitudinal opening is created in the bile duct and a long side-to-side anastomosis is performed. Usually this is done to the extrahepatic portion of the left hepatic duct after it is lowered by dividing the hepatic plate (Fig. 17.15) as described by Hepp (67), referred to as the Hepp-Couinaud approach. This minimizes dissection behind the ducts, thereby making the dissection technically easier and less hazardous; and it decreases the chance of devascularizing the duct at the point of anastomosis. Also it permits a wide anastomosis even when the ducts are not large, as the whole length of the extrahepatic left duct can be used. This approach is particularly suitable for injuries at or just below the bifurcation (types E2 and E3). With type E1 and some E2 injuries the common hepatic duct itself may be used. Right ducts do not lend themselves to this approach as well because they have a short extrahepatic length. Sometimes the end of the right duct is used, but dissection of the left duct provides a guide to the coronal plane in which the intrahepatic right hepatic ducts will be found and these may be exposed by removing liver tissue.

During these procedures exposure is also facilitated by dividing the bridge of tissue between segments III and IV, fully opening the gallbladder fossa, which often collapses with adherence of its walls. If these maneuvers are not sufficient, resecting part of segment IVb and/or V will open the upper porta hepatis (15,68). The latter is an invaluable adjunct in the very difficult cases. Ducts may be sewn individually or be joined to form a single orifice, provided they are not placed on tension when doing so. Fine absorbable sutures are used to construct the anastomosis.

The use of postoperative stents is controversial. There is no evidence that they are helpful if a large caliber mucosa-to-mucosa anastomosis has been achieved. We use them only when very small ducts are anastomosed. Occasionally, the transhepatic tubes are left through the anastomosis for several days to perform postoperative cholangiography.

In cases in which a primary repair has failed, it is not always necessary to perform a fresh hepaticojejunostomy. Sometimes the problem is only a bile leak from an adequate anastomosis, or a slightly stenotic anastomosis. These can often be treated by nonoperative means (14,48) when the stricture is very short, reserving reoperation for the failure of these procedures.

Sometimes biliary reconstruction is not possible or advisable. When ductal reconstruction to a part of the liver is impossible, resection should be performed. Occasionally prior failure of reconstruction leads to secondary biliary cirrhosis and end-stage liver failure, in which case liver transplantation will be required (69). In almost all examples of this unfortunate outcome, high reconstructions have been attempted by surgeons who lacked experience in the procedures.

Treatment of failed repairs with metallic stents gives very poor results in the long term, with 50% of treated patients suffering from repeated cholangitis. Re-repair at specialist centers is far more successful than metallic stenting (20).

OUTCOME OF TREATMENT

Most surgical series of biliary reconstruction cite very good short-term results. However, as is well known from older literature describing ductal injury during open cholecystectomy, there is a progressive re-stenosis rate. Two-thirds of recurrences are diagnosed in the first 2 years after repair but re-stenosis has been described after 10 years. The re-stenosis rate varies from 5% to 28% (70). There is a recent indication that the results in the laparoscopic era may not be as good as these, perhaps because of increased severity of injury. Bauer et al. (3) reported on 30 patients treated surgically and followed for a mean of about 1 year. Results were unsatisfactory in about one-third of the patients (71); 40% required a second procedure or remained symptomatic. The Hepp-Couinaud approach was not used in this group of patients.

In another series consisting of 50 injuries, 25 hepaticojejunostomies were performed; 5 of these patients required further surgery during the short-term follow-up period (6). The main cause of failure was failure to diagnose the full extent of injury preoperatively and extension of injury after repair to ducts that had been "burned." Extension of injury in the first few months may also be due to concomitant vascular injury at the time of laparoscopic injury, as noted, thus our preference to delay repair of complex injuries for several months so that a final level of injury can be established.

Several institutions have reported improved results. Walsh et al. (72) of the Cleveland Clinic reported seven recurrent strictures in 34 patients (20%) who were reexamined for a mean of 3 years (72). Murr et al. (17) of the Mayo Clinic reported 85% excellent results (normal liver function tests and asymptomatic) in a series of 54 patients mostly treated with the Hepp-Couinaud approach. The mean follow-up was 3.7 years. Six patients (11%) were treatment failures, including one postoperative death and five recurrent strictures. Stewart et al. of the University of California at San Francisco reported a treatment failure rate of only 4% in 45 patients, but the length of follow-up was probably relatively short, as this series of laparoscopic injuries was reported in 1995 (20). Lillemoe et al. (65) of Johns Hopkins reported on 59 surgically treated patients with follow-up examinations for a mean of 33 months who had a treatment failure rate (defined similarly to that of the Mayo group) of 8%. We have personally treated 41 biliary injuries since 1992 with a single treatment failure as defined by the Mayo criteria (17).

Valid comparison among series is not easily done because of the lack of standard reporting and the effect of differences in the severity of injuries treated in different series. Injuries above the bifurcation involving several bile ducts have a much worse prognosis than do injuries of the common hepatic duct and the proportion of severe injuries in a series will affect outcome. In the series of Mirza et al. (18), 20 patients underwent surgery; of these 4 have had recurrent bouts of cholangitis, and all of these occurred in the 9 patients who had the more complex E3, E4, or E5 injuries. A similar association between failure and level of injury was noted by Stewart et al. (20).

Reporting of treatment failure is not uniform. Murr et al. (17) have recently suggested a useful classification of outcomes in which there are four grades: excellent (normal liver function tests in an asymptomatic patient), good (mildly abnormal liver function tests in an asymptomatic patient), poor (abnormal liver function tests in a symptomatic patient), and treatment failure (need for a secondary intervention for stricture). We do not consider elevations of the alkaline phosphatase of less than 2 times normal to be abnormal after a Roux-en-Y anastomosis. Also there may be gradations worth considering within the "treatment failure" category, such as failures treatable by percutaneous dilatation; failures requiring reconstruction, resection, or transplantation, each of these being a worsening grade; or failures leading to death. Length of the follow-up is another obvious variable affecting outcome.

In summary, biliary injury is the greatest problem besetting one of this century's greatest advances in biliary surgery, the laparoscopic cholecystectomy. The key to managing this problem lies not in complicated repairs at tertiary centers, but rather in prevention. Prevention requires a commitment to performing meticulous dissections so that only structures that have been unequivocally and conclusively identified are divided.

SUGGESTED READINGS

Davidoff AM, Pappas TN, Murray EA, et al. Mechanisms of major biliary injury during laparoscopic cholecystectomy. Ann Surg 1992;215(3):196–202. Description of the classical injury.

Hepp J. Hepaticojejunostomy using the left biliary trunk for iatrogenic biliary lesions: the French connection. World J Surg 1985;9(3):507–11. Classic article on use of left duct for high injuries.

Lillemoe KD, Pitt HA, Cameron JL. Postoperative bile duct strictures. Surg Clin N Am 1990;70:1355–80. Presentation, management, and results in the open cholecystectomy era.

Murr MM, Gigot JF, Nagorney DM, Harmsen WS, Ilstrup DM, Farnell MB. Long-term results of biliary reconstruction after laparoscopic bile duct injuries. Arch Surg 1999;134(6):604–9. Recent results from a tertiary care center.

Strasberg SM, Hertl M, Soper NJ. An analysis of the problem of biliary injury during laparoscopic cholecystectomy. J Am Coll Surg 1995;180(1):101–25. Review of laparoscopic biliary injuries and their classification.

REFERENCES

1. Savader SJ, Lillemoe KD, Prescott CA, et al. Laparoscopic cholecystectomy-related bile duct injuries: a health and financial disaster. Ann Surg 1997;225:268–73.
2. Woods MS. Estimated costs of biliary tract complications in laparoscopic cholecystectomy based upon Medicare cost/charge ratios. A case-control study. Surg Endosc 1996;10:1004–7.
3. Bauer TW, Morris JB, Lowenstein A, et al. The consequences of a major bile duct injury during laparoscopic cholecystectomy. J Gastrointest Surg 1998;2:61–6.
4. Carroll BJ, Birth M, Phillips EH. Common bile duct injuries during laparoscopic cholecystectomy that result in litigation. Surg Endosc 1998;12:310–3.
5. Asbun HJ, Rossi RL, Lowell JA, Munson JL. Bile duct injury during laparoscopic cholecystectomy: mechanism of injury, prevention, and management. World J Surg 1993;17:547–51.
6. Branum G, Schmitt C, Baillie J, et al. Management of major biliary complications after laparoscopic cholecystectomy. Ann Surg 1993;217:532–40.
7. Ferguson CM, Rattner DW, Warshaw AL. Bile duct injury in laparoscopic cholecystectomy. Surg Laparosc Endosc Percutaneous Tech 1992;2:1–7.
8. Soper NJ, Flye MW, Brunt LM, et al. Diagnosis and management of biliary complications of laparoscopic cholecystectomy. Am J Surg 1993;165:663–9.
9. Vitale GC, Stephens G, Wieman TJ, Larson GM. Use of endoscopic retrograde cholangiopancreatography in the management of biliary complications after laparoscopic cholecystectomy. Surgery 1993;114:806–12. Erratum: Surgery 1994;115:263.
10. Woods MS, Traverso LW, Kozarek RA, et al. Characteristics of biliary tract complications during laparoscopic cholecystectomy: a multi-institutional study. Am J Surg 1994;167:27–33.
11. Roy AF, Passi RB, Lapointe RW, et al. Bile duct injury during laparoscopic cholecystectomy. Can J Surg 1993;36:509–16.
12. Kozarek RA, Ball TJ, Patterson DJ, et al. Endoscopic treatment of biliary injury in the era of laparoscopic cholecystectomy. Gastrointest Endosc 1994;40:10–6.
13. Walker AT, Brooks DC, Tumeh SS, Braver JM. Bile duct disruption after laparoscopic cholecystectomy. Semin Ultrasound CT MR 1993;14:346–55.
14. Wright TB, Bertino RB, Bishop AF, et al. Complications of laparoscopic cholecystectomy and their interventional radiologic management. Radiographics 1993;13:119–28.
15. Strasberg SM, Hertl M, Soper NJ. An analysis of the problem of biliary injury during laparoscopic cholecystectomy. J Am Coll Surg 1995;180:101–25.
16. Adamsen S, Hansen OH, Funch-Jensen P, et al. Bile duct injury during laparoscopic cholecystectomy: a prospective nationwide series. J Am Coll Surg 1997;184:571–8.
17. Murr MM, Gigot JF, Nagorney DM, et al. Long-term results of biliary reconstruction after laparoscopic bile duct injuries. Arch Surg 1999;134:604–9.
18. Mirza DF, Narsimhan KL, Ferraz Neto BH, et al. Bile duct injury following laparoscopic cholecystectomy: referral pattern and management. Br J Surg 1997;84:786–90.
19. McMahon AJ, Fullarton G, Baxter JN, O'Dwyer PJ. Bile duct injury and bile leakage in laparoscopic cholecystectomy. Br J Surg 1995;82:307–13.
20. Stewart L, Way LW. Bile duct injuries during laparoscopic cholecystectomy: factors that influence the results of treatment. Arch Surg 1995;1995:1123–9.
21. Schol FP, Go PM, Gouma DJ. Risk factors for bile duct injury in laparoscopic cholecystectomy: analysis of 49 cases. Br J Surg 1994;81:1786–8.
22. Clavien PA, Sanabria JR, Strasberg SM. Proposed classification of complications of surgery with examples of utility in cholecystectomy. Surgery 1992;111:518–26.
23. Reid SH, Cho SR, Shaw CI, Turner MA. Anomalous hepatic duct inserting into the cystic duct. AJR Am J Roentgenol 1986;147:1181–2.
24. Bernard HR. Laparoscopic cholecystectomy: the New York experience. J Laparoendosc Surg 1993;3:371–4.
25. Russell JC, Walsh SJ, Mattie AS, Lynch JT. Bile duct injuries, 1989–1993. A statewide experience. Connecticut Laparoscopic Cholecystectomy Registry. Arch Surg 1996;131:382–8.
26. Wherry DC, Rob CG, Marohn MR, Rich NM. An external audit of laparoscopic cholecystectomy performed in medical treatment facilities of the Department of Defense. Ann Surg 1994;220:626–34.
27. Buanes T, Mjaland O, Waage A, et al. A population-based survey of biliary surgery in Norway. Relationship between patient volume and quality of surgical treatment. Surg Endosc 1998;12:852–5.
28. Richardson MC, Bell G, Fullarton GM. Incidence and nature of bile duct injuries following laparoscopic cholecystectomy: an audit of 5913 cases. West of Scotland Laparoscopic Cholecystectomy Audit Group. Br J Surg 1996;83:1356–60.
29. Davidoff AM, Pappas TN, Murray EA, et al. Mechanisms of major biliary injury during laparoscopic cholecystectomy. Ann Surg 1992;215:196–202.
30. The Southern Surgeons Club. A prospective analysis of 1518 laparoscopic cholecystectomies. N Engl J Med 1991;324:1073–8. Erratum: N Engl J Med 1991;325:1517–8.
31. Kum CK, Eypasch E, Lefering R, et al. Laparoscopic cholecystectomy for acute cholecystitis: is it really safe? World J Surg 1996;20:43–8.
32. Ponsky JL. Management of complications of laparoscopic cholecystectomy. Endoscopy 1992;24:724–9.
33. Strasberg SM, Sanabria JR, Clavien PA. Complications of laparoscopic cholecystectomy. Can J Surg 1992;35:275–80.
34. Cates JA, Tompkins RK, Zinner MJ, et al. Biliary complications of laparoscopic cholecystectomy. Am Surg 1993;59:243–7.
35. Meyers WC, Peterseim DS, Pappas TN, et al. Low insertion of hepatic segmental duct VII–VIII is an important cause of major biliary injury or misdiagnosis. Am J Surg 1996;171:187–91.
36. Christensen RA, van Sonnenberg E, Nemcek A Jr, D'Agostino HB. Inadvertent ligation of the aberrant right hepatic duct at cholecystectomy: radiologic diagnosis and therapy. Radiology 1992;183:549–53.
37. Berry SM, Ose KJ, Bell RH, Fink AS. Thermal injury of the posterior duodenum during laparoscopic cholecystectomy. Surg Endosc 1994;8:197–200.
38. Funnell IC, Bornman PC, Krige JE, et al. Complete common bile duct division at laparoscopic cholecystectomy: management by percutaneous drainage and endoscopic stenting. Br J Surg 1993;80:1053–4.
39. Brunt LM, Soper NJ. Laparoscopic cholecystectomy; early results and complications. Compl Surg 1993;12:47–53.
40. Moossa AR, Easter DW, Van Sonnenberg E, et al. Laparoscopic injuries to the bile duct. A cause for concern. Ann Surg 1992;215:203–8.
41. Brooks DC, Becker JM, Connors PJ, Carr-Locke DL. Management of bile leaks following laparoscopic cholecystectomy. Surg Endosc 1993;7:292–5.
42. Sanabria JR, Gallinger S, Croxford R, Strasberg SM. Risk factors in elective laparoscopic cholecystectomy for conversion to open cholecystectomy. J Am Coll Surg 1994;179:696–704.
43. Hunter JG. Avoidance of bile duct injury during laparoscopic cholecystectomy. Am J Surg 1991;162:71–6.
44. Fletcher DR, Hobbs MS, Tan P, et al. Complications of cholecystectomy: risks of the laparoscopic approach and protective effects of operative cholangiography: a population-based study. Ann Surg 1999;229:449–57.

45. Carroll BJ, Friedman RL, Liberman MA, Phillips EH. Routine cholangiography reduces sequelae of common bile duct injuries. Surg Endosc 1996;10:1194–7.
46. Kullman E, Borch K, Lindstrom E, et al. Value of routine intraoperative cholangiography in detecting aberrant bile ducts and bile duct injuries during laparoscopic cholecystectomy. Br J Surg 1996;83:171–5.
47. Woods MS, Traverso LW, Kozarek RA, et al. Biliary tract complications of laparoscopic cholecystectomy are detected more frequently with routine intraoperative cholangiography. Surg Endosc 1995;9:1076–80.
48. Adams DB, Borowicz MR, Wootton FD, Cunningham JT. Bile duct complications after laparoscopic cholecystectomy. Surg Endosc 1993;7:79–83.
49. Hawasli A. Does routine cystic duct cholangiogram during laparoscopic cholecystectomy prevent common bile duct injury? Surg Laparosc Endosc Percutaneous Tech 1993;3:290–5.
50. Lorimer JW, Fairfull-Smith RJ. Intraoperative cholangiography is not essential to avoid duct injuries during laparoscopic cholecystectomy. Am J Surg 1995;169:344–7.
51. Wright KD, Wellwood JM. Bile duct injury during laparoscopic cholecystectomy without operative cholangiography. Br J Surg 1998;85:191–4.
52. Park YH, Oskanian Z. Obstructive jaundice after laparoscopic cholecystectomy with electrocautery. Am Surg 1992;58:321–3. Erratum: Am Surg 1992;58:450.
53. Yeh TS, Jan YY, Tseng JH, et al. Value of magnetic resonance cholangiopancreatography in demonstrating major bile duct injuries following laparoscopic cholecystectomy. Br J Surg 1999;86:181–4.
54. Kapoor R, Agarwal S, Calton R, Pawar G. Hepatic artery pseudoaneurysm and hemobilia following laparoscopic cholecystectomy. Indian J Gastroenterol 1997;16:32–3.
55. Genyk YS, Keller FS, Halpern NB. Hepatic artery pseudoaneurysm and hemobilia following laser laparoscopic cholecystectomy. A case report. Surg Endosc 1994;8:201–4.
56. Belkhodja C, Porte H, Quandalle P. [Pedicular traumas during laparoscopic cholecystectomy. Apropos of 5 cases] (in French). Ann Chir 1995;49:149–54.
57. Gigot J, Etienne J, Aerts R, et al. The dramatic reality of biliary tract injury during laparoscopic cholecystectomy. An anonymous multicenter Belgian survey of 65 patients. Surg Endosc 1997;11:1171–8.
58. Mortensen J, Kruse A. Endoscopic management of postoperative bile leaks. Br J Surg 1992;79:1339–41.
59. Marks JM, Ponsky JL, Shillingstad RB, Singh J. Biliary stenting is more effective than sphincterotomy in the resolution of biliary leaks. Surg Endosc 1998;12:327–30.
60. Davids PH, Ringers J, Rauws EA, et al. Bile duct injury after laparoscopic cholecystectomy: the value of endoscopic retrograde cholangiopancreatography. Gut 1993;34:1250–4.
61. Jarnagin WR, Blumgart LH. Operative repair of bile duct injuries involving the hepatic duct confluence. Arch Surg 1999;134:769–75.
62. Geenen DJ, Geenen JE, Hogan WJ, et al. Endoscopic therapy for benign bile duct strictures. Gastrointest Endosc 1989;35:367–71.
63. Millis JM, Tompkins RK, Zinner MJ, et al. Management of bile duct strictures. An evolving strategy. Arch Surg 1992;127:1077–82.
64. van Sonnenberg E, Casola G, Wittich GR, et al. The role of interventional radiology for complications of cholecystectomy. Surgery 1990;107:632–8.
65. Lillemoe KD, Martin SA, Cameron JL, et al. Major bile duct injuries during laparoscopic cholecystectomy. Follow-up after combined surgical and radiologic management. Ann Surg 1997;225:459–68.
66. Gupta N, Solomon H, Fairchild R, Kaminski DL. Management and outcome of patients with combined bile duct and hepatic artery injuries. Arch Surg 1998;133:176–81.
67. Hepp J. Hepaticojejunostomy using the left biliary trunk for iatrogenic biliary lesions: the French connection. World J Surg 1985;9:507–11.
68. Mercado MA, Orozco H, de la Garza L, et al. Biliary duct injury: partial segment IV resection for intrahepatic reconstruction of biliary lesions. Arch Surg 1999;134:1008–10.
69. Robertson AJ, Rela M, Karani J, et al. Laparoscopic cholecystectomy injury: an unusual indication for liver transplantation. Transpl Int 1998;11:449–51.
70. Lillemoe KD, Pitt HA, Cameron JL. Postoperative bile duct strictures. Surg Clin North Am 1990;70:1355–80.
71. Bauer TW, Morris JB, Lowenstein A, et al. The consequences of a major bile duct injury during laparoscopic cholecystectomy. J Gastrointest Surg 1998;2:61–6.
72. Walsh RM, Henderson JM, Vogt DP, et al. Trends in bile duct injuries from laparoscopic cholecystectomy. J Gastrointest Surg 1998;2:458–62.

Chapter

18

Biliary Complications of Liver Transplantation

Paul E. Wise C. Wright Pinson

Liver transplantation has been accepted as the definitive treatment for many end-stage hepatic and biliary disorders (1,2). Early in the liver transplant experience, biliary complications, including bile duct leaks and strictures, were responsible for morbidity and mortality rates ranging from 34% to 50% and 25% to 30%, respectively (3,4). This led Calne to describe the biliary reconstruction as "the technical Achilles' heal of liver transplantation" (3). Since the time of the first liver transplant nearly 40 years ago, significant advances in organ preservation, surgical technique, postoperative care, and immunosuppression have improved the initially high rates of morbidity and mortality associated with the procedure. Despite these advances, biliary tract complications after liver transplantation are still prevalent. Current series report biliary complication rates of 11% to 31% (Table 18.1), and these lead to more than half of the technical liver transplant failures and reoperation in 5% to 20% of patients (5–9). Mortality rates, which are now under 5%, are lower because of today's improved diagnostic and therapeutic techniques used to quickly identify and treat biliary complications. The cost of these complications is significant because of the need for radiologic or endoscopic intervention, reoperation, or retransplantation (8).

Although the biliary anastomosis is usually thought of as the least technically demanding aspect of liver transplantation, the proper operative technique in the creation of the anastomosis plays a critical role in the prevention of complications after liver transplant (9). To improve the outcomes of biliary reconstruction and decrease the complication rates, many techniques of biliary anastomoses have evolved since the early days of liver transplantation. During the initial operative experience, the donor gallbladder was used for the primary anastomosis (e.g., cholecystocholedochostomy, Roux-en-Y cholecystojejunostomy) or as a vascularized conduit (e.g., choledochocholecystocholedochostomy, Roux-en-Y choledochocholecystojejunostomy) to provide additional length between donor and recipient ducts (Fig. 18.1) (10). The use of the donor gallbladder also provided a larger surface area for wider anastomoses without tension. However, the relatively long operative times required, the high stenosis rate (secondary to ischemia), and frequent obstruction leading to cholangitis eventually forced the gallbladder conduit to be abandoned for the simpler choledochocholedochostomy and the Roux-en-Y choledochojejunostomy as the techniques of choice for biliary reconstruction (11).

This chapter addresses the variety of techniques for biliary reconstruction in use today, as well as the biliary complications that can arise from them. In addition, the diagnostic and therapeutic modalities to treat these complications are discussed. A final section is devoted to considerations in the evolving fields of split-liver and living-donor liver transplantation.

TYPES OF BILIARY RECONSTRUCTION

Two techniques, choledochocholedochostomy (CDCD) and Roux-en-Y choledochojejunostomy (CDJ), are commonly used today for biliary tract reconstruction during liver transplantation.

Choledochocholedochostomy

Most surgeons prefer the CDCD as their method of choice for the biliary anastomosis because it allows for shorter operative times, preservation of the sphincter of Oddi mechanism (providing relatively normal physiology), easy access for endoscopic biliary evaluation and treatment, and avoidance of biliary-enteric anastomotic complications (9). This method is used in about 85% of transplants (i.e., when there

Table 18.1. Incidence of biliary complications from selected series

Author	Year	Transplants	Complications				Anastomosis Type (n)	Leaks	Strictures
			Total Rate	Leaks	Strictures	Other			
Grief (5)	1994	1792	11.5%	26.7%	42.9%	30.4%	CDCD (approx. 896)	35 (3.9%)	47 (5.2%)
							CDJ (approx. 896)	22 (2.5%)	45 (5.0%)
Hernandez (6)	1999	300	18%	59%	29.6%	11.4%	CDCD (247)	N/R	N/R
							CDJ (53)	N/R	N/R
O'Connor (7)	1995	220	29.5%	56.9%	23.1%	20%	CDCD (147)	32 (21.8%)	7 (4.8%)
							CDJ (43)	5 (11.6%)	8 (18.6%)
Rossi (9)	1994	219	14.6%	65.6%	25%	9.4%	CDCD (159)	13 (8.2%)	5 (3.1%)
							CDJ (60)	8 (13.3%)	3 (5.0%)
Davidson (8)	1999	100	31%	54.8%	45.2%	0%	CDCD EE (60)	10 (16.7%)	9 (15.0%)
							CDCD SS (40)	7 (17.5%)	5 (12.5%)

Abbreviations: CDCD = choledochocholedochostomy; CDJ = Roux-en-Y choledochojejunostomy; EE = end-to-end; SS = side-to-side.

is no recipient bile duct pathology). It has even been used in selected patients with primary sclerosing cholangitis (PSC), who do not have common duct strictures, without a significant difference in complication rates (12). Because the CDCD reconstruction has certain complications unique to it (such as T-tube exit site leaks and sphincter of Oddi dysfunction), and has significant stenosis and leak rates, controversies persist regarding its technical construction. These controversies include whether to perform the anastomosis as an end-to-end versus side-to-side CDCD, and whether to use a T-tube or other stent to maintain patency of the anastomosis.

We prefer an end-to-end anastomosis performed with interrupted 5–0 polydioxan absorbable sutures around a 6 to 12 French latex T-tube stent. The sutures are precisely placed 2 to 3mm apart and tied down to provide approximation, but not so tight as to strangulate the tissues. Assurance of adequate vascularity at either end of the bile duct is important (4). It is also important to make certain the anastomosis is tension free. We bring the T-tube out through an additional small choledochotomy on the right lateral aspect of the native common duct, a couple of centimeters below the anastomosis. A purse-string suture of 3–0 polydioxan absorbable suture anchors the T-tube, thus preventing a leak and early inadvertent tube dislodgement. A cholangiogram is used to confirm no leaks prior to capping the T-tube 4 to 7 days after the operation. A cholangiogram is repeated at 6 months; if it is normal, the tube is removed (Fig. 18.2).

The formation of the CDCD by the end-to-end versus side-to-side method (see Figs. 18.2 and 18.3) has been debated for the past 10 years. The method of the side-to-side CDCD was first popularized by Neuhaus in 1994 after his results showed a remarkable 0.3% leak rate and a 2.3% total biliary complication rate in a single-center, retrospective analysis of 300 liver transplants (13). Two subsequent retrospective analyses supported his findings of decreased complications with side-to-side versus end-to-end CDCD (14,15). Unfortunately, a prospective, randomized study comparing the two methods showed no difference in morbidity or mortality in 100 patients, including a similar incidence of leaks, strictures, total complications, and need for further intervention (8). Another large comparative review showed slightly fewer complications in the end-to-end anastomosis group (16). The proponents of the side-to-side CDCD believe the advantages of this method are an increased anastomosis size and decreased tension on the anastomosis (15). Problems with the side-to-side CDCD include increased operative time, need for greater length of bile duct to form the necessary overlap for the anastomosis, and the possibility of increased ischemic complications due to increased mobilization and dissection of the bile ducts. Currently, end-to-end anastomosis is strongly favored.

Controversy also surrounds the use of T-tubes or stents for the CDCD. They offer the advantages of allowing observation of bile output and character in the immediate postoperative period as well as providing easy access to the biliary tree for postoperative radiographic evaluation (16). T-tubes and other stents are also believed by some surgeons to reduce stricture formation. A few prospective studies have shown significantly decreased costs and complication rates with the use of T-tubes (17). On the other hand, T-tubes are associated with bile leaks both around the tubes and after removing them (although these leaks can often be managed nonoperatively) (18). Moreover, some studies have linked the use of T-tubes to significant postoperative infections (19), increased cost from "unnecessary" biliary procedures (20), and increased mortality due to anastomotic dehiscence and sepsis (16). The use of T-tubes is still common.

Roux-en-Y Choledochojejunostomy (CDJ)

The CDJ (Fig. 18.4) is the anastomotic procedure of choice when there is underlying biliary disease (such as PSC), when

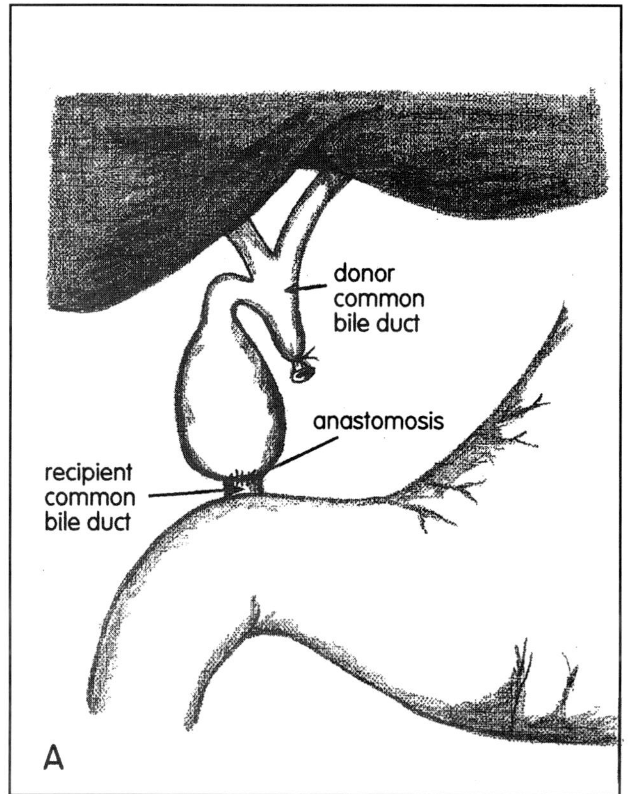

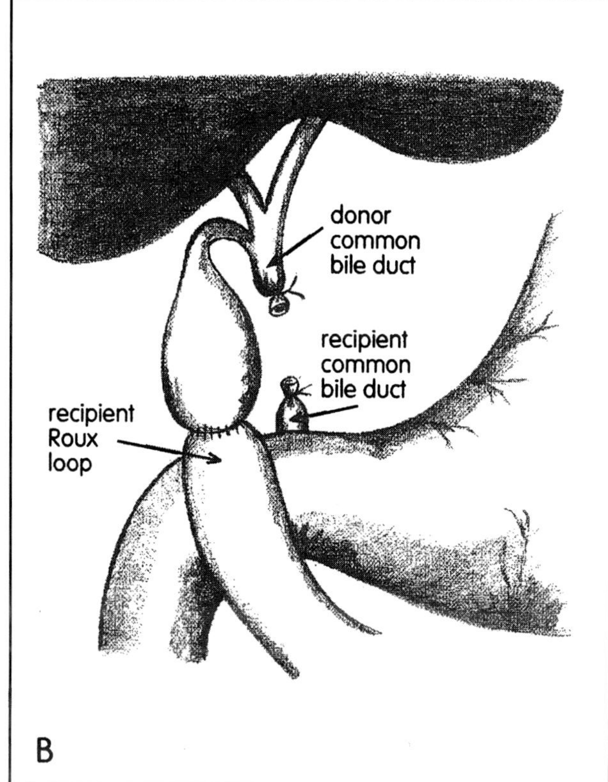

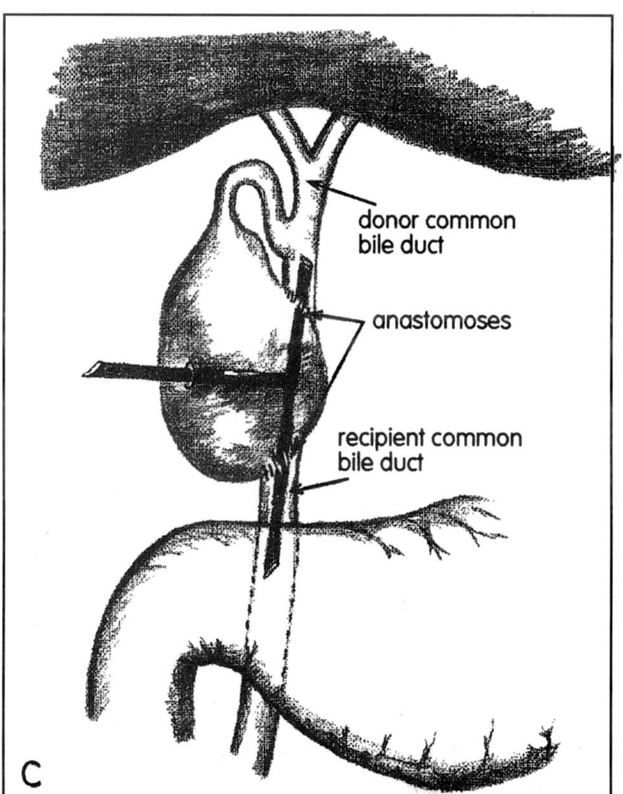

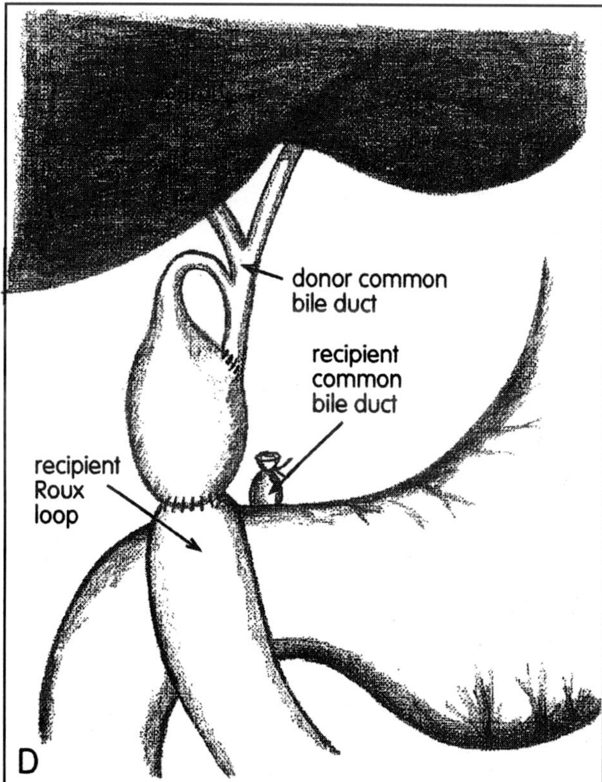

FIGURE 18.1. *Early methods of biliary reconstruction in liver transplantation.* ***(A)*** *Cholecystocholedochostomy.* ***(B)*** *Roux-en-Y cholecystojejunostomy.* ***(C)*** *Choledochocholecystocholedochostomy.* ***(D)*** *Roux-en-Y choledochocholecystojejunostomy.*

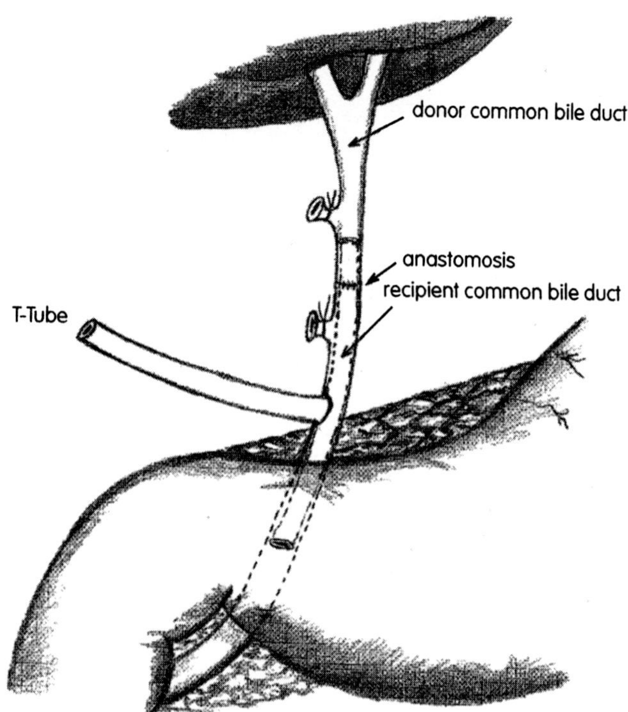

FIGURE 18.2. *Standard end-to-end choledochocholedochostomy (CDCD) over a T-tube.*

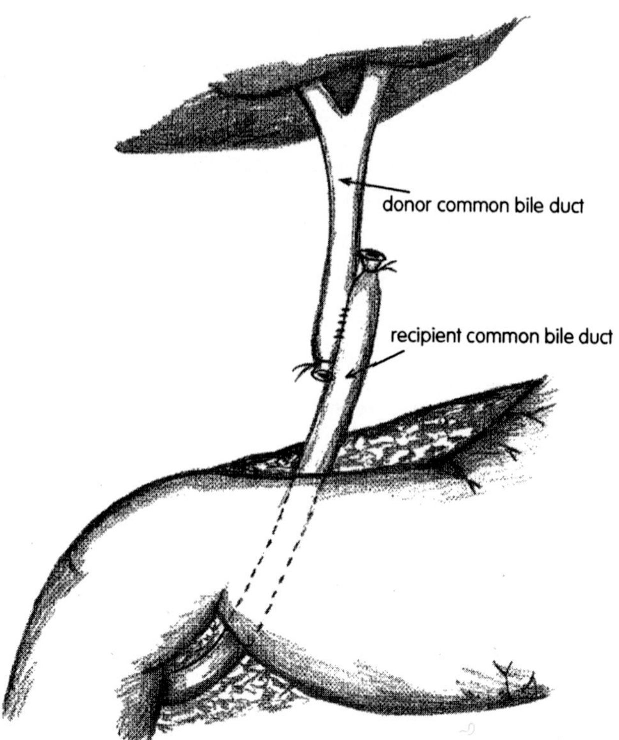

FIGURE 18.3. *Side-to-side choledochocholedochostomy (CDCD).*

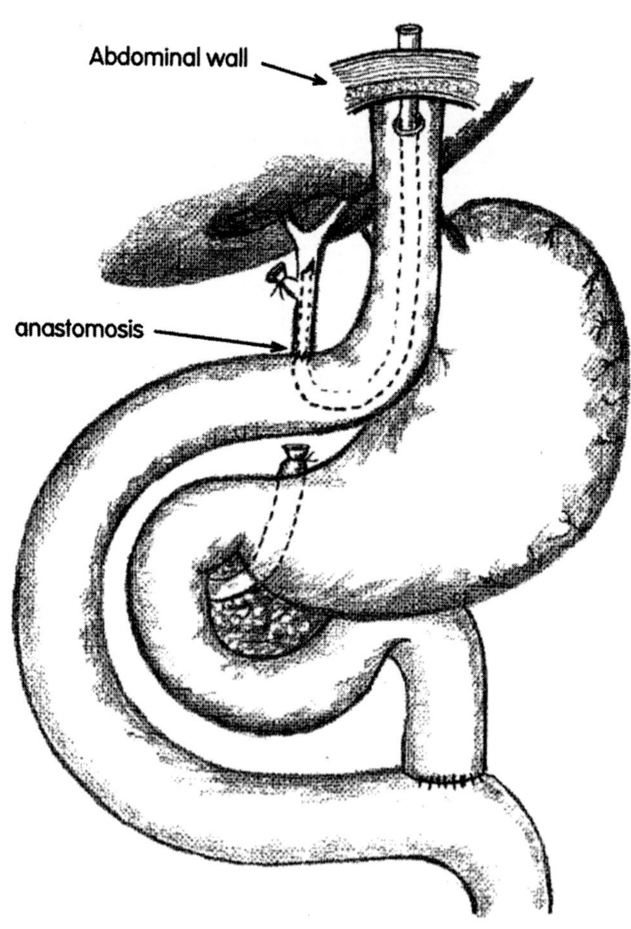

FIGURE 18.4. *Roux-en-Y choledochojejunostomy (CDJ). The end of the Roux loop is tacked to the abdominal wall and marked for potential future radiologic guided access.*

there is a large discrepancy in duct sizes, or in pediatric patients due to small size or atresia of ducts (16). It is also used for patients with cholangiocarcinoma, reduced grafts, split grafts, or retransplants (9). CDJ is rarely used when primary CDCD is an option because of its increased operative time (with a second jejunal anastomosis), difficulty with postoperative endoscopic access to the biliary tree, and increased risk of intestinal complications such as bowel ischemia, perforation, anastomotic hemorrhage, or torsion (11).

Construction of a Roux-en-Y choledochojejunostomy requires a 45- to 60-cm defunctionalized jejunal limb. We perform this biliary anastomosis with 5–0 polydioxan sutures to an antimesenteric jejunostomy several centimeters from the stapled end of the defunctionalized jejunal limb. A Rodney-Smith biliary stent, Turcot stent, or pediatric feeding tube is passed across the anastomosis and out the end of the Roux limb. The end of the Roux limb is marked with a radio-opaque suture and tacked to the abdominal wall. This subfascial, marked loop provides easy access to the biliary reconstruction for percutaneous radiologic methods. The stent is removed 1 to 2 months postoperatively.

Overall complication rates after CDJ are similar to the complication rates after CDCD (7,21). When complications do occur after CDJ, however, they are more difficult to diagnose and manage, more often require reoperation, and can lead to greater morbidity and mortality (22).

ETIOLOGY OF BILIARY COMPLICATIONS

The biliary complications of liver transplantation are believed to occur secondary to technical, immunologic, or vascular factors (8,23). As mentioned above, technical factors involved in the construction of the anastomosis can have a direct effect on the occurrence of complications. The vascular etiologies can be multifactorial and thus more difficult to identify and manage, but they all lead to the same end point of bile duct ischemia. Hepatic artery thrombosis (HAT) is one of the classic causes of biliary ischemia, as the donor duct depends on donor right hepatic arterial blood flow (7). HAT can lead to significant biliary complications that often require retransplantation (5,23,24). Other causes of ischemia are due to microvascular occlusion and include immunologic injury due to viral infection, chronic rejection, or graft ABO incompatibility, cholangitis, or prolonged ischemia during preservation (8,11,25). Finally, use of T-tubes increases the incidence of late biliary leaks.

TYPES OF BILIARY COMPLICATIONS

Approximately two-thirds of the biliary complications after liver transplant are anastomotic and nonanastomotic strictures and leaks (5). Other less common complications include choledocholithiasis, mucocele, hemobilia, and sphincter of Oddi dysfunction (SOD), among others. The timing of these complications varies after the liver transplant (Table 18.2). In a review of 1792 liver transplants, Grief found that approximately 80% of the biliary complications after transplant occurred in the first 6 months (5). Lopez showed that about 50% of complications occur in the first month (21). The incidence of complications after the first year after transplant is less than 4% each year (5). Complications with CDJ usually (70%) occur in the first 30 days, whereas those from CDCD tend to occur later (26). In general, leaks tend to occur in the first month (unless associated with T-tube removal) and strictures tend to occur over the course of several months after transplant (11).

Table 18.2. Timing of biliary tract complications after liver transplantation

Early (<30 Days)	Late (>30 Days)
Bile leak	Bile leak
Anastomotic	After T-tube removal
T-tube exit site	
Biliary stricture	Biliary stricture
Anastomotic (29%)	Anastomotic (71%)
	Nonanastomotic
Obstruction of T-tube	
Sphincter of Oddi dysfunction (11%)	Sphincter of Oddi dysfunction (89%)

Sources: Branch MS, Clavien PA. Biliary complications following liver transplantation. In: Killenberg PG, Clavien PA, eds. Medical care of the liver transplant patient. Malden, MA: Blackwell Science, 1997:193–209; Grief F, Bronsther OL, Van Thiel DH, et al. The incidence, timing, and management of biliary tract complications after orthotopic liver transplantation. Ann Surg 1994;219:40–5.

Strictures

Strictures occur after 8% to 17% of liver transplants (27) and make up the predominance of late biliary complications, occurring an average of a year after transplantation (7). Their spectrum ranges from a slow, gradual narrowing of the biliary tree to severe bile duct obliteration leading to graft failure (11). Usually they are divided into two categories that determine their prognosis: anastomotic and nonanastomotic strictures.

Anastomotic Strictures

Anastomotic strictures (Fig. 18.5) usually appear in the first year after liver transplantation, and are thought to be due to a combination of surgical technique (e.g., narrow anastomosis) and ischemic insult or fibrosis (11). Because HAT can be a causative factor leading to ischemia, hepatic artery patency should be investigated in all cases of strictures. These strictures are most commonly amenable to endoscopic or percutaneous dilation with stent placement for 4 to 12 months (22,28,29). In 12% to 30% of patients, reconstruction of the biliary tract with conversion of a CDCD to a CDJ or hepaticojejunostomy is necessary when stent treatment is unsuccessful (7,28,29). It should also be remembered that, on occasion, a significant mismatch in the size of the donor biliary tract for the recipient can give the appearance of an anastomotic stricture without the true pathology being present or treatment being required.

Nonanastomotic Strictures

Nonanastomotic strictures can occur anywhere throughout the biliary tree, and they can be multiple or singular, localized or diffuse (Fig. 18.6). HAT, ABO incompatibility, and prolonged cold ischemia time beyond 12 hours are factors leading to nonanastomotic strictures (7) (Fig. 18.7). Other causes of microvascular ischemia and eventual stricturing are chronic rejection (vanishing duct syndrome [30]), cytomegalovirus (CMV) infection, and PSC (11). These strictures therefore require full assessment of the hepatic arterial inflow and biliary tree before treatment can be initiated. There is a very high incidence of sludge, stones, and cholangitis with nonanastomotic strictures.

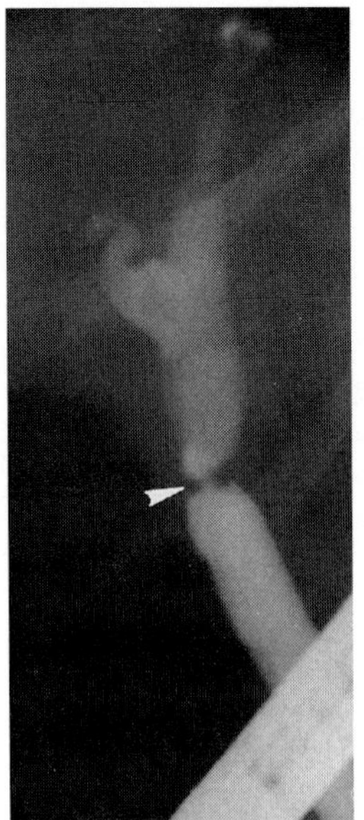
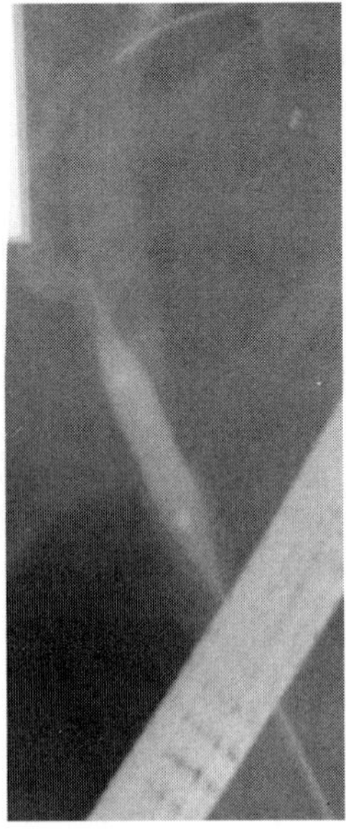
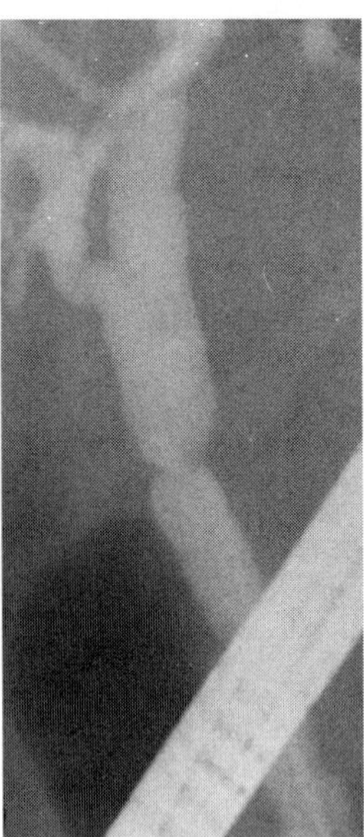

FIGURE 18.5. *Anastomotic stricture. On the left is an obvious narrowing of the anastomosis (arrow). In the middle, the stricture is endoscopically balloon dilated. On the right, the diameter of the stricture has been enlarged.*

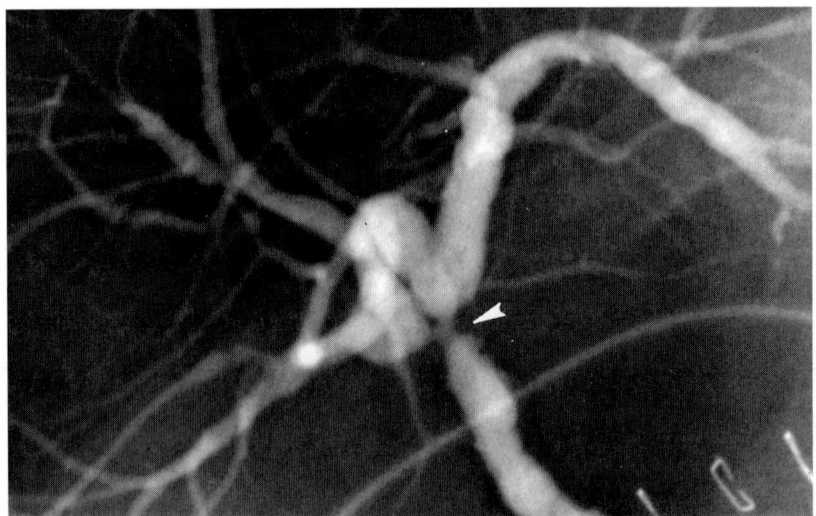

FIGURE 18.6. *Nonanastomotic stricture in the common bile duct bifurcation region (arrow). This patient had hepatic artery thrombosis.*

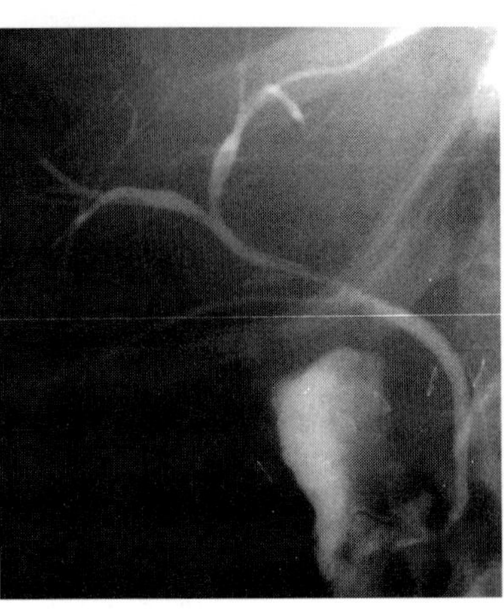
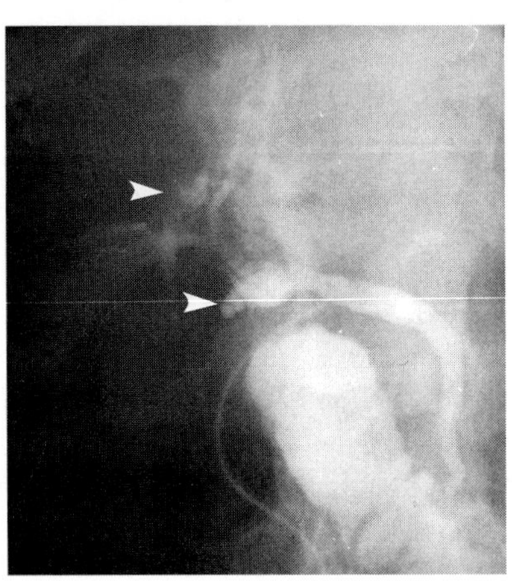

FIGURE 18.7. *Hepatic artery thrombosis. Two cholangiograms from the same patient. The first is immediately postoperatively from liver transplant and the second after the development of hepatic artery thrombosis. This shows the destruction of the biliary tree and development of bile lakes (arrows).*

Treatment for nonanastomotic stricturing depends on the site, and the number and severity of the strictures (22). Asymptomatic strictures can be observed. Antibiotics to control infection are an important adjunct. Singular or intermittent proximal strictures can be treated with percutaneous or endoscopic dilation and stenting (22). For selected patients with isolated bifurcation strictures, in the face of intact hepatic artery inflow, hepaticojejunostomy yields good results (23). In patients with the diffuse form of the disease, most require retransplantation; without this, the mortality rate is 30% to 50% (11). For these patients, palliative metal stenting may be required while awaiting retransplantation.

Bile Leaks

Bile leaks after liver transplantation occur in 3% to 27% of patients (21) at a mean of 50 days (7); they occur at three possible locations (around the tube, anastomotic, or nonanastomotic), and are usually categorized as early or later than 1 month. Early leaks may occur at any location in the biliary tree associated with ischemia and bile duct necrosis (including the anastomosis) or at the T-tube exit site (Fig. 18.8). Early large anastomotic leaks are often due to common bile duct necrosis because the donor duct was too long or overly skeletonized, too many anastomotic sutures are used (causing microvascular occlusion), or there is too much tension on the anastomosis. These leaks can usually be avoided by ensuring adequate flow at the time of hepatic arterial anastomosis, ensuring sufficient blood flow from the cut bile duct ends, and avoiding the use of electrocautery, anastomotic tension, and excessive bile duct dissection (31). Because HAT or hepatic arterial stenosis is present in up to 50% of patients with leaks and bile duct necrosis, hepatic arterial flow should be expeditiously evaluated (11). Limited anastomotic leaks may be treated with short-term percutaneous or endoscopic stenting, and endoscopic sphincterotomy may be useful in treating leaks by decreasing biliary pressures. More than two-thirds of these leaks will eventually require operative repair (7). More extensive anastomotic leaks that are not amenable to endoscopic or percutaneous treatment require surgical revision of the CDCD anastomosis to a CDJ. If CDJ reconstruction already exists, then the duct should be shortened until bleeding is noted from the donor end and then it should be reanastomosed to the Roux limb.

Early leaks can also occur from T-tube sites, which can usually be managed by open T-tube drainage until the surrounding leak has sealed (21). Early leaks can be associated with unrecognized accessory bile ducts or open cystic duct remnants in less than 2% of patients. They can also occur after liver biopsy. These leaks can lead to a biloma that often presents with abdominal pain and/or fever. The biloma can resolve with time if its cause is identified and treated early and there is no infection present. However, bilomas usually require either percutaneous or open surgical drainage as well as repair of the underlying cause, especially if the biloma is infected (11,21).

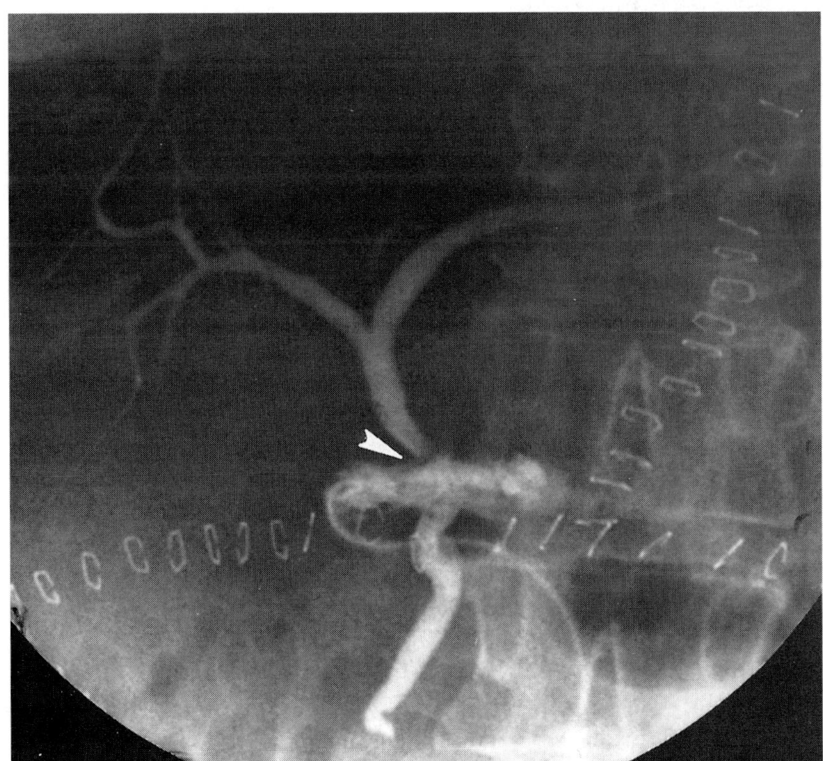

FIGURE 18.8. *Anastomotic bile leak. Cholangiogram demonstrating an anastomotic leak (arrow) proximal to the T-tube.*

Late biliary leaks occur in 10% to 20% of patients after T-tube removal (7) and some groups report T-tube leak rates of up to 33% (16,32). Multivariate analysis of the factors predicting difficulties with T-tube removal have shown only duct wall irregularities to be significantly associated with leaks after T-tube removal. Donor demographics, ischemia time, total steroid dose, SOD, and the length of time the tube was in place did not affect leak rates (32). An intravenous line should be placed prior to T-tube removal in anticipation of treatment for possible peritonitis. Initial treatment of a leak after tube removal is by supportive care and intravenous antibiotics. If there is no improvement after 12 to 24 hours, endoscopic placement of a nasobiliary tube is recommended. Endoscopic nasobiliary stenting is adequate to close leaks in over 90% of cases (11). Laparotomy and suture closure of the T-tube tract is reserved for patients who do not improve after 48 hours.

Miscellaneous Biliary Complications

Stones and Sludge

Choledocholithiasis after liver transplantation is usually secondary to biliary obstruction and stasis, but is occasionally caused by primary cholesterol stones (11) (Fig. 18.9). Sludge is identified in 42% to 60% of liver transplants as thickened, inspissated bile or sloughed epithelium in the bile ducts that can then form firm casts if allowed to condense (33). The casts can lead to biliary obstruction with ascending cholangitis, sepsis, and significant mortality (33,34). Cholangiography is the method for identifying biliary sludge or calculi (33). Treatment choices include daily flushing of the T-tube,

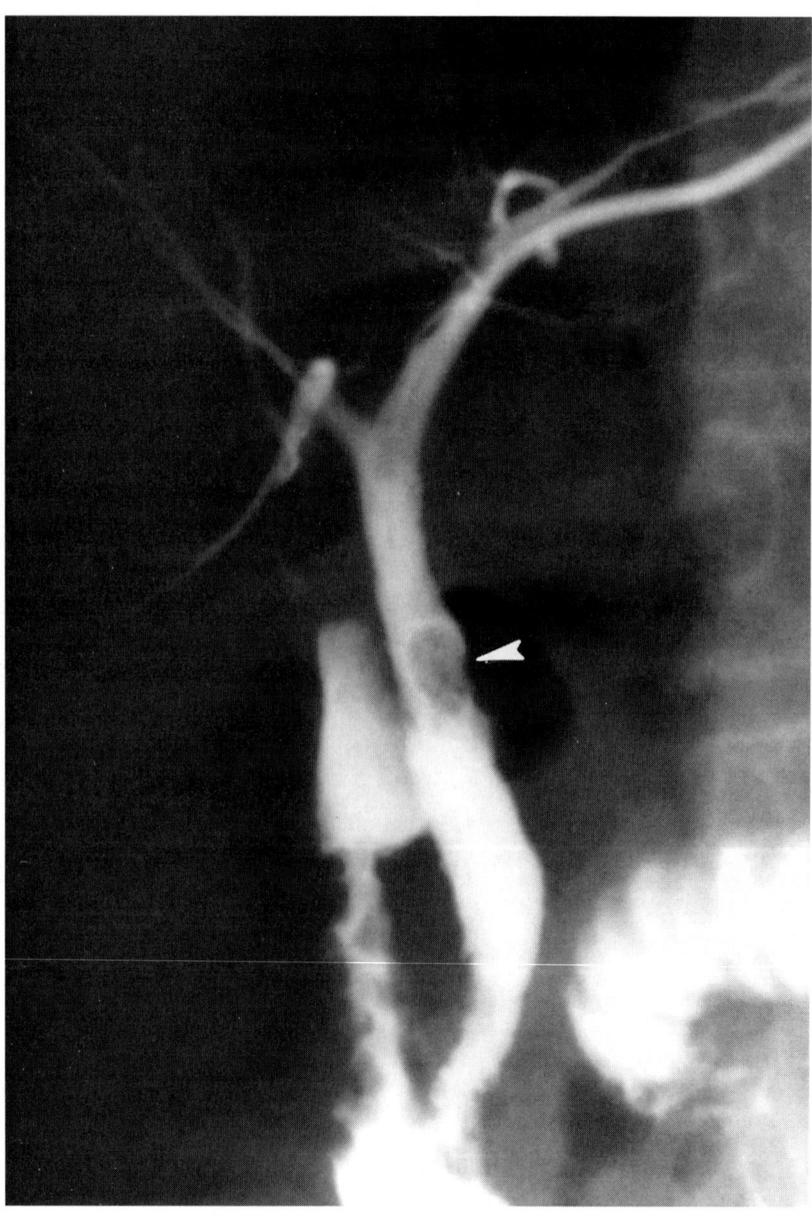

FIGURE 18.9. *Choledocholithiasis. Cholangiogram demonstrating an intraductal stone (arrow) in the mid–common bile duct.*

ursodiol, interventional radiologic chemolysis, endoscopic stone removal (with concomitant stricture dilation/stenting), reoperation, or retransplantation (35).

Mucocele

Mucocele is a rare complication of the cystic duct that can lead to extrinsic compression and obstruction of the bile duct. It is caused by continued epithelial secretion of mucus in a cystic duct that has been ligated at both ends. It can take years to develop (11). The mucocele is identified on radiologic studies as a fluid collection in the porta hepatis. This can be percutaneously drained to alleviate biliary obstruction. Once the obstruction has resolved, the isolated segment of duct may require operative drainage or excision. On rare occasions, operative conversion to a CDJ is required (22).

Sphincter of Oddi Dysfunction

SOD occurs after CDCD and is thought to be due at least in part to denervation and devascularization of the papilla (36). This leads to papillary dysfunction and bile duct dilatation without evidence of stricture. Patients are predisposed to SOD by having pretransplant papillary dysfunction as evidenced by recipient duct dilatation preoperatively (36). The usual onset is a mean of 35 weeks after transplant (with a range of 1 to 330 weeks), and the diagnosis is supported by improvement in serum hepatic enzymes after allowing open T-tube or endoscopic drainage of the bile duct (11). The treatment of choice is either endoscopic sphincterotomy (11) or papillary stenting (36). If ductal dilatation and cholestasis do not resolve, revision to a CDJ or hepaticojejunostomy is necessary (11).

Redundant Duct

Excessive length of bile duct after CDCD reconstruction can lead to kinking and obstruction with possible ensuing cholangitis. This is easily diagnosed on endoscopic or T-tube cholangiography. Stenting for a few weeks will usually resolve this problem by allowing scar tissue to form around the duct and prevent further kinking. Rarely is conversion to CDJ required.

Cholangitis/Liver Abscess

Cholangitis occurs with biliary obstruction or contamination upon manipulation of the biliary tree. The infection is usually from enteric bacteria, but occasionally the organisms involved may be fungal or viral. Treatment is initiated with opening of the T-tube or establishing percutaneous or endoscopic drainage for relief of biliary obstruction. Appropriate treatment with broad spectrum or culture-specific antibiotics is necessary for complete resolution of the cholangitis. Early and aggressive treatment is appropriate to minimize biliary epithelial and graft damage. On rare occasions the cholangitis may become so advanced that an intraparenchymal hepatic abscess may form. This requires direct percutaneous or open surgical drainage of the abscess cavity. The bile duct necrosis and stricturing often accompanying HAT can also lead to intrahepatic abscess formation. Hepatic abscesses in this setting usually require retransplantation.

Cholestasis

Cholestasis can present with abnormal laboratory values mimicking those of mechanical obstruction. Early after transplant it is related to prolonged donor graft ischemia, especially in steatotic livers. Cholestasis can follow episodes of severe rejection due to graft dysfunction. If a liver biopsy is performed, it may show biliary inspissation in the microscopic ducts. Treatment is often institution of ursodiol.

Hemobilia

Significant hemobilia occurs infrequently (<4% in most series [37,38]) after liver biopsy or percutaneous transhepatic cholangiography (PTC). Minor hemobilia can be seen in 10% of percutaneous procedures after liver transplant and is usually self-limited, asymptomatic, and inconsequential. Larger volume bleeds or choledochovenous fistulae can lead to thrombus within the biliary tree. Although bile is a thrombolytic and can lead to the breakdown of a clot within 24 to 48 hours (39), signs of biliary obstruction and cholangitis can result from thrombus in the biliary tree and necessitate further intervention. Occasionally, endoscopy in combination with thrombolytics may be necessary to remove an obstructing clot. If this is unsuccessful, percutaneous or open surgical intervention may be required. If an artery is involved in the etiology of persistent hemobilia (choledochoarterial fistula), it can usually be identified and treated by selective arteriography with coil embolization on either side of the defect.

Neuroma

A few cases of traumatic neuromas obstructing the ducts have been reported, although most are asymptomatic. They consist of a hyperplastic collection of axons that can form at the divided end of the recipient duct and, like the mucocele, can lead to extrinsic compression and obstruction of the biliary tree or hepatic vasculature. Cyclosporine has been implicated in stimulating the axonal growth leading to the neuroma. Treatment requires excision and surgical revision of the biliary anastomosis when symptomatic (40).

Lymphoproliferative Disease

Post-transplant lymphoproliferative disease (PTLD), a pathologic entity involving B cell proliferation and/or lymphoma occurring after 1% to 3% of liver transplants, rarely causes bile duct obstruction and cholangitis. PTLD leading to biliary obstruction requires surgical excision and possible revision of the anastomosis, chemotherapy, and reduction of immunosuppression (41).

DIAGNOSIS AND TREATMENT OF BILIARY COMPLICATIONS

Biliary tract complications are heralded most frequently by asymptomatic sustained elevations of serum bilirubin, alkaline phosphatase, and gamma glutamyltransferase (GGT). These findings can be confused with rejection (11,42), so a liver biopsy may be helpful. For example, in one series, 46% of patients with biliary complication in the first month were initially treated for rejection (5). Some patients will present with abdominal or shoulder pain, nausea, fever, or sepsis. Fluctuating cyclosporine or tacrolimus levels are another less common presentation. Bile from peritoneal drains postoperatively is pathognomonic of a bile leak.

If biliary tract complications are suspected, a cholangiogram is mandatory, whether by T-tube, endoscopic retrograde cholangiography (ERC), or percutaneous transhepatic cholangiography (PTC). ERC and PTC can be used for not only diagnosis but also nonoperative management in many cases.

Endoscopic Evaluation

ERC is useful for the diagnosis and treatment of biliary complications after CDCD. Despite a complication rate of almost 6% (42) (including pancreatitis, gastrointestinal bleeding, and perforation), ERC is performed in some centers more than PTC. Complication rates are not increased in post-transplant patients compared to the general population undergoing endoscopic evaluation. Advantages of ERC include the ability to perform sphincterotomy in addition to balloon dilation, stent placement, and stone retrieval (22,43). Many studies have supported the safety and efficacy of ERC in the management of biliary fistulas and anastomotic strictures with no significant increase in mortality or graft loss (28,29,44,45) (see also Chapters 4 and 6).

Radiologic Evaluation

The radiologic biliary evaluation of a liver transplant patient depends on the type of biliary reconstruction that was performed, the availability of resources, and whether a T-tube or stent is present. If the patient has a T-tube or stent, obtaining the gold standard cholangiogram is relatively simple. Cholangiography has a very high sensitivity and specificity for all types of biliary complications (45–47). If there is no T-tube or stent present or the tube is obstructed, other diagnostic modalities can be used including ultrasound, PTC, ERC, radionuclide scanning, and magnetic resonance cholangiography (MRC) (see also Chapters 3, 5, and 7).

Percutaneous Transhepatic Cholangiography

PTC is required after CDJ if no stent is present. Therapeutic procedures that can be performed via PTC include stricture dilation, stent placement, stone/sludge removal (21), and biliary decompression/drainage for obstruction (45). Because PTC is easier in the presence of a dilated biliary tree, it is a less effective diagnostic modality for biliary leaks than for strictures. Due to the invasive nature of PTC, it has a complication rate of approximately 4%, including biliary fistulae and hemobilia (42).

Ultrasound

Doppler ultrasound has been a standard method for evaluation of the hepatic vasculature and is required when biliary complications are suspected because 10% to 17% will have HAT (5). If the findings are abnormal or uncertain, the ultrasound should be followed by angiography. On the other hand, ultrasound is not as useful for directly identifying specific biliary complications because very advanced pathology is required for it to be diagnostic. Reviews have shown a high level of inaccuracy (50% sensitivity) in early obstruction without ductal dilatation or in bile leaks without biloma formation (45). An abnormal ultrasound is reliable in identifying a significant complication, but a normal ultrasound in no way precludes the presence of underlying pathology (46). Again, a cholangiogram is mandatory.

Radionuclide Scans

Hepatobiliary scintigraphy can be used as a screening test for biliary complications (48). Its sensitivity (95%) in identifying early biliary obstruction is higher than ultrasound, and scintigraphy can identify a bile leak even without biloma formation (49). However, radionuclide scans are not always available due to the limited access to radiotracers; also, their ability to localize a defect is poor (22).

Magnetic Resonance Cholangiography (MRC)

MRC is increasingly available and gaining favor. The ability to diagnose biliary strictures and ductal dilatation is excellent according to two limited studies (42,50). MRC is deficient in the ability to identify cholelithiasis and in diagnosing bile leaks (42).

Surgical Evaluation and Intervention

Surgical exploration is necessary for the identification of pathology that is not identifiable on cholangiography or by other diagnostic methods. Surgical intervention is usually effective in the treatment of strictures and leaks, often when nonsurgical therapeutic methods fail.

SPECIAL CONSIDERATIONS: LIVING-DONOR AND SPLIT-LIVER TRANSPLANTATION

In an attempt to meet the growing indications and demand for liver transplantation in an environment with a relatively stable donor organ pool (especially in the pediatric setting), many centers began performing cadaveric split-liver transplantation and living-donor transplantation approximately 10 years ago (51) (Fig. 18.10). Although the complication rates are now similar to whole organ liver transplantation (13% to 34%) (52,53), there are a few special considerations.

First, because the split grafts and living-related grafts are obtained by division of the liver parenchyma, there is a significant chance for biliary leak from the cut surface. In one series there was a 7% occurrence of biliary leak from the cut surface—all eventually required surgical intervention

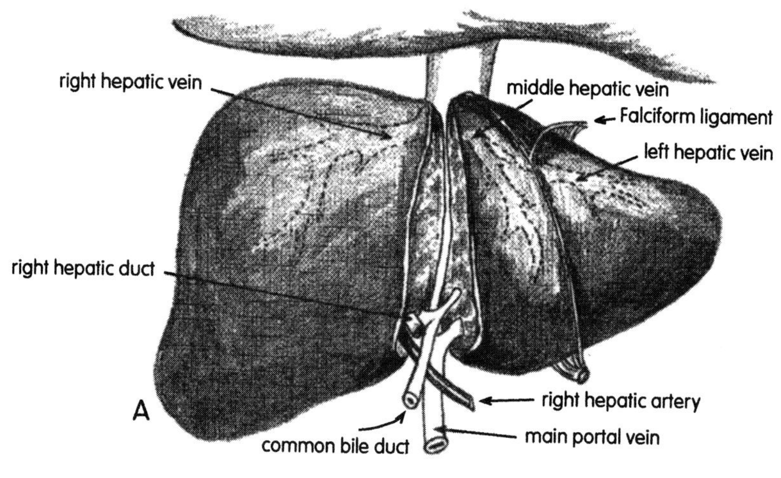

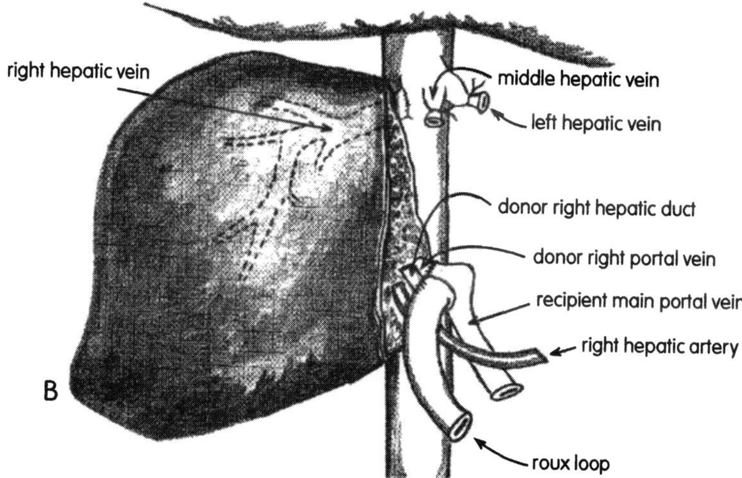

FIGURE 18.10. *Right lobe living-donor liver transplantation.* ***(A)*** *Splitting of the right and left lobes, including biliary tree.* ***(B)*** *Right hepatic lobe graft with Roux-en-Y hepaticojejunostomy biliary reconstruction.*

(53). Therefore, donor cholangiography is used routinely to carefully identify the complete biliary anatomy to help avoid these leaks and also to decrease the chance in the living-donor situation of significant incidental donor bile duct injury that could lead to donor morbidity (52).

A second consideration is that great care must be taken during the "back table" preparation of the liver graft to avoid biliary injury. This complication also requires reoperation and additional jejunal anastomoses to the injured ducts (52). One center has had success in avoiding this complication by using surgical probes and intraoperative ultrasound to determine location and patency of the segmental bile duct branches prior to transplantation. Use of this procedure avoided inadvertent bile duct obstruction in 100% of 60 cases reviewed (54).

Third, in most cases of split-liver and living-related transplantation, the biliary reconstruction must consist of hepaticojejunostomy as there is not enough donor duct to construct a CDCD. When multiple ducts are anastomosed, if possible they are brought together for a single anastomosis. Stents are recommended. The anastomotic stricture rate is reported the same or lower in most living-related series (52,55), possibly because the benefits of a shortened ischemic time are countered by the small size of the ducts anastomosed (52).

SUMMARY

Biliary tract complications occur after 11% to 31% of liver transplantations. More allografts are lost secondary to these complications than those lost due to rejection. Leaks in the early and strictures in the late post-transplant period are the most common complications. When a biliary complication is suspected, cholangiogram, Doppler ultrasound, and liver biopsy should be the exams of choice that are initially considered. Multispecialty therapy including dilation, stenting, or duct debris removal can decrease the need for reoperation or retransplantation. Living-donor and split-liver transplantation encourage more sophisticated techniques to avoid biliary complications.

ACKNOWLEDGMENTS

The authors wish to acknowledge the illustrations by Ms. Patricia Vorndick (Figs. 18.1 through 18.4).

SUGGESTED READINGS

Egawa H, Uemoto S, Inomata Y, et al. Biliary complications in pediatric living related liver transplantation. Surgery 1998;124:901–10. This is a retrospective study from Japan and Canada that reviews 208 living-related liver transplants. The authors provide detailed practical considerations for living-related transplantation and its potential biliary complications.

Grief F, Bronsther OL, Van Thiel DH, et al. The incidence, timing, and management of biliary tract complications after orthotopic liver transplantation. Ann Surg 1994;219:40–5. This retrospective study from the University of Pittsburgh provides detailed information on the incidence and timing of various complications after 1792 orthotopic liver transplants. The authors were thorough in their analysis of the complications after CDCD and CDJ.

Porayko MK, Kondo M, Steer JL. Liver transplantation: late complications of the biliary tract and their management. Semin Liver Dis 1995;15:139–55. This is an excellent overview from the Mayo Clinic of biliary complications and their management. Unlike the title suggests, this summary (with 87 references) provides a thorough evaluation of both early and late complications.

REFERENCES

1. Van Thiel DH. Liver transplantation: a history of the past and present with a vision of the future. In: Maddrey WC, Sorrell MF, eds. Transplantation of the liver. Norwalk: Appleton and Lange, 1995:1–12.
2. Clavien PA, Camargo CA, Croxford R, et al. Definition and classification of negative outcomes in solid organ transplantation. Ann Surg 1994;2220:109–20.
3. Calne RY, McMaster P, Portmann B, et al. Observations on preservation, bile drainage and rejection in 64 human orthotopic liver allografts. Ann Surg 1977;186:282–90.
4. Starzl TE, Putnam CW, Hansbrough JF, et al. Biliary complications after liver transplantation: with special reference to the biliary cast syndrome and techniques of secondary duct repair. Surgery 1977;81:212.
5. Grief F, Bronsther OL, Van Thiel DH, et al. The incidence, timing, and management of biliary tract complications after orthotopic liver transplantation. Ann Surg 1994;219:40–5.
6. Hernandez Q, Ramirez R, Munitiz V, et al. Incidence and management of biliary tract complications following 300 consecutive orthotopic liver transplants. Transplant Proc 1999;31:2407–8.
7. O'Connor TP, Lewis DW, Jenkins RL. Biliary tract complications after liver transplantation. Arch Surg 1995;130:312–7.
8. Davidson BR, Rai R, Kurzawinski TR. Prospective randomized trial of end-to-end versus side-to-side biliary reconstruction after orthotopic liver transplantation. Br J Surg 1999;86:447–52.
9. Rossi G, Lucianetti A, Gridelli B, et al. Biliary tract complications in 224 orthotopic liver transplantations. Transplant Proc 1994;26:3626–8.
10. Rolles K. Biliary tract complications. In: Calne RY, ed. Liver transplantation. London: Grunen and Statton, 1987:473–83.
11. Porayko MK, Kondo M, Steer JL. Liver transplantation: late complications of the biliary tract and their management. Semin Liver Dis 1995;15:139–55.
12. Feith MP, Klompmaker TJ, Maring JK, et al. Biliary reconstruction during liver transplantation in patients with primary sclerosing cholangitis. Transplant Proc 1997;29:560–1.
13. Neuhaus P, Blumhardt G, Bechstein WO, et al. Technique and results of biliary reconstruction using side-to-side choledochocholedochostomy in 300 orthotopic liver transplants. Ann Surg 1994;219:426–34.
14. Golling M, von Frankenberg M, Ioannidis P, et al. Impact of biliary reconstruction on postoperative complications and reinterventions in 1979 liver transplantations. Transplant Proc 1998;30:3180–1.
15. Keck H, Langrehr JM, Knoop M, et al. Reconstruction of the bile duct using the side-to-side anastomosis in 389 orthotopic liver transplants. Transplant Proc 1995;27:1250–1.
16. Rabkin JM, Orloff SL, Reed MH, et al. Biliary tract complications of the side-to-side without T tube versus end-to-end with or without T tube choledochocholedochostomy in liver transplant recipients. Transplantation 1998;65:193–9.
17. Nuno J, Vicente E, Turrion VS, et al. Biliary reconstruction after liver transplantation: with or without T-tube? Transplant Proc 1997;29:564–5.
18. Grande L, Perez-Castilla A, Matus D, et al. Routine use of the T tube in the biliary reconstruction of liver transplantation: is it worthwhile? Transplant Proc 1999;31:2396–7.
19. Ziv BA, Neville L, Davidson B, et al. Infection rates with and without T-tube splintage of common bile duct anastomosis in liver transplantation. Transpl Int 1998;11:123–6.
20. Randall HB, Wachs ME, Somberg KA, et al. The use of the T tube after orthotopic liver transplantation. Transplantation 1996;61:258–61.
21. Lopez RR, Benner KG, Ivancev K, et al. Management of biliary complications after liver transplantation. Am J Surg 1992;163:519–24.
22. Branch MS, Clavien PA. Biliary complications following liver transplantation. In: Killenberg PG, Clavien PA, eds. Medical care of the liver transplant patient. Malden MA: Blackwell Science, 1997:193–209.
23. Schlitt HJ, Meier PN, Nashan B, et al. Reconstructive surgery for ischemic-type lesions at the bile duct bifurcation after liver transplantation. Ann Surg 1999;229:137–45.
24. Margarit C, Hidalgo E, Lazaro JL, et al. Biliary complications due to late hepatic artery thrombosis in adult liver transplant patients. Transpl Int 1998;11(suppl 1):S251–4.
25. Takaya S, Jain A, Yagihashi A, et al. Increased bile duct complications and/or chronic rejection in crossmatch positive human liver allografts. Transplant Proc 1999;31:2028–31.
26. Stratta RJ, Wood RP, Langnas AN, et al. Diagnosis and treatment of biliary tract complications after orthotopic liver transplantation. Surgery 1989;106:675–83.
27. Rieber A, Brambs HJ, Lauchart W. The radiological management of biliary complications following liver transplantation. Cardiovasc Intervent Radiol 1996;19:242–7.
28. Rizk RS, McVicar JP, Emond MJ, et al. Endoscopic management of biliary strictures in liver transplant recipients: effect on patient and graft survival. Gastrointest Endosc 1998;47:128–35.
29. Rossi AF, Grosso C, Zanasi G, et al. Long-term efficacy of endoscopic stenting in patients with stricture of the biliary anastomosis after orthotopic liver transplantation. Endoscopy 1998;30:360–6.
30. Manez R, Bronsther O, Kusne S, et al. Vanishing bile duct syndrome after liver transplantation: alloreactivity or viral reactivity? Transplant Proc 1995;27:2280.
31. Klein S, Savader S, Burdick JF, et al. Reduction of morbidity and mortality from biliary complications after liver transplantation. Hepatology 1991;14:818–23.
32. Shuhart MC, Kowdley KV, McVicar JP, et al. Predictors of bile leaks after T-tube removal in orthotopic liver transplant recipients. Liver Transpl Surg 1998;4:62–70.
33. Barton P, Maier A, Steininger R, et al. Biliary sludge after liver transplantation. 1. Imaging findings and efficacy of various imaging procedures. Am J Radiol 1995;164:859–64.
34. Byun BH, Lee SW, Bae SH, et al. Two cases of common bile duct stone after liver transplantation. J Korean Med Sci 1999;14:97–101.
35. Barton P, Steininger R, Maier A, et al. Biliary sludge after liver transplantation. 2. Treatment with interventional techniques versus surgery and/or oral chemolysis. Am J Radiol 1995;164:865–69.
36. Clavien PA, Camargo CA, Baillie J, Fitz JG. Letter to the editor: sphincter of Oddi dysfunction after liver transplantation. Dig Dis Sci 1995;40:73.
37. Piccinino F, Sagnelli E, Pasquale G, et al. Complications following percutaneous liver biopsy: a multicenter retrospective study on 68,276 biopsies. J Hepatol 1986;2:165–73.
38. Dousset B, Sauvanet A, Bardou M, et al. Selective surgical indications for iatrogenic hemobilia. Surgery 1997:121:37–41.
39. Donovan J. Nonsurgical management of biliary tract disease after transplantation. Gastroenterol Clin North Am 1993;22:317–36.
40. Mentha G, Rubbia-Brandt L, Orci L, et al. Traumatic neuroma with biliary duct obstruction after orthotopic liver transplantation. Transplantation 1999;67:177–9.
41. Navarro F, Pyda P, Pageaux GP, et al. Lymphoproliferative disease after liver transplantation: primary biliary localization. Transplant Proc 1998;30:1486–8.
42. Fulcher AS, Turner MA. Orthotopic liver transplantation: evaluation with MR cholangiography. Radiology 1999;211:715–22.
43. Sherman S, Shaked A, Cryer H, et al. Endoscopic management of biliary fistulas complicating liver transplantation and other hepatobiliary operations. Ann Surg 1993;218:167–75.
44. Sherman S, Jamidar P, Shaked A, et al. Biliary tract complications after orthotopic liver transplantation: endoscopic approach to diagnosis and therapy. Transplantation 1995;60:467–70.
45. Kok T, Van der Sluis A, Klein JP, et al. Ultrasound and cholangiography for the diagnosis of biliary complications after orthotopic liver transplantation: a comparative study. J Clin Ultrasound 1996;24:103–15.
46. Orons PD, Zajko AB. Angiography and interventional procedures in liver transplantation. Radiol Clin North Am 1995;33:541–58.
47. Zemel G, Zajko AB, Skolnick ML, et al. The role of sonography and transhepatic cholangiography in the diagnosis of biliary complications after liver transplantation. Am J Radiol 1988;151:943–6.

48. Kurzawinski TR, Selves L, Farouk M, et al. A prospective study of hepatobiliary scintigraphy and cholangiography for detection of early biliary complications after orthotopic liver transplantation. Br J Surg 1996;83:26–7.
49. Shah AN. Radionuclide imaging in organ transplantation. Radiol Clin North Am 1995;33:473–5.
50. Laghi A, Pavone P, Catalano C, et al. MR cholangiography of late biliary complications after liver transplantation. Am J Radiol 1999;152:1541–6.
51. Grewal HP, Thistlethwaite JR, Loss GE, et al. Complications in 100 living-liver donors. Ann Surg 1998;228:214–9.
52. Egawa H, Uemoto S, Inomata Y, et al. Biliary complications in pediatric living related liver transplantation. Surgery 1998;124:901–10.
53. Reding R, de Goyer JDV, Delbeke I, et al. Pediatric liver transplantation with cadaveric or living related donors: comparative results in 90 elective recipients of primary grafts. J Pediatr 1999;134:280–6.
54. Harihara Y, Makuuchi M, Sakamoto Y, et al. A simple method to confirm patency of the graft bile duct during living-related partial liver transplantation. Transplantation 1997;64:535–7.
55. Lo CM, Fan ST, Liu CL, et al. Adult-to-adult living donor liver transplantation using extended right lobe grafts. Ann Surg 1997;226:261–70.

Chapter 19

Primary Sclerosing Cholangitis

Robert Enns

Primary sclerosing cholangitis (PSC) is a chronic, cholestatic liver disease of unknown etiology characterized by inflammation, destruction, and eventual fibrosis of intrahepatic and extrahepatic bile ducts.

Focal strictures of the biliary tree lead to cholestasis and a characteristic beaded appearance on cholangiography (1–4). The disease may progress silently, or with recurrent episodes of cholangitis characterized by right upper quadrant pain, fever, and jaundice. Eventual progression to cirrhosis with concomitant portal hypertension and liver failure is typical (5–7). PSC is much less common than alcoholic liver disease; nonetheless, because it often affects otherwise relatively healthy young people, it is the fourth most common reason for liver transplantation in the United States (5,8).

Although Delbet first described the syndrome of PSC in 1924, the disease was considered a rare medical curiosity with fewer than 100 cases reported up until 1970 (9,10). With the advent of improved imaging techniques, particularly endoscopic retrograde cholangiography (ERC) in 1974, the numbers of cases diagnosed in many major centers doubled. Subsequent reviews from the Mayo Clinic and Royal Free Hospital in London spurred further interest in the disease as it was demonstrated that the disorder has an association with inflammatory bowel disease (IBD) and typically affects young males (4,11). Increased availability of ERCP has led to a greater number of patients being diagnosed at an earlier stage of disease, which has contributed to an improved understanding of the disorder's classification and pathogenesis, and the clinical, radiographic, and therapeutic modalities appropriate for PSC.

CLASSIFICATION

The early classifications of PSC were very rigid and excluded patients with gallstones, previous biliary tract surgery, inflammatory bowel disease, and retroperitoneal fibrosis. Additionally, progression of disease was required over a 2-year period (12). These strict criteria seem unjustified, and present classification schemes divide sclerosing cholangitis into primary (of unknown etiology) and secondary (with a known or suspected cause). Present criteria for the diagnosis of PSC are shown in Table 19.1 (7). Patients with PSC can be further classified as those with associated liver disease and those without IBD (13).

Typical secondary causes of sclerosing cholangitis include ischemia (arising from operative trauma, hepatic arterial infusion of floxuridine, allograft rejection), recurrent biliary sepsis, cholangiocarcinoma, acquired immunodeficiency syndrome (AIDS), and toxic agents (formaldehyde, absolute alcohol) (14–23). Radiographically, secondary causes of sclerosing cholangitis can resemble PSC but the clinical course and therapeutic options may differ considerably.

PSC has been further classified in various other schemes by several investigators. Caroli and Rosner (24) described an anatomical classification in which the condition is divided according to whether involvement of the biliary tree is diffuse or segmental. Segmental involvement can be further divided into disease that affects the hepatic duct junction, the common hepatic duct, or the common bile duct. Another classification, devised by Longmire (25,26), is based on the disease's clinical course as well as the operative, radiological, and pathological findings in 37 patients at the UCLA Medical Center (Table 19.2). Four distinct groups were identified, of which the most common were diffuse PSC associated with IBD (type 3) and without IBD (type 4). PSC can also be classified according to cholangiographic findings (Table 19.3), which have been reported to predict clinical outcomes (27).

Typically, liver biopsy reveals only a paucity of normal bile ducts and nonspecific fibrosis and inflammation of the

Table 19.1. Criteria for the diagnosis of primary sclerosing cholangitis

1. Presence of typical cholangiographic abnormalities of PSC (involving bile ducts segmentally or extensively).
2. Compatible clinical, biochemical, and hepatic histologic findings (recognizing that they are nonspecific).
3. Exclude the following in most instances
   a. Biliary calculi (unless related to stasis)
   b. Biliary tract surgery (other than simple cholecystectomy)
   c. Congenital abnormalities of the biliary tract
   d. AIDS-associated cholangiopathy
   e. Ischemic strictures
   f. Bile duct neoplasms (unless PSC previously established)
   g. Exposure to irritant chemicals (floxuridine, formalin)
   h. Evidence of another type of liver disease, such as primary biliary cirrhosis or chronic active hepatitis

Source: Porayko MK, LaRusso NF, Wiesner RH. Primary sclerosing cholangitis: a progressive disease? Semin Liver Dis 1991;11:18–25.

Table 19.2. Longmire's classification of primary sclerosing cholangitis

Type	Frequency (%)	Clinical/Radiological Features
1	5–10	Affecting primarily distal common bile duct
2	5–10	Occurring soon after attack of acute necrotizing cholangitis
3	40–50	Chronic diffuse
4	40–50	Chronic diffuse associated with inflammatory bowel disease

Source: Longmire WP Jr. Sclerosing cholangitis. Curr Probl Surg 1977;14:36–43; When is cholangitis sclerosing? Am J Surg 1978;135:312–30.

Table 19.3. Classification of cholangiographic findings in primary sclerosing cholangitis

Type of Duct/Classification	Cholangiographic Appearance
Intrahepatic	
I	Multiple strictures, normal caliber of bile ducts
II	Multiple strictures, saccular dilations, decreased arborization
III	Only central branches filled, severe pruning
Extrahepatic	
I	Slight irregularity of duct contour, no stricture
II	Segmental stricture
III	Stricture of almost the entire length of the duct
IV	Extremely irregular margin, diverticulum outpouchings

Source: Majoie CB, Reeders JW, Sanders JB, et al. Primary sclerosing cholangitis: a modified classification of cholangiographic findings. AJR Am J Roentgenol 1991;157:495–7.

portal tracts (5,11,28). The classic onionskin lesions (Fig. 19.1) are rarely seen on percutaneous biopsy of the liver; therefore, diagnosis has usually been made through cholangiography. Histologically, PSC tends to go through four stages (4,29). Stage 1 is the earliest, characterized by degeneration of epithelial cells in the bile duct and an inflammatory infiltrate localized to the portal triads. In stage 2, fibrosis and inflammation infiltrate the hepatic parenchyma with subsequent destruction of periportal hepatocytes resulting in piecemeal necrosis and loss of bile ducts. In stage 3, cholestasis becomes more prominent and portal-to-portal fibrous septa form. In stage 4, frank cirrhosis develops, with histologic features similar to other causes of cirrhosis. In some patients, findings of large duct obstruction with proliferation and dilatation of interlobular bile ducts may dominate the histologic picture.

PSC has been noted to be associated with a host of other disorders (Table 19.4). The most common association is with IBD, which affects up to 75% of patients with PSC. Of these patients, over 80% have ulcerative colitis and less than 20% have Crohn's disease. Conversely, only 2.5%–7.5% of patients

Table 19.4. Disease associations with primary sclerosing cholangitis

- Inflammatory bowel disease
- Pancreatitis
- Diabetes mellitus
- Retroperitoneal fibrosis
- Sarcoid
- Histiocytosis X
- Hypereosinophilic syndrome
- Sjögren's syndrome
- Reidel's thyroiditis
- Sicca complex
- Celiac disease
- Rheumatoid arthritis

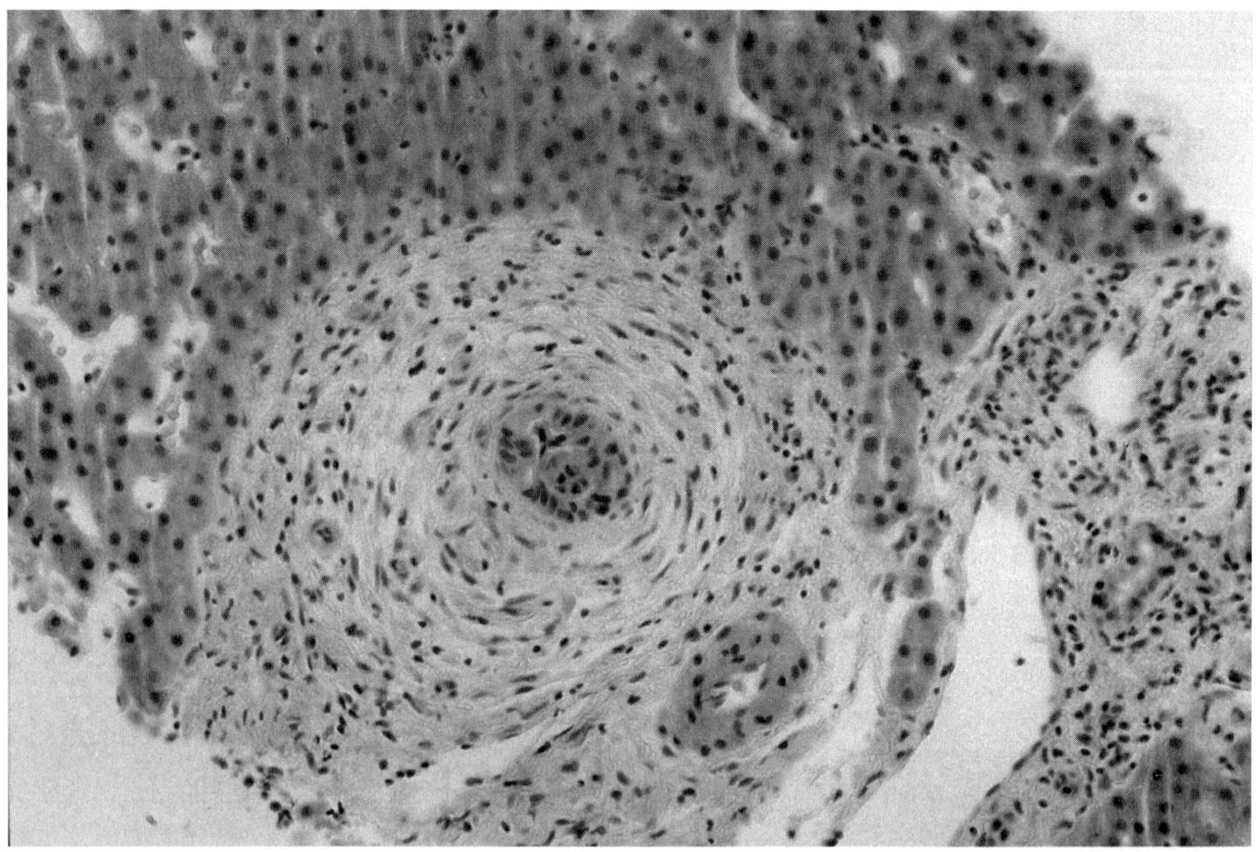

FIGURE 19.1. *Concentric peribiliary fibrosis and inflammation characteristic of early bile duct damage is typical of PSC. It is not usually seen on liver biopsy specimens because it is has a "patchy" distribution, with the highest concentration occurring in the hilum (where biopsies are not usually obtained).*

with ulcerative colitis have or will develop PSC (2–4,28, 30–32). The true prevalence is likely much higher; however, because many patients with ulcerative colitis are asymptomatic and show only minimal elevation in liver enzymes, cholangiography is not performed. In a recent study from Sweden, the prevalence of ulcerative colitis was 170 per 100,000; of these, 3.7% had PSC. This yields a prevalence for PSC of 6.3 per 100,000 inhabitants (33). A subsequent Swedish study demonstrated that 72% of PSC patients had ulcerative colitis, yielding a total prevalence for PSC of 8 per 100,000 inhabitants (34). In contrast to these figures are data from Japan, where only 18% of patients with PSC have IBD (35). Many other disorders, particularly inflammatory disorders, show an association with PSC. These include hypereosinophilic syndrome (20,36–38), Sjögren's syndrome (39), systemic sclerosis (20,40), celiac disease (20,41,42), pancreatitis (43,44), Behçet's syndrome (45), histiocytosis X, sarcoidosis (46–48), sicca complex (49), rheumatoid arthritis (50), systemic mastocytosis (51), histiocytosis X (52,53), and Reidel's thyroiditis (54,55).

All methods of classification attempt to organize the disease process in the hope of determining which subtypes (particularly predominant common bile duct strictures) may be amenable to radiological, endoscopic, and surgical intervention, in contrast with diffuse disease, which may be amenable only to liver transplantation. Classification, particularly histologic, also allows prognostication, which may help identify future transplantation patients in a timely manner.

ETIOLOGY

Although the etiology of PSC is unknown, several mechanisms related to immunological, genetic, toxic, and infectious abnormalities have been proposed as contributing factors (Table 19.5).

Given the close association of PSC with ulcerative colitis, early investigators postulated that recurrent portal bacteremia might be an important factor in the development of the disorder. Recurrent portal infection could lead to chronic biliary tract infection, inflammation, and subsequent fibrosis and classic stricture formation (56). One study even found that portal bacteremia was present in patients who had colonic surgery (57). Subsequent studies, however, could not confirm the findings of portal vein phlebitis (29,56).

Table 19.5. Possible etiologies of primary sclerosing cholangitis

Genetic predisposition
Autoimmune
Portal infection (bacteremia)
Viral infection
Colonic toxins
Copper toxicity
Ischemic injury

Furthermore, if recurrent colitis leads to portal vein phlebitis, colectomy (or at least controlled disease) should have a protective effect. This has not been demonstrated to be true (58). Additionally, hepatic histology does not support portal venous infection because the hallmark of this disorder, portal phlebitis, is mild or absent in most patients with PSC (29). Thus, there is little evidence to support the bacterial infection hypothesis.

If portal bacteremia is not a critical factor, then toxins that might be released from a diseased colon should be considered. Theoretically, toxic bile acids such as lithocholic acid, which arise from bacterial activity within the colon, can be absorbed through a diseased colon with its increased mucosal permeability (59). Lithocholic acid is formed from chenodeoxycholic acid by bacterial 7-α-dehydroxylation in the colon and it has been shown to be hepatotoxic in animals. Unfortunately, abnormalities in bile acid metabolism in PSC or ulcerative colitis patients have not been demonstrated. Furthermore, in human tissue, lithocholic acid is rapidly sulfated and rendered nontoxic, a process that does not occur in animal models (60,61).

Other toxic substances that have been considered more recently are *N*-formylated chemotactic peptides, produced by enteric flora, which have been shown in animal studies to induce fibrosis and damage to major bile ducts through colonic absorption and enterohepatic circulation. Increased biliary excretion of these peptides has been shown in experimentally induced colitis in animal models (62,63). Further investigation to delineate the role of these peptides in the etiology of PSC is required.

The major criticism of the theories of colonic toxins causing PSC comes from studies looking at the natural history of the disorder. It has been demonstrated that the severity of the colitis bears little relation to the development or severity of PSC (30). Furthermore, patients who have a colectomy show no change in their PSC. Some patients develop PSC long after a colectomy or even prior to the onset of their colitis (58). Some patients who develop PSC never have IBD. Antibiotics (which could, theoretically, alter the colonic flora) appear to have little effect on the natural history of PSC (64). Because of these findings, colonic toxins are likely to have only a minor role in the overall etiology of PSC.

Abnormalities of copper metabolism have also been implicated in the pathogenesis of PSC. Several authors have noted that liver samples from patients with PSC show an excess of hepatic copper, which is known to be hepatotoxic (26,65). However, treatment with the chelating agent penicillamine has not been shown to have any benefit (66). Likely, as with many cholestatic disorders, copper accumulation is the result of poor biliary excretion, rather than a primary inciting event critical to the pathogenesis of the disorder (67).

Chronic infection of the biliary tree has been implicated in the pathogenesis of PSC through several observations. Longmire, who noted that some patients appear to develop PSC after an initial episode of acute necrotizing cholangitis, classified this group as a separate category (type 2) of PSC (25,26). Patients with AIDS have been noted to have a sclerosing cholangitis that is felt to be caused by an opportunistic infection (cytomegalovirus, cryptosporidium). Unfortunately, an extensive investigation of 37 PSC patients showed evidence of cytomegalovirus via polymerase chain reaction (PCR) testing of liver tissue in only one patient (68). Experimental cholangitis and biliary atresia can be induced in animal models through infection with reovirus type 3. Early reports suggested that patients with PSC had a significant increase in antibody titers to this virus compared to controls. More recent data, however, show no difference in prevalence or titers of reovirus between controls and PSC patients (69). Rubella can also cause an obliterative cholangitis of the intrahepatic ducts in the fetus, although the histologic picture differs from that of PSC (70). Despite these negative studies, an infectious etiological agent that alters antigenic determinants has yet to be excluded in PSC.

Prompted by the observation of familial aggregates of PSC, genetic predisposition has been increasingly reported (71,72). Several human leukocyte antigens (HLA) molecules, including HLA-B8, HLA-DR2, HLA-DR3, and HLA-DRw52A have been found to be associated with PSC (73,74). Interestingly, HLA-B8 and HLA-DR3 are also known to be associated with other autoimmune diseases, which (as noted below) may play an etiological role in PSC. The DRB3*0101 allele, which encodes HLA-DRw52A, has also been most strongly associated with PSC; it is present in 55% of PSC patients compared to 22% of control subjects. Unfortunately, the finding of HLA-DRw52A in 100% of Caucasian North Americans has not been substantiated in European studies (75–79). Therefore, conflicting data still exist and further research is required to identify possible genetic contributions to the etiology of PSC.

Ischemic arteriolar injury, as can occur with patients who receive intra-arterial infusions of floxuridine, can result in diffuse and focal strictures of the intrahepatic and extrahepatic bile ducts similar to PSC, secondary to obliterative thromboendarteritis (80). Similar findings can be found in polyarteritis nodosa and in those who have hepatic artery thrombosis after liver transplantation (81,82). Although ischemia can cause a biliary disorder typical of PSC, no specific vascular pathology is found in most patients with PSC (83).

Histiocytosis X has been shown in several patients to be associated with PSC. In three patients reported by Thompson et al. (52) both disorders were demonstrated by pathological evaluations to occur in the same patient. The authors suggested that, as the natural history of histiocytosis X is to progress from a proliferative to a fibrous stage, it is a cause of PSC and the two disorders may have a similar pathogenesis.

Despite the absence of antimitochondrial, smooth muscle and nuclear antibodies, accumulating evidence suggests that immune system abnormalities may contribute to the pathogenesis of PSC. Initial support for an autoimmune etiology arose from observations that the disorder occurred in concert with other autoimmune diseases such as ulcerative colitis, Reidel's thyroiditis, rheumatoid arthritis, and sicca complex. The association of PSC with HLA-B8 and HLA-DR3, which are typically linked with autoimmune disorders, also supports an autoimmune pathogenesis. Autoantibodies interacting with nuclei of cells infiltrating the portal tract have been characterized by Chapman et al. (1,78,84,85). They have described anticolon and antiportal tract antibodies, the latter of which is more commonly associated with HLA-B8 and, therefore, more specific for patients with PSC. The antigen in obstructed portal ducts was localized to the nuclei of neutrophils; because the reactivity of the antibody was primarily perinuclear, the antibody was called pANCA. This antibody has been reported in up to 83% of patients with ulcerative colitis and 27% of those with Crohn's disease. The same pattern has been demonstrated in up to 88% of patients with chronic ulcerative colitis and PSC (86,87). The etiological role of pANCA is unclear, but presumably a shared, aberrantly expressed antigenic determinant exists between the biliary tree and the colon that underlies the pathogenesis of the colitis and sclerosis.

Further support for an immunologic pathogenesis of PSC comes from abnormalities noted in both immune complexes and cellular immunity. Most patients with PSC show increased levels of circulating immune complexes, likely reflecting activation of complement through the classic pathway in the serum (88,89). Abnormalities of cellular immunity have also been observed in patients with PSC. In particular, increased expression of intercellular adhesion molecule-1 (ICAM-1) on biliary epithelium has been noted. ICAM-1 may allow T cells to interact with major histocompatibility complex antigens expressed on biliary epithelium, subsequently leading to inflammation and fibrosis. Supporting this is the finding of a significant decrease in circulating CD8 cells (cytotoxic cells), which leads to an increased CD4/CD8 ratio. Within the biliary tree, an increased proportion of CD8 cells has been found specifically in areas of bile duct proliferation, supporting an immune role for PSC (90–92).

Table 19.6. Clinical presentation of primary sclerosing cholangitis

Symptom	Percent of Presentation
Jaundice	75–80
Right upper quadrant pain	50–55
Pruritus	30–35
Fever	20–25
Weight loss	15–20
Fatigue	10–15
Asymptomatic	5–10

Source: Ludwig J, Barham SS, LaRusso NF, et al. Morphologic features of chronic hepatitis associated with primary sclerosing cholangitis and chronic ulcerative colitis. Hepatology 1981;1:632–40.

CLINICAL MANIFESTATIONS

PSC predominantly affects males, with a median onset of 40 years of age but a wide range of 1 to 90 years (4). Pediatric cases show an increased association with immunodeficiency states (10%) and histiocytosis X (15%), and a lesser association with IBD (47%) (93–95). The male predominance occurs primarily in patients with both PSC and ulcerative colitis. PSC has been reported in all races (28). The disorder tends to develop insidiously, with symptoms present in one study for a mean of 52 months (range 0 to 451 months) prior to diagnosis (34). Symptoms of PSC are often nonspecific initially, but jaundice, right upper quadrant pain, pruritus, fever, weight loss, and fatigue subsequently develop (Table 19.6). Atypical presentations of fever of unknown origin or acute supportive cholangitis have been reported. Periodic exacerbations and remissions are typical of the disorder. Exacerbations may be precipitated by gallstones, which form in a strictured biliary tree where normal flow is impeded (96,97). Depending on the location of the stones and the strictures, endoscopic or percutaneous treatment can be useful in removing a nidus of recurrent infection. Unfortunately, many strictures and stones develop in the proximal biliary tree, which may be less amenable to mechanical intervention.

With the increased awareness of PSC, availability of ERCP, and use of laboratory screening, more patients who have asymptomatic elevations in liver enzymes are being diagnosed with this disorder, particularly if they have underlying ulcerative colitis. In particular, asymptomatic elevations of alkaline phosphatase in the setting of chronic ulcerative colitis should raise the suspicion of sclerosing cholangitis and trigger further investigation. Early in the course of PSC, the physical examination is normal. As the disease progresses, the physical stigmata of chronic liver disease (spider angioma, jaundice, palmar erythema) and hepatosplenomegaly may become apparent, as well as the development of portal hypertension, resulting in ascites and variceal bleeding.

LABORATORY EVALUATIONS

Elevation of cholestatic liver enzymes is typical of this disease. Up to 98% of patients will have an increase in the alkaline phosphatase level, although normal alkaline phosphatase levels have occasionally been recorded even in symptomatic patients (98). Most often, the serum alkaline phosphatase is at least twice the upper limit of normal, out of proportion to that of the serum bilirubin. Serum bilirubin levels are also variable (especially early in the course of disease) but inevitably, as the disease progresses, elevations occur in conjunction with a gradual decline in serum albumin. Caution must be used in interpreting isolated findings of low albumin as a negative prognostic factor in PSC, as it may also be decreased by active inflammatory bowel disease in many patients (5). Transient worsening of serum transaminases and bilirubin often occurs during exacerbations of the disease. These will often return to near normal when the episode of fever, chills, or right upper quadrant pain has resolved.

Serum antinuclear, anti-smooth muscle, and antimitochondrial antibodies are negative in over 90% of patients (11,50). One exception may be an uncommon variant of PSC termed "small duct PSC" (where cholangiography is normal) in which there appears to be an overlap with autoimmune hepatitis (99,100). In this disorder, which accounts for only 5% of PSC patients, autoimmune markers may be positive.

Hypergammaglobulinemia is found in about 30% of patients and increased IgM levels are found in 40% to 50% (4,50). Approximately 65% of patients will have a positive pANCA with HLA-DRw52a (DRB3*0101 allele). PANCA is reported to be higher in patients who have both PSC and ulcerative colitis (68% to 83%) than in patients with PSC and Crohn's disease (13% to 27%).

Similar to Wilson's disease and primary biliary cirrhosis, hepatic and urinary copper levels are elevated in PSC (65). The levels appear to correlate with the histologic stage of the disorder, thereby providing prognostic information. Serum copper and ceruloplasmin levels are also elevated in 49% and 71% of patients, respectively (26,66,67).

NATURAL HISTORY

PSC is a progressive disorder with a variable rate of progression. Progression to cirrhosis has occurred as quickly as 8 months, yet other patients have been symptom free after more than 21 years (77). The variability in the progression of the disorder has led to the development of staging systems to provide prognostic information to patients and to allow ample time for arrangements for those who are suitable for liver transplantation. Three large retrospective series have confirmed a median survival (or time to transplantation) of 12 years from the time of diagnosis (2,34,101). The increased use of laboratory screening of patients with IBD for PSC (with liver enzymes) and increased availability of ERCP likely will lead to detection of the disease at an earlier stage and thus the duration of survival may statistically increase.

A subgroup of patients who had no symptoms at the time of diagnosis has also been evaluated. Forty-five patients with no hepatic-related symptoms were followed by the Mayo Clinic for a mean of 6.25 years. Interestingly, 76% demonstrated progression of their liver disease and 31% developed hepatic failure (6). Other studies have found PSC to be more benign; a Norwegian study showed a mean survival of 17 years after initial diagnosis (102,103). Although some of the data conflict, it is clear that for most patients PSC is a progressive disorder that within 10 years will significantly affect their health and, eventually, will lead to hepatic failure and death or require liver transplantation.

Cox multivariate regression analyses have been performed to determine which factors are important in predicting the prognosis for individual patients with PSC. In a Swedish series of 305 patients, age at diagnosis, histologic stage, and serum bilirubin were applied as individual variables to obtain a prognostic index (34). Another regression analysis was performed by the Mayo Clinic: in this study 21 prognostic variables were analyzed individually (in 174 patients with PSC) as predictors in a univariate Cox regression analysis (2). Of these, five variables were determined to be important predictors of survival: age, bilirubin, hemoglobin, presence or absence of IBD, and hepatic histologic stage.

In a third retrospective analysis, a multicenter study evaluated 426 patients with PSC and identified four variables—bilirubin, histologic stage, age, and splenomegaly—as independent variables of prognosis (101,104). A mathematical model to predict survival included these variables:

$$\begin{aligned} R = {} & (0.535 \times \log \text{Bilirubin in mg/dL}) \\ & + (0.486 \times \text{Histologic stage}) + (0.041 \times \text{Age in years}) \\ & + 0.705 \text{ (if splenomegaly was present)} \end{aligned}$$

The survival for 1 and 5 years for low-risk patients (R = 2.35 to 2.46) were 0.98 to 0.92. The 1 and 5 year survival for high-risk patients (R = 5.23 to 5.42) were 0.68 to 0.73 and 0.15 to 0.21, respectively.

Modifications of this formula have also been devised for liver transplantation and shown to be accurate in studies by Kim et al. (105). In this abstract, a modified Mayo score was devised using the formula:

$$\begin{aligned} \text{Risk} = {} & 0.0295 \times \text{Age in years} + 0.5373 \\ & \times \log \text{Bilirubin in milligrams/deciliter} - 0.8389 \\ & \times \text{Albumen} + 0.5380 \times \log \text{Aspartate transaminase} \\ & (\text{IU/L}) + 1.2426 \times \text{Variceal bleeding} \end{aligned}$$

Although somewhat cumbersome, this formula proved particularly important in assessing patients for liver transplantation, as those with low Mayo scores (<4.4) tended to have significantly improved survival following liver transplantation than those with higher scores (>5.3). Furthermore, these same prognostic formulations have also been used to demonstrate that liver transplantation improves overall survival (when compared to predicted survival through the models) (105).

Recently, a comparison between the Mayo Clinic model and age-adjusted Child-Pugh classification has also been performed. This demonstrated that the age-adjusted Child-Pugh score does provide similar accuracy to the Mayo Clinic model. Because it involves less statistical manipulation, it may be easier to use and may help minimize listing criteria for liver transplantation listing selection (106).

Although prognostic models are important and generally help predict the prognosis for individual patients, it is important to realize that some patients have specific strictures (particularly hilar) that are difficult to drain adequately using percutaneous, radiologic, or surgical methods. Usually their serologic laboratory markers elevate them to a high-risk category. Some of these patients may have low-grade histology with no evidence of jaundice, but rather have increasing episodes of sepsis. Some of these patients may be ideally suited for transplantation despite the fact that their Mayo risk score or Child-Pugh score is not markedly elevated. Therefore, despite the use of a very good predictive system, ideally each candidate for transplantation should still be assessed on an individual basis.

DIAGNOSIS

Because histologic findings are not diagnostic in the majority of PSC patients, the gold standard for diagnosis is cholangiography. In the past, operative cholangiography was the primary diagnostic modality; however, currently ERC or percutaneous transhepatic cholangiography (PTC) is the preferred method. Because PTC may be difficult to perform in a nondilated biliary system (with particular difficulty in opacifying small biliary radicals), ERC is the gold standard for diagnosis. Typically, this is performed on a patient with known IBD and cholestatic enzyme elevation (particularly of alkaline phosphatase) (Figs. 19.2 and 19.3). Usually, the patient has had an abdominal ultrasound, which occasionally demonstrates areas of focal biliary dilation.

An ERC in patients with PSC is not without risk; a complication rate of up to 14% has been documented (107). In particular, cholangitis can occur, presumably because focal areas of the biliary tree are poorly drained, resulting in biliary stasis. Because an ERC catheter is not sterile, infection of the biliary tree following an ERC is not uncommon. To decrease this risk, all patients with suspected PSC should receive broad-spectrum antibiotics prior to the procedure. Those who have been demonstrated at ERC to have PSC should receive several days of antibiotics after the procedure. Because most ERCs are done as outpatient procedures, an oral antibiotic is preferable, although parenteral antibiotics can easily be administered prior to the procedure. Ciprofloxacin is effective against most of the typical biliary pathogens (gram-negative bacilli), is well absorbed, and achieves high levels within the biliary tree; thus, it is likely

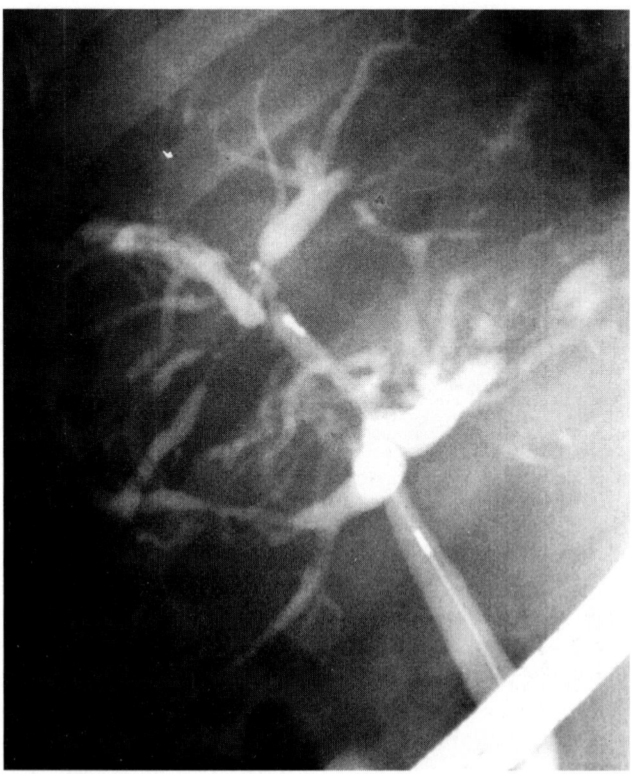

FIGURE 19.2. *Typical intrahepatic strictures in a patient with elevated liver enzymes and known ulcerative colitis.*

the oral antibiotic of choice. A combination of ampicillin and an aminoglycoside or a third-generation cephalosporin can be used if intravenous antibiotics are required.

ERC demonstrates diffuse disease in the majority of PSC patients, with only rare patients having disease limited to the intrahepatic or extrahepatic ducts. Only 1 out of 86 patients reported by MacCarty et al. (108) at the Mayo Clinic had disease limited to the intrahepatic ducts. Lee and Kaplan (5) noted that only 11% of 100 patients with PSC had involvement limited to the intrahepatic ducts and only 2% limited to the extrahepatic ducts. In 20% of patients, however, disease is limited to the intrahepatic and proximal biliary tree, typically not amenable to endoscopic intervention. Diverticular outpouchings of the common bile duct, once considered diagnostic of the disorder, are seen in 25% of patients with PSC (108). In a more recent report by Cameron et al. (109), 24 out of 36 patients with PSC had extensive involvement of the bifurcation, making endoscopic treatment more challenging as well as creating considerable confusion regarding the possibility of cholangiocarcinoma.

A small proportion of patients with IBD have biochemical and histologic findings consistent with PSC but no evidence of typical radiologic abnormalities. This entity, previously known as pericholangitis, is more accurately described as "small-duct PSC" and comprises fewer than 5%

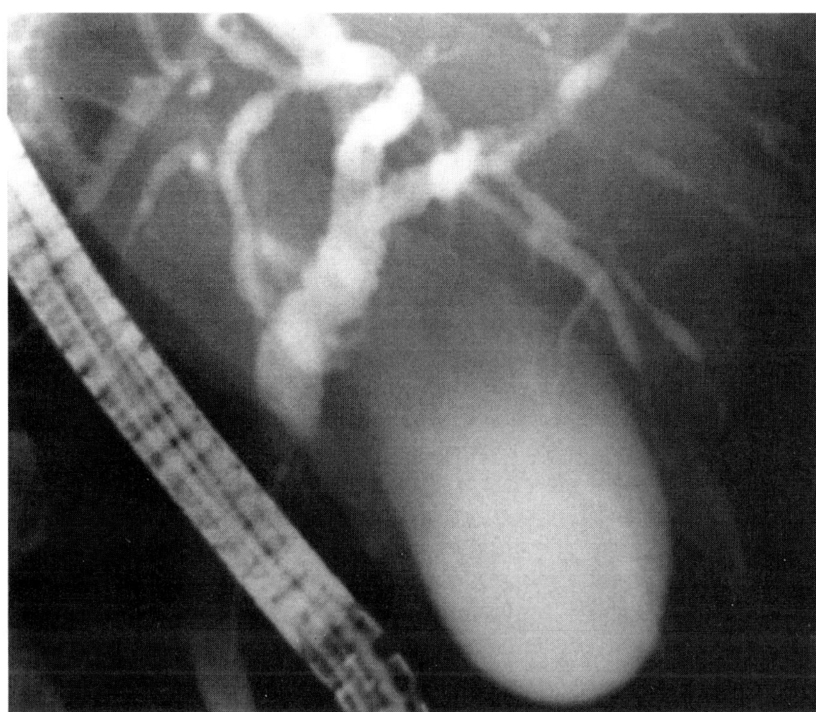

FIGURE 19.3. *Intrahepatic duct strictures occurring in a young male with known acquired immunodeficiency syndrome (AIDS). The cholangiographic picture is similar to PSC (AIDS cholangiopathy).*

of PSC cases overall (99). It has also been described as an "overlap" syndrome with autoimmune hepatitis (100,110).

Pancreatograms have been noted to be abnormal in up to 10% of PSC patients. Stricturing or tapering of the pancreatic duct was noted in 3 of 40 patients with PSC in the Mayo series (108). In a series of 20 PSC patients published by Muller et al. (111), two patients had abnormalities of the choledochopancreatic duct junction, which has been implicated in other biliary disorders such as choledochal cysts and biliary atresia. An unusual amount of pancreatic duct reflux was noted in 43% of patients and overall pancreatic duct abnormalities in up to 50% of patients.

Recently, the advent of magnetic resonance imaging (MRI) has brought a noninvasive testing modality into the diagnostic armamentarium of the gastroenterologist (112). Several studies have demonstrated the usefulness of magnetic resonance cholangiography (MRC) for evaluating the biliary tree for stones, strictures, and other abnormalities (112–119). Single-breath hold sequences with rapid scanning have improved imaging and most strictures, particularly those involving the common bile duct and hilum, can be visualized. If dilatation of the biliary tree is present, imaging sensitivity is improved, but as many patients with PSC have a nondilated biliary tree, diagnostic accuracy is still limited. For those with advanced disease, dilated ducts, and stones, the sensitivity of MRC is likely still high (120–124). Unfortunately, many of these patients still require ERC for therapeutic intervention (stone extraction and stricture dilation) as well as brushings to exclude malignancy, thereby negating some of the benefit of an MRC prior to ERC. If MRC can accurately diagnose patients with mild disease (who do not require therapeutic intervention and in whom malignancy is not a concern) then it would become a very useful diagnostic test. Unfortunately, patients with mild disease typically have diffuse mild intrahepatic duct stricturing, which can be very difficult to diagnose with the present MRC techniques. Attempts to stimulate the biliary tree to enhance dilation of the ducts through the use of cholecystokinin may improve the diagnostic sensitivity of MRC but further studies are required to draw concrete conclusions.

Table 19.7. Medical treatments evaluated in primary sclerosing cholangitis

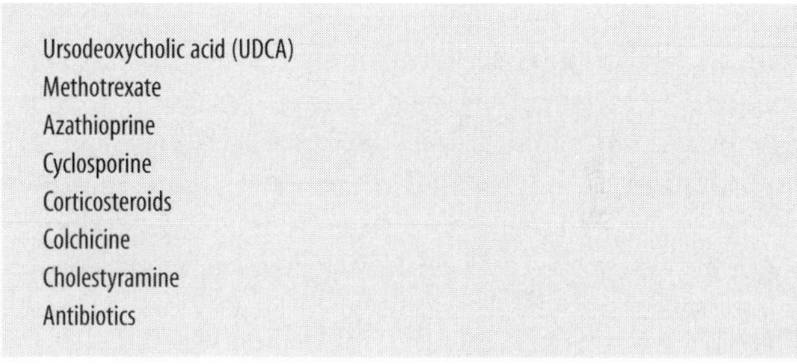

Treatment
Ursodeoxycholic acid (UDCA)
Methotrexate
Azathioprine
Cyclosporine
Corticosteroids
Colchicine
Cholestyramine
Antibiotics

THERAPY

Although a variety of antifibrotic, anti-inflammatory, and immunosuppressive medications have been used to treat PSC (Table 19.7), none of them has demonstrated effectiveness in altering the natural history of the disease. Of critical importance is understanding a fundamental difference between sclerotic biliary tract disorders and disorders of a hepatocellular nature. Hepatocytes have a remarkable ability to regenerate, and, when the inciting agent (i.e., fulminant viral hepatitis) is removed, is treated, or spontaneously disappears, patients can fully recover despite a major hepatic insult. On the other hand, when patients with PSC (or other sclerotic biliary disorders) scar their biliary tree, this results in a permanent loss of function with limited ability for regeneration. Once the serum bilirubin starts to climb, a seemingly irreversible, medically untreatable disorder is present and liver transplantation is the only viable alternative. Ideally, medical therapy should be directed at the underlying cause of PSC (which is unknown) and administered early in the course of the disease when the patient is asymptomatic (5,125). Furthermore, medical therapy is difficult to evaluate because the disease has a slow progression with spontaneous fluctuations in severity. This means that larger, lengthy, multicenter, randomized controlled trials are required for accurate assessment of response to therapy.

Treatment of the disorder is therefore divided into medical therapy for PSC, symptom control, complication therapy, and monitoring for malignancy.

Because PSC is presumed to have an autoimmune etiology, it would be logical to expect that steroids would have a beneficial effect. Only uncontrolled trials are available to assess the effectiveness of corticosteroids. Sivak et al. (126) treated 10 patients with early PSC with prednisone without significant biochemical improvement. Burgert et al. (127) found conflicting data, with some improvement in biochemical testing in 10 patients with documented PSC. Although some of these uncontrolled trials have suggested improvement in PSC in those who took corticosteroids, there is little support for their routine use. PSC develops in some patients who have been exposed to, or are taking, corticosteroids (for IBD), thereby suggesting its lack of benefit. Furthermore, steroids enhance osteoporosis, for which these patients are already at risk. Lastly, in another, more recent, combined trial of prednisone (10 mg daily) and colchicine (0.6 mg twice daily), when compared to a historic control group, improvement in biochemical tests results and alteration in the progression of the disease could not be demonstrated (128). For these reasons, corticosteroids, outside of a clinical trial, cannot be recommended as therapy for PSC.

Given early evidence of its possible benefit in hepatic fibrosis and cirrhosis, colchicine has been used in several studies (129–131). Unfortunately, in studies by Lindor et al. (when it was used in combination with prednisone) and in other case reports, colchicine has not been shown to be useful (128). This has been confirmed in a randomized trial from Sweden where colchicine (1 mg a day) was compared with placebo in 84 patients with PSC. At the 3-year follow-up there were no differences in clinical symptoms, serum biochemistry, liver histology, or survival between the two groups.

Topical corticosteroids have been administered through a nasobiliary drain inserted during ERC. Three anecdotal studies have demonstrated a benefit (132–134), but the only controlled trial, from the Royal Free Hospital in London, showed no benefit when compared to a placebo group (135). Furthermore, the bile of treated patients rapidly became colonized with enteric flora and they had a higher incidence of bacterial cholangitis. Therefore, topical steroids are not recommended.

Methotrexate yielded promising results in an uncontrolled trial of 10 PSC patients (136). Unfortunately, when the investigators performed a prospective double-blind randomized control trial (methotrexate 15 mg a week vs placebo) in 24 patients with PSC, the only significant change was a fall (31%) in the serum alkaline phosphatase in those receiving methotrexate. There was no improvement in symptoms, histology, serum albumin, bilirubin, or transaminases. Complications of methotrexate were minimal, with only a single episode of *Campylobacter enterocolitis* infection and one leukopenic episode, related to bacterial cholangitis, reported. Because many patients in this study had advanced disease (7 of the 12 receiving methotrexate had cirrhosis), it is possible that a positive effect in early stage PSC could have been missed (137). A larger trial in early stage PSC is required to definitively determine the role of methotrexate in this disease. Unfortunately, given its toxicity and the lack of benefit of methotrexate added to ursodeoxycholic acid (UDCA) in 19 patients with PSC by Lindor et al. (138), it is unlikely that a larger trial can be justified.

Because hepatic copper levels are increased in all patients with cholestatic liver disorders, penicillamine was tested in a well-designed, randomized, placebo-controlled trial of 70 patients at the Mayo Clinic. As expected, urinary excretion of copper increased with concomitant reduction in hepatic copper concentrations; however, after 3 years there were no beneficial effects on symptoms, biochemical results, liver histology, disease progression, or survival. In addition, significant toxicity, such as proteinuria and pancytopenia leading to permanent discontinuation of penicillamine, was noted in 21% of patients, thereby discouraging any further use of this agent in PSC (66).

Enthusiasm for the use of UDCA stems from the theory that replacing toxic bile acids such as lithocholic acid with UDCA may decrease hepatic damage. UDCA may also have an immunologic effect by decreasing the expression of class 1 antigens, and a choleretic effect by increasing bile flow (139). Numerous uncontrolled trials demonstrated a beneficial effect (primarily biochemically with improvement of alkaline phosphatase). Symptom improvement was variable and liver histology usually not available (138,140,141). In controlled studies (Table 19.8), typically between 13 mg/kg and 15 mg/kg of UDCA were used. The study durations varied, but ranged from 12 months to 30 months. In the first randomized, double-blind, controlled trial of UDCA in PSC, Beuers et al. (142) placed six patients on UDCA and eight on placebo for a period of 12 months. After 6 months there was an improvement in serum alkaline phosphatase

Table 19.8. Placebo controlled trials of ursodeoxycholic acid in primary sclerosing cholangitis

Reference	Number of Patients	Study Duration (months)	Alk Phos Improved	Bilirubin Improved	Symptom Improved	Histology Improved	Percentage with Early Disease
Beuers (142)	14	12	Yes	Yes	No	Yes	57%
Lo (196)	23	24	Trend	No	No	No	74%
Van Thiel (197)	48	18	No	Yes	N/A	N/A	N/A
Bansi (198)	23	12	Yes	No	No	N/A	30%
Lindor (147)	105	35	Yes	Yes	No	No	N/A

and aminotransferases in the treatment group, but it took up to 12 months to demonstrate an improvement in the serum bilirubin. Hepatic histology improved, particularly of portal and parenchymal inflammation. Unfortunately, symptoms did not improve. Similar results were seen by Stiehl and colleagues, who had to terminate the placebo-controlled arm because the majority of patients experienced a twofold rise in aminotransferases after 3 months. Improvement with UDCA was documented in biochemical and histologic analysis but not with symptoms (143–146).

In a larger trial by Lindor (147), 105 patients were randomized to treatment or placebo, and the follow-up was for up to 6 years. Treatment with UDCA had no effect on time to transplantation, death, or evolution of cirrhosis. Although there was significant improvement in liver biochemistry, this was not reflected by improvement in liver histology or symptoms.

From these studies, it can be concluded that there is a beneficial effect of UDCA on serum transaminases and alkaline phosphatase; unfortunately, it does not appear to improve hepatic histology or symptoms, prolong survival, or affect evolution of cirrhosis or time to transplantation. When UDCA is combined with aggressive endoscopic intervention (dilation of amenable biliary strictures), actual survival rates have been longer than predicted (142,148).

Only long-term studies will determine whether the biochemical improvement produced by UDCA results in improved outcome and survival. Although UDCA has minimal side effects, the current lack of clinical benefit demonstrated by multiple studies suggests that it cannot be regarded as an effective treatment for PSC.

Other immunosuppressive drugs have been tried in a number of studies. No controlled trials are available for azathioprine but in one uncontrolled study two patients improved (149), while in the other case report the patient deteriorated (150). Cyclosporine has been used in a randomized clinical trial involving 34 patients with PSC, most with coexisting ulcerative colitis. After 2 years of therapy, the ulcerative colitis had improved but there was no beneficial effect demonstrated on serum biochemistry. Regarding histology, there was progression of disease in 9 out of 10 patients on placebo and in only 11 out of 20 on therapy. The incidence of side effects was relatively low and included paresthesias and hypertrichosis, but no serious renal toxicity was noted (151,152).

Tacrolimus (FK-506) has been used in one open study in 10 patients with PSC. After 360 days, there was evidence of biochemical improvement in all patients (153). A randomized controlled clinical trial is required to confirm these results.

In summary, numerous medical therapies have been used for PSC and, although several treatment modalities apparently result in biochemical improvement, there appears to be no convincing evidence that these medications yield a sustained clinical benefit. Therefore, outside of a clinical trial, their use is not recommended.

MANAGEMENT OF COMPLICATIONS OF PSC

Associated complications of PSC include fatigue, pruritus, steatorrhea, and fat-soluble vitamin deficiency and its complications, including osteoporosis. Fatigue often parallels progression of disease and can be disabling; however, no medical treatment has been demonstrated to be effective in ameliorating this symptom.

The pruritus can be intense, leading to a diminished quality of life as well as skin and systemic infections arising from excoriations. The pathogenesis of itching may be related to the increased availability of endogenous opiate ligands at central receptors. Although therapy for pruritus associated with cholestatic liver diseases typically starts with cholestyramine, other medical therapies include activated charcoal, rifampin, phenobarbital, plasmapheresis, and opiate antagonists (naloxone, nalmefene) (Table 19.9). Cholestyramine is a nonabsorbable resin that binds bile acids and therefore results in increased fecal excretion of bile by inhibiting enterohepatic circulation. The dose is typically 12–24 grams per day, but as over 50% of patients receiving the drug are troubled by constipation and nausea, compliance is often poor. In primary biliary cirrhosis, rifampicin has been demonstrated to be more effective in reducing pruritus than phenobarbital. Unfortunately, up to 10% of patients get

Table 19.9. Treatments used for pruritus

Resins
Cholestyramine
Colestipol
Antibiotics
Rifampicin
Metronidazole
Enzyme inducers
Rifampicin
Phenobarbitone
Antihistamines
Opiate antagonists
Naloxone
Anabolic steroids
Stanozolol
Other
Primrose oil
Phototherapy
Plasmapheresis
Liver transplantation

drug-induced hepatitis from rifampicin, necessitating discontinuation of this medication (154–156). Opiate antagonists such as naloxone are occasionally useful in ameliorating pruritus but they are awkward to use and can be expensive.

Cholestasis eventually results in significant changes in fat malabsorption. Although chronic pancreatitis and celiac disease have been associated with PSC and can contribute to fat malabsorption, most patients with PSC have steatorrhea secondary to decreased bile acid concentrations within the small intestine. Fat-soluble vitamins (A, D, E, and K) are typically malabsorbed and patients can occasionally develop night blindness, osteomalacia, and coagulopathy. Patients should be screened for these deficiencies and supplemental therapy supplied as required (157).

Osteoporosis is a common problem in cholestatic liver disease. In 50% of PSC patients undergoing transplantation, the bone density levels are below the fracture threshold. One-third of liver transplant patients with PSC will develop vertebral compression fractures. Bone mineral densities do not correlate with serum bilirubin or 25-hydroxyvitamin D, fecal fat, or the presence or absence of ulcerative colitis. As in PBC, the etiology of the osteoporosis is unknown and therapy has not been fully evaluated (139,158). Dual-energy x-ray absorptiometry and dual-photon absorptiometry are noninvasive techniques that provide an excellent quantification of the bone mass. Antiresorptive agents such as the newer biphosphonates (etidronate, pamidronate, alendronate) may avoid the osteopenic complications but further clinical trials in this area are necessary.

The end stages of PSC are often associated with portal hypertension resulting in esophageal varices, ascites, and encephalopathy. These complications can be managed in the usual fashion for patients with end-stage liver disease with a few exceptions. Particular caution should be maintained in patients undergoing systemic surgical shunting for difficult to control esophageal or gastric varices. With the advent of cyanoacrylate ("glue") for fundal varices and transjugular intrahepatic portosystemic shunts, it is uncommon for patients to require surgical decompression. Some reports have suggested that if patients have had previous biliary surgery, future liver transplantation was compromised (109). Two recent reports have suggested the contrary, that previous biliary surgery was not associated with a decreased survival after liver transplantation (159,160). Cirrhotic patients require careful postoperative management and a combined, multidisciplinary team approach. If biliary surgery is required, consultation with the local liver transplantation team would be appropriate before it is performed to ensure that future liver transplantation is not compromised.

A troublesome complication of portal hypertension that occurs in those patients who have undergone proctocolectomy is bleeding from peristomal varices. This bleeding can be severe, with therapy of sclerosants only providing temporary relief. TIPS or surgical portosystemic shunts can control bleeding, but because most of these patients have severe portal hypertension, liver transplantation should always be considered (161).

ENDOSCOPIC MANAGEMENT OF PSC

Although bacterial cholangitis is an unusual presentation of PSC, once the biliary tree has been manipulated (percutaneously, endoscopically, or surgically) it becomes contaminated with gram-negative organisms and recurrent biliary sepsis is common. If dominant strictures are present, several major endoscopy centers have demonstrated that endoscopic therapy is successful in relieving sepsis and improving biochemical tests (Table 19.10). In 1987, the Milwaukee group reported on 10 patients with PSC in whom a total of 19 Gruentzig-type balloon dilations were performed. In those with high grade strictures, endoprostheses were inserted. Strictures treated endoscopically were typically at the level of the hilum, or common bile or hepatic duct (Fig. 19.4). The number of hospitalizations decreased from 2.5 to 0.2 per year, and over a follow-up period of 19 months both the serum bilirubin and alkaline phosphatase decreased significantly (from 6.9 to 2.7 mg/dL and 959 to 385 IU/L, respectively). Three patients died: one from a cholangiocarcinoma, one from bleeding peristomial varices, and one from an unknown cause. Only one complication of endoscopic therapy was noted in this series: a single case of mild pancreatitis (162).

Subsequently, Cotton et al. (163) reported a 32% reduction in bilirubin levels and 29% reduction in alkaline phosphatase after a mean follow-up of 6 months in 17 PSC patients treated with a combination of endoscopic dilation, endoprosthesis, and biliary sphincterotomy. In 1991, the Mil-

Table 19.10. Therapeutic endoscopic series in patients with primary sclerosing cholangitis

Author	Number of Patients	Use of Nasobiliary Tube	Follow-up (months)	Mean Bilirubin Decrease	Mean Alk Phos Decrease	Radiology Stricture Score	Subsequent Hospital Admission Rate
Wagner (167)	12	Yes	23	73%	46%	Improved	N/A
Johnson (164)	35	No	24	60%	15%	Improved	Decreased
Gaing (165)	16	Yes	52	60%	35%	Improved	N/A
Lee (107)	53	Yes (8/53)	31	50%	50%	Improved	N/A
van Milligen de Wit (199)	25	No	25	80%	50%	Improved	N/A

waukee group expanded their previous cohort to 35 patients with a mean follow-up of 24 months. They used a combination of dilating catheters and hydrostatic balloon dilators to dilate dominant strictures. In addition, biliary stents were inserted in 11 patients who could not be dilated adequately. Typically, the stents were removed in 2 to 3 months and dilation was performed during a second ERC. They demonstrated that the number of hospitalizations, total serum bilirubin level, and average radiological stricture score all decreased significantly in patients treated endoscopically (164).

Lee et al. (107) subsequently reviewed the Duke experience by evaluating the results of 85 ERCPs in 53 patients with PSC. Overall, 77% of patients had improvement in their clinical symptoms, liver function tests, or cholangiograms. From the patients' point of view, of 50 patients available for evaluation, 28 felt better, 21 the same, and one felt worse following the therapeutic ERCP. These procedures are done with broad-spectrum antibiotics before the ERC and for a minimum of 24 hours after the procedure. Dilating balloons are typically held in position for 30 to 60 seconds until the "waist" is obliterated (107).

There are several problems with ERC in patients with PSC. First, as noted by Gaing et al. (165) in 1993, approximately 50% of patients will have disease that is primarily intrahepatic in nature, thereby making it more difficult to treat endoscopically. With advancing radiologic techniques such as MRC, it might be reasonable to consider screening patients with PSC with MRC to determine if there is disease that is amenable to endoscopic therapy. Provided that MRC is sensitive and specific for the location of endoscopically amenable strictures, it could avoid diagnostic ERCs in selected patients. Second, the complication rate following an ERC in a patient with PSC may be as high as 15%. This is primarily accounted for by ascending cholangitis. Preoperative and postoperative antibiotics should be administered in all patients with known and suspected PSC to avoid this complication. Third, strictures in PSC must

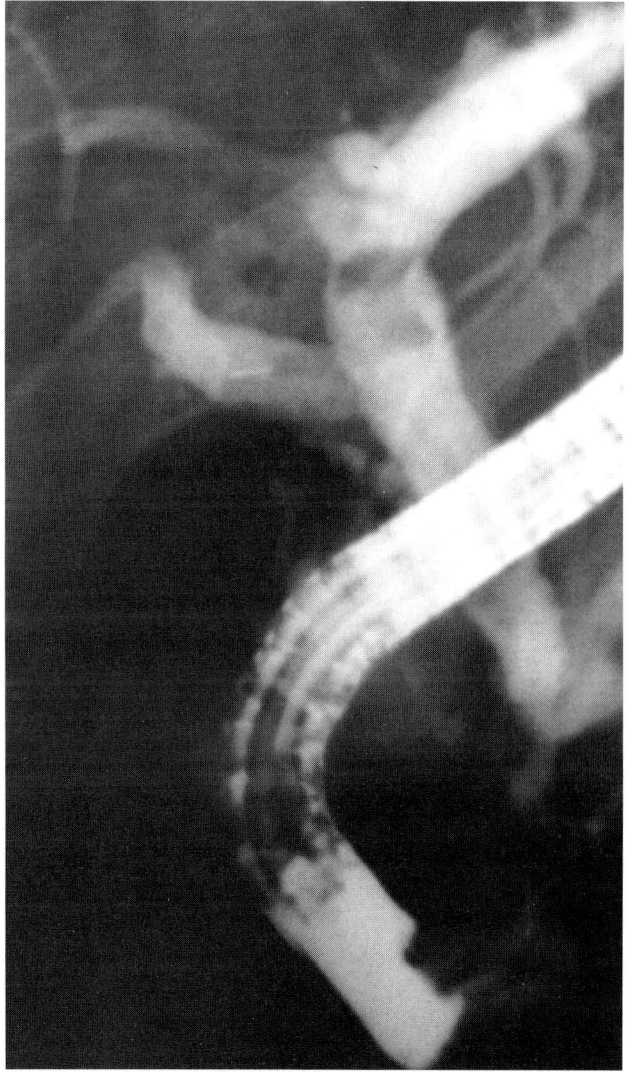
(A)

FIGURE 19.4. ***(A)*** *Distal biliary stricture secondary to PSC with proximal stone formation.* ***(B)*** *The stricture was dilated with subsequent common bile duct stone extraction.*

(B)

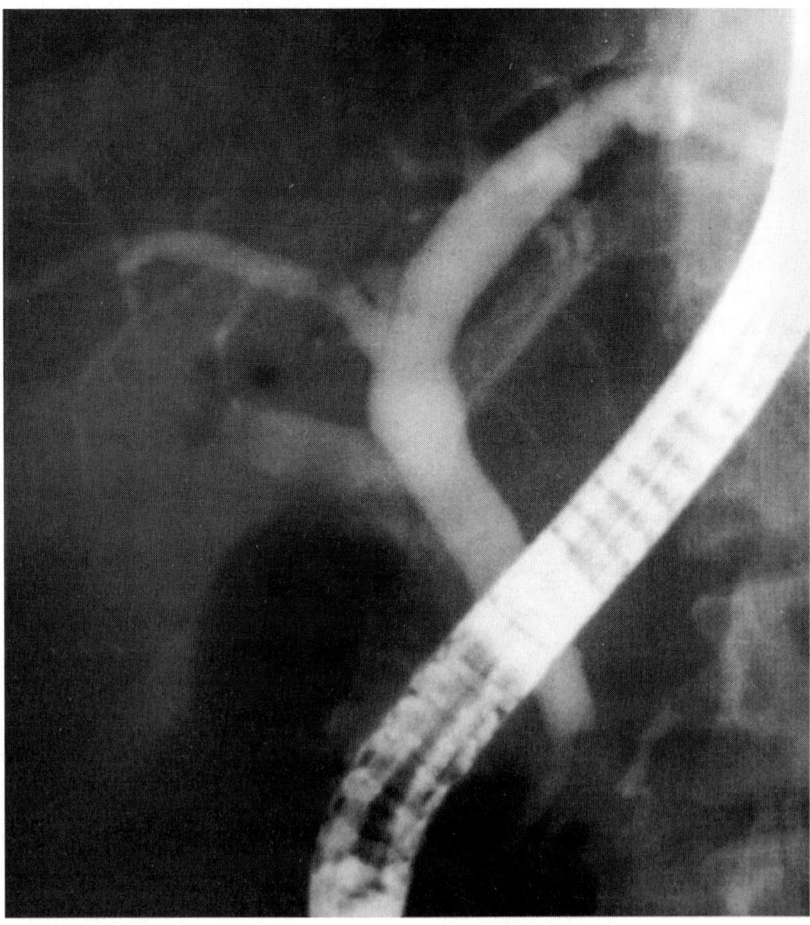

FIGURE 19.4. *Continued*

always be evaluated for the presence of malignancy. Even with aggressive brushing sampling, only a 50% to 60% sensitivity is obtained. A combination of serologic tumor markers (e.g., CEA, CA 19-9) with repeated brushings may increase the diagnostic yield of cholangiocarcinoma in this disease. Last, although there are reports of possible prolongation of survival with endoscopic therapy (166), convincing evidence of this or increased survival until transplantation has not been demonstrated in most patients with PSC treated endoscopically.

Recent investigators have looked at the use of nasobiliary lavage following endoscopic therapy. Wagner et al. (167) followed 12 patients with dominant strictures from PSC treated with hydrostatic balloon dilation and nasobiliary drainage and followed their progress for up to 50 months. Eight patients demonstrated biochemical improvement with only three requiring liver transplantation. No major complications were reported.

Present methods of endoscopic therapy have not been controlled or randomized and clearly have significant bias. However, the results demonstrated by multiple authors have proven a major role for ERC therapy of PSC by demonstrating significant biochemical and radiological improvement in selected patients (see Table 19.10). Although the diagnostic potential of MRC may be great, the therapeutic role of ERC in PSC is not going to be replaced in the near future. It must be remembered, however, that published results have been produced by experts at experienced biliary centers and these results may not be generalizable to smaller centers.

CHOLANGIOCARCINOMA

Up to 15% of patients with PSC may eventually develop cholangiocarcinoma (see Chapters 2 and 20) (2,34,101,168, 169). The patients at highest risk appear to be those with long-standing cirrhosis and ulcerative colitis (170). Bile duct carcinomas have been difficult to diagnose because no single test has proven both sensitive and specific for the disorder (171). Ultrasound and computerized tomography (CT) have a low sensitivity for the diagnosis of primary bile duct tumors. The advent of duplex ultrasonography and bolus-enhanced CT scans may increase sensitivity up to 80% (172,173). Biliary brushings of the stricture have a variable yield of between 50% and 80% (77,174–179).

Tumor markers such as serum CEA have not been shown to be sensitive, with a sensitivity of only 53% being reported

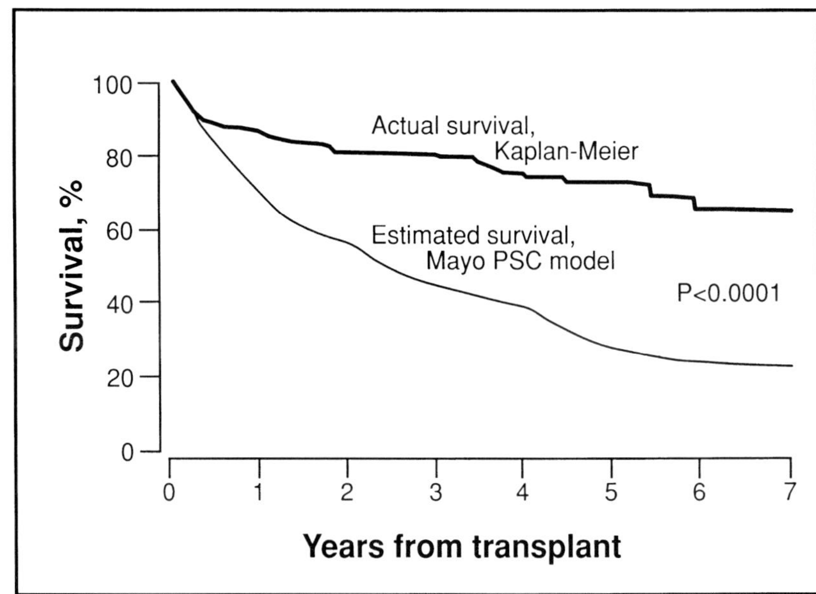

FIGURE 19.5. *Estimated survival after liver transplantation (based on Kaplan-Meier analysis) in patients with PSC compared with estimates of survival without liver transplantation. Liver transplantation increases survival significantly. (Abu-Elmagd KM, Malinchoc M, Dickson ER, et al. Efficacy of hepatic transplantation in patients with primary sclerosing cholangitis. Surg Gynecol Obstet 1993;177:335–44.)*

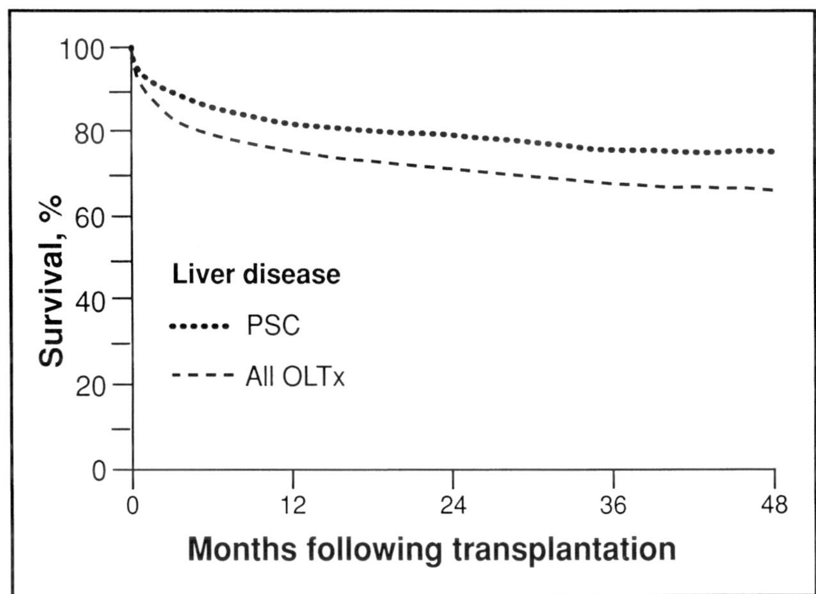

FIGURE 19.6. *Survival in patients undergoing liver transplantation for PSC in comparison to overall survival for all indications of orthotopic liver transplantation. Patients undergoing liver transplantation for PSC have significantly improved survival. (Wiesner RH. Managing complications of PSC and monitoring disease progression. Contemp Intern Med 1994;6:37–46.)*

in one group of 15 patients with cholangiocarcinoma (11 occult tumors) (178). Serum levels of CA 19-9 appear to be slightly more sensitive and specific, although it has not been found to be predictive of cholangiocarcinoma in patients with advanced disease (the group most likely to develop this tumor) (180,181). Ramage et al. (178) have shown that the calculation of a serum tumor index (CEA × 40 + carbohydrate antigen [CA] 19-9) was 86% accurate in diagnosing cholangiocarcinoma in PSC patients and probably is the best laboratory-based method to raise suspicion of a malignant lesion. Biliary CEA, which can be detected through bile aspirates, also has been suggested as a possible marker for cholangiocarcinoma (173). Unfortunately, it is also elevated in patients with intrahepatic cholelithiasis, which is relatively common in PSC. Biliary CEA is also mildly elevated in PSC itself making its accuracy in assessing cholangiocarcinoma in PSC questionable.

The prognosis for cholangiocarcinoma in the setting of PSC is poor, with a reported survival of less than 12 months (168,182). However, in patients with the incidental finding of cholangiocarcinoma in the explanted liver (with regional lymph nodes clear of disease), long-term survival similar to those undergoing transplant without cholangiocarcinoma has been reported. Therefore, those patients who are diagnosed with cholangiocarcinoma preoperatively may be expected to have a poor prognosis; however, those with cholangiocarcinoma discovered incidentally may have a long survival (159).

LIVER TRANSPLANTATION

The treatment of choice for end-stage PSC is liver transplantation (Fig. 19.5). The reported 1- and 3-year survival rates are 85% and 75%, respectively (159,183,184). Patients with PSC undergoing liver transplantation have significantly improved survival when compared to patients undergoing liver transplantation for all indications (Fig. 19.6) (139). One of the challenges facing today's hepatologists is not only the timing of the transplant, but determining when patients should be referred to transplant centers to optimize the results and minimize resource use. Clearly, transplantation may be required for the usual complications of cirrhosis such as recurrent variceal bleeding, diuretic-resistant ascites, and hepatic encephalopathy. Unlike other causes of cirrhosis, however, symptoms particular to PSC such as wasting, fatigue, pruritus, recurrent bacterial cholangitis, and jaundice without evidence of cholangiocarcinoma often prompt referral to transplant centers. In an era where organs such as livers are in short supply, it is often difficult to accommodate potential recipients (even if they are excellent candidates) and various strategies for transplant assessment are used.

A number of complications particular to PSC patients do occur after transplant. PSC patients seem to have a higher incidence of chronic ductopenic rejection after liver transplantation compared with PBC (159,184). In addition, colon cancer in patients with PSC and ulcerative colitis represents a significant cause of late mortality after liver transplantation; therefore, surveillance every 6 to 12 months by colonoscopy is recommended (185–191). Nonanastomotic biliary strictures, not associated with recurrent PSC, have been reported with increasing frequency after liver transplantation and can be difficult to manage (192). Although definitive criteria for the diagnosis of PSC recurrence have not been established for the period after liver transplantation, some patients appear to develop a similar postoperative syndrome. Other conditions such as ischemia, cytomegalovirus infection, and chronic ductopenic rejection must also be considered in the differential diagnosis of post-transplant PSC (5,193–195).

SUMMARY

Primary sclerosing cholangitis is a chronic cholestatic disorder of unknown etiology, commonly associated with IBD and characterized by destruction of intrahepatic and/or extrahepatic biliary ducts. The disease tends to present with abdominal pain, elevated liver enzymes, jaundice, and cholangitis. Although its natural history is variable from patient to patient, several models have been developed to help predict survival and enable timely arrangements for liver transplantation. No medical therapies have demonstrated prolonged survival or duration until transplantation. Several studies have demonstrated that endoscopic therapy can be very successful, especially if dominant strictures occur within the distal biliary tree. In some patients endoscopic therapy may decrease the future need for hospitalization from cholangitis. The complication of cholangiocarcinoma must always be considered when dealing with a dominant biliary stricture. Brushings at the time of endoscopy and tumor marker evaluation are critical to making an early diagnosis of these mitotic lesions, which are often difficult to find. Other complications such as osteoporosis, vitamin deficiencies, and those related to portal hypertension should be treated aggressively to minimize future morbidity and mortality. Ultimately, most patients will require liver transplantation, for which survival rates are excellent.

SUGGESTED READINGS

Boberg KM, Lundin KE, Schrumpf E. Etiology and pathogenesis in primary sclerosing cholangitis. [Review] [127 refs]. Scand J Gastroenterol Suppl 1994;204:47–58. Although the etiology of PSC is unknown, this article reviews the theories regarding etiology and pathogenesis in a comprehensive, logical fashion.

Dickson ER, Murtaugh PA, Wiesner RH, et al. Primary sclerosing cholangitis: refinement and validation of survival models. Gastroenterology 1992;103:1893–901 and Farrant JM, Hayllar KM, Wilkinson ML, et al. Natural history and prognostic variables in primary sclerosing cholangitis. Gastroenterology 1991;100:1710–7. Two key papers evaluating the natural history and prognostic variables (i.e., bilirubin, age, splenogmegaly, histological stage) for survival of patients with PSC. The prediction of survival is critical for the timing of liver transplantation.

Goss JA, Shackleton CR, Farmer DG, et al. Orthotopic liver transplantation for primary sclerosing cholangitis. A 12-year single center experience. Am Surg 1997;225:472–81. In this article the results of orthotopic liver transplantation in 127 PSC patients are presented. A 5-year actuarial patient survival was up to 85%, with incidental cholangiocarcinomas not affecting patient survival significantly.

Lee JG, Schutz SM, England RE, et al. Endoscopic therapy of sclerosing cholangitis. Hepatology 1995;21:661–7. One of the key articles retrospectively reviewing the results of endoscopic therapy in 85 patients with PSC. This clearly demonstrated, at least in the short term, that patient's improved radiologically, biochemically and tended to feel better when endoscopic therapy was used in appropriate patients.

Mitchell SA, Chapman RW. Review article: the management of primary sclerosing cholangitis. [Review] [43 refs]. Aliment Pharmacol Ther 1997;11:33–43. This review article from 1997 evaluated the medical therapy for PSC in a concise fashion. Key trials with all immunosuppressive medication and UDCA are reviewed with clarity.

REFERENCES

1. Chapman RW. Aetiology and natural history of primary sclerosing cholangitis—a decade of progress? Gut 1991;32:1433–5.
2. Wiesner RH, Grambsch PM, Dickson ER, et al. Primary sclerosing cholangitis: natural history, prognostic factors and survival analysis. Hepatology 1989;10:430–6.
3. Lindor KD, Wiesner RH, MacCarty RL, et al. Advances in primary sclerosing cholangitis. Am J Med 1990;89:73–80.
4. Chapman RW, Arborgh BA, Rhodes JM, et al. Primary sclerosing cholangitis: a review of its clinical features, cholangiography, and hepatic histology. Gut 1980;21:870–7.
5. Lee YM, Kaplan MM. Primary sclerosing cholangitis. N Engl J Med 1995;332:924–33.
6. Porayko MK, Wiesner RH, LaRusso NF, et al. Patients with asymptomatic primary sclerosing cholangitis frequently have progressive disease. Gastroenterology 1990;98:1594–602.

7. Porayko MK, LaRusso NF, Wiesner RH. Primary sclerosing cholangitis: a progressive disease? Semin Liver Dis 1991;11:18–25.
8. Garagliano CF, Lilienfeld AM, Mendeloff AI. Incidence rates of liver cirrhosis and related diseases in Baltimore and selected areas of the United States. J Chronic Dis 1979;32:543–54.
9. Delbet P. Retrecissement du choledoque: cholecysto-duodenostomie. Bull Mem Soc Natl Chir 1924;50:1144.
10. White TT, Hart MJ. Primary sclerosing cholangitis. Am J Surg 1987;153:439–43.
11. Wiesner RH, LaRusso NF. Clinicopathologic features of the syndrome of primary sclerosing cholangitis. Gastroenterology 1980;79:200–6.
12. Myers RN, Cooper JH, Padis N. Primary sclerosing cholangitis. Complete gross and histologic reversal after long-term steroid therapy. Am J Gastroenterol 1970;53:527–38.
13. Whelton MJ. Sclerosing cholangitis. Clin Gastroenterol 1973;2:163–73.
14. Batts KP. Ischemic cholangitis. Mayo Clin Proc 1998;73:380–5.
15. Bird GL, Kennedy DH, Forrest JA. AIDS-related cholangitis: diagnostic features and course in four patients. Scott Med J 1995;40:53–4.
16. Buscombe JR, Miller RF, Ell PJ. Hepatobiliary scintigraphy in the diagnosis of AIDS-related sclerosing cholangitis. Nucl Med Commun 1992;13:154–60.
17. Campos LT. A randomized trial of intrahepatic infusion of fluorodeoxyuridine with dexamethasone versus fluorodeoxyuridine alone in the treatment of metastatic colorectal cancer. Cancer 1993;71:875–6.
18. Castellano G, Moreno-Sanchez D, Gutierrez J, et al. Caustic sclerosing cholangitis. Report of four cases and a cumulative review of the literature. Hepatogastroenterolopy 1994;41:458–70.
19. Cello JP. Acquired immunodeficiency syndrome cholangiopathy: spectrum of disease. Am J Med 1989;86:539–46.
20. Dowsett JF, Miller R, Davidson R, et al. Sclerosing cholangitis in acquired immunodeficiency syndrome. Case reports and review of the literature. Scand J Gastroenterol 1988;23:1267–74.
21. Forbes A, Blanshard C, Gazzard B. Natural history of AIDS related sclerosing cholangitis: a study of 20 cases. Gut 1993;34:116–21.
22. Fukuzumi S, Moriya Y, Makuuchi M, Terui S. Serious chemical sclerosing cholangitis associated with hepatic arterial 5FU and MMC chemotherapy. Eur J Surg Oncol 1990;16:251–5.
23. Lemmer ER, Robson SC, Jaskiewicz K, et al. Malignant obstructive cholangiopathies mimicking primary sclerosing cholangitis. J Clin Gastroenterol 1994;19:86–8.
24. Caroli J, Rosner D. Chronic sclerosing cholangitis. In: Bockus HK, ed. Gastroenterology. Philadelphia: WB Saunders, 1976:668–73.
25. Longmire WP Jr. Sclerosing cholangitis. Curr Probl Surg 1977;14:36–43.
26. Longmire WP Jr. When is cholangitis sclerosing? Am J Surg 1978;135:312–30.
27. Majoie CB, Reeders JW, Sanders JB, et al. Primary sclerosing cholangitis: a modified classification of cholangiographic findings. AJR Am J Roentgenol 1991;157:495–7.
28. Lillemoe KD, Pitt HA, Cameron JL. Primary sclerosing cholangitis. Surg Clin North Am 1990;70:1381–402.
29. Ludwig J, Barham SS, LaRusso NF, et al. Morphologic features of chronic hepatitis associated with primary sclerosing cholangitis and chronic ulcerative colitis. Hepatology 1981;1:632–40.
30. Fausa O, Schrumpf E, Elgjo K. Relationship of inflammatory bowel disease and primary sclerosing cholangitis. Semin Liver Dis 1991;11:31–9.
31. Rabinovitz M, Gavaler JS, Schade RR, et al. Does primary sclerosing cholangitis occurring in association with inflammatory bowel disease differ from that occurring in the absence of inflammatory bowel disease? A study of sixty-six subjects. Hepatology 1990;11:7–11.
32. Stockbrugger RW, Olsson R, Jaup B, Jensen J. Forty-six patients with primary sclerosing cholangitis: radiological bile duct changes in relationship to clinical course and concomitant inflammatory bowel disease. Hepatogastroenterology 1988;35:289–94.
33. Olsson R, Danielsson A, Jarnerot G, et al. Prevalence of primary sclerosing cholangitis in patients with ulcerative colitis. Gastroenterology 1991;100:1319–23.
34. Broome U, Olsson R, Loof L, et al. Natural history and prognostic factors in 305 Swedish patients with primary sclerosing cholangitis. Gut 1996;38:610–15.
35. Kashihara T, Sibamoto S, Fujimoro, et al. Two cases of primary sclerosing cholangitis and review of the recent literature. Gastrointest Endosc 1992;32:1194–204.
36. Grauer L, Padilla VM, Bouza L, Barkin JS. Eosinophilic sclerosing cholangitis associated with hypereosinophilic syndrome. Am J Gastroenterol 1993;88:1764–69.
37. Ichikawa N, Taniguchi A, Akama H, et al. Sclerosing cholangitis associated with hypereosinophilic syndrome. Intern Med 1997;36:561–4.
38. Scheurlen M, Mork H, Weber P. Hypereosinophilic syndrome resembling chronic inflammatory bowel disease with primary sclerosing cholangitis. J Clin Gastroenterol 1992;14:59–63.
39. Nieminen U, Koivisto T, Kahri A, Farkkila M. Sjögren's syndrome with chronic pancreatitis, sclerosing cholangitis, and pulmonary infiltrations. Am J Gastroenterol 1997;92:139–42.
40. Fraile G, Rodriguez-Garcia JL, Moreno A. Primary sclerosing cholangitis associated with systemic sclerosis. Postgrad Med J 1991;67:189–92.
41. Fracassetti O, Delvecchio G, Tambini R, et al. Primary sclerosing cholangitis with celiac sprue: two cases. J Clin Gastroenterol 1996;22:71–2.
42. Hay JE, Wiesner RH, Shorter RG, et al. Primary sclerosing cholangitis and celiac disease. A novel association. Ann Intern Med 1988;109:713–17.
43. Imrie CW, Brombacher GD. Sclerosing cholangitis: a rare etiology for acute pancreatitis. Int J Pancreatol 1998;23:71–5. See comments.
44. Kazumori H, Ashizawa N, Moriyama N, et al. Primary sclerosing pancreatitis and cholangitis. Int J Pancreatol 1998;24:123–7.
45. Hisaoka M, Haratake J, Nakamura T. Small bile duct abnormalities and chronic intrahepatic cholestasis in Behcet's syndrome. Hepatogastroenterology 1994;41:267–70.
46. Alam I, Levenson SD, Ferrell LD, Bass NM. Diffuse intrahepatic biliary strictures in sarcoidosis resembling sclerosing cholangitis. Case report and review of the literature. Dig Dis Sci 1997;42:1295–301.
47. Das D, Smith A, Warnes TW. Hepatic sarcoidosis and renal carcinoma. J Clin Gastroenterol 1999;28:61–3.
48. Ilan Y, Rappaport I, Feigin R, Ben-Chetrit E. Primary sclerosing cholangitis in sarcoidosis. J Clin Gastroenterol 1993;16:326–8.
49. Montefusco PP, Geiss AC, Bronzo RL, et al. Sclerosing cholangitis, chronic pancreatitis, and Sjögren's syndrome: a syndrome complex. Am J Surg 1984;147:822–6.
50. Lillemoe KD, Pitt HA, Cameron JL. Sclerosing cholangitis. Adv Surg 1988;21:65–92.
51. Baron TH, Koehler RE, Rodgers WH, et al. Mast cell cholangiopathy: another cause of sclerosing cholangitis. Gastroenterology 1995;109:1677–81.
52. Thompson HH, Pitt HA, Lewin KJ, Longmire WP Jr. Sclerosing cholangitis and histiocytosis X. Gut 1984;25:526–30.
53. Leblanc A, Hadchouel M, Jehan P, et al. Obstructive jaundice in children with histiocytosis X. Gastroenterology 1981;80:134–9.
54. De Boer WA. Riedel's thyroiditis, retroperitoneal fibrosis, and sclerosing cholangitis: diseases with one pathogenesis? (letter). Gut 1993;34:714.
55. Laitt RD, Hubscher SG, Buckels JA, et al. Sclerosing cholangitis associated with multifocal fibrosis: a case report. Gut 1992;33:1430–2.
56. Palmer KR, Duerden BI, Holdsworth CD. Bacteriological and endotoxin studies in cases of ulcerative colitis submitted to surgery. Gut 1980;21:851–4.
57. Brooke BN, Dykes PW, Walker F. A study of liver disorder in ulcerative colitis. Postgrad Med J 1961;37:245–51.
58. Cangemi JR, Wiesner RH, Beaver SJ, et al. Effect of proctocolectomy for chronic ulcerative colitis on the natural history of primary sclerosing cholangitis. Gastroenterology 1989;96:790–4.
59. Palmer RH. Bile acids, liver injury and liver disease. Arch Intern Med 1972;130:606–17.
60. Cowen AE, Korman MG, Hofmann AF, et al. Metabolism of lithocholate in healthy man. Biotransformation and biliary excretion of intravenously administered lithocholate, lithocholyglycine, and their sulphates. Gastroenterology 1975;69:59–66.
61. Siegel JH, Barnes S, Morris JS. Bile acids in liver disease associated with inflammatory bowel disease. Digestion 1977;15:469–81.
62. Hobson CH, Butt TJ, Ferry D, et al. Enterohepatic circulation of bacterial chemotactic peptide in rats with experimental colitis. Gastroenterology 1988;94:1006–13.
63. Lichtman SN, Sartor RB, Keku J, Schwab JH. Hepatic inflammation in rats with experimental small intestinal bacterial overgrowth. Gastroenterology 1990;98:414–23.
64. Mistilis SP, Skyring AP, Goulston SJ. Effect of long-term tetracycline therapy, steroid therapy and colectomy in pericholangitis associated with ulcerative colitis. Australas Ann Med 1965;14:286–94.
65. Gross JBJ, Ludwig J, Wiesner RH, et al. Abnormalities in tests of copper metabolism in primary sclerosing cholangitis. Gastroenterology 1985;89:272–8.
66. LaRusso NF, Wiesner RH, Ludwig J, et al. Prospective trial of penicillamine in primary sclerosing cholangitis. Gastroenterology 1988;95:1036–42.
67. Wiesner RH, LaRusso NF, Ludwig J, et al. Comparison of the clinicopathologic features of primary sclerosing cholangitis and primary biliary cirrhosis. Gastroenterology 1985;88:108–14.

68. Mehal WZ, Hattersley AT, Chapman RW, Fleming KA. A survey of cytomegalovirus (CMV) DNA in primary sclerosing cholangitis (PSC) liver tissues using a sensitive polymerase chain reaction (PCR) based assay. J Hepatol 1992;15:396–9.
69. Minuk GY, Paul RW, Lee PWK. The prevalence of antibodies to reovirus type 3 in adults with idiopathic cholestatic liver disease. J Med Virol 1985;16:55–60.
70. Lindor KD, Wiesner RH, LaRusso NF. Recent advances in the management of primary sclerosing cholangitis. Semin Liver Dis 1987;7:322–7.
71. Jorge AD, Esley C, Ahumada J. Family incidence of primary sclerosing cholangitis associated with immunologic diseases. Endoscopy 1987;19:114–17.
72. Record CO, Shilkin KB, Eddleston AL, Williams R. Intrahepatic sclerosing cholangitis associated with a familial immunodeficiency syndrome. Lancet 1973;2:18–20.
73. Donaldson PT, Doherty DG, Hayllar KM, et al. Susceptibility to autoimmune chronic active hepatitis: human leukocyte antigens DR4 and A1-B8-DR3 are independent risk factors. Hepatology 1991;13:701–6.
74. Schrumpf E, Fausa O, Forre O, et al. HLA antigens and immunoregulatory T cells in ulcerative colitis associated with hepatobiliary disease. Scand J Gastroenterol 1982;17:187–91.
75. Farrant JM, Doherty DG, Donaldson PT, et al. Amino acid substitutions at position 38 of the DR beta polypeptide confer susceptibility to and protection from primary sclerosing cholangitis. Hepatology 1992;16:390–5.
76. Zetterquist H, Broome U, Einarsson K, Olerup O. HLA class II genes in primary sclerosing cholangitis and chronic inflammatory bowel disease: no HLA-DRw52a association in Swedish patients with sclerosing cholangitis. Gut 1992;33:942–6.
77. Ponsioen CI, Tytgat GN. Primary sclerosing cholangitis: a clinical review. Am J Gastroenterol 1998;93:515–23.
78. Chapman RW. Role of immune factors in the pathogenesis of primary sclerosing cholangitis. Semin Liver Dis 1991;11:1–4.
79. Prochazka EJ, Terasaki PI, Park MS, et al. Association of primary sclerosing cholangitis with HLA-DRw52a. N Engl J Med 1990;322:1842–4.
80. Ludwig J, Kim CH, Wiesner RH, Krom RA. Floxuridine-induced sclerosing cholangitis: an ischemic cholangiopathy? Hepatology 1989;9:215–18.
81. Kemeny MM, Battifora H, Blayney DW, et al. Sclerosing cholangitis after continuous hepatic artery infusion of FUDR. Ann Surg 1985;202:176–81.
82. Terblanche J, Allison HF, Northover JM. An ischemic basis for biliary strictures. Surgery 1983;94:52–7.
83. Ludwig J, LaRusso NF, Wiesner RH. The syndrome of primary sclerosing cholangitis. Prog Liver Dis 1990;9:555–66.
84. Chapman RW. The immunology of primary sclerosing cholangitis. Springer Semin Immunopathol 1990;12:121–8.
85. Snook JA, Chapman RW, Fleming K, Jewell DP. Anti-neutrophil nuclear antibody in ulcerative colitis, Crohn's disease and primary sclerosing cholangitis. Clin Exper Immunol 1989;76:30–3.
86. Duerr RH, Targan SR, Landers CJ, et al. Neutrophil cytoplasmic antibodies: a link between primary sclerosing cholangitis and ulcerative colitis. Gastroenterology 1991;100:1385–91.
87. Klein R, Eisenburg J, Weber P, Seibold F, Berg PA. Significance and specificity of antibodies to neutrophils detected by western blotting for the serological diagnosis of primary sclerosing cholangitis. Hepatology 1991;14:1147–52.
88. Alberti-Flor JJ, de Medina M, Jeffers L, et al. Elevated levels of immunoglobulins and immune complexes in the bile of patients with primary sclerosing cholangitis. Am J Gastroenterol 1986;81:325–8.
89. Bodenheimer HCJ, LaRusso NF, Thayer WRJ, et al. Elevated circulating immune complexes in primary sclerosing cholangitis. Hepatology 1983;3:150–4.
90. Adams DH, Hubscher SG, Shaw J, et al. Increased expression of intercellular adhesion molecule 1 on bile ducts in primary biliary cirrhosis and primary sclerosing cholangitis. Hepatology 1991;14:426–31.
91. Adams DH, Mainolfi E, Burra P, et al. Detection of circulating intercellular adhesion molecule-1 in chronic liver diseases. Hepatology 1992;16:810–14.
92. Lindor KD, Wiesner RH, LaRusso NF, Homburger HA. Enhanced autoreactivity of T-lymphocytes in primary sclerosing cholangitis. Hepatology 1987;7:884–8.
93. Sisto A, Feldman P, Garel L, et al. Primary sclerosing cholangitis in children: study of five cases and review of the literature. Pediatrics 1987;80:918–23.
94. el-Shabrawi M, Wilkinson ML, Portmann B, et al. Primary sclerosing cholangitis in childhood. Gastroenterology 1987;92:1226–35.
95. Johnson DA, Cattau ELJ, Hancock JE. Pediatric primary sclerosing cholangitis. Dig Dis Sci 1986;31:773–7.
96. Kaw M, Silverman WB, Rabinovitz M, Schade RR. Biliary tract calculi in primary sclerosing cholangitis. Am J Gastroenterol 1995;90:72–5. See comments.
97. Pokorny CS, McCaughan GW, Gallagher ND, Selby WS. Sclerosing cholangitis and biliary tract calculi—primary or secondary? Gut 1992;33:1376–80.
98. Balasubramaniam K, Wiesner RH, LaRusso NF. Primary sclerosing cholangitis with normal serum alkaline phosphatase activity. Gastroenterology 1988;95:1395–8.
99. Wee A, Ludwig J. Pericholangitis in chronic ulcerative colitis: primary sclerosing cholangitis of the small bile ducts? Ann Intern Med 1985;102:581–7.
100. Ludwig J. Small-duct primary sclerosing cholangitis. Semin Liver Dis 1991;11:11–17.
101. Farrant JM, Hayllar KM, Wilkinson ML, et al. Natural history and prognostic variables in primary sclerosing cholangitis. Gastroenterology 1991;100:1710–17.
102. Aadland E, Schrumpf E, Fausa O, et al. Primary sclerosing cholangitis: a long-term follow-up study. Scand J Gastroenterol 1987;22:655–64.
103. Helzberg JH, Petersen JM, Boyer JL. Improved survival with primary sclerosing cholangitis. A review of clinicopathologic features and comparison of symptomatic and asymptomatic patients. Gastroenterology 1987;92:1869–75.
104. Dickson ER, Murtaugh PA, Wiesner RH, et al. Primary sclerosing cholangitis: refinement and validation of survival models. Gastroenterology 1992;103:1893–901.
105. Kim WR, Lindor KD, Poterucha JJ, et al. The Mayo risk score increases rapidly in the terminal phase of primary sclerosing cholangitis (abstract). Gastroenterology 1998;114:A1274.
106. Shetty K, Rybicki L, Carey WD. The Child-Pugh classification as a prognostic indicator for survival in primary sclerosing cholangitis. Hepatology 1997;25:1049–53.
107. Lee JG, Schutz SM, England RE, et al. Endoscopic therapy of sclerosing cholangitis. Hepatology 1995;21:661–7.
108. MacCarty RL, LaRusso NF, Wiesner RH, Ludwig J. Primary sclerosing cholangitis: findings on cholangiography and pancreatography. Radiology 1983;149:39–44.
109. Cameron JL, Pitt HA, Zinner MJ, et al. Resection of hepatic duct bifurcation and transhepatic stenting for sclerosing cholangitis. Ann Surg 1988;207:614–22.
110. Boberg KM, Schrumpf E, Fausa O, et al. Hepatobiliary disease in ulcerative colitis. An analysis of 18 patients with hepatobiliary lesions classified as small-duct primary sclerosing cholangitis. Scand J Gastroenterol 1994;29:744–52.
111. Muller EL, Miyamoto T, Pitt HA, Longmire WP Jr. Anatomy of the choledochopancreatic duct junction in primary sclerosing cholangitis. Surgery 1985;97:21–7.
112. Barish MA, Yucel EK, Ferrucci JT. Magnetic resonance cholangiopancreatography. N Engl J Med 1999;341:258–64.
113. Ho JT, Yap CK. Magnetic resonance cholangiopancreatography: value of using the half-Fourier acquisition single-shot turbo spin-echo (HASTE) sequence. Ann Acad Med Singapore 1999;28:366–70.
114. Fulcher AS, Turner MA. Benign diseases of the biliary tract: evaluation with MR cholangiography. Semin Ultrasound CT MR 1999;20:294–303.
115. Varghese JC, Farrell MA, Courtney G, et al. A prospective comparison of magnetic resonance cholangiopancreatography with endoscopic retrograde cholangiopancreatography in the evaluation of patients with suspected biliary tract disease. Clin Radiol 1999;54:513–20.
116. Deviere J, Matos C, Cremer M. The impact of magnetic resonance cholangiopancreatography on ERCP. Gastrointest Endosc 1999;50:136–40.
117. Yamakawa K, Satake H, Naganawa S, et al. [MR-cholangiopancreatography using three-dimensional Fourier transfer fast asymmetric spin-echo method (3DFT-FASE)—clinical evaluation] (Japanese). Nippon Rinsho 1998;56:2825–9.
118. Ichikawa T, Hanaoka H, Nitatori T, et al. [Breath-hold MR cholangiopancreatography with 2D and 3D-FASE sequence at 0.5 tesla: evaluation based on measurements of signal intensity ratio and contrast-to-noise ratio] (Japanese). Nippon Rinsho 1998;56:2817–24.
119. Lee MG, Jeong YK, Kim MH, et al. MR cholangiopancreatography of pancreaticobiliary diseases: comparing single-shot RARE and multislice HASTE sequences. AJR Am J Roentgenol 1998;171:1539–45.
120. Durieu I, Pellet O, Simonot L, et al. Sclerosing cholangitis in adults with cystic fibrosis: a magnetic resonance cholangiographic prospective study. J Hepatol 1999;30:1052–6.
121. Ernst O, Asselah T, Talbodec N, Sergent G. MR cholangiopancreatography: a promising new tool for diagnosing primary sclerosing cholangitis. AJR Am J Roentgenol 1997;168:1115–16.

122. Ernst O, Asselah T, Sergent G, et al. MR cholangiography in primary sclerosing cholangitis. AJR Am J Roentgenol 1998;171:1027–30.
123. Ito K, Mitchell DG, Outwater EK, Blasbalg R. Primary sclerosing cholangitis: MR imaging features. AJR Am J Roentgenol 1999;172:1527–33.
124. Revelon G, Rashid A, Kawamoto S, Bluemke DA. Primary sclerosing cholangitis: MR imaging findings with pathologic correlation. AJR Am J Roentgenol 1999;173:1037–42.
125. Kaplan MM. Medical approaches to primary sclerosing cholangitis. Semin Liver Dis 1991;11:56–63.
126. Sivak MVJ, Farmer RG, Lalli AF. Sclerosing cholangitis: its increasing frequency of recognition and association with inflammatory bowel disease. J Clin Gastroenterol 1981;3:261–6.
127. Burgert SC, Brown BP, Kirkpatrick RB, et al. Positive corticosteroid response in patients with primary sclerosing cholangitis (abstract). Gastroenterology 1984;86:A1037.
128. Lindor KD, Wiesner RH, Colwell LJ, et al. The combination of prednisone and colchicine in patients with primary sclerosing cholangitis. Am J Gastroenterol 1991;86:57–61.
129. Leiser A, Kadish U. Beneficial effect of colchicine in a case of sclerosing cholangitis. Am J Med Sci 1986;291:416–18.
130. Rojkind M, Kershenobich D. Effect of colchicine on collagen, albumin and transferrin synthesis by cirrhotic rat liver slices. Biochim Biophys Acta 1975;378:415–23.
131. Rojkind M, Uribe M, Kershenobich D. Colchicine and the treatment of liver cirrhosis. Lancet 1973;1:38–9.
132. Jeffrey GP, Reed WD, Laurence BH, Shilkin KB. Primary sclerosing cholangitis: clinical and immunopathological review of 21 cases. J Gastroenterol Hepatol 1990;5:135–40.
133. Grijm R, Huibregtse K, Bartelsman J, et al. Therapeutic investigations in primary sclerosing cholangitis. Dig Dis Sci 1986;31:792–8.
134. Craig PI, Williams SJ, Hatrield ARW, et al. Endoscopic management of primary sclerosing cholangitis (abstract). Gut 1990;31:1182A.
135. Allison MC, Burroughs AK, Noone P, Summerfield JA. Biliary lavage with corticosteroids in primary sclerosing cholangitis. A clinical, cholangiographic and bacteriological study. J Hepatol 1986;3:118–22.
136. Knox TA, Kaplan MM. Treatment of primary sclerosing cholangitis with oral methotrexate. Am J Gastroenterol 1991;86:546–52.
137. Knox TA, Kaplan MM. A double-blind controlled trial of oral-pulse methotrexate therapy in the treatment of primary sclerosing cholangitis. Gastroenterology 1994;106:494–9. See comments.
138. Lindor KD, Jorgensen RA, Anderson ML, et al. Ursodeoxycholic acid and methotrexate for primary sclerosing cholangitis: a pilot study. Am J Gastroenterol 1996;91:511–15.
139. Wiesner RH. Current concepts in primary sclerosing cholangitis. Mayo Clin Proc 1994;69:969–82.
140. Chazouilleres O, Poupon R, Capron JP, et al. Ursodeoxycholic acid for primary sclerosing cholangitis. J Hepatol 1990;11:120–3.
141. O'Brien CB, Senior JR, Arora-Mirchandani R, et al. Ursodeoxycholic acid for the treatment of primary sclerosing cholangitis: a 30-month pilot study. Hepatology 1991;14:838–47. Erratum. Hepatology 1992;15:566.
142. Beuers U, Spengler U, Kruis W, et al. Ursodeoxycholic acid for treatment of primary sclerosing cholangitis: a placebo-controlled trial. Hepatology 1992;16:707–14.
143. Stiehl A. Ursodeoxycholic acid in the treatment of primary sclerosing cholangitis. Ann Med 1994;26:345–9.
144. Stiehl A. Ursodeoxycholic acid therapy in treatment of primary sclerosing cholangitis. Scand J Gastroenterol Suppl 1994;204:59–61.
145. Stiehl A, Walker S, Stiehl L, et al. Effect of ursodeoxycholic acid on liver and bile duct disease in primary sclerosing cholangitis. A 3-year pilot study with a placebo-controlled study period. J Hepatol 1994;20:57–64.
146. Stiehl A. Ursodeoxycholic acid in the treatment of primary sclerosing cholangitis. Ital J Gastroenterol 1996;28:178–80.
147. Lindor KD. Ursodiol for primary sclerosing cholangitis. Mayo Primary Sclerosing Cholangitis-Ursodeoxycholic Acid Study Group. N Engl J Med 1997;336:691–5. See comments.
148. Stiehl A, Rudolph G, Sauer P, Benz C, et al. Efficacy of ursodeoxycholic acid treatment and endoscopic dilation of major duct stenoses in primary sclerosing cholangitis. An 8-year prospective study. J Hepatol 1997;26:560–6.
149. Javett SL. Azathioprine in primary sclerosing cholangitis. Lancet 1971;1:810.
150. Wagner A. Azathioprine treatment in primary sclerosing cholangitis. Lancet 1971;2:663–4.
151. Sandborn WJ, Tremaine WJ. Cyclosporine treatment of inflammatory bowel disease. Mayo Clin Proc 1992;67:981–90.
152. Sandborn WJ, Wiesner RH, Tremaine WJ, LaRusso NF. Ulcerative colitis disease activity following treatment of associated primary sclerosing cholangitis with cyclosporin. Gut 1993;34:242–6.
153. Van Thiel DH, Carroll P, Abu-Elmagd K, et al. Tacrolimus (FK 506), a treatment for primary sclerosing cholangitis: results of an open-label preliminary trial. Am J Gastroenterol 1995;90:455–9.
154. Mitchell SA, Chapman RW. Review article: the management of primary sclerosing cholangitis. Aliment Pharmacol Ther 1997;11:33–43.
155. Bachs L, Pares A, Elena M, et al. Effects of long-term rifampicin administration in primary biliary cirrhosis. Gastroenterology 1992;102:2077–80.
156. Bachs L, Pares A, Elena M, et al. Comparison of rifampicin with phenobarbitone for treatment of pruritus in biliary cirrhosis. Lancet 1989;1:574–6.
157. Jorgensen RA, Lindor KD, Sartin JS, et al. Serum lipid and fat-soluble vitamin levels in primary sclerosing cholangitis. J Clin Gastroenterol 1995;20:215–19.
158. Hay JE, Lindor KD, Wiesner RH, et al. The metabolic bone disease of primary sclerosing cholangitis. Hepatology 1991;14:257–61.
159. Goss JA, Shackleton CR, Farmer DG, et al. Orthotopic liver transplantation for primary sclerosing cholangitis. A 12-year single center experience. Ann Surg 1997;225:472–81.
160. Narumi S, Roberts JP, Emond JC, et al. Liver transplantation for sclerosing cholangitis. Hepatology 1995;22:451–7.
161. Wiesner RH, LaRusso NF, Dozois RR, Beaver SJ. Peristomal varices after proctocolectomy in patients with primary sclerosing cholangitis. Gastroenterology 1986;90:316–22.
162. Johnson GK, Geenen JE, Venu RP, Hogan WJ. Endoscopic treatment of biliary duct strictures in sclerosing cholangitis: follow-up assessment of a new therapeutic approach. Gastrointest Endosc 1987;33:9–12.
163. Cotton PB, Nickl N. Endoscopic and radiologic approaches to therapy in primary sclerosing cholangitis. Semin Liver Dis 1991;11:40–8.
164. Johnson GK, Geenen JE, Venu RP, et al. Endoscopic treatment of biliary tract strictures in sclerosing cholangitis: a larger series and recommendations for treatment. Gastrointest Endosc 1991;37:38–43.
165. Gaing AA, Geders JM, Cohen SA, Siegel JH. Endoscopic management of primary sclerosing cholangitis: review, and report of an open series. Am J Gastroenterol 1993;88:2000–8.
166. Johnson GK, Beblawi I, Geenen JE, et al. Endoscopic treatment of patients with primary sclerosing cholangitis may improve survival: a long term follow up (abstract). Gastroenterology 1998;114:A544.
167. Wagner S, Gebel M, Meier P, et al. Endoscopic management of biliary tract strictures in primary sclerosing cholangitis. Endoscopy 1996;28:546–51.
168. Rosen CB, Nagorney DM. Cholangiocarcinoma complicating primary sclerosing cholangitis. Semin Liver Dis 1991;11:26–30.
169. Rosen CB, Nagorney DM, Wiesner RH, et al. Cholangiocarcinoma complicating primary sclerosing cholangitis. Ann Surg 1991;213:21–5.
170. Fausa O, Schrumpf E. Cholangiocarcinoma occurs with high frequency in primary sclerosing cholangitis (abstract). Scand J Gastroenterol 1989;24:59A.
171. van Leeuwen DJ, Reeders JW. Primary sclerosing cholangitis and cholangiocarcinoma as a diagnostic and therapeutic dilemma. Ann Oncol 1999;10(suppl 4):89–93.
172. Campbell WL, Ferris JV, Holbert BL, et al. Biliary tract carcinoma complicating primary sclerosing cholangitis: evaluation with CT, cholangiography, US, and MR imaging. Radiology 1998;207:41–50.
173. Nakeeb A, Lipsett PA, Lillemoe KD, et al. Biliary carcinoembryonic antigen levels are a marker for cholangiocarcinoma. Am J Surg 1996;171:147–52.
174. Ponsioen CY, Vrouenraets SM, van Milligen de Wit AW, et al. Value of brush cytology for dominant strictures in primary sclerosing cholangitis. Endoscopy 1999;31:305–9.
175. Keiding S, Hansen SB, Rasmussen HH, et al. Detection of cholangiocarcinoma in primary sclerosing cholangitis by positron emission tomography. Hepatology 1998;28:700–6. See comments.
176. Miros M, Kerlin P, Walker N, et al. Predicting cholangiocarcinoma in patients with primary sclerosing cholangitis before transplantation. Gut 1991;32:1369–73.
177. Nesbit GM, Johnson CD, James EM, et al. Cholangiocarcinoma: diagnosis and evaluation of resectability by CT and sonography as procedures complementary to cholangiography. AJR Am J Roentgenol 1988;151:933–8.
178. Ramage JK, Donaghy A, Farrant JM, et al. Serum tumor markers for the diagnosis of cholangiocarcinoma in primary sclerosing cholangitis. Gastroenterology 1995;108:865–9.
179. Lee JG, Leung JW, Baillie J, et al. Benign, dysplastic or malignant—making sense of endoscopic bile duct brush cytology: results in 149 consecutive patients. Am J Gastroenterol 1995;90:722–6.
180. Nichols JC, Gores GJ, LaRusso NF, et al. Diagnostic role of serum CA 19-9

for cholangiocarcinoma in patients with primary sclerosing cholangitis. Mayo Clin Proc 1993;68:874–9.
181. Fisher A, Theise ND, Min A, et al. CA19-9 does not predict cholangiocarcinoma in patients with primary sclerosing cholangitis undergoing liver transplantation. Liver Transpl Surg 1995;1:94–8.
182. Angulo P, Lindor KD. Primary sclerosing cholangitis. Hepatology 1999;30:325–32.
183. Langnas AN, Grazi GL, Stratta RJ, et al. Primary sclerosing cholangitis: the emerging role for liver transplantation. Am J Gastroenterol 1990;85:1136–41.
184. McEntee G, Wiesner RH, Rosen C, et al. A comparative study of patients undergoing liver transplantation for primary sclerosing cholangitis and primary biliary cirrhosis. Transplant Proc 1991;23:1563–4.
185. Higashi H, Yanaga K, Marsh JW, et al. Development of colon cancer after liver transplantation for primary sclerosing cholangitis associated with ulcerative colitis. Hepatology 1990;11:477–80.
186. Marchesa P, Lashner BA, Lavery IC, et al. The risk of cancer and dysplasia among ulcerative colitis patients with primary sclerosing cholangitis. Am J Gastroenterol 1997;92:1285–8.
187. Bleday R, Lee E, Jessurun J, et al. Increased risk of early colorectal neoplasms after hepatic transplant in patients with inflammatory bowel disease. Dis Colon Rectum 1993;36:908–12.
188. D'Haens GR, Lashner BA, Hanauer SB. Pericholangitis and sclerosing cholangitis are risk factors for dysplasia and cancer in ulcerative colitis. Am J Gastroenterol 1993;88:1174–8.
189. Fabia R, Levy MF, Testa G, et al. Colon carcinoma in patients undergoing liver transplantation. Am J Surg 1998;176:265–9.
190. Gurbuz AK, Giardiello FM, Bayless TM. Colorectal neoplasia in patients with ulcerative colitis and primary sclerosing cholangitis. Dis Colon Rectum 1995;38:37–41.
191. Loftus EVJ, Aguilar HI, Sandborn WJ, et al. Risk of colorectal neoplasia in patients with primary sclerosing cholangitis and ulcerative colitis following orthotopic liver transplantation. Hepatology 1998;27:685–90.
192. Feller RB, Waugh RC, Selby WS, et al. Biliary strictures after liver transplantation: clinical picture, correlates and outcomes. J Gastroenterol Hepatol 1996;11:21–5.
193. Boyer TD. Does primary sclerosing cholangitis recur after liver transplantation? No! Liver Transpl Surg 1997;3:S24–5.
194. Graziadei IW, Wiesner RH, Batts KP, et al. Recurrence of primary sclerosing cholangitis following liver transplantation. Hepatology 1999;29:1050–6.
195. Sebagh M, Farges O, Kalil A, et al. Sclerosing cholangitis following human orthotopic liver transplantation. Am J Surg Pathol 1995;19:81–90.
196. Lo SK, Hermann R, Chapman RW, et al. Ursodeoxycholic acid in primary sclerosing cholangitis: a double-blind placebo controlled trial (abstract). Hepatology 1992;16:92A.
197. Van Thiel DH, Wright HI, Gravaler JS. Ursodeoxycholic acid therapy for primary sclerosing cholangitis: preliminary report of a randomized controlled trial (abstract). Hepatology 1992;16:62A.
198. Bansi D, Chrisitie J, Fleming K, Chapman R. High-dose ursodeoxycholic acid in primary sclerosing cholangitis: a randomized double-blind placebo-controlled trial (abstract). Gastroenterology 1996;110(suppl 4):A1146.
199. van Milligen de Wit AW, van Bracht J, Rauws EA, et al. Endoscopic stent therapy for dominant extrahepatic bile duct strictures in primary sclerosing cholangitis. Gastrointest Endosc 1996;44:293–9.

Chapter

20

Cholangiocarcinoma

Markus Selzner Pierre-Alain Clavien

The diagnosis and treatment of cholangiocarcinoma has been a constant challenge since its first description by Altmeier in 1957 (1). In 1965 Klatskin (2) reported the first series of patients with cholangiocarcinoma of the hepatic hilum, and introduced the concept of radical resection of the diseased bile duct. However, at this time surgery was associated with high morbidity and mortality rates. In addition, due to the lack of adequate diagnostic techniques the disease was usually diagnosed late with no options for curative treatment. Although cholangiocarcinoma is a slow-growing cancer with a tendency for late metastases, the infiltrating spread pattern and the close proximity to vital structures has prevented an attempt of curative therapy in most centers until recently. The last decade has brought new developments in radiology, gastroenterology, and surgery as well as a hope for a curative treatment in a large number of patients.

ETIOLOGY

Cholangiocarcinomas are found in 0.01% to 0.2% of all autopsies and about 4500 new cases are reported in the United States each year (3,4). It mostly affects elderly patients above 60 years with a slight male predominance, although occasionally young people present with a bile duct cancer. Different conditions, such as cholangitis, stones, and biliary stasis, have been associated with an increased frequency of cholangiocarcinomas. For example, patients with primary sclerosing cholangitis (PSC) have a 6% to 30% chance of developing a cholangiocarcinoma during their life, and between 10% and 30% of all patients undergoing liver transplantation for PSC have an occult cholangiocarcinoma at the time of transplantation. Furthermore, 2% to 25% of patients with choledochal cysts and 5% of patients with hepatolithiasis develop biliary cancer. Therefore, cholestasis should be treated when possible, for example, by resection of even asymptomatic choledochal cysts (5,6) (see Chapter 16).

CLASSIFICATION

The vast majority of cholangiocarcinomas are mucus-secreting adenocarcinomas. A detailed description of the different histologic types is presented in Chapter 2. The most common site is the confluence of the left and right main hepatic bile ducts (perihilar, 67% of cases) (7). The tumor has a tendency to spread along the bile ducts and perineural sheets. Distant metastases are rare and are found in only half of autopsies in patients who died from bile duct cancer. The tumor typically forms annular structures in the bile ducts and can ulcerate.

Different classifications have been used to describe cholangiocarcinomas. Anatomically, bile duct cancer can be divided into intrahepatic and extrahepatic diseases. The vast majority of cholangiocarcinomas (94%) are extrahepatic. The extrahepatic tumors are further divided according to their location within the extrahepatic bile duct into upper third, middle third, and lower third (7) (Fig. 20.1). However, this descriptive division does not reflect clinical prognosis and treatment options. Currently, the more frequently used classification is the Bismuth classification, which describes the extrahepatic bile duct cancer in perspective to the bile duct bifurcation, and has direct implications on the surgical strategy (8) (Fig. 20.2). Bismuth I tumors are below the hepatic bifurcation, and can be treated by bile duct resection alone. Bismuth II tumors reach the bifurcation. They require usually a caudate lobe resection. Bismuth IIIa are carcinomas, which reach the second intrahepatic division of the right main bile duct. Bismuth IIIb tumors involve the second division of the left main bile duct. Both Bismuth

IIIa and IIIb tumors require either left or right hemihepatectomy together with the bile duct resection. Finally, Bismuth IV tumors infiltrate bile ducts beyond the second bile duct division on both sides; Bismuth IV tumors are usually not amenable to surgical therapy.

Finally, the TNM (tumor/node/metastasis) staging system is often used and describes the lymph node involvement, the extent of tumor infiltration, and the presence of distant metastases. Several studies have used this classification to predict clinical outcome (see Chapter 2). According to the TNM-system, stage I tumors are limited to the muscular layer of the bile duct, whereas stage II tumors involve periductal tissues. Stage III tumors are defined by lymph node involvement, and stage IV tumors either have distant metastases or invade surrounding structures.

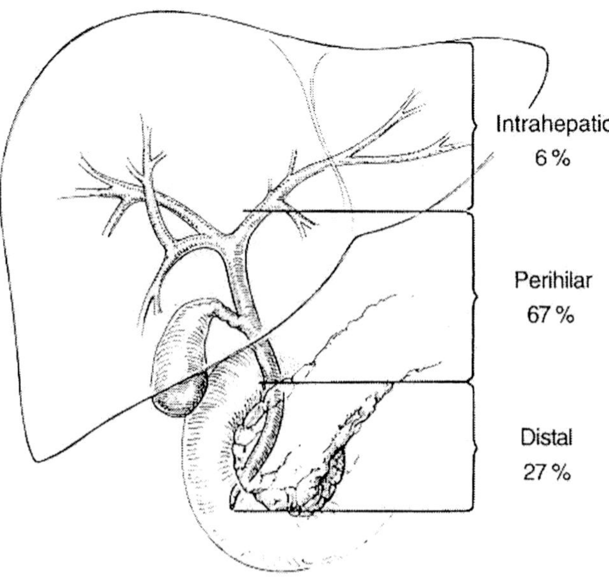

FIGURE 20.1. *Distribution of cholangiocarcinomas within the biliary tree.*

CLINICAL PRESENTATION

The key feature of cholangiocarcinomas is the development of a biliary obstruction with cholestasis. The patients present with jaundice, together with pale stool, dark urine, and pruritus. Unspecific symptoms such as malaise, anorexia, weight loss, and unexplained fever can accompany or precede the development of jaundice. Caution is necessary as cholangiocarcinomas occasionally coexist with gallstone disease, which might be falsely accepted as the cause of obstruction. On the other hand, cholangiocarcinomas proximal to the bifurcation or intrahepatic carcinomas will not cause jaundice, as only 10% to 20% of unobstructed functioning liver tissue is sufficient to effectively eliminate the bilirubin. Alkaline phosphatase is a sensitive marker of early bile duct obstruction, and cholangiocarcinoma should be considered in the differential diagnosis when patients present with an isolated elevation of the alkaline phosphatase.

Biliary obstruction can result in important secondary problems. First, patients with cholestasis are predisposed for the development of cholangitis. Bile culture in patients with biliary obstruction has revealed bacterial contamination in 32% of the patients. *Klebsiella* spp, *Escherichia coli*, and *Streptococcus faecalis* are the most frequent organisms (4). Effective drainage of the biliary tree and antibiotic coverage when any manipulation of the bile duct is performed is critical. A second common problem is dehydration and malnutrition in patients who have severe cholestasis due to nausea, vomiting, and general malaise. Adequate rehydration and nutritional support is important to avoid severe postoperative complications.

DIAGNOSIS

The radiologic evaluation of the biliary tree has dramatically improved over the last decade, as discussed in more detail in Chapters 3 and 5. The first step is an abdominal ultrasound. The dilatation of the bile ducts is easily visualized, and the localization of the biliary stenosis can be determined. At the

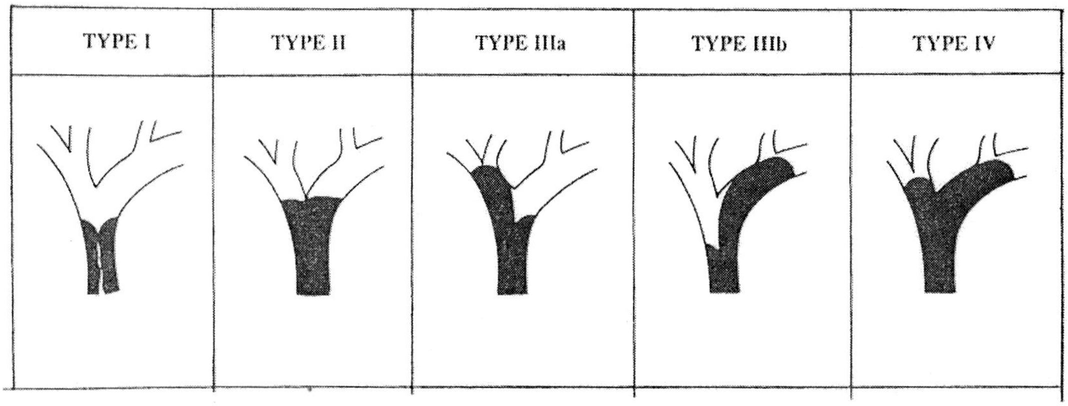

TYPE I | TYPE II | TYPE IIIa | TYPE IIIb | TYPE IV

FIGURE 20.2. *Bismuth classification of cholangiocarcinoma.*

same time, the patency of the main hepatic artery and portal vein and their branches can be evaluated by Doppler ultrasound. Then, a multiphasic helical computed tomography (CT) should be performed to further evaluate local invasion of the tumor and possible distant metastasis. If the tumor is located at the bifurcation or above and is associated with an elevated bilirubin, a percutaneous transhepatic cholangiography (PTC) with the placement of drains in both sides of the biliary tree should be performed to visualize the upper limit of the biliary stricture, relieving the cholestasis and providing critical information for evaluating the tumor's respectability. If the cholangiocarcinoma is located in the middle or lower bile duct, an endoscopic retrograde cholangiography (ERCP) is preferable. Tumor specimens can be obtained either by endoscopic brushing or by CT or ultrasound guided needle biopsy. An angiography is usually not performed, and should be restricted to situations in which vascular involvement remains unclear on other less invasive tests (see Chapters 3 and 5). Magnetic resonance cholangiography (MRC) is a new technique that provides noninvasive visualization of the bile ducts. Although the role of MRC in comparison to PTC or ERCP remains to be established, it has a significant advantage in children or when the other diagnostic modality cannot be performed. With future developments, this technique is likely to rapidly become a routine diagnostic test. In a recent report (9), positron-emission tomography (PET) scanning was recommended as a diagnostic tool for the detection of cholangiocarcinomas, in particular in the setting of primary sclerosing cholangitis. However, while we have had excellent results with the PET scan for the diagnosis of metastatic colon cancer to the liver, our experience for cholangiocarcinomas has been associated with a high frequency of false-positive and false-negative findings. Currently, we do not perform PET scans for the evaluation of bile duct cancer. Finally, an intraoperative ultrasound is routinely performed at the time of surgery to determine the extent of intrahepatic tumor growth.

TREATMENT

Resection

The natural history of patients with cholangiocarcinoma is dismal, and 5-year survival is exceptional (10). The only therapeutic option offering a chance of cure is resection. Preoperative considerations and patient selection are discussed in Chapter 8. Several prognostic factors have been described in univariate analysis for patient survival after resection of cholangiocarcinomas. The most common include resection margin, lymph node status, vascular involvement, tumor size, and histologic type (7,11–14). However, in multivariate analysis only tumor-free margins, the absence of positive secondary lymph nodes, and no distant metastasis are consistently associated with significant survival benefits. The importance of local lymph node infiltration remains controversial. Different groups have reported no survival difference in patients with or without tumor infiltration of the local lymph nodes after curative resection (15,16).

Intrahepatic cholangiocarcinomas represent 15% to 20% of all primary liver tumors and about 6% of all cholangiocarcinomas (6). Obstructive jaundice only occurs late in the disease process, and therefore most patients are diagnosed with advanced disease. Only 15% to 50% of the patients are resectable at the time of diagnosis (5,7,12,17). Liver resection, usually anatomic hemihepatectomy or extended hemihepatectomy, is necessary to achieve tumor negative margins. Liver resection for cholangiocarcinoma is associated with an operative mortality of 2% to 3% in specialized centers (6). Complete tumor resection with negative margins is associated with 1-, 3-, and 5-year survival rates of 50% to 70%, 30% to 40%, and 10% to 30%, respectively (5,7,18). If curative resection cannot be achieved, patient survival beyond 2 years is exceptional (5,7,11).

Extrahepatic cholangiocarcinomas represent about 94% of all bile duct cancers. Typically, the patients present with obstructive jaundice early in the course of the disease. However, the infiltrative growth pattern and the close proximity to the portal vein and the hepatic artery results in a low respectability rate ranging between 20% and 40% (3,4). The tumor is considered nonresectable in presence of massive involvement of the main portal vein or the hepatic artery, involvement of the hepatic artery or the portal vein in both hemilivers, involvement of the main hepatic duct on one side and the main hepatic artery or the portal vein branch on the contralateral side, or intrahepatic metastases present on both sides of the liver.

Curative resection is the strongest predictor of outcome, and it can be performed in experienced centers with a mortality of less than 5% (7,8,19). In recent reports the mortality rates have been no different in patients with local bile duct resection versus combined bile duct and liver resection (7,15). Curative resection either as local bile duct resection or combined with liver resection results in 3- and 5-year survivals between 40% and 50% and between 20% and 40%, respectively (14,20–22) (Table 20.1) (7,8,11, 14–16,19,21,23–32). Resection with tumor positive margins (R1) is associated with 3- and 5-year survivals of 18% and 9%, respectively (21,23,24), while the median survival after explorative laparotomy is only 6 months (23,27,33) (see Table 20.1).

If the tumor is at the bile duct bifurcation or above, bile duct resection should be combined with a liver resection to achieve clear margins (see Chapter 8). Caudate lobe infiltration has been documented between 30% and 95% of patients with tumors at the bifurcation or above (20,26,34). Therefore, for tumors at the level of the bifurcation or above the caudate lobe should be resected. A significantly improved 5-year survival was reported by Sugiura et al. (16) in patients treated with caudate lobe resection when compared to patients treated with bile duct resection alone (46% vs 12%). If the tumor is proximal to the bifurcation, a left

Table 20.1. Results of curative resection for hilar cholangiocarcinoma in series of the last decade

Reference	Number of Patients	Mortality (%)	Survival			
			3 Years	5 Years	10 Years	Median (months)
Tsuzuki (23)	25	4	NA	31%	NA	NA
Teleky (24)	21	10	52%	NA	NA	34
Baer (25)	21	4	NA	NA	NA	36
Bismuth (8)	23	0	25%	NA	NA	26
Tashiro (26)	34	8	60%	30%	NA	NA
Sugiura (16)	83	8, 4	NA	33%	NA	NA
Washburn (27)	59	10	NA	NA	NA	23
Su (11)	49	10	NA	15%	NA	14
Nakeeb (7)	109	4	NA	17%	NA	20
Klempnauer (19)	151	10	NA	28%	16%	NA
Harrison (28)	32	3	NA	42%	NA	59
McMasters (29)	40	0	NA	NA	NA	22
Nagino (30)	138	10	43%	26%	12%	NA
Launois (31)	40	13	46%	27%	NA	NA
Gulik (15)	10	0	NA	NA	NA	17
Neuhaus (21)	80	8	NA	37%	NA	NA
Kosuge (14)	65	6	NA	52%	26%	NA
Miyazaki (32)	93	10	NA	26%	NA	NA
Total	1073	6	45%	30%	18%	28

Abbreviations: NA = not available.

or right hemihepatectomy should be added to the local bile duct resection depending on the side of infiltration.

Tumors of the middle or distal bile duct are less common and mostly require a partial pancreaticoduodenectomy with or without partial gastrectomy (Whipple procedure) (see Chapter 8). The resectability of distal bile duct tumors ranges between 50% and 70% and is mostly limited by invasion of the portal vein or the superior mesenteric artery. Partial pancreaticoduodenectomy can be performed with a mortality of below 5% in specialized centers today (7,35). Curative resection of distal cholangiocarcinomas is associated with a 5-year survival between 20% and 30% (4,7).

The indications for resection of the portal vein or hepatic artery remain controversial (Chapter 8). Nimura et al. (20) reported an acceptable mortality of 8% and a 5-year survival of 41% after combined bile duct and portal vein resection for cholangiocarcinoma. However, other authors (19,31) have reported less favorable results, with a 5-year survival below 5% after extensive vascular resection. The indication for extensive surgery including resection and reconstruction of the portal vein and the hepatic artery has to be made on a case-by-case basis and depends on the patient's age and the extension of tumor growth. We recommend limited vascular resection if complete tumor clearance can be achieved in the young patient. In contrast, in case of significant comorbidities or if an extensive involvement of the portal triad is present, we do not perform extensive procedures.

Chemotherapy and Radiotherapy

Cholangiocarcinomas respond poorly to either chemotherapy or radiation therapy. The use of chemotherapy and radiotherapy alone or in combination with surgery remains controversial. Prospective randomized studies comparing various therapeutic modalities are rare, making evaluating the different strategies difficult. Chemotherapy and radiotherapy are often combined in patients with cholangiocarcinomas (see below). The different regimens are discussed in more detail in Chapters 7 and 10. Three different scenarios are possible for the use of chemoradiation: first, as a neoadjuvant treatment prior to resection; second, as an adjuvant treatment after a curative or noncurative resection; and third, as a palliative treatment.

Neoadjuvant treatment of cholangiocarcinomas has been investigated by a few groups (29,36,37). In a retrospective study (29) 9 patients who received preoperative 5-fluorouracil (5-FU) and external beam radiation were compared with 31 patients who underwent resection only. In all patients with neoadjuvant chemoradiation a curative resection (R0) was possible, whereas only 54% of the patients who underwent surgery alone were resectable. Unfortunately, patient or tumor-free survival was not investigated in this study. Urego et al. (36) reported on 61 patients receiving 5-FU and external beam for cholangiocarcinoma, 23 of them as neoadjuvant treatment prior to resection or transplantation. In a univariate analysis the only predictor of outcome was curative resection. Chemotherapy or the radiation dose did not correlate with survival.

The role of chemoradiotherapy as an adjuvant treatment after either curative or noncurative resection is still debated. In a retrospective study Pitt et al. (38) compared 23 patients receiving adjuvant external beam radiation after resection of a cholangiocarcinoma with 27 patients treated with surgery only. Again, the only predictor of outcome was curative resection. Radiotherapy had no impact on survival in patients receiving curative surgery. Others have confirmed these results and in the absence of a randomized study there are no data indicating a benefit of adjuvant treatment after an R0-resection (37,39). In contrast, a few studies have reported a benefit for adjuvant chemoradiotherapy for patients with tumor-positive margins after surgery. Verbeek (40) found in a retrospective study of 64 patients improved median survival (27 months vs 8 months) in patients treated with chemoradiation after noncurative resection. Currently, we recommend postoperative chemotherapy (5-FU) in combination with external beam radiation in the presence of positive margin after resection or lymph node involvement.

The most common indication for chemotherapy and radiotherapy of cholangiocarcinomas is palliative treatment. In a prospective randomized study Glimelius et al. (41) compared a group of patients receiving leucovorin and 5-FU with patients receiving supportive care only. Although there was no difference in patient survival, the investigators reported better quality of life in the group receiving palliative chemotherapy. Similarly, radiotherapy can improve bile drainage in patients with nonresectable cholangiocarcinoma. Two studies reported a reduction of jaundice with radiotherapy when compared to supportive care alone. However, palliative radiation did not result in prolonged survival in both series. The indication for palliative chemotherapy and radiotherapy has to be discussed with each patient. Although it is unlikely to prolong survival, selected patients might have an improvement of quality of life from palliative treatment.

Liver Transplantation

Liver transplantation was originally thought to be the ideal treatment for primary liver tumors, offering complete tumor removal. However, the results of liver transplantation for cholangiocarcinoma have been disappointing, with a 5-year survival of only 17% and a median survival of only 15 months (42). However, a recent report suggested encouraging results by the use of a multimodality approach with innovative neoadjuvant radiation therapy and liver transplantation in a selected group of patients with cholangiocarcinoma (Gores, personal communication). However, the long-term outcome of this group of patients remains to be determined. Thus, while cholangiocarcinoma is a contraindication for liver transplantation in most centers, neoadjuvant strategies and better diagnostic techniques may lead to new therapeutic approaches in the near future. However, it is widely accepted that patients with an occult intrahepatic cholangiocarcinoma, which is found incidentally during transplantation, have a similar outcome when compared to patients without malignancies (42).

Palliative Treatment

The treatment of obstructive jaundice is the main focus in patients with unresectable cholangiocarcinoma. Different surgical strategies exist, such as surgical bypass, operative intubation, and endoscopic or percutaneous drainage. Controlled studies comparing the different procedures are not available. The choice of each therapeutic approach depends on the extensiveness of the disease and the patient's condition. Various surgical drainage procedures are discussed in Chapter 8.

Surgical bypass is an attractive strategy in patients whose tumors are found to be unresectable during exploration. A hepaticojejunostomy results in a temporary relief of jaundice in 90% of the patients (33), whereas intrahepatic bypass procedures are less successful. A surgical bypass procedure should be performed only by an experienced surgeon. However, extensive surgery should be avoided because even palliative bypass procedures are associated with a mortality rate of 9%.

Advances in endoscopic and percutaneous techniques during the last decade offer new and safer access to the biliary tree. Stents can be inserted in 90% of the patients with obstructive jaundice. Cholangitis, the most frequent complication after stent placement, occurs in 7% of the cases and is associated with a 30-day mortality of 10% (43). The various techniques of biliary drainage are often combined with palliative chemotherapy or radiation. As mentioned above, at this point there are no data indicating prolonged survival by palliative chemoradiation. However, the patency of the biliary drainage might be prolonged and some authors have reported improved quality of life for patients via palliative chemotherapy and radiotherapy.

SUGGESTED READINGS

Blumgart LH, Benjamin IS. Cancer of the bile ducts. In: Blumgart LH, ed. Surgery of the liver and the biliary tree, 1st ed. Edinburgh: Churchill Livingstone, 1988:967–95. This chapter gives an extensive overview of various etiologies, the natural history and the treatment options for cholangiocarcinoma.

Broelsch CE. Atlas of liver surgery. New York: Churchill Livingston, 1993. This atlas very nicely illustrates the different steps of bile duct and liver resection for cholangiocarcinoma. Excellent drawings are used.

Nakeeb A, Pitt HA, Sohn TA, et al. Cholangiocarcinoma: a spectrum of intrahepatic, perihilar, and distal tumors. Ann Surg 1995;224:463–75. The authors reviewed their extensive experience with the surgical treatment of cholangiocarcinoma. Prognosis, treatment options, and outcome for different tumor localizations were carefully analyzed.

REFERENCES

1. Altmeier W, Gall E, Zinninger M, Hoxworth P. Sclerosing carcinoma of the major intrahepatic (hilar) bile ducts. Arch Surg 1957;75:450–61.
2. Klatskin G. Adenocarcinoma of the hepatic bifurcation within the porta hepatis. Am J Med 1965;38:241–56.

3. Kuvshinoff B, Fong Y, LH. B. Proximal bile duct tumors. Surg Oncol Clin North Am 1996;5:317–31.
4. Blumgart L. Cancer of the bile ducts. In: Blumgart L, ed. Surgery of the liver and biliary tract. New York: Churchill Livingston, 1994;2:829–53.
5. Ahrendt S, Cameron JL, Pitt HA. Current management of patients with perihilar cholangiocarcinoma. Adv Surg 1997;30:427–52.
6. Selzner M, Clavien PA. Resection of liver tumors: special emphasis on neoadjuvant and adjuvant therapy. In: Clavien PA, ed. Malignant liver tumors: current and emerging therapies. Malden, MA: Blackwell Science, 1999:137–49.
7. Nakeeb A, Pitt HA, Sohn TA, et al. Cholangiocarcinoma. Ann Surg 1996;224:463–75.
8. Bismuth H, Nakache R, Diamond T. Management strategies in resection for hilar cholangiocarcinoma. Ann Surg 1992;215:31–8.
9. Keiding S, Hansen S, Rasmussen H, et al. Detection of cholangiocarcinoma in primary sclerosing cholangitis by positron emission tomography. Hepatology 1998;28:700–6.
10. Farley DR, Weaver AL, Nagorney DM. Natural history of unresected cholangiocarcinoma: patient outcome after noncurative resection. Mayo Clin Proc 1995;70:425–9.
11. Su CH, Tsay SH, Wu CC, et al. Factors influencing postoperative morbidity, mortality, and survival after resection for hilar cholangiocarcinoma. Ann Surg 1996;223:384–94.
12. Klempnauer J, Ridder GJ, Werner M, et al. What constitutes long term survival after surgery for hilar cholangiocarcinoma? Cancer 1997;79:26–34.
13. Kayahara M, Nagakawa T, Tsukioka Y, et al. Neural invasion and nodal involvement in distal bile duct cancer. Hepatogastroenterology 1994;41:190–4.
14. Kosuge T, Yamamoto J, Shimada K, et al. Improved surgical results for hilar cholangiocarcinoma with procedures including major hepatic resection. Ann Surg 1999;230:663–71.
15. Gulik T, Gerhards M, Vries J, et al. Local resection of biliopancreatic cancer. 1999:243–6.
16. Sugiura Y, Nakamura S, Iida S, et al. Extensive resection of the bile ducts combined with liver resection for cancer of the main hepatic duct junction: a cooperative study of the Keio Bile Duct Cancer Study Group. Surgery 1994;115:445–51.
17. Cherqui D, Tantawi B, Alon R, et al. Intrahepatic cholangiocarcinoma. Arch Surg 1995;130:1073–8.
18. Cameron JL, Pitt HA, Zinner MJ, et al. Management of proximal cholangiocarcinomas by surgical resection and radiotherapy. Am J Surg 1990;159:91–8.
19. Klempnauer J, Ridder G, Wasielewski R, et al. Resectional surgery of hilar cholangiocarcinoma: A multivariate analysis of prognostic factors. J Clin Oncol 1997;15:947–54.
20. Nimura Y, Hayakawa N, Kamiya J, et al. Hepatic segmentectomy with caudate lobe resection for bile duct carcinoma of the hepatic hilus. World J Surg 1990;14:535–44.
21. Neuhaus P, Jonas S, Bechstein W, et al. Extended resection for hilar cholangiocarcinoma. Ann Surg 1999;230:808–19.
22. Pinson W, Rossi R. Extended right hepatic lobectomy, left hepatic lobectomy, and skeletonization resection for proximal bile duct cancer. World J Surg 1988;12:52–9.
23. Tsuzuki T, Ueda M, Kuramochi S, et al. Carcinoma of the main hepatic junction: Indications, operative morbidity and mortality, and long-term survival. Surgery 1990;108:495–501.
24. Teleky B, Funovics J, Herbst F, Fritsch A. Chirurgische Therapie des proximalen Gallengangskarzinoms. Langenbecks Arch Chir 1991;376:286–90.
25. Baer H, Stain S, Dennison A, et al. Improvements in survival by aggressive resections of hilar cholangiocarcinomas. 1992:20–7.
26. Tashiro S, Tsuji T, Kanemitsu K, et al. Prolongation of survival for carcinoma at the hepatic duct confluence. Surgery 1993;113:270–8.
27. Washburn W, Lewis W, Jenkins R. Aggressive surgical resection for cholangiocarcinoma. Arch Surg 1995;130:270–6.
28. Harrison LE, Brennan MF, Newman E, et al. Hepatic resection for noncolorectal, nonneuroendocrine metastases: a fifteen-year experience with ninety-six patients. Surgery 1997;121:625–32.
29. McMasters K, Tuttle T, Leach S, et al. Neoadjuvant chemoradiation for extrahepatic cholangiocarcinoma. Am J Surg 1997;174:605–9.
30. Nagino M, Nimura Y, Kamiya J, et al. Segmental liver resection for hilar cholangiocarcinoma. Hepatogastroenterology 1998;45:7–13.
31. Launois B, Terblanche J, Lakehal M, et al. Proximal bile duct cancer: high resectability rate and 5-tear survival. Ann Surg 1999;230:266–75.
32. Miyazaki M, Ito H, Nakagawa K, et al. Parenchyma-presercing hepatectomy in the surgical treatment of hilar cholangiocarcinoma. J Am Coll Surg 1999;189:575–83.
33. Schlitt H, Weimann A, Klempnauer J, et al. Perihilar hepaticojejunostomy as palliative treatment for irresectable malignant tumors of the liver hilum. Ann Surg 1999;229:181–6.
34. Mizumoto R, Kawarada Y, Suzuki H. Surgical treatment of hilar carcinoma of the bile duct. Surg Gynecol Obstet 1986;162:153–8.
35. Nakayama F, Miyazaki K, Naggafuchi K. Radical surgery for middle and distal thirds bile duct cancer. World J Surg 1988;12:60–3.
36. Urego M, Flickinger J, Carr B. Radiotherapy and multimodality management of cholangiocarcinoma. Int J Rad Oncol Biol Phys 1999;44:121–6.
37. Gonzales D, Gouma D, Rauws E, et al. Role of radiotherapy, in particular intraluminal brachytherapy, in the treatment or proximal bile duct carcinoma. Ann Oncol 1999;10:S215–20.
38. Pitt H, Nakeeb A, Abrams R, et al. Perihilar cholangiocarcinoma: Postoperative radiotherapy does not improve survival. Ann Surg 1995;221:788–98.
39. Shiina T, Mikuriya S, Uno T, et al. Radiotherapy of cholangiocarcinoma: the roles for primary and adjuvant therapies. Cancer Chemother Pharmacol 1992;31:S115–18.
40. Verbeek P, Leeuwen D, Heyde M, Gonzales D. Does additive radiotherapy after hilar resection improve survival of cholangiocarcinoma? Ann Chir 1990;45:350–4.
41. Glimelius B, Hoffman K, Sjoden P, et al. Chemotherapy improves survival and quality of life in advanced pancreatic and biliary cancer. Ann Oncol 1996;7:593–600.
42. Pichlmayr R, Lamesch P, Weimann A, et al. Surgical treatment of cholangiocellular carcinoma. World J Surg 1995;19:83–8.
43. Polydorou A, Cairns S, Dowsett J. Palliation of proximal malignant biliary obstruction by endoscopic endoprosthesis insertion. Gut 1991;32: 685–9.

Section 3.3

Diseases of the Small Bile Ducts

Chapter

21

Primary Biliary Cirrhosis and Other Diseases of the Small Bile Ducts

E. Jenny Heathcote

DISEASE OF THE SMALL BILE DUCTS

Primary Biliary Cirrhosis

Primary biliary cirrhosis was first reported by Addison and Gull in 1851 when they described six patients with jaundice, vitiligo, and xanthoma (1), but the term "primary biliary cirrhosis" (PBC) was first introduced into the literature in 1950 by Ahrens (2). It was he who suggested that the primary organ affected was the liver. The histopathologic features of PBC were first clearly described by Scheuer in 1967 (3). The pathological hallmark of PBC is inflammatory destruction of the interlobular bile ducts (sometimes granulomatous) with progressive bile duct loss, fibrosis, and eventual cirrhosis. Also in the 1960s Doniach (4) and her colleagues described serum antibodies to mitochondria (AMA) which were non–species-specific but nevertheless relatively specific for humans with PBC. Mitochondrial antibodies have stood the test of time and remain the hallmark of this disease. The histologic findings of primary biliary cirrhosis may be found in patients who have no symptoms and even normal liver biochemistry, but who test positive for AMA (5). Data indicate that inappropriate presentation of nucleotide sequences common to the enzymes of the inner membrane of mitochondria are expressed on the apical membrane of biliary epithelial cells (BEC) (6). It is possible that these enzymes, or part thereof, may be the antigen that initiates a destructive immune response. Recently an animal model for PBC has been described but has not yet been confirmed by others (7).

Acquired Vanishing Bile Duct Syndromes

The first well-recognized case of drug-induced jaundice causing progressive disease and eventual cirrhosis was reported many years ago, and since then there have been numerous subsequent case reports, particularly disease attributed to chlorpromazine (8). A wide range of medications cause a cholestatic hepatitis that upon resolution may be followed by silent progressive small bile duct injury. The term "disappearing ducts" or the "vanishing bile duct syndromes" (VBDS) was not adopted until relatively recently (9). There is a wide spectrum of causes of VBDS, the most common of these are immune (e.g., PBC as described above), although vascular injury, malignancies, and infections as well as drug reactions may also cause progressive loss of the intrahepatic, interlobular bile ducts. In some instances no identifiable cause can be found, thus they are called "idiopathic" (10).

Congenital Diseases Involving the Intrahepatic Bile Ducts

There are children who are found to have abnormalities of liver biochemistry, with or without jaundice, who do not have a history compatible with neonatal hepatitis and do not have biliary atresia. Some evidence of intra-uterine or perinatal viral infection may be found in some (11). It was Alagille (12) who described a syndrome which he called arterio hepatic dysplasia. The children described by Alagille typically had reduced numbers of intrahepatic bile ducts. There are congenital causes of cholestasis that present with much more rapidly progressive intrahepatic bile duct injury, liver failure, and death (13). Now several forms of progressive familial intrahepatic cholestasis (types 1, 2, and 3) are recognized, defined by the specific canalicular transporter defect present (14). Cystic fibrosis, the most common genetic defect of children, frequently involves the liver. This is not surprising, as the hepatic biliary epithelial cells express the cystic fibrosis transmembrane regulator (CFTR) and hence the chloride ion channel at the level of the BEC is abnormal (15).

Since the introduction of regular screening of liver biochemistry in healthy people, clinically silent cholestasis is detected much more frequently than it was several decades ago. With the advent of ultrasonography, then endoscopic retrograde cholangiopancreatography (ERCP), and now magnetic resonance cholangiography (MRC), it has become much easier to determine whether the cholestatic patient has extrahepatic or intrahepatic biliary disease. The purpose of this chapter is to provide a comprehensive review of only those liver diseases that affect the intrahepatic biliary system.

PRIMARY BILIARY CIRRHOSIS

Clinical Presentation

As is the case with all diseases limited to the intrahepatic bile ducts, it is most unusual for jaundice to be the first manifestation of primary biliary cirrhosis, unless patients present very late in the course of their illness (Table 21.1).

Primary biliary cirrhosis predominantly affects women at a ratio of 9:1. The rather subjective symptom of *fatigue* is a common presenting complaint and may be the only clinical feature of someone affected by PBC (16). This fatigue appears to be central in origin in that it is not worsened or brought on by physical exercise, neither is it relieved by rest. Fatigue is a symptom that is common to patients with many forms of liver disease and to most chronic diseases in general. There is no correlation between the degree of fatigue and age, or the duration or severity of liver disease, so it appears to be an extrahepatic manifestation of PBC (17).

Chronic cholestasis, especially with pruritus, causes a progressive increase in skin *pigmentation*. Patients with cholestasis from any cause may report *pruritus*. But neither fatigue nor pruritus is universally present in subjects diagnosed with PBC. The cause of pruritus related to cholestasis remains unknown. This symptom tends to diminish with the progression of the disease. Evidence suggests that bile contains the pruritogen because biliary diversion or use of the anion exchange resin cholestyramine, which binds bile in the gut, effectively ameliorates this symptom. Repeated plasmapheresis will also reduce the symptom of pruritus. As pruritus generally occurs prior to the development of jaundice, patients with PBC may present to a dermatologist or even a psychiatrist before it is realized that their problem is hepatic in origin.

Table 21.1. Complications of primary biliary cirrhosis

Increased skin pigmentation/xanthoma
Variceal hemorrhage
Osteoporosis
Hepatocellular carcinoma
Hepatic decompensation
Associated autoimmune diseases

It is quite common for persons with underlying PBC to present initially with symptoms of another *autoimmune disease*, such as Sjögren's syndrome, rheumatoid arthritis, scleroderma, Raynaud's syndrome, or full-blown CREST (calcinosis, Raynaud's phenomenon, esophageal dysmotility, sclerodactyly, and telangiectasia) syndrome (18). A history of hypothyroidism is present in up to 25% of patients with PBC, and celiac disease is present in 6%. Other quite rare associated manifestations include vitiligo, glomerulonephritis, and granulomatous pneumonitis. There is an association between PBC and sarcoidosis, but only the latter affects the skin and the bones (19).

The primary pathogenesis of PBC is in the portal triads of the liver. There is often a great deal of inflammation present, which may damage the portal venous radicals and cause them to become obliterated. Thus, a noncirrhotic portal hypertension develops that leads to the development of esophageal varices. For this reason, initial presentation with variceal hemorrhage is reported in early PBC and may not be associated with other signs of hepatic decompensation, especially if there is no cirrhosis present (20).

Now that bone mineral density tests can detect osteopenia/osteoporosis well before symptoms from fractures occur, it is recognized that one-third of patients with PBC are osteoporotic; in 11% of these patients, the condition is severe. Although osteoporosis is often worse after menopause, it may be present before that point (21). The cause is unknown; vitamin D metabolism is normal and absorption of calcium and other fat-soluble vitamins is only minimally altered. The pathology is a combination of a decrease in the deposition of new bone and an increase in resorption.

As the liver manufactures cholesterol and its major excretory route is the biliary tract, elevated levels of serum cholesterol are common in patients with cholestasis of any origin, and skin xanthoma may be present.

Patients with PBC are at an increased risk of developing hepatocellular carcinoma once cirrhosis is present (22).

As many individuals with PBC are asymptomatic when they are first diagnosed, abnormalities in the serum biochemistry may be all that are initially identified during a routine check-up. The biochemical abnormalities common to all forms of cholestasis are an elevation in serum alkaline phosphatase, gamma glutamyltransferase (GGT), and five prime nucleotidase (5′NT) levels with or without elevation in conjugated bilirubin. Whereas an isolated elevation in serum alkaline phosphatase does not necessarily indicate a hepatic disorder, the presence of an elevated GGT value in the absence of the use of enzyme inducers (such as alcohol or drugs) indicates a hepatic source for the enzyme changes.

PBC Diagnosis

The finding of PBC is based on a composite of the history and physical findings, a liver biochemical profile that indicates cholestasis (generally anicteric), and a positive antimitochondrial antibody test in serum (Table 21.2). Approximately 95% of patients with PBC test positive for AMA (23). This antibody is very rarely found in association with any other disease. The exception is autoimmune hepatitis, in which approximately 2% to 3% of patients may test positive for AMA. The usual technique used to detect AMA is via immunofluorescent staining of rat stomach and kidney tissue. False-positive results are occasionally seen in patients who really have type 2 autoimmune hepatitis; they will test positive for antibody to kidney microsomes, which may be misread as mitochondria. Rarely, in other unrelated disorders a false-positive AMA may be seen in patients with anticardiolipin antibodies. A more specific enzyme-linked immunosorbent assay (ELISA) test for AMA can now be used because the substrates for AMA (inner mitochondrial enzymes of the 7 oxoacid dehydrogenase family) have been identified. The highly sensitive and very specific immunoblotting technique is mostly confined to research laboratories. A liver biopsy is not essential to confirm the diagnosis but is generally performed if only to determine the degree of fibrosis present. The typical bile duct lesion on histologic examination is seen in Figure 21.1.

Table 21.2. Diagnostic hallmarks of primary biliary cirrhosis

Mitochondrial antibody in serum
Elevation in serum alkaline phosphatase and gamma glutamyltransferase ± elevated conjugated bilirubin
Inflammatory destruction of interlobular bile ducts (sometimes granulomatous) on needle biopsy of the liver

Natural History of PBC

One small study has reported a 10-year follow-up of patients who underwent liver biopsy when the only abnormality was a positive AMA test in serum. This study indicated that all of the patients subsequently developed abnormal liver biochemical tests but at an unpredictable rate (24). It is likely that some patients never progress beyond the asymptomatic phase. Indeed those patients found to be AMA positive but with otherwise normal tests were older than those patients who present with symptomatic disease.

Unlike most other autoimmune diseases, PBC has not been described in children and AMA is never detected in children. Patients with PBC may present in their 20s, but most are diagnosed between the ages of 40 and 55 years. Prior to the introduction of therapy, the median survival of symptomatic patients with PBC was 8 years, median survival being 12 years or longer for those without symptoms (25). To date no markers have been identified to predict which asymptomatic patients will develop symptomatic disease (26).

There are several excellent formulas that can be used to predict the timing of the onset of liver failure once the patient has become symptomatic. As no invasive procedures are required, measurement of the serum bilirubin and/or the Mayo risk score assessment have become the two most frequently used prognostic indices (27). The components of the Mayo Risk Score include age, height of serum bilirubin, serum albumin, coagulation time, and the presence or absence of edema. It has been observed that when the score is 4 or less, esophageal varices are unlikely to be present (28). As liver transplantation is the only known cure for this disease, it is very important to be able to accurately determine when liver failure is likely to occur, at which point liver transplant becomes essential.

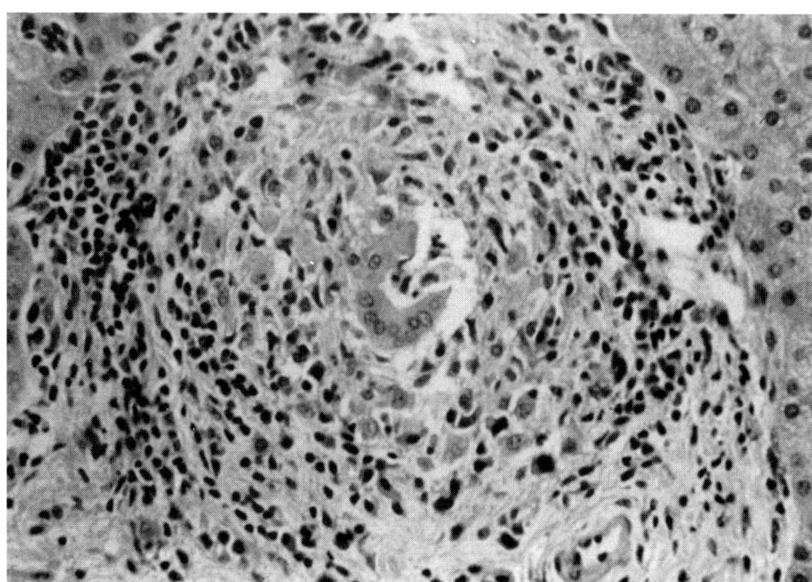

FIGURE 21.1. *Inflammatory bile duct lesion typical of PBC duct invasion by chronic inflammatory cells (lymphocytes).*

It is now recognized that PBC is not as rare as was once thought. It is unclear whether the apparent increase in the reporting of this disease is due to increased physician awareness or whether the incidence of the disease is truly increasing. It affects all racial groups but is particularly prevalent in persons of northern European extraction where the prevalence appears to be 240 to 329 per million (29).

Therapy of PBC

There are three major aspects to the therapy of PBC: treating symptoms, taking necessary preventive measures, and applying specific therapies for the disease.

Symptomatic Therapy

The symptom that most commonly affects patients with PBC is *fatigue*, present in about 70% of patients. Our lack of knowledge with regards to its causes is extremely frustrating, as this prevents us from enhancing the patient's vitality.

Pruritus is a symptom that is frequently ignored by physicians who fail to recognize it and can be extremely distressing—it may interrupt sleep, alienate the patient socially, and can become so severe as to induce suicidal ideation. The first line of treatment for pruritus due to cholestasis is oral administration of the anion exchange resin cholestyramine, which is most effective when given just prior to and after breakfast, when it presumably has the greatest chance to bind bile. Unfortunately, this resin also binds many drugs, in particular digoxin, thyroxin (8), the oral contraceptive pill, and ursodeoxycholic acid (UDCA). Thus, patients must be advised to take no medications within 4 hours of cholestyramine ingestion. The most common side effects of cholestyramine include abdominal bloating and constipation.

Rifampin (in a dose of 150 mg twice daily) completely eradicates pruritus in 50% of those affected, but is hepatotoxic in up to 15% and occasionally nephrotoxic. Patients also need to be reminded that rifampin will stain their urine and other body secretions. Rifampin also causes an unconjugated hyperbilirubinemia. Rifampin induces the cytochrome P450 system and hence may alter the metabolism of other drugs.

Opioid antagonists also appear to effect a dramatic reduction in the pruritus of cholestasis. Endogenous opioid levels in serum are high in patients with PBC and these likely exert a central effect. Treatment of pruritus with opioid antagonists is always associated with unpleasant symptoms of withdrawal; thus, the lowest tolerable dose of naltrexone should be employed initially and only tried in patients whose pruritus is resistant to cholestyramine and/or rifampin. There are many anecdotal reports of other methods whereby pruritus may be relieved; the least toxic is exposure to ultraviolet light without sunblock. On the rare occasions when a patient suffers from intractable pruritus, liver transplantation is the only cure for the symptom.

A few patients with PBC experience the development of unsightly *xanthelasma*, generally around the eyes. Occasionally these deposits of cholesterol may be found on the palms, elbows, and heels. Patients should be discouraged from undergoing plastic surgery as the xanthoma rapidly returns. These deposits tend to disappear with progression of the disease. They may be a marker of hypercholesterolemia but this is not universal. A very rare complication is a xanthomatous neuropathy, which may be temporarily relieved with plasmapheresis.

Preventive Therapy

It is not entirely clear whether the osteoporosis that accompanies PBC can in fact be prevented. As in the general population, there is a genetic component to the development of osteoporosis; but in all patients with cholestasis, advice regarding adequate nutrition is appropriate. All patients should consume calcium (1500 mg per day) and vitamin-D (1000 IU per day). A retrospective study of hormone-replacement therapy (HRT) in postmenopausal women with PBC suggests that HRT is both safe and effective in reducing osteoporosis.

There is a great deal of controversy about the use of bisphosphonates and their effectiveness in reducing the rate of osteoporosis in PBC. It is well recognized that bisphosphonates can slow the rate of osteoporosis in patients who require corticosteroid therapy and this has also been observed in PBC patients who are receiving corticosteroids (30). There are now two brief reports that suggest that etidronate is ineffective in preventing osteoporosis in PBC and that alendronate may be more effective.

Rarely PBC patients with previously silent osteoporosis may present with spontaneous fractures, generally of the vertebra. It is recommended that such patients undergo immediate liver transplantation. Although the osteoporosis may worsen during the first 6 months after the transplant, a marked improvement is seen thereafter (31). This suggests that some "toxic" factor in cholestasis may be responsible for the osteoporosis, but that factor remains unknown.

It is important in patients who have overt jaundice that they also be prescribed supplements of the other fat-soluble vitamins: vitamins A, E, and K. Since the introduction of liver transplantation to treat PBC, it is rare for patients to become deeply jaundiced, but when present it will be associated with marked steatorrhea and massive weight loss. Supplementation of the diet with medium-chain triglycerides (which are most unpalatable) may maintain the patient's weight.

As with all patients who are found to have large esophageal varices, prophylactic nonselective β blockade is recommended.

Specific Therapies for PBC

There is no medical therapy that cures PBC. Immunosuppressive drugs assessed in randomized control trials have not been shown to be effective. Such trials have tested azathioprine, cyclosporine, chlorambucil, prednisolone, and methotrexate. Three trials of the antifibrotic agent colchicine also have been conducted. In all three studies an improvement in liver function, namely albumin and coagulation profile, was observed, but in none was the sample size large enough to assess the effect of treatment on survival.

As the natural progression of PBC is relatively slow and the majority of patients now diagnosed are asymptomatic, it is necessary to study many patients for many years to give the studies sufficient power to determine whether a certain drug improves survival. To date only UDCA, a hydrophilic bile acid, has been assessed in a sufficiently large number of patients to determine whether this agent is truly effective. There have been four large studies using UDCA. Three of these trials used the same dose (13–15 mg/kg per day) and have combined their raw data on over 500 patients. A beneficial effect on survival was observed when patients were treated for up to 4 years with the trial dosage of UDCA (32), although clearly some patients respond much better than others. It has now been shown that those patients with PBC (without cirrhosis) treated with UDCA appear to have a 10-year survival, which is no different from an age and gender matched population (33). Overall the greatest effect on short-term survival was seen in those patients with more severe disease, for whom UDCA treatment delayed the need for transplantation. It would appear that treatment before transplant does not have a detrimental effect on the patients' post-transplant outcome (34), despite the patients being older when they eventually come to need a transplant.

Liver transplantation remains the only cure for PBC, and this patient group has the highest post-transplant survival of all patients who receive a liver allograft (35). Recurrence of PBC in the allograft probably does occur, but the lesion may be hard to distinguish from chronic allograft rejection (36).

OTHER DISEASES OF THE SMALL BILE DUCTS

Table 21.3 lists the causes of vanishing bile duct syndrome (VBDS).

Drug-Induced VBDS

Patients who present with a cholestatic hepatitis that causes jaundice and pruritus following ingestion of a drug (just one dose may be sufficient) are at risk of subsequent intrahepatic bile duct damage. This damage does not occur following ingestion of a drug that induces only a bland cholestasis (that is, one not associated with any inflammation, as may be seen following estrogen therapy). An increasing number of drugs have been recognized to induce long-term bile duct injury (8). This duct injury only develops after the initial jaundice fades (Fig. 21.2). In those who are progressing to intrahepatic bile duct loss, typically the levels of alkaline phosphatase and gamma-glutamyl transpeptidase, the serum markers of cholestasis, begin to climb as the serum bilirubin falls. Despite this, the patient frequently remains asymptomatic and anicteric. The prognosis is generally excellent in that only very rarely do such patients develop progressive liver failure and require liver transplantation.

Cross sensitivity may be seen between drugs such as trimethoprim sulfamethoxazole and dapsone. Patients may respond similarly to more than one medication. It may be that these patients have a unique polymorphism of the gene for one of their cytochrome P450 drug-metabolizing enzymes, and this may be responsible for the development of a "toxic" metabolite. Occasionally the patient may have been exposed to the drug on a previous occasion but no jaundice was noted although, abnormal liver tests would have been present, if the tests were performed. Worsening of the response following a second exposure suggests that

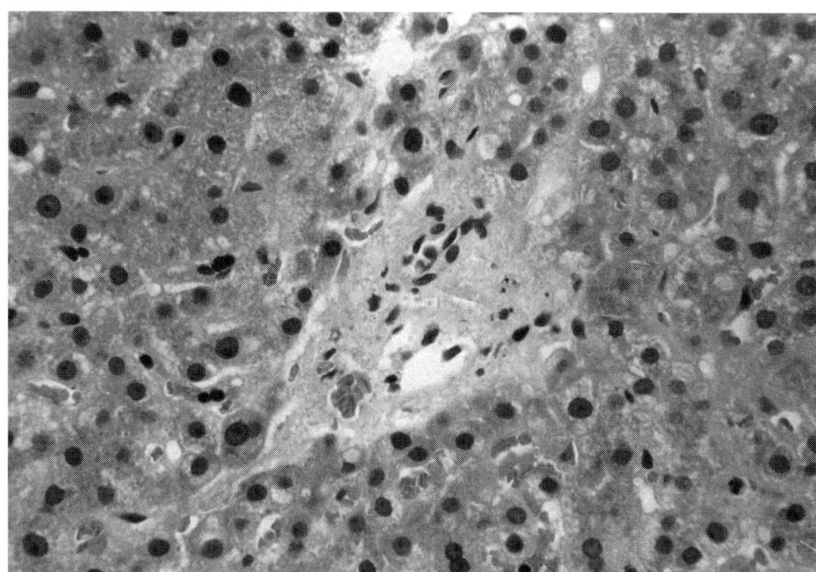

FIGURE 21.2. *Absent bile ducts in the portal tract 9 months after an acute antibiotic-induced cholestatic hepatitis (ERCP normal).*

Table 21.3. Causes of vanishing bile duct syndrome (ductopenia)

Congenital
Alagille syndrome (and nonsyndromatic)
Cystic fibrosis
Duct plate abnormalities
Progressive familial intrahepatic cholestasis (PFIC)
Malignant
Cholangiocarcinoma
Histocytosis X
Lymphoma
Mastocytosis
Immune
Primary biliary cirrhosis (PBC)
Primary sclerosing cholangitis (PSC)
Graft-versus-host disease
Allograft rejection
Sarcoid
Infectious
Cytomegalovirus
Recurrent biliary sepsis
Parasites
Ischemic
Hepatic artery thrombosis
Paroxysmal nocturnal hemoglobinuria (PNH)
Surgical
Vasculitis
Toxic
Drugs

the damage may be immune mediated. An HLA association with certain hepatic drug reactions has recently been described (37).

Immunologic VBDS

Graft-versus-host disease (GVHD) of the liver can develop acutely following bone marrow transplantation, although the pattern of illness is generally more chronic (38,39). It is common for other manifestations of GVHD (affecting the skin and/or bowel) to be present when there is GVHD of the liver, but this is not universal. As with PBC, the liver, salivary ducts, and possibly the pancreatic ducts may be affected. Liver biochemical abnormalities vary, ranging from a mild transaminitis to a biochemical pattern more typical of cholestasis, sometimes with jaundice.

Jaundice is quite common following bone marrow transplantation, and often there is more than one factor operating at once. A liver biopsy is essential to be sure whether GVHD of the liver is present (Fig. 21.3). A confident diagnosis of GVHD will initiate the institution of immunosuppressive therapy.

Patients with GVHD of the liver may range from being asymptomatic to suffering from profound pruritus with or without jaundice. The latter may sometimes be so severe as to be accompanied by steatorrhea that makes the immunosuppressive therapy ineffective by the oral route. Fortunately, progressive liver failure and death from chronic GVHD are rare. If the jaundice is prolonged, silent severe osteoporosis is common, and its severity is enhanced by the need for long-term immunosuppressive therapy.

To date there has been one published randomized control trial of UDCA in patients undergoing bone marrow transplantation. Surprisingly, the effect of UDCA was greatest in reducing early veno-occlusive disease of the liver but the sample size was not sufficiently large to show an effect of treatment on the outcome of hepatic GVHD (40). As UDCA not only enhances transport of hydrophobic bile acids across the liver cell and canalicular membrane (41) but also appears to have immunoregulatory properties that include the reduction in bile acid–induced apoptosis of hepatocytes (42), this drug is frequently used after bone marrow transplantation in spite of the lack of conclusive proof that it either prevents or effectively reduces the severity of GVHD of the liver.

Chronic liver allograft rejection may cause a vanishing bile duct syndrome and the first-line therapy is with potent immunosuppressive drugs. FK 506 is generally the treatment of choice (43). It is rare for such patients to have symptoms of cholestasis such as pruritus. There have been no trials of other therapies aside from immunosuppressive treatments. Progressive bile duct loss generally requires a new liver graft.

Sarcoidosis of the liver is most often asymptomatic and generally causes nonprogressive disease. Multiple granuloma, both in the parenchyma and the portal tracts, are found. Rarely do the granuloma in the portal tracts cause bile duct destruction, and only then is the pathology almost indistinguishable from PBC (44). The granuloma appear different, in that they are commonly fibrotic and their distribution within the liver is dissimilar to that seen in PBC. Unless PBC is coexistent, the serum tests for AMA will be negative.

Secondary Sclerosing Cholangitis

Primary sclerosing cholangitis generally involves both the extrahepatic and the intrahepatic bile ducts (see Chapter 19). There are, however, many secondary causes of sclerosing cholangitis that are sometimes limited to the intrahepatic duct system. These rare causes include systemic mastocytosis (45), paroxysmal nocturnal hemoglobinuria, and possibly retroperitoneal fibrosis. Ischemic injury to the bile duct causes marked damage to the extrahepatic and intrahepatic biliary system. Postoperative damage to a small branch of the hepatic artery (such as during a cholecystectomy) may cause intrahepatic bile duct loss confined to the ischemic segment (Fig. 21.4), but hepatic artery thrombosis (as seen after a liver transplant) will affect the entire biliary tree (46).

Chronic infection of the biliary tree may cause damage to the intrahepatic bile ducts, although usually the large intrahepatic ducts are involved. The infectious agents include

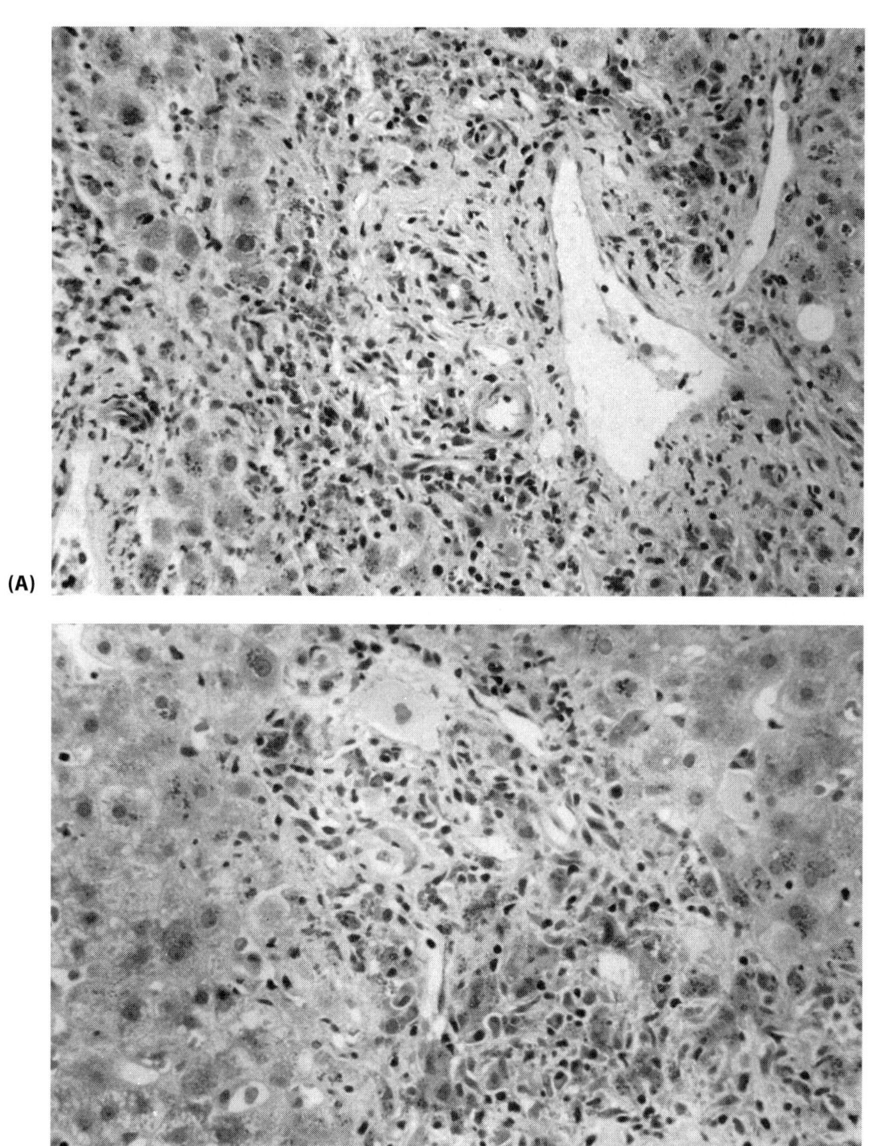

FIGURE 21.3. ***(A)*** *Duct injury following a bone marrow transplant, likely a result of graft-versus-host disease.* ***(B)*** *Portal infiltrate following a bone marrow transplant, likely a result of graft-versus-host disease of the liver.*

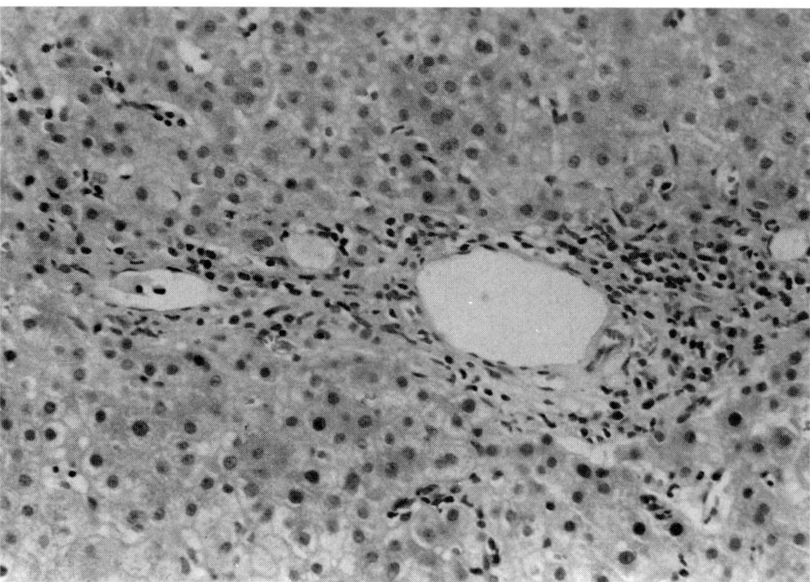

FIGURE 21.4. *Ductopenia secondary to inadvertent ligation of an aberrant branch of the hepatic artery during cholecystectomy.*

the protozoal organisms *Clonorchis sinensis*, Fasciola hepatica, or cryptosporidiosis (47). Bacterial infection of the liver may give rise to a picture that transiently resembles sclerosing cholangitis, but it is completely reversible following drainage and adequate antibiotic therapy (48).

It is disputed as to whether infection with cytomegalovirus (CMV) can cause a paucity of the intrahepatic bile ducts. Overwhelming infection with CMV is most commonly observed in immunosuppressed patients, particularly those undergoing organ transplantation. In the case of liver transplantation it is almost impossible to discern whether intrahepatic bile duct injury is related to chronic allograft rejection and/or CMV infection (49).

Malignancies

Several malignancies may cause the intrahepatic bile ducts to disappear, either as a result of direct invasion—for example, cholangiocarcinoma—or as part of a nonmalignant manifestation of the disease. Abnormal liver tests have been described in patients with hypernephroma; the liver tests return to normal once the tumor is removed. Although direct lymphomatous involvement of the liver may cause cholestasis, VBDS has been described even when all evidence of the lymphoma has gone (50). The patient may succumb to rapidly progressive cholestatic liver disease.

Direct Toxicity

A number of toxic compounds can damage both the intrahepatic and extrahepatic biliary systems. Chemotherapy introduced into the liver via the hepatic artery (e.g., floxuridine) may cause severe sclerosis of the biliary tree (51). Inadvertent leakage of caustic agents used to treat hydatid disease of the liver may also damage the local bile ducts (52). Clearly, in these circumstances there is no diagnostic dilemma.

Intrahepatic Cholestasis Presenting in Childhood Progressing Through to Adulthood

The management of children with lung and pancreatic disease secondary to cystic fibrosis has markedly improved. As a result, the long-term complications, particularly of the liver, have become a major issue for individuals with cystic fibrosis who survive into adulthood. Typically such patients have a focal biliary cirrhosis secondary to plugging of the intrahepatic bile ducts with viscous, proteinaceous material (Fig. 21.5). Treatment with UDCA has been advocated; liver biochemical tests improve following the introduction of UDCA, but no study has been conducted on a sufficient sample size for long enough to show whether UDCA improves survival (53). Whether a "form fruste" of cystic fibrosis may be responsible for idiopathic ductopenia remains unknown.

Both syndromatic (Alagille syndrome) or nonsyndromatic bile duct paucity generally, but not always, present in childhood. Many patients survive into adulthood, and although often anicteric, they may suffer from chronic pruritus. Cirrhosis also may be present. Occasionally the disease is not diagnosed until adulthood when some other manifestation of the syndrome is detected, such as peripheral pulmonary artery stenosis or "butterfly" vertebra (widely separated pedicles and malformed neural arch).

Clearly the spectrum of disease severity in this condition varies greatly. The childhood condition of progressive familial intrahepatic cholestasis (PFIC) is caused by a mutation in the MDR3 gene, which controls the transport of phospholipid across the canalicular membrane. PFIC leads to such severe damage to the intrahepatic bile ducts that these

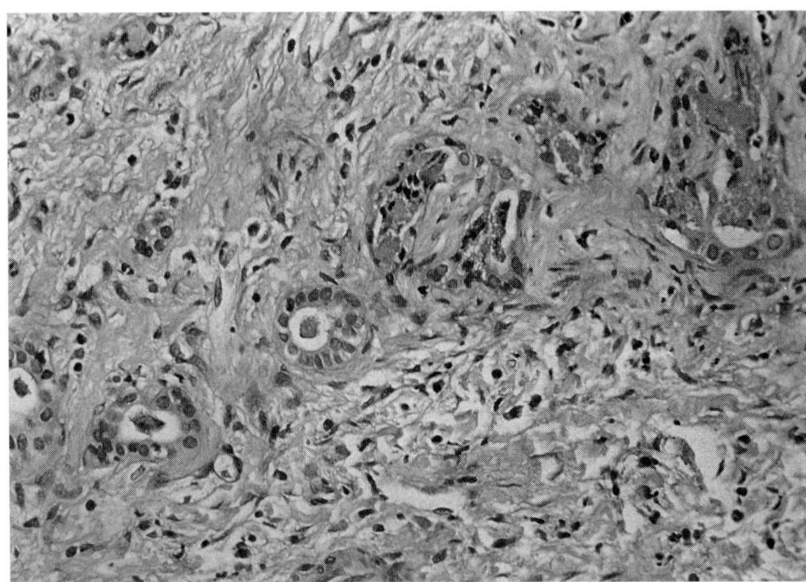

FIGURE 21.5. *Intrahepatic bile duct lesions in a patient with cystic fibrosis.*

children do not survive into adulthood unless a liver transplant is performed (54).

Therapy for Vanishing Bile Duct Syndromes

As with PBC, therapeutic endeavors for VBDS need to focus on control of symptoms, prevention of complications, and treatment of the specific disease. With children, it is particularly important to improve their nutritional status with dietary supplementation so that their growth will not be stunted. Symptomatic and preventative therapy are the same as described for PBC.

Clearly the treatment for each individual disease depends on its etiology. In the case of genetic disorders, these cannot currently be reversed. Treatment of PFIC with UDCA causes a remarkable improvement in cholestasis. Also biliary diversion has been used to relieve pruritus (55). Although UDCA treatment for other causes of small duct diseases of the liver seems logical and is frequently used (56), as yet there have been no appropriate clinical trials to support its use.

SUMMARY

For PBC, there is a highly sensitive and specific serum marker, AMA. For other conditions in adults, a diagnosis of intrahepatic bile duct injury may be difficult, and an obvious etiology may not always be found. Examination of adequate amounts of liver tissue is the only reliable method to diagnose a patient as having a vanishing bile duct syndrome. It has been said that the definition of VBDS can only be made when 20 or more portal tracts are available for examination and 50% of those tracts have missing bile ducts (56). In some diseases, such as PBC, the lesions may be very patchy; hence it is essential that sufficient portal tracts be available for examination (57).

Both the clinician and the pathologist need to know what they are looking for to ensure that the diagnosis is not missed, as overt signs of cholestasis such as "bile lakes" on liver biopsy, are usually absent. The clinical, biochemical, and histologic manifestations of disease of the intrahepatic bile ducts may be very subtle, so a high index of suspicion needs to be maintained.

SUGGESTED READINGS

Degott C, Feldmann G, Larrey D, et al. Drug-induced prolonged cholestasis in adults: a histological semiquantitative study demonstrating progressive ductopenia. Hepatology 1992;15:244–51. Drug-induced cholestasis causing damage to the intrahepatic bile ducts is much more common than appreciated—usually the drug history has been missed!

Dickson ER, Grambsch PM, Fleming TR, et al. Prognosis in primary biliary cirrhosis: model for decision making. Hepatology 1989;10:1–7. This is the classic article which describes how the Mayo Risk Score was generated from a large population of patients with PBC (before the era of liver transplantation). This model has stood the "test of time" as a very reliable marker of prognosis in PBC.

Ferrara JLM, Deeg HJ. Graft-versus-host disease. N Engl J Med 1991;324:667–74. Graft versus host disease following bone marrow transplantation takes many forms and connot be accurately diagnosed without a liver biopsy as the biochemical pattern is so variable and there may be many other ongoing medical problems which complicate the diagnosis.

Poupon RE, Lindor KD, Cauch-Dudek K, et al. Combined analysis of randomized controlled trials of ursodeoxycholic acid in primary biliary cirrhosis. Gastroenterology 1997;113:884–90. This is the definitive study which combines the raw data (i.e., not a meta-analysis) from three large, randomized, controlled trials of UDCA in PBC which indicates that when treatment is given for up to 4 years there was a survival benefit, in treated patients (this could not be seen at 2 years).

REFERENCES

1. Addison T, Gull W. On a certain affection of the skin, vitiligoidea—α plana, β tuberosa. Guy's Hosp Rev 1851;7:265–76.
2. Ahrens EH, Rayne MA, Kunkle HG, et al. Primary biliary cirrhosis. Medicine 1950;29:299–364.
3. Scheuer PJ. Primary biliary cirrhosis. Proc R Soc Med 1967;60:1257–60.
4. Doniach D, Roitt IM, Walker JG, Sherlock S. Tissue antibodies in primary biliary cirrhosis, active chronic (lupoid) hepatitis, cryptogenic cirrhosis and other liver diseases and their clinical implications. Clin Exp Immunol 1966;1:237–62.
5. Mitchison HC, Bassendine MF, Hendrick A, et al. Positive antimitochondrial antibody but normal alkaline phosphatase: is this primary biliary cirrhosis? Hepatology 1986;6:1279–84.
6. Joplin R, Lindsay JG, Johnson GD, Strain A, Neuberger J. Membrane dihydrolipoamide acetyltransferase (E2) on human biliary epithelial cells in primary biliary cirrhosis. Lancet 1992;339:93–4.
7. Jones DEJ, Palmer JM, Yeaman SJ, et al. Breakdown of tolerance to pyruvate dehydrogenase complex in experimental autoimmune cholangitis: a mouse model of primary biliary cirrhosis. Hepatology 1999;30:65–70.
8. Degott C, Feldmann G, Larrey D, et al. Drug-induced prolonged cholestasis in adults: a histological semiquantitative study demonstrating progressive ductopenia. Hepatology 1992;15:244–51.
9. Sherlock S. The syndrome of disappearing intrahepatic bile ducts. Lancet 1987; 1:493–6.
10. Ludwig J, Wiesner RH, LaRusso NF. Idiopathic adulthood ductopenia. A cause of chronic cholestatic liver disease and biliary cirrhosis. J Hepatol 1988;7: 193–9.
11. Heathcote J, Deodhar KP, Scheuer P, Sherlock S. Intrahepatic cholestasis in childhood. N Engl J Med 1976;295:801–5.
12. Alagille D, Odievre M, Gautier M, Dommergues JP. Hepatic ductular hypoplasia associated with characteristic facies, vertebral malformations, retarded physical, mental and sexual development, and cardiac murmur. J Pediatr 1975; 86:63–71.
13. Alonso EM, Snover DC, Montag A, et al. Histologic pathology of the liver in progressive familial intrahepatic cholestasis. J Pediatr Gastroenterol Nutrit 1994; 18:128–33.
14. Jansen PLM, Muller MM. Progressive familial intrahepatic cholestasis types 1, 2, and 3. Gut 1998;42:766–7.
15. Colombo C, Battezzati PM, Podda M. Hepatobiliary disease in cystic fibrosis. Semin Liver Dis 1994;14:259–67.
16. Witt-Sullivan H, Heathcote J, Cauch K, et al. The demography of primary biliary cirrhosis in Ontario, Canada. Hepatology 1990;12:98–105.
17. Cauch-Dudek K, Abbey S, Stewart DE, Heathcote EJ. Fatigue in primary biliary cirrhosis. Gut 1998;43:705–10.
18. Inoue K, Hirohara J, Nakano T, et al. Prediction of prognosis of primary biliary cirrhosis in Japan. Liver 1995;15:70–7.
19. Keefe EB. Sarcoidosis and primary biliary cirrhosis: literature review and illustrative case. Am J Med 1987;83:977–80.
20. Kew MC, Varma RR, Dos Santos HA, et al. Portal hypertension in primary biliary cirrhosis. Gut 1971;12:830–4.
21. Springer JE, Cole DEC, Rubin LA, et al. Vitamin D receptor genotypes as independent genetic predictors of decreased bone mineral density in primary biliary cirrhosis. Gastroenterology 2000;118:145–51.
22. Nijhawan PK, Therneau TM, Dickson ER, Lindor KD. Incidence of cancer in primary biliary cirrhosis: the Mayo experience. Hepatology 1999;29:1396–8.
23. Sherlock S, Scheuer PJ. The presentation and diagnosis of 100 patients with primary biliary cirrhosis. N Engl J Med 1973;289:674–8.
24. Mitchison HC, Bassendine MF, Hendrick A, et al. Positive antimitochondrial antibody but normal alkaline phosphatase: is this primary biliary cirrhosis? Hepatology 1986;6:1279–84.
25. Mahl T, Shockcor W, Boyer JL. Primary biliary cirrhosis: survival of a large

cohort of symptomatic and asymptomatic patients followed for 24 years. J Hepatol 1994;20:707–13.
26. Springer J, Cauch-Dudek K, O'Rourke K, et al. Asymptomatic primary biliary cirrhosis: a study of its natural history and prognosis. Am J Gastroenterol 1999;94:47–53.
27. Dickson ER, Grambsch PM, Fleming TR, et al. Prognosis in primary biliary cirrhosis: model for decision making. Hepatology 1989;10:1–7.
28. Angulo P, Lindor KD, Therneau TM, et al. Utilization of the Mayo risk score in patients with primary biliary cirrhosis receiving ursodeoxycholic acid. Liver 1999;19:115–21.
29. Metcalf JV, Bhopal RS, Gray J, et al. Incidence and prevalence of primary biliary cirrhosis in the city of Newcastle upon Tyne, England. Int J Epidemiol 1997;26:830–6.
30. Wolfhagen FHJ, van Buren HR, denOuden JW, et al. Cyclical etidronate in the prevention of bone loss in corticosteroid-treated primary biliary cirrhosis. A prospective, controlled pilot study. J Hepatol 1997;26:325–30.
31. Eastell R, Dickson ER, Hodgson S, et al. Rates of vertebral bone loss before and after liver transplantation in women with primary biliary cirrhosis. Hepatology 1991;14:296–300.
32. Poupon RE, Lindor KD, Cauch-Dudek K, et al. Combined analysis of randomized controlled trials of ursodeoxycholic acid in primary biliary cirrhosis. Gastroenterology 1997;113:884–90.
33. Poupon RE, Bonnand AM, Chretien Y, et al. Ten-year survival in ursodeoxycholic acid-treated patients with primary biliary cirrhosis. Hepatology 1999;29:1668–71.
34. Heathcote EJ, Stone J, Cauch-Dudek K, et al. The effect of pre-transplant ursodeoxycholic acid therapy on outcome of liver transplantation in patients with primary biliary cirrhosis. Liver Transpl Surg 1999;5:1–7.
35. Ricci P, Therneau TM, Malinchoc M, et al. A prognostic model for the outcome of liver transplantation in patients with cholestatic liver disease. Hepatology 1997;25:672–7.
36. Hubscher SG, Buckels JAC, Elias E, et al. Vanishing bile-duct syndrome following liver transplantation—is it reversible? Transplantation 1991;51:1004–10.
37. Hautekeete ML, Horsmans Y, Van Waeyenberge C, et al. HLA association of amoxicillin-clavulanate-induced hepatitis. Gastroenterology 1999;117:1181–6.
38. Yeh KH, Hsieh HC, Tang JL, et al. Severe isolated acute hepatic graft-versus-host disease with vanishing bile duct syndrome. Bone Marrow Transpl 1994;14:319–21.
39. Ferrara JLM, Deeg HJ. Graft-versus-host disease. N Engl J Med 1991;324:667–74.
40. Fried RH, Murakami CS, Fisher LD, et al. Ursodeoxycholic acid treatment of refractory chronic graft-versus-host disease of the liver. Ann Intern Med 1992;116:624–9.
41. Jazrawi RP, Caestecker JS, Goggin PM, et al. Kinetics of hepatic bile acid handling in cholestatic liver disease: effect of ursodeoxycholic acid. Gastroenterology 1994;106:134–42.
42. Rodrigues CM, Fan G, Ma X, et al. A novel role for ursodeoxycholic acid in inhibiting apoptosis by modulating mitochondrial membrane perturbation. J Clin Invest 1998;101:2790–9.
43. Klintmalm GB, Gibbs JF, McMillan R, et al. Rejection: FK 506 for rescue or maintenance? Transpl Proc 1993;25:1914–5.
44. Murphy JR, Sjögren MH, Kikendall JW, et al. Small duct abnormalities in sarcoidosis. J Clin Gastroenterol 1990;12:555–61.
45. Mican JM, Di Bisceglie AM, Fong TL, Travis WD, et al. Hepatic involvement in mastocytosis: clinicopathologic correlations in 41 cases. Hepatology 1995;22:1163–70.
46. Margarit C, Hidalgo E, Lazaro JL, et al. Biliary complications secondary to late hepatic artery thrombosis in adult liver transplant patients. Transpl Int 1998;11:S251–4.
47. Leung JW, Yu AS. Hepatolithiasis and biliary parasites. Baillieres Clin Gastroenterol 1997;11:681–706.
48. Steinhart H, Heathcote J, Stone R, Simons M. Multiple hepatic abscesses: cholangiographic changes simulating sclerosing cholangitis and resolution following percutaneous drainage. Am J Gastroenterol 1990;85:306–8.
49. Lao WC, Lee D, Burroughs AK, et al. Use of polymerase chain reaction to provide prognostic information on human cytomegalovirus disease after liver transplantation. J Med Virol 1997;51:152–8.
50. Hubscher SG, Lumley MA, Elias E. Vanishing bile duct syndrome: a possible mechanism for intrahepatic cholestasis in Hodgkin's lymphoma. Hepatology 1993;17:70–7.
51. Hohn D, Melnick J, Stagg R, et al. Biliary sclerosis in patients receiving hepatic arterial infusions of floxuridine. J Clin Oncol 1985;3:98–102.
52. Belghiti J, Benhamou JP, Houry S, et al. Caustic sclerosing cholangitis. A complication of the surgical treatment of hydatid disease of the liver. Arch Surg 1986;121:1162–5.
53. Lindblad A, Glaumann H, Strandvik B. A two-year prospective study of the effect of ursodeoxycholic acid on urinary bile acid excretion and liver morphology in cystic fibrosis-associated liver disease. Hepatology 1998;27:166–74.
54. Jacquemin E, Hermans D, Myara A, et al. Ursodeoxycholic acid therapy in pediatric patients with progressive familial intrahepatic cholestasis. Hepatology 1997;25:519–23.
55. Rebhandl W, Felberbauer FX, Turnbull J, et al. Biliary diversion by use of the appendix (cholecystoappendicostomy) in progressive familial intrahepatic cholestasis. J Pediatr Gastroenterol Nutr 1999;28:217–19.
56. O'Brien CB, Shields DS, Saul SH, Reddy KR. Drug-induced vanishing bile duct syndrome: response to ursodiol. Am J Gastroenterol 1996;91:1456–7.
57. Tadrous PJ, Goldin RD. How many portal tracts are necessary to make a diagnosis of significant bile duct loss (SBDL)? J Pathol 1997;181:11A.

Chapter

22

Intrahepatic Cholestasis

ANDREW STOLZ NEIL KAPLOWITZ

Cholestatic liver injury has multiple causes, all of which require vastly different diagnostic and therapeutic approaches. In this chapter, we review a diverse group of nonsurgical diseases that can mimic the presentation of other cholestatic liver diseases discussed elsewhere in this book. To understand how these diverse disorders can cause cholestatic liver injury, we concisely review the current understanding of the key proteins that constitute the normal hepatic uptake and biliary excretory pathways. In human disease and animal models, the molecular regulation of these key transport proteins in response to cholestatic liver injury has provided detailed insight into the pathophysiological mechanisms in different cholestatic conditions. The clinical presentation, evaluation, treatment, and medical conditions associated with cholestasis follow a review of the normal biliary physiology. A review of drug-induced cholestasis is also provided, as an inability to recognize this important etiology can lead to persistent exposure to the offending agent and unnecessary diagnostic or therapeutic interventions. We anticipate that enhanced understanding of molecular mechanisms of cholestatic liver disease should lead to new therapeutic strategies for these widely different diseases in the future.

MECHANISMS FOR HEPATIC BILE FORMATION

The cellular organization of the liver, combined with the unique endothelial structure of the sinusoids, is ideally suited for the efficient sinusoidal uptake and efflux of molecules by the hepatocyte as well as their biliary excretion into the canaliculus, the most proximal portion of the biliary system (1–4). The hepatocytes, like other epithelial cells such as the enterocyte, are polarized cells with distinct membrane domains exposed to either the sinusoidal surface (referred to as basal or sinusoidal domain) or the canaliculus (referred to as the apical or canalicular domain). The membrane between these regions forms the lateral domain. Cords of hepatocytes, two cells thick, are attached at their sinusoidal and apical domains by gap junctions, generating a physical barrier between the vascular sinusoidal space and biliary excretory pathway. Ions and water can travel between these gaps, and disruption of these anchors between hepatocytes can lead to regurgitation of biliary components into the vascular space during cholestatic conditions. Bile formation requires the maintenance of these cell-to-cell contacts as well as vectorial uptake at the sinusoidal membrane followed by secretion of biliary components at the canalicular membrane.

Animal studies have revealed that the origin of bile flow is divided into bile acid dependent and independent bile flow. Bile salts are the predominant solute in bile; along with sodium ions, bile salts are responsible for water movement into the canalicular space predominantly by paracellular pathways between adjacent hepatocytes. Bile salts are also essential for biliary phospholipid excretion, which is extracted from the outer leaflet of the canalicular membrane forming micelles in the presence of bile salts. An absence of bile salts leads to significant reduction in bile formation and phospholipid excretion. A bile acid independent bile flow also exists in which an efflux of organic anions and the important peptide antioxidant, glutathione, coupled with its cleavage by gamma glutamyltransferase and dipeptidases into its component amino acids, generates an osmotic gradient promoting water movement into the canalicular space (5). Bicarbonate secretion is another important component whose contribution is highly species dependent (6).

The bile canalicular space generated by adjacent hepatocytes eventually empties at the periphery of the lobule into ductules lined by cholangiocytes, which further modify the ion and bicarbonate content in bile, as regulated by secretin. A cholehepatic shunt between the hepatocytes and cholangiocytes has been proposed to explain the bicarbonate-rich biliary excretion caused by infusion of unconjugated bile salts such as ursodeoxycholate in animals. The role this plays in normal bile flow is controversial. It is postulated that certain unconjugated bile salts secreted by hepatocytes are reabsorbed by cholangiocytes in protonated form (leaving bicarbonate behind) and then returned to the hepatocytes in a repetitive recycling that leads to enhanced bicarbonate secretion associated with a hypercholeresis (7). In addition to fluid and electrolyte movement, mechanical contraction of canalicular membrane by microfilaments network located at the apical domain of hepatocytes also promotes bile flow by a "squeezing action" on the canalicular space.

Within the last decade, identification of the cellular transport proteins mediating sinusoidal uptake and biliary secretion of the key solutes has greatly expanded our understanding of the cellular mechanism for bile formation and its dysregulation in cholestatic conditions. We will review the key transport proteins, listed in Table 22.1 and illustrated in Figure 22.1, at each domain. The altered regulation of these transporters in response to cholestatic stimuli is now known to play a key role in the development and maintenance of cholestasis (8–10).

Sinusoidal Membrane

Uptake of bile acids by the sinusoidal membrane is a key step in the enterohepatic circulation of bile salts, in which approximately 95% of the bile acid pool is efficiently recovered by the intestine and resecreted by the liver (11). Initial characterization of bile acid uptake in isolated hepatocytes and enriched sinusoidal plasma membrane vesicles identified both sodium-dependent and sodium-independent transport systems for bile salts. In addition, hydrophobic secondary bile acids or unconjugated bile acids may also enter into the hepatocytes by passive diffusion. Using an expression cloning strategy, investigators have identified a specific sodium-dependent bile salt transporter as well as sodium-independent organic anion transporters, some of which can also mediate sodium-independent bile acid uptake.

Sodium-Dependent Bile Acid Transporter

The sodium-dependent taurocholate carrier protein, ntcp, is a 55-kd glycoprotein composed of 362 amino acids in the

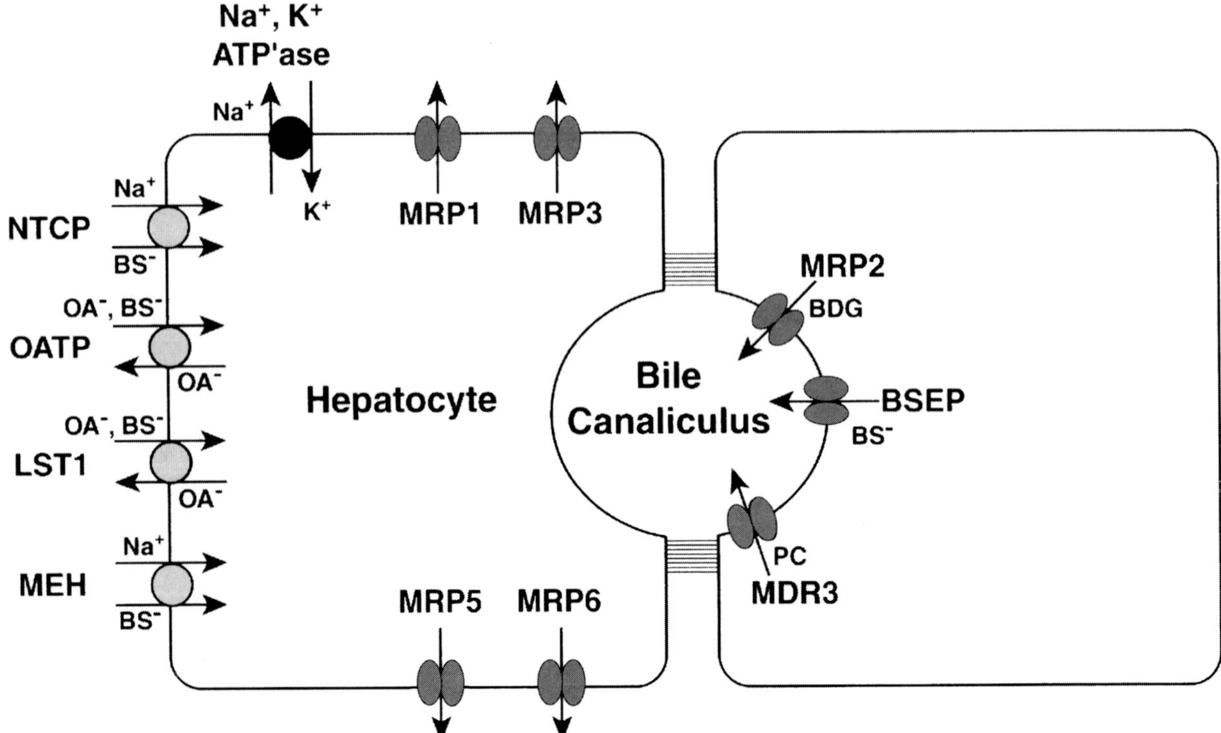

FIGURE 22.1. *Transport proteins of the basolateral (sinusoidal) and canalicular surface of human hepatocytes. Proteins involved in the hepatocellular uptake of organic anions include Na^+-taurocholate cotransporting polypeptide (NTCP) and microsomal epoxide hydrolase (MEH) (secondary active unidirectional transporters), and organic anion transporting polypeptides (OATP1 and 2) (bidirectional antiporters). Multidrug resistant proteins (MRP), bile salt export pump (BSEP), multidrug-resistant (MDR) gene product are unidirectionally primary active transporters involved in efflux. Na^+,K^+ ATPase is responsible for maintaining the low sodium, high potassium within the cell. BS^- = bile salts, OA^- = organic anions, PC = phosphatidylcholine, LST1 = OATP2.*

Table 22.1. Molecular and functional characteristics of hepatocyte membrane transporters

Transporter	Species	AA	Domain	Transport Features	Model Substrates
ntcp	Rat	362	Sinusoidal	Uni	Bile acids, conjugated sex steroids, T_4
NTCP	Human	349	Sinusoidal	Uni	Bile acids
mEH	Rat	413	Sinusoidal/ intracellular	Uni	Cholate, taurocholate
oatp1	Rat	670	Sinusoidal	Bi	Bromosulfophthalein, bile acids, conjugated sex steroids, ouabain
oatp2	Rat	671	Sinusoidal	Bi	Digoxin, taurocholate
lst-1	Rat	652	Sinusoidal	Bi	Taurocholate, HMG-Co reductase inhibitors
OATP	Human	670	Sinusoidal	Bi	Bromosulfophthalein, bile acids, conjugated sex steroids, ouabain
OATP2 (LST-1)	Human	691	Basolateral	Bi	Taurocholate, HMG-Co reductase inhibitors
bsep	Rat	1321	Canaliculus	Uni	Taurocholate, bile acids
BSEP	Human	1321	Canaliculus	Uni	Taurocholate, bile acids
MDR3	Human	1279	Canaliculus	Uni	Phosphatidylcholine
mrp2	Rat	1541	Canaliculus	Uni	Leukotriene C4, GSH conjugates, conjugated bilirubin
MRP2	Human	1545	Canaliculus	Uni	Leukotriene C4, GSH conjugates, conjugated bilirubin
mrp3	Rat	1523	Basolateral	Uni	Bile acids, conjugated sex steroids
mrp6	Rat	1502	Basolateral	Uni	Not determined

Note: Species, amino acid (AA), and location (domain) of rat and human hepatic transporters (9,28). Transport features refers to ability of transporter to function as a unidirectional (Uni) or bidirectional (Bi) transporter.

rat; it strictly mediates sodium-dependent bile salt transport, favoring taurine-conjugated trihydroxy-bile acids (12). This protein is exclusively expressed in the hepatocyte at the sinusoidal domain throughout the hepatic acinus. Like other sodium co-transporters, the concentrative uptake of bile salt is thermodynamically favored by coupling to a significant outside-to-inside sodium gradient maintained by the Na^+,K^+ ATPase activity, ensuring efficient uptake of bile salts at the sinusoidal surface. Two sodium ions are transported for each molecule of bile salt. Activity of the ntcp transporter is regulated by its levels of expression at the sinusoidal surface and by gene transcription, which is an active area of investigation (3,10). Increased cyclic adenosine monophosphate (cAMP) rapidly increases content of ntcp at the sinusoidal membrane by modulating an intracellular pool of transporters, which is dependent on microfilament activity (13). The ntcp expression is rapidly lost in primary cultured hepatocytes and all tumor-derived liver cell lines, suggesting tight regulation of this transporter; however, it has been identified in human hepatocellular carcinoma samples. Elevated serum levels of bile acids are associated with decreased expression, whereas increased expression of the transporter gene has been noted postpartum due to prolactin (14,15). Increased bile acid flux does not regulate its expression in the rat (16). Teleologically, decreased expression of ntcp protects the liver in cholestasis in the face of elevated serum bile salts by reducing the hepatic accumulation and potential toxicity of an increased concentration of intrahepatic bile salts. Human ntcp is a 349 amino acid protein that shares 77% sequence identity with the rat (17). Of note, ntcp shares 50% sequence identity with the sodium-dependent ileal bile acid transporter (ibat), which is expressed at the lumenal (apical) domain of the enterocyte (18). The ibat transporter has also been identified in the apical domain of large cholangiocytes (where it participates in cholehepatic shunting) and in renal tubule cells (19,20). Microsomal epoxide hydrolase (MEH), a key enzyme in the detoxification of reactive epoxides expressed at both the plasma membrane and endoplasmic reticulum in rat, has also been implicated as a sodium-dependent bile acid transporter as its expression in a cell line can confer sodium-dependent bile salt uptake (21). MEH expression seems to favor glycine-conjugated bile acids.

Organic Anion and Sodium-Independent Bile Salt Transport

In addition to sodium-dependent bile salt transport, dihydroxy-bile acids and unconjugated bile acids can enter hepatocytes via a sodium-independent transport mechanism. An organic anion transporter (oatp1) was identified in the rat liver by the use of an expression cloning strategy for uptake of sulfobromophthalein (SBP), an organic anion (22). This transporter, composed of 670 amino acids, can function as an organic anion exchanger, promoting uptake of organic anions into the liver by exchanging them with efflux of other anions such as bicarbonate and glutathione (23,24). Bile salts are also efficient substrates for this transporter (25). In the rat, oatp2 has been identified in the mid-zone to perivenous region suggesting that it is a backup system for oatp1, which is uniformly expressed in the liver (26). A liver-specific member, referred to as either LST-1 or OATP2 in humans, shares 43% identity with oatp1 and can transport taurocholate in a sodium-independent fashion (27,28). This liver-selective expression suggests that it may be responsible for the majority of sodium-independent bile acid uptake in humans. Molecular cloning of other oatp family members reveals a complex pattern of substrate specificity and distinct organ distribution in different species, suggesting that these transporters are involved with organ-specific uptake of specific organic anions such as steroids (9).

Transcellular Movement

Little is known about the transcellular movement of the key constituents of bile (29). Intracellular binding proteins with high affinity for bile acids, organic anions, fatty acids, and phosphatidylcholine have been identified but their physiological function is still speculative (2,30). These proteins are assumed to target their hydrophobic ligands to different intracellular components of the cell, including their respective canalicular transporters. Vesicular-mediated transport of bile acids has also been implicated based on increased transcellular movement of bile acids in response to cAMP and enhanced phospholipid excretion in response to infused bile acids. These effects may also be a result of increased insertion of canalicular transporters into the membrane. Detailed studies with fluorescent bile acids have failed to demonstrate evidence for vesicular transport in isolated hepatocytes, although these modified bile acids may not accurately reflect the processing of bile salts (31).

Canalicular Excretion

Canalicular membrane transport is the rate-limiting step in the vectorial movement of biliary constituents from the sinusoidal space into bile. Excretion of biliary components occurs across a relative concentration gradient of 100- to 1000-fold excess, requiring an active transport process. Prior biochemical characterization of transport activity in canalicular enriched plasma membrane vesicles has recently been advanced by the molecular identification of specific canalicular transporters. Detailed analysis of these individual transporters, coupled with loss of activities in rare human cholestatic syndromes and genetically engineered mice, has revealed their role in normal biliary physiology. To date, all the canalicular transporters involved with biliary excretion are members of the diverse ATP-binding cassette (ABC) class of membrane transporters, in which transport of substrate depends on ATP hydrolysis (32). These proteins share a common ATP-binding domain with substrate specificity dictated by other domains of the transporter. Major subclasses within this super gene family, whose members play essential roles in biliary excretion, include the multidrug resistant (MDR) proteins or P-glycoprotein, and the multidrug resistant protein (MRP). Another key gene involved with bile formation is a recently identified P-type ATPase referred to as FIC 1, which is responsible for Byler disease and benign recurrent intrahepatic cholestasis (BRIC) (33). We will review these key ATP-dependent transporters and their role in the excretion of biliary components.

Canalicular Bile Salt Transporter

As bile salt transport is increased by ATP hydrolysis, ABC transporters of unknown function were screened as a potential bile salt transporter (34,35). Using this strategy, investigators considered a rat gene similar to rat P-glycoprotein that is exclusively expressed in the hepatocyte at the canalicular domain; it was shown to mediate ATP-dependent taurocholate transport in recombinant expression studies (36). This transporter, now referred to as bile salt excretory peptide (bsep), is composed of 1321 amino acids and shares 70% identity to the P-glycoprotein. The gene is located on chromosome 2 q24 in humans, which is identical to a shared chromosomal region identified in children with a rare progressive familial intrahepatic cholestasis (PFIC 2), thus further confirming its essential role in biliary excretion of bile acids (see the discussion of familial disorders below) (37,38). Kinetic features, coupled with unique expression at the canalicular domain of the hepatocytes and absence in PFIC 2, indicate that this is the major, if not the sole, bile acid transporter in the canaliculus.

Regulation of bsep transport activity occurs at both the transcriptional and, more importantly, the post-translational level in which its redistribution from the subcanalicular endosomal pool to canalicular domain can be rapidly enhanced during high bile salt loads. Trafficking between these pools is regulated by second messengers, including cAMP and PI3 kinase products, that enhance insertion into the membrane (39,40). This rapid regulation of expression at the canalicular membrane permits dynamic modulation of transport activity coupled to flux of bile acids by altering the relative density of transporter.

Canalicular Phospholipid Flippase

In addition to bile salts, phospholipids such as phosphatidylcholine and cholesterol are significant components of bile. Elimination of murine mdr2, which corresponds to MDR3 in humans, by gene knockout technology leads to almost complete elimination of phosphatidylcholine in the bile with a progressive cholangitis in mice (30, 41). This ABC transporter is postulated to function as a "flippase," transferring the energetically unfavorable movement of phosphatidylcholine from the inner leaflet to the outer leaflet of the canalicular membrane. Once at the outer leaflet, phosphatidylcholine is extracted from the membrane by the high concentration of bile salts present in the canalicular space. Inability to translocate the phospholipid to the outer leaflet in the mdr2 knockout mice leads to bile salts freely interacting with the luminal membrane of ductules, causing a detergent-induced cholangiopathy (42). In these mdr2-deficient mice, progressive injury from the lack of buffering of bile salts leads to a progressive cholangiopathy and eventual hepatocellular tumor formation. The human counterpart is discussed below.

Canalicular Organic Anion Transporter

A multispecific organic anion transporter whose substrates include conjugated bilirubin, originally referred to as cMOAT, was initially characterized in enriched canalicular membrane preparations whose activity was enhanced by ATP hydrolysis (43). In humans, Dubin-Johnson syndrome is associated with persistent conjugated hyperbilirubinemia and retention of hepatic pigment without other manifestations of cholestatic liver injury, suggesting specific loss of cMOAT. These patients have a classical SBP-retention pattern in which a delayed regurgitation of SBP-conjugates in the serum occurs after initial clearance, indicating a deficiency in biliary efflux. Rodent models of this disease also exist, allowing for detailed analysis of bile composition (44). Mrp2, a member of the MRP subfamily of the ABC transporters, was shown to be responsible for bilirubin diglucuronide transport; mutation in the gene was found in both human and animal models of Dubin-Johnson syndrome (45). This 1545 amino acid protein is expressed predominantly in the apical domain of hepatocytes as well as the proximal tubule of the kidney and duodenum, and it is one of six mrp family members cloned to date (46). A peculiar feature of the animal models (TR^- and EHBR rats) is the lack of biliary GSH, indicating that mrp2 is essential for hepatic GSH excretion, a major contributor of bile salt independent bile flow (24).

Other members of the Mrp family are also implicated in having roles in the biliary excretion of organic anions. Mrp1 is minimally expressed in the rat liver but may be upregulated during cholestasis at the basolateral domain. Mrp3, which is located at the basolateral surface of hepatocytes, is upregulated in rats lacking mrp2, suggesting an alternative pathway for the elimination of organic anions across the basolateral surface (46). MRP3 is upregulated in patients with primary biliary cirrhosis as well, suggesting a compensatory pathway in response to chronic cholestasis (6). Mrp3 is able to transport bile acids and their sulfated and glucuronidated conjugates, which could provide another elimination route for retained bile salts in cholestatic disorders. Also, MRP3 is expressed on the basolateral aspect of human cholangiocytes where it might participate in cholehepatic shunting and provide another means for the elimination of bile salts in cholestatic conditions. In addition to the liver, mrp3 is extensively expressed in the small intestine.

Mrp4 is not expressed in the liver and mrp5 has low levels of expression in the liver. Mrp6 is well expressed in the liver and has been localized to the basolateral membrane and therefore may mediate efflux from the liver into the sinusoidal space during normal and cholestatic conditions. The substrates of mrp6 have not been characterized. Differential regulation of these family members during cholestasis with reduction of apical mrp2 expression and induction of Mrps located at the basolateral membrane provide alternative routes for efflux of biliary-excreted compounds from hepatocytes into blood, thereby protecting hepatocytes from toxic accumulation and allowing these substances to be excreted by the kidney.

FIC-1 P Type Aminophospholipid Transporter

Rare disorders of progressive familial intrahepatic cholestasis provide a unique opportunity to identify genes associated with bile formation by searching for shared chromosomal regions within selected affected populations. Linkage analysis of Byler disease in an Amish population and benign recurrent intrahepatic cholestasis in a small Dutch fishing village revealed that both these disorders shared the same chromosomal region at 18q21–22 (37). Subsequent identification of the FIC-1 gene at this locus and the discovery of mutations within it in both clinical syndromes reveal that both diseases are due to varying degrees of loss of activity of FIC-1 protein (33). This protein shares amino acid sequence identity with an amino-phospholipid P-type ATPase that mediates transfer of aminophospholipids from the outer to the inner leaflet of membranes similar to the flippase activity of MDR3. The protein is expressed in small intestine and pancreas with lower expression in the liver, which in the rat is limited to cholangiocytes. The mechanism by which the defect in this gene leads to impairment of bile formation is unknown, but its high level of expression in the intestine and the increased level of secondary bile salts in the serum of these patients suggest that intestinal malabsorption of bile salts may lead to secondary cholestasis due to production of cholestatic factors by intestinal bacteria.

REGULATION OF KEY HEPATIC TRANSPORTERS IN EXPERIMENTAL CHOLESTATIC CONDITIONS

Animal models have been developed to mimic the different types of clinical cholestatic syndromes that can occur with either sepsis, bile duct obstruction, or high estrogen levels as found in pregnancy (6). The response of the different transporters to each type of cholestatic injury will be reviewed and their potential consequences will be considered (Table 22.2).

Effect of Estrogens

High doses of circulating estrogens have been implicated in both intrahepatic cholestasis of pregnancy and oral contraceptive–associated cholestasis (47). Because the concentration of ethinyl estradiol, a synthetic estrogen, has been reduced in current oral contraceptive pills, this is now a rare cause of drug-induced cholestatic liver injury. However, intrahepatic cholestasis of pregnancy is likely to be due in part to high levels of circulating estrogen or their metabolites such as the estradiol 17β glucuronide (which is known to be cholestatic). Treatment with the synthetic estrogen ethinyl estradiol (EE) in rats has led to decreased bile flow and reduced excretion of organic anions, including bile salts and bilirubin, in the absence of any morphologic changes; this is referred to as bland cholestasis. Estrogen-induced cholestasis is complicated by multiple effects on membrane fluidity, expression and location of key transporters, as well as decreased enzymatic activity of the Na^+,K^+ ATPase, a key regulator for sodium-dependent co-transport processes. Increased permeability across tight junctions has also been implicated in contributing to cholestasis (47).

Estrogens affect transport activity at both sinusoidal and canalicular domain. Decreased ATP-dependent transport of organic anions and bile acids occurs in canalicular membranes from EE-treated animals. Decreased mrp2 and bsep protein expression in rats without alteration in mRNA levels was found after EE treatment, indicating a post-translational dysregulation (47,48). At the sinusoidal domain, decreased Na^+,K^+ ATPase activity was noted without any corresponding decrease in mRNA or protein levels, indicating a functional change in enzymatic activity that may be due to the secondary increase in membrane fluidity. Decreased sodium-dependent taurocholate uptake activity was associated with a progressive loss of both ntcp protein and gene expression as well as oatp1 protein and gene expression (6,9). These effects observed in the rats may mirror similar mechanisms that contribute to cholestasis of pregnancy in humans.

Effect of LPS/Endotoxin/Cytokines

Cholestasis associated with sepsis is a well-described clinical entity that can be reproduced in animal models by a single-dose administration of endotoxin, the lipopolysaccharide (LPS) component of the outer membrane of gram-negative bacteria. In rats treated with LPS, bile salt independent bile flow decreases with reduced expression of mrp2 in the canalicular membrane and slowly recovers after 3 to 4 days. Uptake of organic anions from the basolateral and canalicular membrane fractions isolated from LPS-treated animals are reduced without altered transport kinetics, indicating a decrease in total number of transporters (10,49). No changes in P-glycoprotein were found, indicating a selective down-regulation of the mrp2 canalicular transporter. Decreased expression of the ntcp protein and gene was also found,

Table 22.2. Regulation of hepatic transporters by cholestasis in rats

	LPS		Estrogen		BDO		TNFα	
Gene	mRNA	Protein	mRNA	Protein	mRNA	Protein	MRNA	Protein
ntcp	↓↓↓	↓↓↓	↓↓↓	↓↓	↓↓	↓↓↓	↓↓	↓↓
oatp1	nc	↓↓↓	↓↓↓	↓	↓↓	↓↓	nd	nd
bsep	↓↓	↓↓	nc	↓↓	↓↓	↓	nd	nd
mrp2	↓↓↓	↓↓↓	nc	↓↓↓	↓↓↓	↓↓↓	nd	nd
mrp3	nd	nd	nd	nd	↑↑↑	↑↑↑	nd	nd
Na^+, K^+ ATPase	nc*	nc*	nc	nc	nc*	nc*	nd	nd

* Alpha subunit of the Na^+,K^+ ATPase.
BDO = bile duct obstruction; nc = no change; nd = not determined.

Sources: Trauner M, Meier PJ, Boyer JL. Molecular regulation of hepatocellular transport systems in cholestasis. J Hepatol 1999;31:165–78; Kullak-Ublick GA. Regulation of organic anion and drug transporters of the sinusoidal membrane. J Hepatol 1999;31:563–73; Simon FR, Fortune J, Iwahashi M, et al. Ethinyl estradiol cholestasis involves alterations in expression of liver sinusoidal transporters. Am J Physiol 1996;271:G1043–52; Lee JM, Trauner M, Soroka CJ, et al. Expression of the bile salt export pump is maintained after chronic cholestasis in the rat. Gastroenterology 2000;118:163–72.

which is mediated by the proximal regulatory element in the ntcp gene.

Regulation of different transporters in response to LPS injection is mediated by cytokine response. Pretreatment of animals with steroids prior to LPS prevents reduction in mrp2 expression by decreasing the activation of the NF-kB pathway, a key regulator for the induction of cytokines. Treatment with anti-TNF (tumor necrosis factor) antibody also abrogates cholestatic response. Treatment with interleukin 1 (IL-1) or TNF-α can also mimic effects of LPS on ntcp gene expression, whereas IL-6 treatment leads to reduced taurocholate uptake by reduction of the Na^+,K^+ ATPase activity without affecting ntcp expression (49). Thus, specific cytokines can contribute to cholestasis by modulating different components of the normal excretory pathway and provide targets for future treatments for cholestatic disorders.

Effect of Bile Duct Obstruction

Animal models of acute bile duct obstruction mimic biliary tract obstructions due to stones, tumors, or stricture. In rats, acute obstruction of the common bile duct leads to retention of biliary content within the hepatocytes, further contributing to cholestatic syndrome (16). Accumulation of secondary, hydrophobic bile acid species can also reduce bile formation, increasing the cholestatic insult. Absence of bile salts in the intestinal lumen can also promote translocation of bacterial LPS. NTCP (14) gene expression is inversely correlated with serum bilirubin levels, suggesting that increased biliary content in the serum can downregulate gene expression. Downregulation of NTCP in this setting would protect the hepatocyte from further accumulation of toxic bile acids. Rat oatp1 is transiently downregulated in bile duct obstruction whereas oatp2 is unaffected. Rat lst-1, corresponding to human OATP2, is downregulated in bile duct obstruction. In contrast to the downregulation of ntcp and oatp1 in the rat, human OATP is upregulated in primary biliary cirrhosis (9). Canalicular transporters are differentially affected by cholestasis in humans. In canalicular-enriched membrane from obstructed rats, both mrp2 and, to a lesser extent, bsep have decreased protein expression which correlates with their mRNA levels (48).

CLINICAL APPROACHES TO INTRAHEPATIC CHOLESTASIS AND SPECIFIC CONDITIONS

Cholestatic disease clinically means hepatobiliary disease predominantly caused by and manifested by impaired bile secretion, usually without major liver destruction. Thus, acute and chronic viral hepatitis and alcoholic hepatitis and cirrhosis commonly cause jaundice; this undoubtedly represents failure of bile secretion, but occurs in the setting of marked parenchymal cell death (elevated ALT) and abnormal synthetic function (coagulopathy and low serum albumin). Cholestatic conditions typically are associated with increased serum bile acids, markedly abnormal serum alkaline phosphatase, and variable conjugated hyperbilirubinemia.

When bilirubin is normal to about 3 mg/dL, we refer to this as anicteric cholestasis; this is typical of primary biliary cirrhosis, primary sclerosing cholangitis, chronic pancreatitis–associated common bile duct stricture, and infiltrative diseases of the liver. Otherwise, when jaundice is present, it is referred to as icteric cholestasis. Because bile acids are the major solute that determines osmotic bile secretion, retention and elevation of bile acids in serum is a hallmark of cholestasis. Selective defects in bilirubin metabolism and transport, such as the MRP2-deficiency of Dubin-Johnson syndrome, cause noncholestatic jaundice, which is not accompanied by increased serum bile acids.

Conceptually, cholestasis can occur because of mechanical obstruction due to diseases of bile ducts: macroscopic extrahepatic ducts (stones, stricture, intrinsic or extrinsic neoplasms) or destruction of microscopic intrahepatic ducts (primary biliary cirrhosis, autoimmune cholangiopathy, sarcoidosis, drug-induced vanishing duct syndrome). Alternatively, cholestasis can occur at the level of the hepatocanaliculus as a result of a selective impairment in bile secretion, which is the focus of the rest of this chapter (Table 22.3).

The work-up of cholestasis is covered elsewhere in this volume (Chapters 3, 4, and 5). Suffice it to say that once extrahepatic duct obstruction has been excluded, one is working in the realm of intrahepatic cholestasis. In adults, a limited number of associated or causative conditions are pertinent, most of which will be obvious on clinical grounds: pregnancy, BRIC, sepsis, alcohol, postviral hepatitis, drugs, total parenteral nutrition, paraneoplastic syndrome, and amyloidosis, along with the vanishing duct diseases (e.g., primary biliary cirrhosis, sarcoid). From a diagnostic point of view, patients presenting with intrahepatic cholestasis should have blood cultures, viral hepatitis serology panel, serum mitochondrial antibody, and if there is suspicion of infiltrative processes, imaging of the liver and abdomen. It is important

Table 22.3. Intrahepatic cholestasis

Congenital/Inherited: PFIC 1, 2, 3
Benign recurrent intrahepatic cholestasis
Pregnancy
Sepsis
Viral hepatitis
Alcoholic fatty liver
Total parenteral nutrition
Lymphoma and paraneoplastic syndrome
Amyloidosis
Drug

Note: Exclusive of intrahepatic duct disease: PBC, sarcoid, cystic, PSC, autoimmune cholangiopathy.

to remember that neoplasms that infiltrate the liver can produce anicteric cholestasis but rarely cause jaundice.

Genetic Disorders Presenting with Cholestatic Syndrome

Rare genetic disorders of progressive familial intrahepatic cholestasis clearly demonstrate the key function of these transporters, and the clinical presentation of these disorders illustrates the loss of their activity. Subtle changes in functional activity of these key transporters lead to reduced but not absent activity; or the loss of a normal copy of the gene (heterozygous conditions) may be an important risk factor for development of cholestatic syndrome in response to clinical conditions such as sepsis or possibly drug-induced cholestatic liver injury.

Progressive familial intrahepatic cholestatic (PFIC) syndromes commonly present with distinctive pathological and laboratory features and a normal biliary anatomy during early childhood (2,50). Biliary atresia is the major cause of cholestasis in this age group, whereas PFIC syndromes represent a distinct minority. If untreated, these patients may develop progressive liver injury that will require transplantation. It is important to identify genetic disorders in the bile acid synthetic pathway, in which toxic accumulation of normal precursors occurs and are poorly transported by the canalicular transport system. Molecular identification of accumulated bile acid precursors by mass spectroscopy of the urine is highly effective at identifying these rare patients. The PFIC disorders have recently been classified by the identity of the specific genes mutated (Table 22.4), along with other disorders of the excretory pathway.

PFIC-1: Byler Syndrome/Disease

Byler disease, initially observed in descendants of the large Amish family of Jacob Byler, is characterized by recurrent episodes of jaundice that become persistent, accompanied by severe pruritus and elevated serum and reduced biliary levels of bile salts (51,52). Patients with this disease who are not direct descendants of Byler are referred to as having Byler syndrome. Byler patients have intermittent diarrhea and failure to develop due to fat malabsorption. A unique feature of these patients is that they have normal levels of serum gamma glutamyl transpeptidase, which differentiates this condition from other progressive cholestatic syndromes in children (50). Byler patients develop progressive liver disease within the first decade of life and require liver transplantation.

Benign Recurrent Intrahepatic Cholestasis

The diagnosis of BRIC should always be considered in patients who have recurrent episodes of cholestasis in the absence of bile duct obstruction, or infiltrative or chronic liver disease. Because mutations in the FIC-1 gene are found in both BRIC and PFIC-1, the severity of cholestatic liver disease reflects the relative activity of the FIC-1 transporter (33). Both BRIC and PFIC-1 are inherited as autosomal recessive diseases. BRIC initially presents in childhood or during early adolescence and recurs throughout adulthood. During cholestatic episodes, patients present with a 1- to 2-week prodrome of pruritus and anorexia before the onset of jaundice, which can last from 1 to 3 months and spontaneously resolves. Viral illness, pregnancy, or winter has been temporally associated with the onset of cholestatic episodes but often no precipitating event can be identified. Diets rich in fatty acids and oral contraceptives have also been implicated as precipitating factors. In between episodes, patients have a contracted bile acid pool, which is enriched with conjugates of secondary bile acids (53). Treatment with rifampin, cholestyramine, or ursodeoxycholate may hasten resolution of cholestatic episodes but not prevent their occurrences (50). Like PFIC-1 patients, BRIC patients have elevated serum alkaline phosphatase levels with normal serum gamma glutamyltranspeptidase levels, which differentiates BRIC from other cholestatic syndromes in adults. These recurrent cholestatic episodes do not cause chronic

Table 22.4. Hereditary disorders of liver transporters causing jaundice

Gene		Chromosome	Genetic Defect
Progressive familial intrahepatic cholestasis (PFIC)			
PFIC 1 (Byler disease)	FIC 1	18q21–22	Mutations in gene
PFIC 2	BSEP	2q24	Mutation in gene, absent protein
PFIC 3	MDR 3	7q21	Mutation in gene, absent protein
Benign recurrent intrahepatic cholestasis	FIC 1	18q21–22	Mutations in gene
Dubin-Johnson syndrome	MRP2	10q23–24	Mutation in gene, absent protein

Adapted from Trauner M, Meier PJ, Boyer JL. Molecular regulation of hepatocellular transport systems in cholestasis. J Hepatol 1999;31:165–78.

liver injury or fibrosis. In the future, genetic testing may be used to confirm the diagnosis of BRIC.

PFIC-2

PFIC-2 was originally identified in rare familial pediatric cholestatic disorders that presented with a serum chemistry similar to Byler disease but affected individuals lacked the commonly shared PFIC-1 region (54). These patients had a more aggressive cholestatic syndrome soon after birth with rapidly developing liver failure that required transplantation; they were unresponsive to ursodeoxycholate therapy (50). Linkage analysis revealed a shared chromosomal region in afflicted patients at position 2q24, the same location as the BSEP gene (37,38). Subsequent studies in these patients confirmed mutations in the BSEP gene leading to absence of protein expression (55). The absence of the characteristic elevation in the serum GGT levels in severe cholestasis and the minimal ductal injury observed in liver biopsies indicate that bile salts within the biliary tree are essential for the duct injuries associated with increased serum GGT levels.

PFIC-3

Patients who have a similar pattern of cholestatic liver disease as seen in PFIC-1 and -2 but have elevated serum GGT levels were recently shown to have mutations in both alleles of human MDR3 gene that mediates phospholipid flippase activity (50,56). These patients, as in the corresponding mdr2 knockout mice, have severe ductal injury due to lack of buffering of bile salts by phospholipids (42). Histologically, these patients have portal fibrosis with ductular proliferation and inflammatory infiltrate despite patency of the bile ducts. Clinically, these patients present at later stages than PFIC-1 and -2 patients and have more symptoms related to cirrhosis such as portal hypertension.

TPN-Associated Cholestatic Syndromes

Long-term total parenteral nutrition (TPN), especially in neonates, is associated with a nonobstructive cholestatic syndrome and can lead to liver failure. Correlation between incidence of cholestasis and TPN in adults is complicated by any underlying conditions and the different indications for TPN support (57,58). In adults, cholestasis is the predominant hepatic abnormality that occurs after TPN therapy lasting 3 weeks or longer; it presents as increased alkaline phosphatase levels, occasionally associated with serum bilirubin elevation. The liver biopsy typically reveals canalicular bile plugs in periportal or perivenous zones in combination with mild portal triaditis. The cholestasis is attributed to multiple etiological factors directly related to the TPN solution or to underlying clinical conditions. Increased uptake of amino acids by the liver in combination with decreased excretion of normal biliary constituents and steatosis secondary to the high carbohydrate concentration of the TPN solution are risk factors considered to be responsible for cholestasis. Lack of oral intake with loss of the normal enterohepatic circulation of bile salts is associated with a 10-fold increase in TPN-associated cholestasis. In these patients, greater production of cholestatic secondary bile acids is another factor. Patients with ileal dysfunction, such as with Crohn's disease, are also at greater risk, further indicating that the lack of a normal enterohepatic circulation is an important factor. Intercurrent sepsis is another risk factor and by itself may cause cholestasis as previously described.

Cessation of TPN leads to resolution of the cholestasis in most cases. Alternatively, reduction in carbohydrate content of TPN, treatment with oral antibiotics, and small enteral feeding to promote the enterohepatic circulation can be tried while closely monitoring cholestatic markers. In anecdotal case reports, ursodeoxycholic acid (UDCA) treatment has improved TPN-associated cholestasis.

It is important to recognize that these patients are also at increased risk for formation of biliary sludge and gallstones leading to cholecystitis and/or cholangitis that can present as right upper quadrant pain and fever associated with increased alkaline phosphatase levels and jaundice. Prompt recognition and imaging of the liver and biliary system is required to make the diagnosis and initiate treatment.

Cholestasis of Pregnancy

Intrahepatic cholestasis of pregnancy (ICP) is a rare disease of unknown cause which may be recurrent in 40% to 60% of cases (59). Patients typically present in the second half of their pregnancy initially with pruritus occasionally accompanied by jaundice which rapidly resolves in the postpartum period. Increased levels of serum bile acids (which is predominately conjugated cholic acid), bilirubin, and moderately increased alkaline phosphatase and GGT are found. No long-term sequelae have been noted for the mother, but the fetus is at increased risk of premature delivery, fetal distress, and perinatal mortality. In clinical studies, treatment with UDCA has been associated with improved fetal outcome (60).

These patients are also at risk for oral contraceptive–induced jaundice. The cause of the disease is unknown, but an increased incidence of ICP has been noted with multiparous women, who have higher estrogen levels; this suggests that a possible mechanism for this disorder lies in a defect in estrogen metabolism, leading to an increased production of the cholestatic estradiol 17β glucuronide. Interestingly, cholestasis of pregnancy was also observed in a heterozygote carrier of the MDR3 mutation, suggesting that heterozygote mutations in key hepatic transport genes may also be responsible for cholestasis of pregnancy (61).

Widely different rates of ICP are noted in different countries. Chile and Sweden have the highest rates, so genetic factors are clearly important. Recently, the incidence of ICP has decreased in both these countries.

Viral Hepatitis and Cholestatic Liver Disease

Jaundice with acute or chronic viral hepatitis is caused by the loss of the parenchymal function as a result of hepatocellular necrosis and/or fibrosis. Rarely, viral hepatitis may present with cholestasis as the predominant clinical feature and is most frequently found in adults with a hepatitis A virus (HAV) infection (62). Unlike children in whom HAV is often a subclinical and anicteric illness, adults can present with severe cholestatic syndrome mimicking chronic bile duct obstruction. Patients complain of pruritus, fever, diarrhea, and weight loss; the symptoms may last 1 to 4 months. A relapsing course can occur in which an initial apparent improvement that lasts 3 to 5 weeks with normal serum chemistries is followed by a recurrence of cholestatic serum markers and symptoms for an additional 4 to 6 weeks. Liver biopsies reveal intraductal cholestasis and portal tract inflammation associated with paucity of bile ducts.

In anecdotal case reports of HAV, treatment with oral prednisone decreased jaundice and improved cholestatic symptoms. This treatment is not recommended for other viral hepatitides. HAV in adults should always be considered in the differential diagnosis of intrahepatic cholestasis. Rarely, other causes of acute and chronic viral hepatitis can present with predominantly cholestatic features. Case reports of cholestasis accompanying chronic hepatitis C virus infection, acute cytomegalovirus in immunocompetent individuals, and Epstein-Barr virus infection have also been reported (63,64).

Cholestatic Syndrome with Ethanol

Occasionally, patients who have alcoholic liver disease may present with a cholestatic syndrome in the absence of cirrhosis or alcoholic hepatitis. Initial reports have associated alcoholic intrahepatic cholestasis with marked steatosis (65,66). Patients present with malaise, anorexia, and hepatomegaly with a cholestatic pattern of serum liver tests. Compared to patients presenting with alcoholic hepatitis, these patients tended to have poorer nutritional status, greater alcohol consumption, and a worse prognosis. Treatment consists of nutritional supplementation and supportive care after imaging of the liver to eliminate biliary obstruction or infiltrative disease. Chief histologic features of alcoholic cholestatic liver are macrovesicular fat with some microvesicular fat in centrolobular hepatocytes, portal tracts infiltrated with inflammatory cells, and proliferating bile ducts. Fibrosis extending from the portal tract into the liver acinus is routinely found without Mallory bodies and minimal focal necrosis. In one large Veteran's Administration cooperative study, the retrospective review of patients with cholestatic features on liver biopsy was associated with increased serum alkaline phosphatase levels and significantly decreased survival compared to patients without cholestatic features (67).

Sepsis-Associated Cholestatic Syndromes

Cholestatic liver disease accompanying systemic sepsis is a well-recognized clinical syndrome and is hypothesized to be caused by increased cytokine production. The development of jaundice with sepsis is a poor prognostic indicator because of the gravity of the underlying infection. Cholestatic liver disease can be caused by fungal infections and gram-positive and gram-negative bacterial infections. Sepsis is the predominant clinical feature in these patients, who do not complain of right upper quadrant pain or pruritus. The levels of serum alkaline phosphatase are routinely elevated (but only mildly) with conjugated hyperbilirubinemia occurring to a variable degree. Occasionally, 10-fold or greater increased serum alkaline phosphatase levels in the absence of jaundice have been reported (68). In one study, cholestasis and increasing hyperbilirubinemia were associated with multi-system failure and increased mortality (69).

No specific therapy for the cholestasis is necessary in these patients after excluding the liver or biliary system as the site of infection; cholestasis resolves with treatment of the underlying infection. Jaundice without increased alkaline phosphatase levels may be a herald of impending sepsis (70). Liver biopsies in patients with cholestasis associated with severe sepsis reveal inspissated bile with dilated and proliferating portal and periportal bile ductules. Cholestasis has also been reported in toxic shock syndrome, accompanied by increased levels of serum bile acids, mild transaminases, and hypoalbuminemia.

Paraneoplastic Cholestasis

Cytokines play a key role in mediating cholestasis associated with sepsis. Increased cytokine production associated with neoplastic diseases is now presumed to be responsible for rare cholestatic disorders associated with malignancy in which there is no bile duct obstruction or infiltration of the liver parenchyma. Anecdotal case reports of patients with Hodgkin's disease and other lymphomas have noted an increase in alkaline phosphatase and bilirubin levels in the absence of infiltrative disease (71). Stauffer's syndrome, a paraneoplastic syndrome associated with renal cell carcinoma which presents with cholestasis, fever, increased acute phase reactants and anemia, is associated with increased serum IL-6 levels. Experimental treatment with anti-IL-6 antiserum in these patients leads to a temporary decrease in alkaline phosphatase; they return to their elevated levels after cessation of treatment, indicating that IL-6 was responsible for cholestasis (72). Patients treated with IL-2 were also found to develop reversible cholestasis, as evidenced by increased levels of serum bile acids, bilirubin, and alkaline phosphatase, all of which returned to normal after completion of treatment (73). It is likely that excess cytokines are also responsible for other paraneoplastic cholestatic syndromes.

Amyloidosis

Although amyloid infiltrates are commonly found in the liver, patients rarely present with jaundice. Hepatomegaly associated with amyloid has been attributed to the associated congestive heart failure and not the liver infiltration. Rarely, amyloidosis may initially present as intrahepatic cholestasis (74). Histologically, these patients present with perisinusoidal deposition of amyloid paralleled by advanced hepatocellular atrophy with varying degrees of bile stasis. Patients with amyloidosis exhibit low serum gamma globulin levels in contrast to elevated serum globulin levels found in chronic liver disease.

Drug-Induced Cholestasis

A wide variety of drugs can cause cholestatic liver disease. Aside from the bland cholestasis (no inflammation) seen with androgens and estrogens, which probably occurs in individuals with a genetic predisposition to cholestasis, drug-induced cholestasis tends to exhibit portal tract inflammation and bile duct injury along with variable parenchymal inflammation and necrosis/apoptosis. Indeed, many of the drugs that induce clinical cholestasis with jaundice, pruritus, and marked increased alkaline phosphatase levels also are associated with moderate to marked parenchymal destruction as reflected in elevated alanine aminotransferase (ALT). Thus, the same drug in some individuals will produce predominantly cholestasis, but in others mixed cholestasis/hepatitis, and in some predominantly hepatitis (75). Table 22.5 lists drugs that either usually produce predominantly cholestasis or most often produce cholestasis but with variable and sometimes predominant hepatitis. The jaundice in this condition tends to resolve very slowly after discontinuing the drug, sometimes lasting for months and even evolving into a vanishing duct/biliary cirrhosis condition (Table 22.6).

A very high proportion of the drugs that produce clinical cholestatic disease seem to do so on an immunoallergic basis; this is based on early onset in the first few weeks of therapy and the concomitant appearance of fever, rash, eosinophilia, and in some instances positive rechallenge. In some instances the drugs—for example, antibiotics such as erythromycins or Augmentin—may be given for a course of 1 to 2 weeks and the cholestatic syndrome appears up to 3 to 4 weeks after discontinuing the drug.

Whether or not features of allergy are present, the pathophysiology is uncertain. However, the target of many of

Table 22.5. Some drugs that can lead to cholestasis

Cholestatic Injury Characteristic	Cholestatic or Hepatocellular Injury
Ajmaline	Allopurinol
Amoxicillin-clavulanate	Antidepressants (Tricyclic, tetracyclic)
Anabolic steroids	Captopril
Benoxaprofen	Carbamazepine
Benzodiazepines	Cimetidine
Butyrophenones	Clozapine
Carbimazole	Droxicam
Cloxacillin	Enalapril
Cyproheptadine	Fluconazole
D-Proxaphene	Gold compounds
Danazol	Hydralazine
Dicloxacillin	Itraconazole
Erythromycins	Ketoconazole
Flucloxacillin	Naproxen
Griseofulvin	Nitrofurantoin
Methimazole	Phenylbutazone
Oral contraceptives	Phenytoin
Penicillamine	Piroxicam
Phenothiazines	Ranitidine
Sulfonylureas (most)	Sulfonamides
Thiabendazole	Sulfamethoxazole-trimethoprim
Thioxanthines	Sulindac
Ticlopidine	Zidovudine
Troleandomycin	
Xenalamine	

Reprinted with permission from Zimmerman HJ, ed. Hepatotoxicity: the adverse effects of drugs and other chemicals on the liver. Philadelphia: Lippincott Williams & Wilkins, 1999.

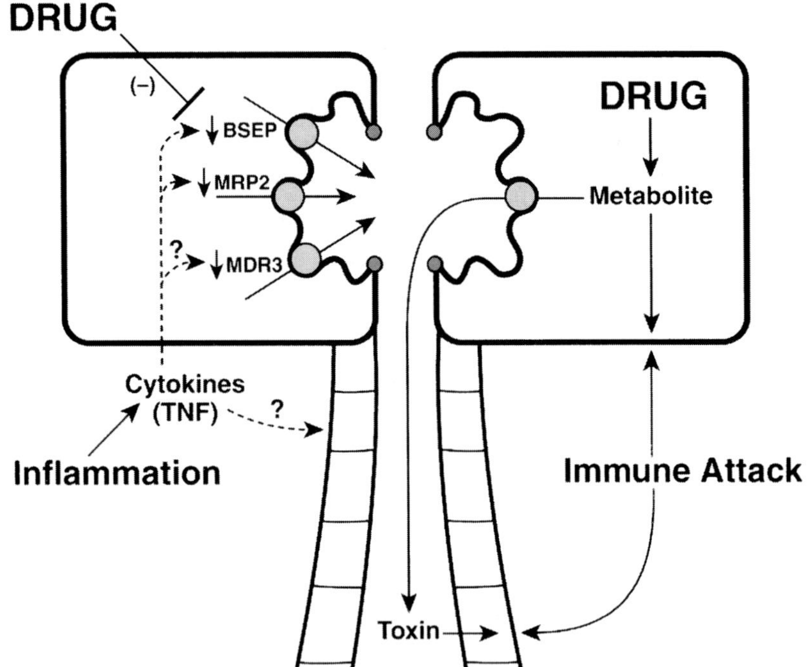

FIGURE 22.2. *Pathogenesis of drug-induced cholestasis. Drugs can inhibit canalicular BSEP (e.g., cyclosporin A, rifampicin), be converted to toxic metabolites that might elicit an immune response directed at hepatocytes or bile ducts (via secretion), or an associated inflammatory response that might lead to cytokine-mediated downregulation of hepatocyte export pumps.*

Table 22.6. Drugs incriminated in chronic cholestasis

Aceprometazine (with meprobamate)	Erythromycins
Ajmaline and related drugs	Estradiol
Amineptine	Flucloxacillin
Amitriptyline	Glycyrrhiza
Amoxicillin-clavulanic acid	Haloperidol
Ampicillin	Imipramine
Arsenicals, organic	Methyltestosterone
Azathioprine	Norethandrolone
Barbiturates	Phenytoin
Carbamazepine	Prochlorperazine
Carbutamide	Sulfamethoxazole-trimethoprim
Chlorothiazide	Terbinafine
Chlorpromazine	Tetracycline
Cimetidine	Thiabendazole
Clindamycin	Ticlopidine
Cyamemazine	Tiopronin
Cyclohexylpropionate	Troleandomycin
Cyproheptadine	Xenalamine

Reprinted with permission from Zimmerman HJ, ed. Hepatotoxicity: the adverse effects of drugs and other chemicals on the liver. Philadelphia: Lippincott Williams & Wilkins, 1999.

these immunologic reactions appears on circumstantial evidence to be the bile ductules, which are often associated with inflammation and not infrequently with progressive destruction (Fig. 22.2). However, parenchymal inflammation and cytokines may contribute by downregulating the various hepatic transporters leading to impaired bile acid and organic anion secretion. In theory, this could be more likely to be clinically manifest in patients with a genetic predisposition, such as heterozygotes for defects in the transporters. This might account for many of the drugs commonly inducing mild anicteric liver test abnormalities but rarely causing overt liver disease. In addition, BSEP-mediated bile acid transport is competitively inhibited by cyclosporin A (76–78), rifamycin SV, and rifampicin, glibenclamide, whereas only cyclosporine among this group inhibits MRP2 (78). Sulindac also inhibits canalicular bile acid transport (79). Interestingly ethinylestradiol-17β-glucuronide is secreted into bile by MRP2 and then transinhibits BSEP (78). Another intriguing possibility with limited proof is that toxic but stable metabolites of certain drugs, which are secreted into bile, exert toxic effects on the bile duct system.

SUGGESTED READINGS

Jacquemin E, Hadchouel M. Genetic basis of progressive familial intrahepatic cholestasis. J Hepatol 1999;31:377–81. This is an up-to-date and concise review of the clinical features of progressive familial cholestatic syndromes, which have recently been classified by the identification of mutations in key canalicular and hepatic transporters. This review is recommended as an initial introduction to the molecular classification of this rapidly advancing field and as a good preparation for a review of the original literature.

Trauner M, Meier PJ, Boyer JL. Molecular regulation of hepatocellular transport systems in cholestasis. J Hepatol 1999;31:165–78. Excellent review of the current understanding of bile formation and the features of hepatic transporters and their regulation in human and animal models of cholestatic liver disease. The material presented in this review article provides detailed and current knowledge about the principal membrane transporters required for bile formation and their regulation in whole animals and cell culture systems. This article is suggested for those readers who want an introduction to this area or are interested in the basic biology of these membrane transporters.

REFERENCES

1. Arias IM, Che M, Gatmaitan Z, et al. The biology of the bile canaliculus, 1993. Hepatology 1993;17:318–29.

2. Bahar RJ, Stolz A. Bile acid transport. Gastroenterol Clin North Am 1999;28: 27–58.
3. Muller M, Jansen PL. Molecular aspects of hepatobiliary transport. Am J Physiol 1997;272:G1285–303.
4. Meier PJ. Molecular mechanisms of hepatic bile salt transport from sinusoidal blood into bile. Am J Physiol 1995;269:G801–12.
5. Ballatori N, Truong AT. Glutathione as a primary osmotic driving force in hepatic bile formation. Am J Physiol 1992;263:G617–24.
6. Trauner M, Meier PJ, Boyer JL. Molecular regulation of hepatocellular transport systems in cholestasis. J Hepatol 1999;31:165–78.
7. Hofmann AF. Current concepts of biliary secretion. Dig Dis Sci 1989;34(suppl 12):S16–20.
8. Koopen NR, Muller M, Vonk RJ, et al. Molecular mechanisms of cholestasis: causes and consequences of impaired bile formation. Biochim Biophys Acta 1998;1408:1–17.
9. Kullak-Ublick GA. Regulation of organic anion and drug transporters of the sinusoidal membrane. J Hepatol 1999;31:563–73.
10. Gartung C, Matern S. Molecular regulation of sinusoidal liver bile acid transporters during cholestasis. Yale J Biol Med 1997;70:355–63.
11. Carey MC, Duane WC. Enterohepatic circulation. In: Arias IM, Boyer JL, Fausto N, et al., eds. The liver: biology and pathobiology. 3rd ed. New York: Raven Press, 1994:719–67.
12. Hagenbuch B, Stieger B, Foguet M, et al. Functional expression cloning and characterization of the hepatocyte Na^+/bile acid cotransport system. Proc Natl Acad Sci U S A 1991;88:10629–33.
13. Mukhopadhayay S, Ananthanarayanan M, Stieger B, et al. cAMP increases liver Na^+-taurocholate cotransport by translocating transporter to plasma membranes. Am J Physiol 1997;273:G842–8.
14. Shneider BL, Fox VL, Schwarz KB, et al. Hepatic basolateral sodium-dependent-bile acid transporter expression in two unusual cases of hypercholanemia and in extrahepatic biliary atresia. Hepatology 1997;25:1176–83.
15. Ganguly TC, Liu Y, Hyde JF, et al. Prolactin increases hepatic Na^+/taurocholate co-transport activity and messenger RNA post partum. Biochem J 1994;303: 33–6.
16. Gartung C, Schuele S, Schlosser SF, Boyer JL. Expression of the rat liver Na^+/taurocholate cotransporter is regulated in vivo by retention of biliary constituents but not their depletion. Hepatology 1997;25:284–90.
17. Hagenbuch B, Meier PJ. Molecular cloning, chromosomal localization, and functional characterization of a human liver Na^+/bile acid cotransporter. J Clin Invest 1994;93:1326–31.
18. Wong MH, Oelkers P, Craddock AL, Dawson PA. Expression cloning and characterization of the hamster ileal sodium-dependent bile acid transporter. J Biol Chem 1994;269:1340–7.
19. Lazaridis KN, Pham L, Tietz P, et al. Rat cholangiocytes absorb bile acids at their apical domain via the ileal sodium-dependent bile acid transporter. J Clin Invest 1997;100:2714–21.
20. Christie DM, Dawson PA, Thevananther S, Shneider BL. Comparative analysis of the ontogeny of a sodium-dependent bile acid transporter in rat kidney and ileum. Am J Physiol 1996;271:G377–85.
21. von Dippe P, Amoui M, Stellwagen RH, Levy D. The functional expression of sodium-dependent bile acid transport in Madin-Darby canine kidney cells transfected with the cDNA for microsomal epoxide hydrolase. J Biol Chem 1996;271:18176–80.
22. Jacquemin E, Hagenbuch B, Stieger B, et al. Expression cloning of a rat liver Na^+-independent organic anion transporter. Proc Natl Acad Sci U S A 1994; 91:133–7.
23. Satlin LM, Amin V, Wolkoff AW. Organic anion transporting polypeptide mediates organic anion/HCO_3^- exchange. J Biol Chem 1997;272:26340–5.
24. Ballatori N, Rebbeor JF. Roles of MRP2 and oatp1 in hepatocellular export of reduced glutathione. Semin Liver Dis 1998;18:377–87.
25. Meier PJ, Eckhardt U, Schroeder A, et al. Substrate specificity of sinusoidal bile acid and organic anion uptake systems in rat and human liver. Hepatology 1997;26:1667–77.
26. Reichel C, Gao B, Van Montfoort J, et al. Localization and function of the organic anion-transporting polypeptide Oatp2 in rat liver. Gastroenterology 1999;117:688–95.
27. Hsiang B, Zhu Y, Wang Z, et al. A novel human hepatic organic anion transporting polypeptide (OATP2). Identification of a liver-specific human organic anion transporting polypeptide and identification of rat and human hydroxymethylglutaryl-CoA reductase inhibitor transporters. J Biol Chem 1999;274:37161–8.
28. Abe T, Kakyo M, Tokui T, et al. Identification of a novel gene family encoding human liver-specific organic anion transporter LST-1. J Biol Chem 1999;274: 17159–63.
29. Erlinger S. Do intracellular organelles have any role in transport of bile acids by hepatocytes? J Hepatol 1996;24(suppl 1):88–93.
30. Cohen DE. Hepatocellular transport and secretion of biliary phospholipids. Semin Liver Dis 1996;16:191–200.
31. El-Seaidy AZ, Mills CO, Elias E, Crawford JM. Lack of evidence for vesicle trafficking of fluorescent bile salts in rat hepatocyte couplets. Am J Physiol 1997;272:G298–309.
32. Dean M, Allikmets R. Evolution of ATP-binding cassette transporter genes. Curr Opin Genet Dev 1995;5:779–85.
33. Bull LN, van Eijk MJ, Pawlikowska L, et al. A gene encoding a P-type ATPase mutated in two forms of hereditary cholestasis. Nature Genet 1998;18:219–24.
34. Suchy FJ, Sippel CJ, Ananthanarayanan M. Bile acid transport across the hepatocyte canalicular membrane. FASEB J 1997;11:199–205.
35. Lomri N, Fitz JG, Scharschmidt BF. Hepatocellular transport: role of ATP-binding cassette proteins. Semin Liver Dis 1996;16:201–10.
36. Gerloff T, Stieger B, Hagenbuch B, et al. The sister of P-glycoprotein represents the canalicular bile salt export pump of mammalian liver. J Biol Chem 1998; 273:10046–50.
37. Strautnieks SS, Kagalwalla AF, Tanner MS, et al. Identification of a locus for progressive familial intrahepatic cholestasis PFIC2 on chromosome 2q24. Am J Hum Genet 1997;61:630–3.
38. Strautnieks SS, Bull LN, Knisely AS, et al. A gene encoding a liver-specific ABC transporter is mutated in progressive familial intrahepatic cholestasis. Nat Genet 1998;20:233–8.
39. Gatmaitan ZC, Nies AT, Arias IM. Regulation and translocation of ATP-dependent apical membrane proteins in rat liver. Am J Physiol 1997;272: G1041–9.
40. Misra S, Ujhazy P, Varticovski L, Arias IM. Phosphoinositide 3-kinase lipid products regulate ATP-dependent transport by sister of P-glycoprotein and multidrug resistance associated protein 2 in bile canalicular membrane vesicles. Proc Natl Acad Sci U S A 1999;96:5814–9.
41. Smit JJ, Schinkel AH, Oude Elferink RP, et al. Homozygous disruption of the murine mdr2 P-glycoprotein gene leads to a complete absence of phospholipid from bile and to liver disease. Cell 1993;75:451–62.
42. Mauad TH, van Nieuwkerk CM, Dingemans KP, et al. Mice with homozygous disruption of the mdr2 P-glycoprotein gene. A novel animal model for studies of nonsuppurative inflammatory cholangitis and hepatocarcinogenesis. Am J Pathol 1994;145:1237–45.
43. Oude Elferink RP, Bakker CT, Roelofsen H, et al. Accumulation of organic anion in intracellular vesicles of cultured rat hepatocytes is mediated by the canalicular multispecific organic anion transporter. Hepatology 1993;17:434–44.
44. Jansen PL, Groothuis GM, Peters WH, Meijer DF. Selective hepatobiliary transport defect for organic anions and neutral steroids in mutant rats with hereditary-conjugated hyperbilirubinemia. Hepatology 1987;7:71–6.
45. Paulusma CC, Bosma PJ, Zaman GJ, et al. Congenital jaundice in rats with a mutation in a multidrug resistance-associated protein gene. Science 1996;271: 1126–8.
46. Borst P, Evers R, Kool M, Wijnholds J. The multidrug resistance protein family. Biochim Biophys Acta 1999;1461:347–57.
47. Simon FR, Fortune J, Iwahashi M, et al. Ethinyl estradiol cholestasis involves alterations in expression of liver sinusoidal transporters. Am J Physiol 1996;271: G1043–52.
48. Lee JM, Trauner M, Soroka CJ, et al. Expression of the bile salt export pump is maintained after chronic cholestasis in the rat. Gastroenterology 2000;118: 163–72.
49. Green RM, Beier D, Gollan JL. Regulation of hepatocyte bile salt transporters by endotoxin and inflammatory cytokines in rodents. Gastroenterology 1996;111:193–8.
50. Jacquemin E, Hadchouel M. Genetic basis of progressive familial intrahepatic cholestasis. J Hepatol 1999;31:377–81.
51. Clayton RJ, Iber FL, Ruebner BH, McKusick VA. Byler disease. Fatal familial intrahepatic cholestasis in an Amish kindred. Am J Dis Child 1969;117:112–24.
52. Jacquemin E, Dumont M, Bernard O, et al. Evidence for defective primary bile acid secretion in children with progressive familial intrahepatic cholestasis (Byler disease). Eur J Pediatr 1994;153:424–8.
53. Bijleveld CM, Vonk RJ, Kuipers F, et al. Benign recurrent intrahepatic cholestasis: altered bile acid metabolism. Gastroenterology 1989;97:427–32.
54. Kagalwalla AF, Al Amir AR, Khalifa A, et al. Progressive familial intrahepatic cholestasis (Byler's disease) in Arab children. Ann Trop Paediatr 1995;15:321–7.
55. Jansen PL, Strautnieks SS, Jacquemin E, et al. Hepatocanalicular bile salt export pump deficiency in patients with progressive familial intrahepatic cholestasis. Gastroenterology 1999;117:1370–9.
56. de Vree JM, Jacquemin E, Sturm E, et al. Mutations in the MDR3 gene cause progressive familial intrahepatic cholestasis. Proc Natl Acad Sci U S A 1998;95: 282–7.

57. Fein BI, Holt PR. Hepatobiliary complications of total parenteral nutrition. J Clin Gastroenterol 1994;18:62–6.
58. Quigley EM, Marsh MN, Shaffer JL, Markin RS. Hepatobiliary complications of total parenteral nutrition. Gastroenterology 1993;104:286–301.
59. Reyes H, Simon FR. Intrahepatic cholestasis of pregnancy: an estrogen-related disease. Semin Liver Dis 1993;13:289–301.
60. Palma J, Reyes H, Ribalta J, et al. Ursodeoxycholic acid in the treatment of cholestasis of pregnancy: a randomized, double-blind study controlled with placebo. J Hepatol 1997;27:1022–8.
61. Jacquemin E, Cresteil D, Manouvrier S, et al. Heterozygous non-sense mutation of the MDR3 gene in familial intrahepatic cholestasis of pregnancy Lancet 1999;353:210–1.
62. Schiff ER. Atypical clinical manifestations of hepatitis A. Vaccine 1992;10(suppl 1):S18–20.
63. Edoute Y, Baruch Y, Lachter J, et al. Severe cholestatic jaundice induced by Epstein-Barr virus infection in the elderly. J Gastroenterol Hepatol 1998;13: 821–4.
64. Serna-Higuera C, Gonzalez-Garcia M, Milicua JM, Munoz V. Acute cholestatic hepatitis by cytomegalovirus in an immunocompetent patient resolved with ganciclovir. J Clin Gastroenterol 1999;29:276–7.
65. Glover SC, McPhie JL, Brunt PW. Cholestasis in acute alcoholic liver disease. Lancet 1977;2:1305–7.
66. Morgan MY, Sherlock S, Scheuer PJ. Acute cholestasis, hepatic failure, and fatty liver in the alcoholic. Scand J Gastroenterol 1978;13:299–303.
67. Nissenbaum M, Chedid A, Mendenhall C, Gartside P. Prognostic significance of cholestatic alcoholic hepatitis. VA Cooperative Study Group #119. Dig Dis Sci 1990;35:891–6.
68. Maldonado O, Demasi R, Maldonado Y, et al. Extremely high levels of alkaline phosphatase in hospitalized patients. J Clin Gastroenterol 1998;27:342–5.
69. te Boekhorst T, Urlus M, Doesburg W, et al. Etiologic factors of jaundice in severely ill patients. A retrospective study in patients admitted to an intensive care unit with severe trauma or with septic intra-abdominal complications following surgery and without evidence of bile duct obstruction. J Hepatol 1988;7:111–7.
70. Franson TR, Hierholzer WJ Jr, LaBrecque DR. Frequency and characteristics of hyperbilirubinemia associated with bacteremia. Rev Infect Dis 1985;7:1–9.
71. Watterson J, Priest JR. Jaundice as a paraneoplastic phenomenon in a T-cell lymphoma. Gastroenterology 1989;97:1319–22.
72. Blay JY, Rossi JF, Wijdenes J, et al. Role of interleukin-6 in the paraneoplastic inflammatory syndrome associated with renal-cell carcinoma. Int J Cancer 1997;72:424–30.
73. Fisher B, Keenan AM, Garra BS, et al. Interleukin-2 induces profound reversible cholestasis: a detailed analysis in treated cancer patients. J Clin Oncol 1989;7:1852–62.
74. Peters RA, Koukoulis G, Gimson A, et al. Primary amyloidosis and severe intrahepatic cholestatic jaundice. Gut 1994;35:1322–5.
75. Zimmerman HJ, ed. Hepatotoxicity: the adverse effects of drugs and other chemicals on the liver. Philadelphia: Lippincott Williams & Wilkins, 1999.
76. Kassianides C, Nussenblatt R, Palestine AG, et al. Liver injury from cyclosporine A. Dig Dis Sci 1990;35:693–7.
77. Klintmalm GBG, Iwatsuki S, Starzl TE. Cyclosporin A hepatotoxicity in 66 renal allograft recipients. Transplantation 1981;32:488–9.
78. Stieger B, Fattinger K, Madon J. Drug- and estrogen-induced cholestasis through inhibition of the hepatocellular bile salt export pump (Bsep) of rat liver. Gastroenterology 2000;118:422–30.
79. Bolder U, Trang NV, Hagey LR. Sulindac is excreted into bile by a canalicular bile salt pump and undergoes a cholehepatic circulation in rats. Gastroenterology 1999;117:962–71.

Chapter 23

Biliary Diseases in Infants and Children

William R. Treem   Michael A. Skinner

Biliary disease is found less commonly in infants and children compared to adults. However, cholestasis and direct hyperbilirubinemia are quite common manifestations of liver and systemic diseases in neonates and infants. Almost any insult affecting the liver of the infant will result in neonatal cholestasis, jaundice, liver enzyme elevations, and biliary stasis. Systemic infections, fasting, the use of parenteral nutrition, ischemia, and many drugs commonly used to treat infants will provoke bile canalicular injury, decreased bile flow, and cholestasis. In addition, there are specific inherited genetic syndromes and inborn errors of metabolism that are unique to infants and children and can profoundly affect biliary function from the level of the canalicular membrane to the level of the common bile duct. Defects affecting the synthesis and transport of bile acids or the development of the interlobular bile ducts and small intrahepatic ductules can inhibit bile flow just as profoundly as lesions resulting in the obstruction of extrahepatic bile ducts. In other words, shutting off the faucet can produce as marked an effect as kinking the hose.

Thus, the clinician is faced with a special challenge when confronted with a young patient who exhibits direct hyperbilirubinemia and other signs of cholestatic jaundice. A decision must be made whether the patient has intrahepatic or extrahepatic cholestatic disease. This branch point in the decision tree must be reached rapidly because extrahepatic obstruction can have devastating effects on the infant's liver if not quickly relieved. As some of the most common causes of biliary disease in adults such as cholelithiasis, cholecystitis, sclerosing cholangitis, and primary biliary cirrhosis are less prevalent in children, a knowledge of the unique infectious, immunologic, metabolic, and genetic syndromes affecting biliary secretion in the pediatric liver is essential to construct a differential diagnosis. This chapter reviews both extrahepatic and intrahepatic biliary disease affecting the infant and the older child. It will emphasize diseases and syndromes unique to the pediatric population, and also discuss the differences in presentation, natural history, and management of those entities that affect both children and adults.

BILIARY DISEASES IN NEONATES AND INFANTS

Biliary Atresia

Biliary atresia is a condition in which there is idiopathic obliteration or progressive destruction of the extrahepatic bile ducts. The disease occurs in approximately 1 in 10,000 live births worldwide, with about 400 to 600 new cases diagnosed in the United States each year. In one population-based study, the incidence of biliary atresia was significantly higher in nonwhite infants compared with white infants (1). The condition is the most common cause of chronic cholestasis in infancy, and is the most frequent etiology of chronic liver failure requiring liver transplant in childhood (2). Because early surgical treatment is associated with improved outcome, it is critical that the diagnosis of biliary atresia be established as early as possible.

Pathology and Etiology

The etiology and pathogenesis of biliary atresia are unknown. The condition is characterized by an inflammatory and fibrosing process of the extrahepatic biliary tract leading to segmental or total duct luminal closure. In untreated patients, there is cholestasis and progressive liver failure ultimately resulting in hepatic cirrhosis. Characteristic histopathologic findings in the liver include ductular proliferation, canalicular and cellular bile stasis, and perilobular or portal fibrosis. It is thought that the clinical course and pathologic findings may represent a final pathway resulting from at least several different inciting factors.

There are apparently two distinct clinical varieties of biliary atresia (3). The *embryonic* form is characterized by an early onset of neonatal jaundice with no recovery after the period of expected physiologic jaundice, and is associated with congenital anomalies in about 10% to 20% of cases. The most common associated anomalies include abnormalities in the gastrointestinal and cardiac systems. In a smaller group of patients, there are findings associated with the heterotaxia syndromes such as polysplenia, asplenia, intestinal malrotation, *situs inversus*, and cardiac defects (4). The *perinatal* form of biliary atresia occurs in about two-thirds of cases, and is usually associated with a transient jaundice-free period after the recovery of the infant from physiologic jaundice. There are usually no associated congenital anomalies. Often, some remnants of the extrahepatic biliary tree persist in the perinatal form of the disease, but are not present with the embryonic form of biliary atresia. The two subtypes of biliary atresia are thought to differ pathophysiologically. The embryonal form is postulated to result from a process starting in utero, whereas the perinatal variety is thought to result from some postnatal insult.

The proposed etiologic mechanisms for biliary atresia are listed in Table 23.1. There is a paucity of precise information regarding the molecular mechanisms responsible for the syndrome. In general, it is thought that there is some inciting event that injures the bile ducts and initiates acute and chronic inflammation preceding the development of periductular fibrosis and luminal obliteration (2). Then there is the release of inflammatory mediators and cytokines by the bile duct epithelial cells and neighboring dendritic cells to amplify the inflammation and deposition of collagen, ultimately inducing cirrhosis. It is likely that the local leakage of toxic bile acids, resulting from the initial duct injury and subsequent obstruction, further contributes to hepatocyte injury and liver failure (5). Thus, the whole process results from a complex interchange between some initial insult to the extrahepatic biliary tree and the subsequent inflammatory process. The relative contributions of the initiating factor and the inflammatory response to the development of biliary atresia remain elusive.

The occasional clustering of biliary atresia cases supports an infectious etiology for the disease, and viral etiologies have been sought in a number of studies. Reovirus has been implicated by the finding of serologic reactivity to reovirus type 3 in a subset of patients, and reovirus-like particles have been found in the porta hepatis of at least one affected child (6). Subsequent studies have disputed whether reovirus is implicated in human biliary atresia (7). In a more recent report, the prevalence of cytomegalovirus infection was significantly higher in infants with biliary atresia than nonaffected infants (8). Another study described the finding of group C rotaviral RNA in 10 of 20 children with biliary atresia, but in none of 12 infants with cholestatic jaundice of other etiologies (9). Although time-space clustering of biliary atresia may also be consistent with some toxic exposure causing the disease, no evidence for a toxic etiology exists.

Table 23.1. Proposed etiologies of biliary atresia

Viral infection
Toxin exposure
Developmental defect
Immunological defect
Abnormal fetal biliary circulation

There are several lines of evidence suggesting that host/genetic factors play a role in the development of biliary atresia. For example, there are rare reports of the disease occurring in siblings. Moreover, the coincidence of biliary atresia and other anatomic anomalies in the neonatal form of the disease suggests that there may be an underlying abnormality in biliary system development. It has been postulated that in some cases biliary atresia may result in an arrest in the normal process of embryonic ductal remodeling, which is essential for the development of patent ducts (10). The primary maldevelopment of bile ducts as an etiology of biliary atresia is further supported by the existence of a transgenic mouse model in which there is the coincidence of situs inversus with bile duct abnormalities reminiscent of biliary atresia (11). Finally, there are probably cases in which the final destruction of the bile ducts responsible for phenotypic biliary atresia is caused by an abnormal immune response to some initial injury to the ducts. There is an increased incidence of biliary atresia in children having certain HLA types, suggesting that idiosyncratic factors in the immune system may play a pathogenetic role in the disease (12). Although, the cause of biliary atresia remains elusive, it is likely that there are a number of conditions in which a combination of environmental, infectious, inflammatory, and host immune factors result in the maldevelopment or destruction of the bile ducts, resulting in phenotypic biliary atresia.

Clinical Manifestations and Diagnosis

The patient must be diagnosed with biliary atresia as early as possible to allow early surgical reestablishment of biliary drainage before there is irreversible sclerosis of the intrahepatic bile ducts (13). Unfortunately, it is often difficult to unequivocally diagnose biliary atresia noninvasively because the clinical and laboratory findings are nonspecific. In general, the diagnosis should be excluded in any child who is jaundiced after the age of 14 days. Clinical findings at presentation include scleral icterus, hepatosplenomegaly, and acholic stools. In the first 3 months of life, infants with biliary atresia usually maintain adequate nutrition and weight gain. Later in the course of untreated biliary atresia, evidence of portal hypertension may be seen. Biochemical evidence of conjugated hyperbilirubinemia is present, and owing to synthetic liver disease or poor absorption of fat-soluble vitamins, a coagulopathy may be present. It should be emphasized that physical and laboratory findings are non-specific for establishing the exact cause of cholestatic jaundice in the newborn.

Several diagnostic studies must be performed to exclude biliary atresia. A suggested diagnostic schema is listed in Table 23.2. Abdominal ultrasound in infants with biliary atresia will usually demonstrate an absent or contracted gallbladder with no dilatation of the bile ducts. In some cases, polysplenia may be recognized. Because intrahepatic causes of cholestasis will demonstrate similar ultrasonographic findings, the sensitivity of ultrasound for biliary atresia is only about 85%, and the specificity is less than 80%. Cholescintigraphy (DISIDA scan) can exclude biliary atresia if there is unequivocal excretion of the radionuclide in the intestine. However, the absence of excretion does not prove the diagnosis; patients with intrahepatic cholestatic syndromes will also fail to reliably absorb and excrete the radionuclide. The accuracy of radionuclide scanning in excluding biliary atresia in children with other causes of cholestatic jaundice is about 70% to 90% (14). In many cases, percutaneous biopsy and histologic evaluation of the liver will be required to ascertain whether surgical exploration is indicated. The sensitivity of liver biopsy in evaluating neonatal jaundice is greater than 90% and the specificity is about 75% (15). Obstructive causes of cholestasis are suggested by the histologic findings of portal bile ductular proliferation, bile plugging, periportal bridging fibrosis, and multinucleated giant hepatocytes (15).

Surgical Management and Outcome

The first effective surgical procedure for establishing bile drainage in patients with biliary atresia was Kasai's hepatic portoenterostomy, first described in 1959 (16). The advent of liver transplantation has further improved the survival of children with biliary atresia. The first step at surgery is to perform a cholangiogram to definitively establish or exclude the diagnosis of biliary atresia. Most surgeons attempt to access the gallbladder with a catheter and inject radio-opaque dye under fluoroscopy. In many cases, the gallbladder will be shrunken and fibrotic and there will be no lumen, which is strongly indicative of biliary atresia. The gallbladder can then be removed from its fossa and the cystic duct followed down to the common bile duct, which will generally be quite sclerotic with no evidence of ductular patency. Some surgeons have initially performed the cholangiogram using laparoscopic techniques. If cholangiography demonstrates the patency of the cystic duct and extrahepatic and intrahepatic bile ducts, the diagnosis of biliary atresia is excluded. The surgical procedure should be completed and the patient should be managed medically. If ductal hypoplasia is present, the surgeon may be tempted to perform a procedure to improve drainage—this temptation should be resisted. Rather, a bile sample should be collected and subjected to the appropriate biochemical studies to help establish the diagnosis.

After demonstrating the presence of biliary atresia, a portoenterostomy should be constructed. The dissection into the porta hepatis begins with the division of the common bile duct distal to the junction with the cystic duct. This fibrotic extrahepatic duct is then used for traction and the dissection is then advanced into the hilum of the liver. Care should be taken to carefully identify the left and right branches of the portal vein that should be retracted posteriorly and inferiorly. The fibrous ductal structure will generally widen into a cone at the hilum and extend posteriorly behind the portal vein bifurcation. The fibrous cone should be amputated flush with the hepatic parenchyma at the posterior surface of the portal vein. The dissected fibrous cone should be sent for frozen section analysis to document the presence of bile ductules. If these are not present, the dissection will have to continue slightly up into the hepatic parenchyma. There will often be some capillary bleeding during the course of this dissection. Electrocautery should be used only minimally and the bleeding can usually be controlled by placing a gauze sponge into the area while the Roux limb is created. The drainage is most commonly performed using a 35- to 40-cm Roux-en-Y jejunal limb and using a single layer anastomosis between the bowel loop and the hepatic parenchyma surrounding the amputated ductal plate at the liver hilum. Some surgeons place an intussuscepting anti-reflux valve in the Roux limb to decrease the incidence of postoperative cholangitis. Recent studies have demonstrated the incidence of cholangitis is unaffected by the creation of such a valve (17).

In a recent large study of 266 patients treated with the Kasai procedure, the failure rate of the procedure (progression to liver transplant or death) was 33% at 1 year, 45% at 5 years, and 65% at 10 years (17). Twenty-one percent of the patients were still alive without transplantation following their Kasai procedure 20 years after the surgery. Risk factors for failure included patients who had corrective surgery at an age greater than 71 days, and the presence of bile ductules less than 150 microns in diameter at the site of the portoenterostomy. Overall, multiple studies have

Table 23.2. Recommended evaluation schema in the infant with jaundice

1. Document conjugated hyperbilirubinemia in any infant with prolonged jaundice after age 14 days.
2. Exclude known medically treatable causes of neonatal cholestasis.
3. Perform an abdominal ultrasound.
4. Perform a hepatobiliary scintigraphy (HIDA, DISIDA scan).
5. Perform a liver biopsy.
6. Perform a surgical exploration and cholangiogram.

Source: Modified from Bates MD, Bucuvalas JC, Alonso MH, Ryckman FC. Biliary atresia: pathogenesis and treatment. Semin Liver Dis 1998;18:281–93.

demonstrated that in about one-third of patients there is inadequate bile flow immediately after the Kasai portoenterostomy. These children will require an early liver transplant (18–20). In another third of patients with biliary atresia, even if there is initially adequate bile flow and resolution of the jaundice, there will ultimately develop progressive liver disease, which will ultimately require orthotopic liver transplantation (17,20). In many studies, the long-term survival following liver transplantation for biliary atresia is on the order of 70% (21,22). The shortage of donor organs has in part been alleviated by the increasing use of living-related donors and split livers from adult cadaver donors (23).

Spontaneous Biliary Perforation

Although spontaneous biliary perforation is rare, it is the most common cause of jaundice requiring surgery in infancy, excluding biliary atresia (24). The origins of this condition are unknown but it is postulated there is a congenital weakness in the wall of the bile ducts or elevated pressure related to distal obstruction of unknown etiology. Most cases of spontaneous bile duct perforation present within the first 2 months of life, although cases have been described as late as 19 months of age (25). The presenting signs and symptoms include jaundice with abdominal distention and bile peritonitis. These findings generally induce surgical exploration, and there is either a localized collection of bile or generalized bile throughout the peritoneal cavity. A cholangiogram through the gallbladder should be obtained to ascertain where the leak has occurred. If identified, the leaks are typically within the cystic duct or in the common bile duct near the junction of the cystic duct and the common bile duct. Common duct obstruction may be present. Cystic duct leaks are managed with cholecystectomy. To manage common bile duct or unidentified bile leaks, many investigators have concluded that external drainage of bile fluid collections is adequate treatment. However, other reports have recorded a failure of management with this treatment alone, and some patients have required second and third operations to establish adequate drainage of bile from the liver (26). Complications associated with inadequate drainage include death, cirrhosis, and portal vein thrombosis. In light of these occurrences, it seems reasonable to perform a cholecystostomy drainage at the very least in addition to external drainage for the management of spontaneous bile leak. Then if a postoperative cholangiogram does not demonstrate adequate patency of the bile ducts, early consideration should be given to a Roux-en-Y hepaticojejunostomy for definitive management.

Choledochal Cyst

Choledochal cysts of the common bile duct are exceedingly rare and have been categorized according to their anatomic appearance. The most common subtype is type 1, which is a fusiform dilatation of the common bile duct (Fig. 23.1). Type 2 is a simple diverticulum of the common bile duct, and type 3 is a choledochocele. These are quite rare, as are types 4 and 5 which include the combination of common bile duct and intrahepatic bile duct dilatation and solitary hepatic duct dilatation (Caroli's disease), respectively. The classic presenting symptom triad in patients with choledochal cysts includes obstructive jaundice, abdominal pain, and the presence of a palpable abdominal mass. These findings are actually quite rare. Choledochal cysts in infancy are usually diagnosed during the course of an evaluation for unremitting obstructive jaundice. In older children, the diagnosis is generally made after an extended evaluation for

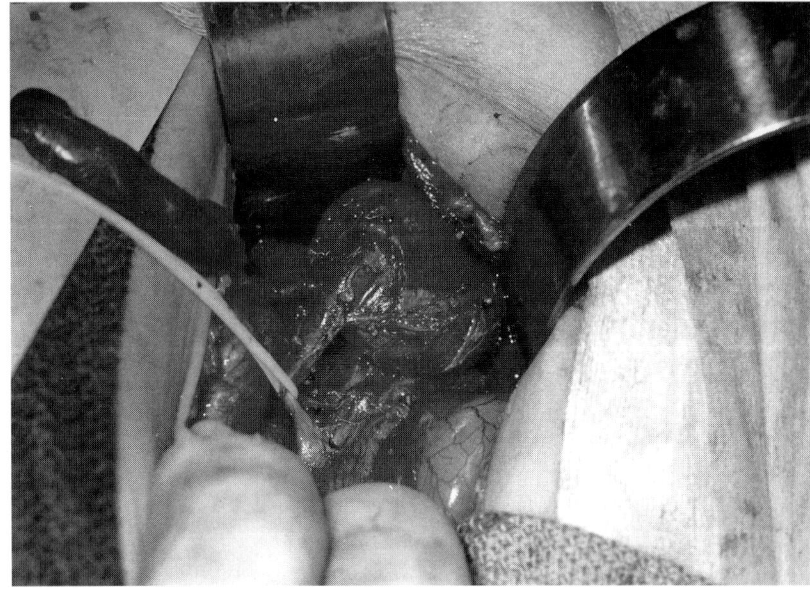

FIGURE 23.1. *Intraoperative photograph of a type I fusiform choledochal cyst in a 1-month-old infant.*

intermittent abdominal pain, occasional jaundice, or pancreatitis. Indeed, pancreatitis can be the presenting manifestation, and any child with newly diagnosed pancreatitis should undergo an evaluation for choledochal cyst (Fig. 23.2).

There are considerable differences in the modes of presentation in patients in the newborn age group compared to older children (27). In particular, infants almost uniformly have unremitting jaundice with or without a palpable mass, whereas the older children are more likely to present with abdominal pain. Moreover, there is increased fibrosis in the livers of newborns operated on for choledochal cysts when compared to older children. Indeed, these infants have such severe obstructive hepatopathy that, in rare cases, their course following surgery will be progressive, much like biliary atresia; in some cases liver transplantation is ultimately required (27). In rare cases, there may be spontaneous perforation of the choledochal cyst, and the condition may initially present with bile peritonitis (28) (Fig. 23.3). In such patients, the diagnosis can usually not be distinguished from spontaneous perforation of the bile duct prior to surgical exploration. The diagnosis of choledochal cyst is established by ultrasound and/or endoscopic retrograde cholangiopancreatography (ERCP). With the advent of small (7.5 mm external diameter) side-viewing endoscopes, ERCP can be readily performed even in infants. Magnetic resonance cholangiopancreatography (MRCP) can also be performed in children; in small studies, MRCP findings appear to agree with the diagnoses established by ERCP. Although MRCP avoids invasive endoscopic techniques, both ERCP and MRCP usually require general anesthesia to ensure adequate immobility, pain control, and airway management, especially in young children and infants.

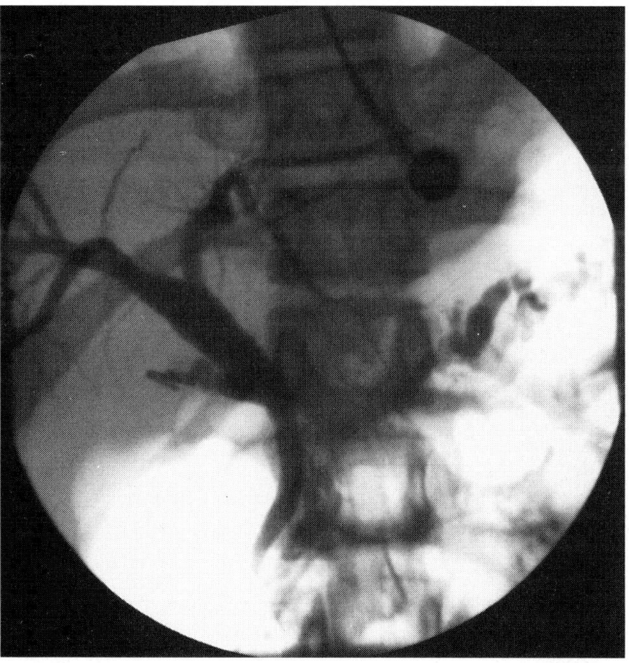

FIGURE 23.2. *ERCP of a 13-year-old child demonstrating a fusiform choledochal cyst and chronic pancreatitis with a dilated pancreatic duct.*

The pathologic evaluation of resected choledochal cysts reveals dense, fibrous tissue in the wall with inflammation and patchy ulceration of mucosa and submucosa (Fig. 23.4). There is usually a considerable amount of inflammation, and occasional metaplasia of the mucosal cells. The metaplastic changes are more commonly seen in older patients and the mucosal lining may be completely absent in patients with advanced cases.

The etiology of choledochal cysts remains speculative. The most frequently postulated causative mechanism relates to the increased incidence of the common channel between the pancreatic and common bile duct, as is seen in many, but not all, patients with choledochal cysts. It is thought that some component of a distal obstruction in association with the reflux of pancreatic enzymes into the common bile duct results in the ductal dilatation seen pathologically. Although this is an attractive hypothesis, not all patients with choledochal cysts have anomalous pancreatic or biliary junctions. Moreover, many patients who have a long common channel do not develop clinical cysts. A number of choledochal cysts have been described that have distal sclerosis and obliteration of the common bile duct, suggesting that choledochal cyst may be a forme fruste of biliary atresia. Taken together, research on the etiology of choledochal cysts suggests that this condition actually is a spectrum of disorders arising from either a congenital anomaly or some acquired insult to the biliary tree.

Surgical resection is the accepted management for choledochal cysts. Whereas cystenterostomy was historically used to reestablish biliary drainage, this procedure was associated with the later development of cholangiocarcinoma and has therefore been abandoned. In most cases, and particularly in young infants, the cyst can then be easily dissected from the surrounding tissues, resected, and the biliary tract can be reconstructed with a Roux-en-Y hepaticojejunostomy. If the cysts extend up into the right and left hepatic ducts into the liver parenchyma, the anastomosis can be performed at the level of the liver parenchyma. In most cases, intrahepatic cysts will spontaneously resolve once adequate drainage is established. Other authors have suggested that drainage may be reestablished more physiologically by reconstructing an interposition length of jejunum between the common hepatic duct and the duodenum (29). In patients in whom there is much inflammation between the cyst and the other structures of the porta hepatis, it may be impossible to dissect the cyst free from the portal vein and hepatic artery without injuring these structures. In such instances, the adherent outer wall of the cyst can be left in place and a dissection plane can be developed around the mucosal lining posteriorly to excise the cyst.

The outcome is usually excellent for children after choledochal cyst excision with hepaticojejunostomy. In one study

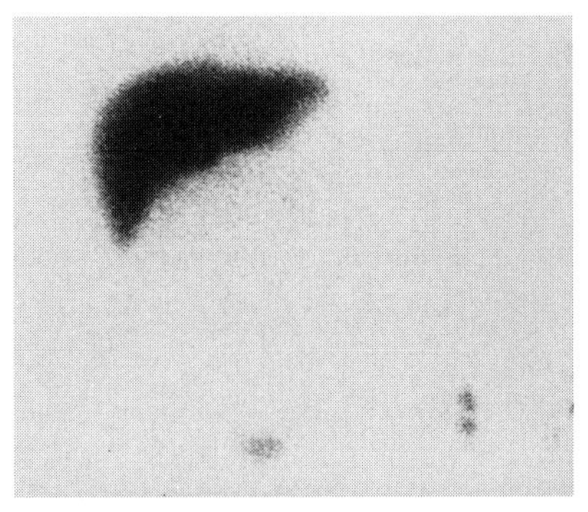
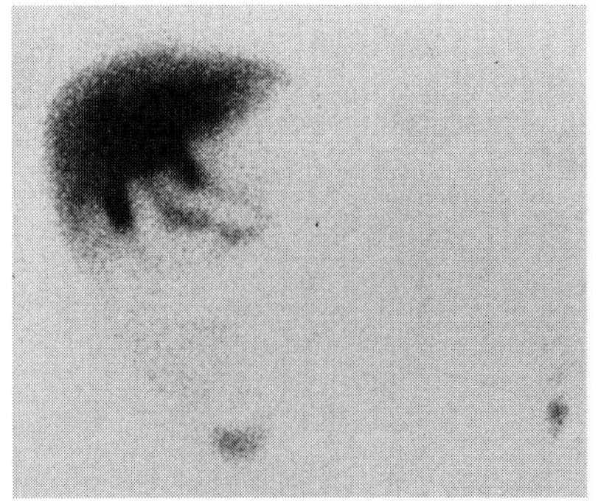
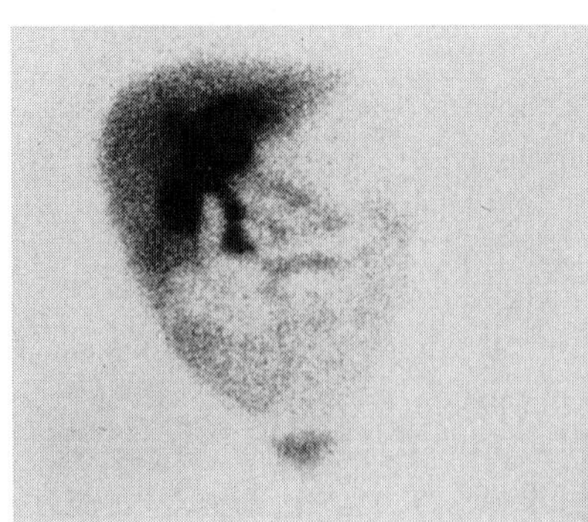
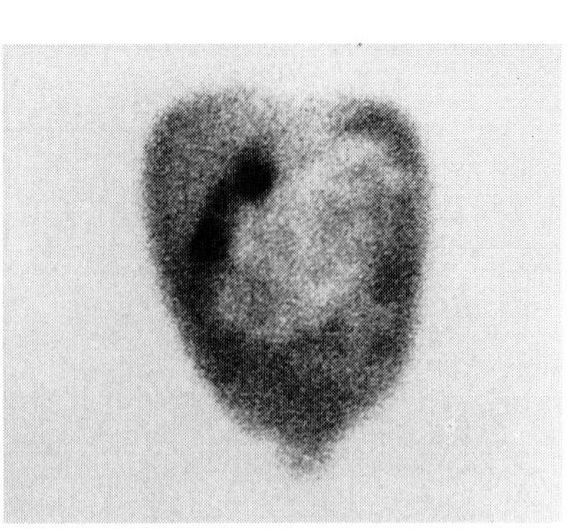

FIGURE 23.3. *Technetium-99m DISIDA hepatobiliary scan in a 3-year-old child with abdominal pain, vomiting, and peritoneal signs. Liver enzymes were mildly elevated and pancreatic enzymes markedly elevated. Top left panel shows normal hepatic uptake 20 minutes after injection. Top right shows initial puddling of activity in the porta hepatis and visualization of a separate gallbladder at 40 minutes after injection. Bottom left shows diffuse blush of activity at 50 minutes after injection filling the lower abdomen; and the bottom right panel shows persistent activity in the porta hepatitis and gallbladder and diffuse activity in the peritoneal cavity at 3.5 hours after injection. (From Treem WR, et al. Spontaneous rupture of a choledochal cyst: clues to diagnosis and etiology. J Pediatr Gastroenterol Nutr 1991;13:301–306.)*

(A)
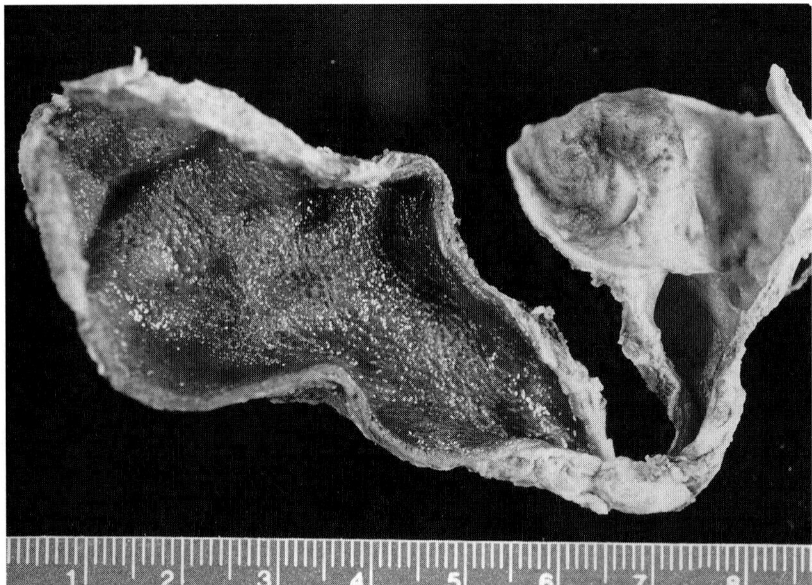

(B)
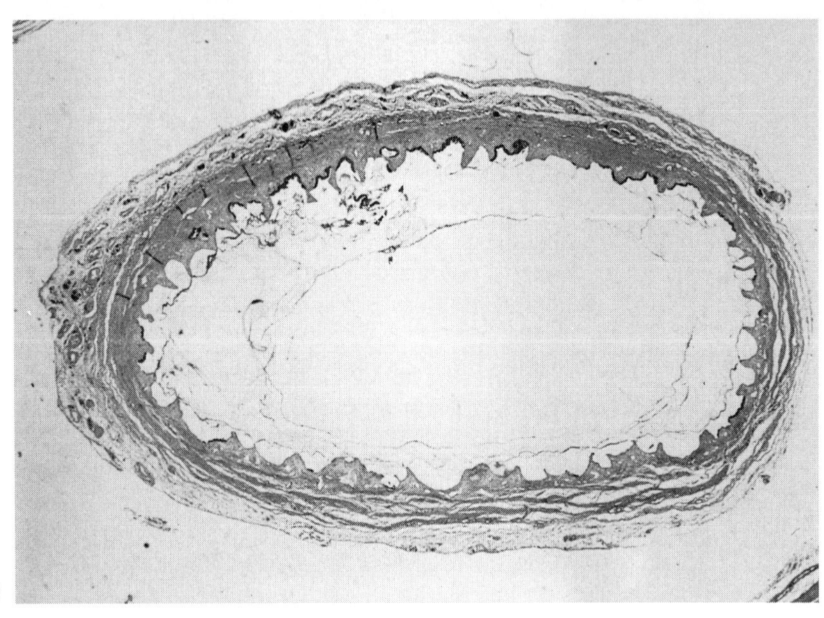

FIGURE 23.4. ***(A)*** *Photograph of a resected fusiform choledochal cyst.* ***(B)*** *Pathologic specimen, of the choledochal cyst demonstrating mural fibrosis and patchy luminal ulceration of mucosa.*

of 41 patients who were examined for a mean of 8.5 years following their procedure, the complications included the development of hepatic duct stones with cholangitis in 5% of patients and the development of a stricture with stone development in 2% (30). None of these patients developed cholangiocarcinoma.

Paucity of Intrahepatic Bile Ducts

Table 23.3 lists conditions that can be associated with a paucity of interlobular bile ducts in infants and children. The normal ratio of interlobular bile ducts to the number of portal tracts is between 0.9 and 1.8 in term infants, and slightly lower in infants prior to 30 weeks' gestation when the intrahepatic ducts are not fully developed. A ratio of less than 0.5 suggests a pathologic diagnosis of bile duct paucity (31). Some conditions associated with paucity are now known to be inherited, including Alagille syndrome, cystic fibrosis, α_1-antitrypsin deficiency, Zellweger syndrome, inborn errors in bile acid metabolism, and trisomies 18, 21, and partial trisomy 11. Others are part of the manifestation of systemic infections with pathogens such as cytomegalovirus, rubella, and syphilis. Still others are the end result of immune-mediated damage of biliary ductular epithelium, such as the lesions seen in chronic graft-versus-host disease, allograft rejection, and some forms of drug hepatotoxicity. Although these lesions do not ordinarily result in abnormalities of the extrahepatic biliary tree, their clinical presentation may mimic biliary obstruction, especially in infants. Thus their recognition is imperative when planning a diagnostic and therapeutic approach for the infant with cholestatic jaundice. This section highlights genetic diseases unique to infants and children, which can manifest themselves as neonatal cholestasis with a paucity of interlobular bile ducts.

Table 23.3. Conditions associated with paucity of interlobular bile ducts in childhood

Inherited
Alagille Syndrome
Cystic fibrosis
α_1-Antitrypsin deficiency
Zellweger syndrome (absent peroxisomes)
Trisomy 18, 21, 11
Inborn errors in bile acid synthesis
Infectious
Cytomegalovirus
Rubella
Syphilis
Immunologic
Graft-versus-host disease
Allograft rejection
Drug-induced hepatotoxicity

Syndromic Paucity of the Interlobular Bile Ducts (Alagille Syndrome)

Alagille syndrome (AGS), or syndromic paucity of the interlobular bile ducts, is the most common form of familial cholestatic liver disease and generally presents in infants less than 6 months of age with jaundice and failure to thrive (32). Its prevalence is estimated at 1 in 100,000 live births; this is probably an underestimate, because cases were ascertained on the basis of the finding of neonatal liver disease and some patients may not manifest overt liver disease in infancy. Five major clinical features have been recognized defining the "syndromic" nature of the disease (Table 23.4), including:

1. A paucity of intralobular bile ducts
2. Peripheral pulmonary artery hypoplasia or stenosis, either isolated or associated with complex cardiac anomalies
3. A birth defect of the anterior chamber of the eye consisting of a thickening of Schwalbe's line, also called posterior embryotoxon, and accompanied in some by attachment of iris strands to Descemet's membrane (Axenfeld anomaly)
4. Spinal butterfly or hemivertebral arch defects
5. Dysmorphic facies characterized by a broad forehead, widely spaced and deep-set eyes, prominent nasal tip, and a pointed chin giving the face a triangular appearance.

Other less common features affecting less than 50% of patients include renal disease (most commonly renal tubular acidosis), pancreatic insufficiency, developmental delay, and intracranial bleeding. Unilateral or bilateral renal artery stenosis leading to renovascular hypertension 3.5 to 28.0 years after the initial diagnosis has been reported in some patients in conjunction with other major artery abnormalities (33). Approximately 15% of patients are born small for gestational age, and growth retardation (defined as length

Table 23.4. Clinical manifestations of Alagille syndrome

Major
Paucity of interlobular bile ducts
Peripheral pulmonary artery stenosis (+/– other cardiac anomalies)
Posterior embryotoxon (+/– Axenfeld's anomaly, pigmentary retinopathy)
Vertebral arch defects
Dysmorphic facies
Less Common
Renal disease (RTA, renal artery stenosis)
Pancreatic insufficiency
Growth retardation
Developmental delay
Intracranial bleeding

RTA = renal tubular acidosis.

and weight below the 5th percentile in the first 3 years of life) is present in the majority.

The genetic abnormality responsible for most cases of Alagille syndrome has recently been elucidated (34). Inheritance is autosomal dominant with nearly complete penetrance but extremely variable expression (35). Jagged 1 (JAG1), on the short arm of chromosome 20 (20p12), has been identified as the AGS disease gene; and currently JAG1 mutations distributed across the entire coding region of the gene are detected in about 70% of patients with AGS (36). The JAG1 gene encodes a cell surface protein that functions as a ligand in the Notch signaling pathway. The Notch transmembrane receptor is a key signaling molecule that functions in many cell types throughout development to regulate cell fate decisions (37). It is not known precisely how mutations in JAG1 affect cellular differentiation in the liver, heart, kidney, skeletal system, eye, and other tissues, or how this defective gene leads to the loss of interlobular bile ducts and in some cases progressive cholestatic liver disease. As yet, no clear genotype–phenotype correlations have been found. In fact, patients with either point mutations in JAG 1 or complete deletions of the gene have been found who only manifested isolated right sided cardiac defects (tetralogy of Fallot, pulmonic stenosis) without liver disease (38). Based on the genetic mutation present, it is not possible to predict which patients will progress to end-stage liver disease.

Most symptomatic patients with AGS present in infancy with manifestations of liver disease ranging from mild cholestasis and jaundice to progressive liver failure. At some point in the course, hepatomegaly is almost universally present and splenomegaly is found in 70% of patients. The cholestasis may be sufficiently severe to cause acholic stools and failure of excretion of the isotope used in hepatobiliary scanning thus mimicking the findings in patients with biliary atresia. Markedly elevated levels of gamma glutamyltransferase (GGT), alkaline phosphatase, and serum bile acids with normal or mildly elevated aminotransferases are characteristic laboratory findings in these patients. Hypercholesterolemia and hypertriglyceridemia are observed in the majority of patients; later, in the early school age years, xanthomas are present in about half. Severe pruritus is a cause of significant morbidity in about half the children during the first decade of life, but typically improves with time thereafter. Fat-soluble vitamin deficiencies are inevitable and will result in rickets or pathologic fractures, ophthalmoplegia, ataxia, pigmentary retinopathy, skin changes, night blindness, and coagulopathy if not aggressively treated.

Paucity of interlobular bile ducts is the characteristic lesion seen in liver biopsies but may be absent in the youngest patients (Fig. 23.5). This implies that paucity develops with time and suggests that bile ducts are formed but either are destroyed, atrophy, or do not continue to develop postnatally to form terminal branches that supply newly formed lobules. A cross-sectional analysis of the prevalence of paucity as it relates to age at biopsy was recently performed and showed that only 60% of infants less than 6 months of age showed this finding as compared to 95% of infants older than 6 months (32). In fact, some of the youngest patients had biopsy specimens showing cholestasis, portal inflammation, fibrosis, and occasional bile ductular proliferation, again causing confusion with the findings in biliary atresia patients. Cholangiography performed via ERCP or intraoperatively can usually resolve this dilemma by showing an intact extrahepatic biliary tree in patients with AGS. However, approximately one-third of infants studied in this way will have small or hypoplastic common bile ducts, and in some, the proximal biliary tree is not visualized, leading to the mistaken assumption that they have biliary atresia and the performance of a Kasai procedure (hepatoportoenterostomy). At least 21 such patients have been reported and 13 have required liver transplantation within the first decade of life (32,39,40). This is a much

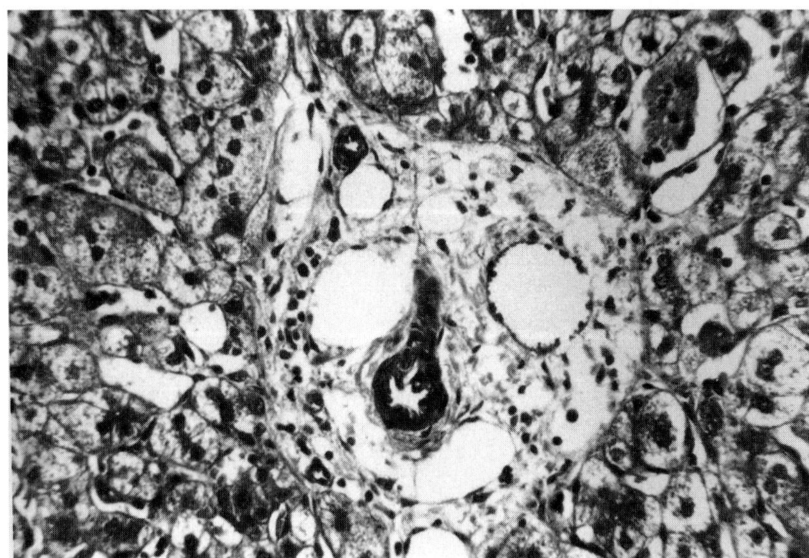

FIGURE 23.5. *Percutaneous liver biopsy from an infant with Alagille syndrome showing a portal area with a muscular artery, multiple sections of a portal venous branch, but no evidence of an interlobular bile duct.*

higher percentage than that seen in AGS patients who do not undergo the Kasai procedure. It remains unclear whether AGS patients who undergo the Kasai procedure belong to a subpopulation for whom transplantation is more likely or whether the progression of their liver disease is hastened by the surgical procedure. Because no benefit can be seen after this surgery, the Kasai procedure should be avoided in patients with AGS.

The prognosis for most children with AGS has been considered good, with improvement in cholestasis, pruritus, xanthomas, and malabsorption with time. However, now that patients are being examined into adulthood, this relatively benign prognostic assessment may change. A study of a small group of AGS patients who had survived into adulthood has shown latent development of hepatic and combined hepatic and kidney failure, the development of pancreatic insufficiency, and death from hepatocellular carcinoma (41). Hepatocellular carcinoma has been reported in other patients with AGS, with the tumor detected between the ages of 2 to 31 years. A recent report documented only a 50% probability of transplant-free survival in 26 children with AGS (39).

An analysis of clinical and laboratory features at the time of presentation shows that only the presence of major structural congenital heart disease in infancy is specifically associated with increased mortality (32). Other series have reported patients who died of intracranial hemorrhage and renal failure. No presenting features predict which infants will develop progressive liver disease and cirrhosis or severe chronic cholestasis leading to unacceptable morbidity. In most recently published series, between 20% and 47% of patients undergo liver transplantation for indications of progressive liver synthetic dysfunction accompanied by growth failure, intractable pruritus, osteodystrophy and pathologic fractures, and significant variceal bleeding. Recent reports record a 75% to 100% post-transplant survival rate in these patients (32,39,42), with considerable improvement in growth parameters and bone density, and the disappearance of pruritus and xanthomas (43).

Small numbers of patients with AGS have undergone biliary diversion procedures for intractable pruritus with the use of a 10-cm properistaltic jejunal segment anastomosed to the side of the gallbladder and terminating as an end stoma for the collection and discard of bile (44–46). Approximately half of these patients have had sustained relief from their pruritus and xanthomas since their diversion procedure. These patients have not had progression of their liver disease, suggesting that this surgical procedure may be an alternative to transplantation in certain AGS patients.

As in patients with cystic fibrosis, treatment with ursodeoxycholic acid (UDCA) has resulted in initial biochemical (AST, ALT, GGT) and symptomatic (pruritus) improvement in a small number of patients with AGS but no clear sustained improvement in these parameters, and no change in quantitative tests of hepatic function (47).

Progressive Familial Intrahepatic Cholestasis

Perhaps the greatest recent advances in our understanding of pediatric cholestatic liver disease have come in the area of defining inherited defects in bile acid synthesis or bile acid transport. Because bile acids are the driving force for bile flow at the level of the canalicular membrane, a defect in bile acid synthesis or transport would be expected to severely impair bile flow. Such defects manifest themselves in infants as neonatal jaundice and cholestasis with certain biochemical and histologic features, which offer clues to their diagnosis (Table 23.5).

Inborn Errors in Bile Acid Metabolism

Infants with autosomal recessive inborn errors of bile acid metabolism present with jaundice, direct hyperbilirubinemia, steatorrhea, failure to thrive, pale but generally not completely acholic stools, and signs of fat-soluble vitamin deficiencies including bleeding diathesis, pathologic fractures, and hyporeflexia (48). In untreated patients, death from complications of cirrhosis before 5 years of age is common. However, early intervention with oral bile acid replacement therapy can reverse the progression to hepatic failure (49). In contrast to most causes of neonatal cholestasis, infants with these disorders may have a normal or only minimally elevated levels of GGT, no pruritus, low serum

Table 23.5. Progressive familial intrahepatic cholestasis: clinical, biochemical, and histologic features

Name	GGT	Pruritus	Bile Acids	Histology	Gene/ Chromosome	Defect
Byler disease (PFIC-1)	Low	+	High	bland intracanalicular cholestasis, mild portal inflammation	FIC-1 18q21	?
Byler syndrome (PFIC-2)	Low	+	High	neonatal giant-cell hepatitis	BSEP 2q24	Bile salt export pump
MDR-3 deficiency (PFIC-3)	High	+	High	ductular proliferation, portal inflammatory infiltrate	MDR-3 ?	Phospholipid transport
BRIC	Low	+	High	intracanalicular bile plugs	FIC-1 18q21	?
Inborn errors of bile acid synthesis	Low	–	Low	variable, giant-cell hepatitis	?	3B-OH dehydrogenase deficiency

levels of primary bile acids, and low serum cholesterol. The lack of elevated GGT levels is likely due to the absence of normally synthesized hydrophobic bile acids with detergent properties, which are responsible for partially solubilizing the canalicular membrane when they accumulate in obstructive cholestatic syndromes, thus liberating GGT from the membrane. Because of the inborn error in bile acid metabolism, no such bile acids are synthesized and GGT does not accumulate in the blood.

The liver biopsy in these patients shows a periportal inflammatory infiltrate, giant cells, hepatocellular and canalicular bile stasis, mild hepatocellular necrosis, and usually, minimal fibrosis. Serum bile acids (glycocholate), which are expected to be elevated in conditions associated with neonatal direct hyperbilirubinemia, are often reported as normal. The diagnosis is made by analyzing urine or plasma via fast atom bombardment mass-spectrometry which detects abnormal unsaturated dihydroxycholestanoic and trihydroxycholestanoic bile acid metabolites. Deficiency in the enzyme 3-beta-hydroxysteroid dehydrogenase leads to a block in the synthesis of both primary bile acids, cholate and chenodeoxycholate, and accumulation of metabolites produced from 7-alpha-hydroxycholesterol. These metabolites are hepatotoxic. Alternatively, failure of bile-acid–dependent bile flow can lead to hepatocyte damage, possibly as a result of the accumulation of toxic compounds normally eliminated in the bile.

Byler Disease

Byler disease was first described in the Amish community in the direct descendants of Jacob Byler. The clinical features of the disease usually include progressive and sometimes episodic intrahepatic cholestasis starting in infancy, low serum GGT levels in spite of elevations in alkaline phosphatase, poor growth, fat and fat-soluble vitamin malabsorption, and pruritus. A bland-appearing liver biopsy is characterized by intracanalicular bile plugs and minimal hepatocyte giant cell transformation and portal fibrosis. A characteristic coarse particulate appearance of canalicular bile is seen on transmission electron microscopy (50,51).

Chenodeoxycholic acid in bile is extremely low in these patients in whom cholic acid predominates; but in the serum and urine chenodeoxycholic acid is the major bile acid. These features suggest a defect in the canalicular transport of bile acids. Later in life, these patients exhibit growth failure, wheezing (25%), severe epistaxis in the absence of coagulopathy or thrombocytopenia (75%), and cholelithiasis (30% to 40%) (52). In contrast to patients with Alagille syndrome, these children do not develop xanthomas. Progressive portal tract fibrosis and bridging are seen with advancing age, and death from cirrhosis and liver failure is likely in childhood or early adolescence. Liver transplantation has been successful with no recurrences. Some children respond well to a surgically created partial biliary diversion, implying that abnormalities in the regulation of the enterohepatic circulation of toxic bile salts are responsible for progressive hepatic damage. Children who have a disorder similar to Byler disease but are not members of the original Amish kindred are said to have Byler syndrome.

The gene for Byler disease has been mapped to the region of chromosome 18q21-q22 (53). Progressive familial intrahepatic cholestasis (PFIC) caused by a lesion in this region has been designated PFIC-1. The gene for benign recurrent intrahepatic cholestasis (BRIC) has been mapped to the same locus (54). This gene (called FIC1) encodes a P-type ATPase, which is likely involved with ATP-dependent aminophospholipid transport. FIC1 is expressed in several epithelial tissues (biliary, pancreas, intestine), and is found more strongly in small intestine than in liver (55). Its protein product is likely to play an essential role in the enterohepatic circulation of bile acids. Liver transplantation may therefore be only partly corrective in patients with PFIC-1. Persistent diarrhea, perhaps related to a defect in intestinal reabsorption of bile acids, has been reported in children who have undergone liver transplantation for this disease.

Progressive Familial Intrahepatic Cholestasis-2 (PFIC-2)

A form of PFIC not linked to chromosome 18q21-q22 was recently described, primarily in Middle Eastern and European populations (56,57). The gene responsible for this form of PFIC has been mapped to chromosome 2q24 and this disorder has been termed PFIC-2. This gene encodes the human bile salt export pump (BSEP) which is mainly responsible for the transport of bile acids across the canalicular membrane. As a result of mutations in this gene, patients with PFIC-2 do not express BSEP on the canalicular membrane and have a marked reduction in biliary bile acid secretion and bile flow (58). Bile acids retained in hepatocytes cause progressive liver damage, and a fraction leaks into the blood, causing markedly elevated serum bile acids. Again, because bile acids never enter bile ducts and never release GGT from biliary epithelium, there is no elevation of GGT even in the presence of severe cholestasis and elevated serum alkaline phosphatase.

At presentation in infancy, patients exhibit jaundice and direct hyperbilirubinemia and the liver biopsy findings show extensive neonatal "giant-cell" hepatitis rather than the bland intracanalicular cholestasis seen in patients with PFIC-1. There is diffuse lobular disarray, Kupffer cells are swollen, and there are many leukocytes as well as hematopoietic cells scattered through the sinusoids. The coarse granular bile seen in the canalicular spaces of patients with PFIC-1 is replaced by fine filamentous bile. This disease is often rapidly progressive, resulting in portal-to-portal bridging fibrosis and cirrhosis within the first few years of life. Liver transplantation is often necessary and life-saving for these patients.

Progressive Familial Intrahepatic Cholestasis-3 (PFIC-3)

A third type of progressive familial intrahepatic cholestasis has recently been described that differs from the other two because of the presence of an elevated serum GGT level in the presence of severe progressive intrahepatic cholestasis presenting in the first year of life and progressing rapidly to hepatic failure (59). The gene responsible for this defect is a multidrug resistant gene (MDR-3) located on the canalicular membrane and responsible for transporting phospholipid across the membrane into bile (60). Knockout mice with this defect are incapable of secreting phospholipids into bile and develop severe, progressive nonsuppurative cholangitis (61). Bile in these patients is characterized by extremely low phospholipid levels and a predominance of monomeric nonmicellar bile salts. Phospholipids in bile normally protect bile–ductule epithelial cells from the toxicity of bile salts by forming mixed micelles (62). The detergent properties of the nonmicellar bile salts are presumed to cause canalicular injury, cholangitis, and eventually biliary cirrhosis.

Liver biopsies from these infants show periportal inflammation, extensive bile duct proliferation, feathery degeneration of hepatocytes, and fibrosis. The mothers of some of these patients have had recurrent episodes of cholestasis and pruritus during pregnancy, suggesting that the heterozygote state for this autosomal recessively inherited defect is sufficient to express cholestasis under the altered hormonal conditions of pregnancy. About 50% of children with this defect will respond to treatment with UDCA. The therapeutic use of UDCA is based on the hypothesis that this nontoxic hydrophilic bile acid could reverse the potential hepatotoxicity of endogenous bile acids, increase their excretion from the hepatocyte, and inhibit their return to the liver via the enterohepatic circulation (63,64). For those who do not respond to UDCA therapy, partial biliary diversion can be considered; or if liver disease has progressed to cirrhosis and liver failure, liver transplantation can be undertaken.

BILIARY DISEASES IN CHILDREN AND ADOLESCENTS

Cholelithiasis and Cholecystitis

Cholelithiasis is increasingly being recognized in pediatric patients. The risk factors for cholelithiasis are listed in Table 23.6. Recent studies have documented an apparent increase in the incidence of symptomatic gallstone disease in children who do not have any of the recognized risk factors (65). Although the exact cause for the increased incidence of symptomatic cholelithiasis in childhood is unknown, potential factors include the increased use of total parenteral nutrition, an increased prevalence of obesity in the pediatric population, and the increasing reliance on abdominal ultrasound in the evaluation of children with nonspecific abdominal pain (65). The gallstones noted in children and adolescents having no antecedent risk factor are usually of the cholesterol variety, whereas pigment stones are usually seen in association with hematologic disorders.

Table 23.6. Risk factors for cholelithiasis

Hemolytic diseases
Sickle-cell anemia
Thalassemia major
Hereditary spherocytosis
Parenteral nutrition
Ileal resection
Pregnancy
Oral contraceptives
Neonatal factors
Prematurity
Necrotizing enterocolitis
Parenteral nutrition

Clinical Presentation and Diagnosis

Symptomatic gallstones may be present in children of any age, ranging from the unborn fetus to the adolescent. Risk factors for gallstones in the neonatal period include parenteral nutrition, history of bowel resection, and prematurity. In neonatal patients, the condition may frequently be asymptomatic or patients may present with jaundice and sepsis related to gangrene of the gallbladder (66). Infants and children with acute cholecystitis may have right upper quadrant pain and tenderness and may be febrile. Adolescent patients may present with the classic symptoms of biliary colic such as right upper quadrant pain following meals in association with nausea, vomiting, and intolerance of fatty foods. Moreover, the occasional child will present atypical abdominal pain, and a thorough gastroenterologic evaluation will be unrevealing except for the presence of gallstones. If all other common etiologies of abdominal pain have been ruled out in these patients, it is reasonable to consider the pain related to biliary colic. In rare cases, children will present with common bile duct obstruction, obstructive jaundice, elevated liver enzymes, and acholic stools. Occasionally, gallstone pancreatitis will be the first clinical manifestation of symptomatic cholelithiasis.

Abdominal ultrasound is the most accurate modality for the diagnosis of cholelithiasis and choledocholithiasis. In addition, the findings associated with acute cholecystitis, such as gallbladder wall thickening, pericholecystic fluid, and an ultrasound Murphy's sign (pain over the gallbladder increased by pressure with the ultrasound transducer) may be diagnostically important. Cholescintigraphy (DISIDA) may be useful to document cystic duct obstruction and cholecystitis, but this test is less useful in the chronically ill patients owing to the nonvisualization of the gallbladder in such patients. Plain abdominal radiographs may demonstrate radio-opaque gallstones in about 40% of children (67), reflecting a higher incidence of pigmented gallstones in children relative to adults.

Children with sickle cell disease have an increased risk of cholelithiasis, owing to increased hemoglobin degradation to bilirubin. Gallstones are found in 20% of patients with sickle cell disease and an additional 16% of patients may have biliary sludge without gallstones. In a recent study of the natural history of biliary sludge in children with sickle cell disease, 80% of children either had a cholecystectomy or had progression to frank cholelithiasis over a period of 4 years (68). Thus, patients with sickle cell disease are at risk of developing symptomatic gallstones and should be followed closely so that surgical management can be instituted prior to the development of complications.

Management

In neonates, the factors leading to the development of gallstones are often self-limiting. Spontaneous resolution of gallstones in infants has been reported in a number of studies. Therefore, in the absence of symptoms, it is reasonable to follow infants with cholelithiasis and await resolution. Some authors advocate cholecystectomy if calcified stones are present, because such stones are less likely to spontaneously resolve (67). Surgical management is mandatory in the rare infant with acute cholecystitis or gangrenous cholecystitis or in the baby with jaundice or cholangitis related to common bile duct obstruction. Owing to the small size of the structure, surgical manipulation of the common bile duct is difficult. One method to clear the common duct consists of placing a cholecystostomy tube that may be used to irrigate the distal duct. In addition, choledochotomy with stone removal or transduodenal sphincterotomy may be considered. In the absence of symptoms, common bile duct stones should be observed. Recent reports have documented the successful use of ERCP in infants and, if available, this may be a very good option for the management of symptomatic common bile duct stones (69,70).

Laparoscopic cholecystectomy has become the standard for management of symptomatic cholelithiasis. The safety of the procedure in children has been well established and the aspects of the technique unique to children have been well described (71). The principal advantage of laparoscopic cholecystectomy is decreased pain and decreased hospital stay relative to the open procedure. In most cases, children can be discharged the day following the operative procedure. Intraoperative cholangiography can be performed to evaluate for the presence of common bile duct stones.

The treatment of common bile duct stones in children is controversial. At issue is whether ERCP should be performed prior to laparoscopic cholecystectomy in patients suspected of having common bile duct stones or whether ERCP should be performed postoperatively based on the results of intraoperative cholangiography. To address this issue, a recent study was conducted to assess the usefulness of ERCP prior to laparoscopic cholecystectomy (72). In this report, clinical criteria suggesting the presence of common bile duct stones were used to determine whether children were subjected to ERCP prior to laparoscopic cholecystectomy; 6 of 14 children suspected of having common duct stones had no abnormalities demonstrated at ERCP (72). Thus, to prevent unnecessary ERCP, most pediatric surgeons elect to perform a laparoscopic cholecystectomy and obtain an intraoperative cholangiogram if there is a suspicion of common bile duct stones. Then, if the stones cannot be flushed through the duct during the course of the operation, ERCP can be obtained postoperatively. In some centers, it is possible to perform ERCP in the operating room immediately following the laparoscopic cholecystectomy, reducing the need for another anesthetic. One potential disadvantage of performing ERCP after the cholecystectomy is that in cases where ERCP is not successful at relieving the obstruction, the patient will need to undergo a formal laparotomy after the laparoscopic cholecystectomy to explore the common bile duct. In practice, ERCP is successful at relieving the common bile duct obstruction in the vast majority of cases.

The incidence of choledocholithiasis in childhood is relatively rare. In one large study of 131 children undergoing laparoscopic cholecystectomy for cholelithiasis, only 14 (10.7%) were suspected of having choledocholithiasis preoperatively.

Acalculous Gallbladder Disease

Congenital Anomalies of the Gallbladder

Congenital agenesis of the gallbladder occurs with a frequency of approximately 1 in 10,000 live births. Absence of the gallbladder may be found as an isolated anomaly or in association with other malformations. The embryonic form of biliary atresia (described above) is associated with the absence of the gallbladder, situs inversus, asplenia or polysplenia, and congenital heart defects. Imperforate anus, genitourinary anomalies, anencephaly, bicuspid aortic valves, and cerebral aneurysms have all been associated with agenesis of the gallbladder (73).

Heterotopic tissue of foregut origin may also be found within the gallbladder wall including most commonly gastric or hepatic mucosa, and more rarely ectopic adrenal, pancreatic, and thyroid tissue (74). These ectopic foci are seldom of clinical significance. Other rare congenital anomalies include gallbladder duplications or a single gallbladder divided into multiple chambers by longitudinal septae, presumably secondary to incomplete resolution of its solid phase. Small diverticula off the body of the gallbladder may also be seen. Because these diverticula promote bile stasis, gallstones may form.

Hydrops of the Gallbladder

Acute hydrops is defined by marked gallbladder distention in the absence of stones, bacterial infection, obstruction of the extrahepatic biliary system, or a congenital anomaly (Fig. 23.6). The absence of a significant inflammatory component distinguishes hydrops from acalculous cholecystitis (75). Conditions associated with gallbladder hydrops in neonates include sepsis, total parenteral nutrition, α_1-antitrypsin deficiency, and fasting; and in children the associated conditions include Kawasaki syndrome, streptococcal pharyngitis, viral hepatitis, staphylococcal infection, Henoch-Schönlein purpura, Sjögren's syndrome, and nephrotic syndrome. Many of these entities share a vasculitic process as a

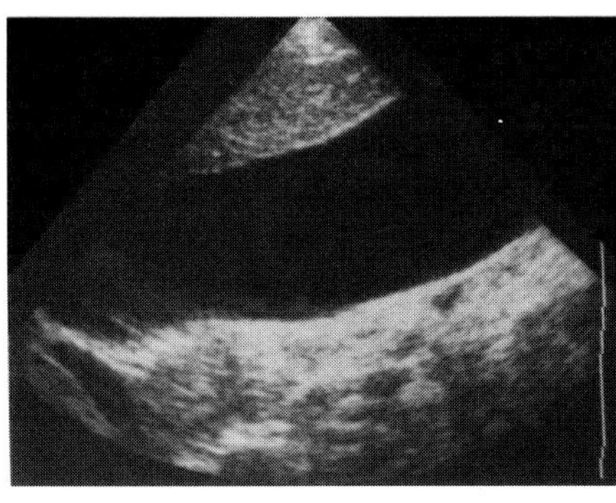
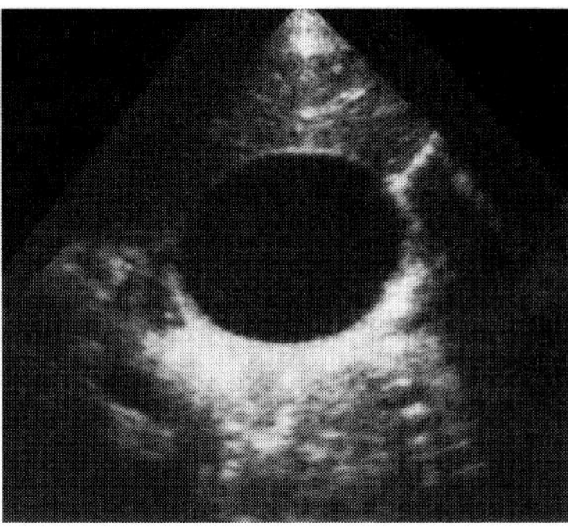

FIGURE 23.6. *Hydrops of the gallbladder in a patient with Kawasaki's disease.*

Table 23.7. Acute and chronic cholecystitis in childhood

	Acute	Chronic
Age	Neonates → children	Older children (age 7–18)
Predisposing conditions	Previous surgery, burns, trauma, transfusions, HUS, cystic fibrosis, leukemia, cirrhosis	None
Associated infections	*Salmonella*, *Leptospirosis*, RMSF, CMV, *Aspergillus*,* *Candida*,* *Giardia*,* *Cryptosporidium*,* gram-negative cholangitis	None
Clinical symptoms	Fever, RUQ pain, vomiting, ↑WBC, ↑LFT	RUQ pain, nausea, vomiting, no fever, normal WBC and LFT
Ultrasound findings	Gallbladder distention, sludge, wall thickening	Normal
Hepatobiliary scan	Nonvisualization of gallbladder	Abnormal gallbladder uptake and delayed emptying

* Seen in immunocompromised hosts.
Abbreviations: CMV = cytomegalovirus, HUS = hemolytic uremic syndrome, LFT = liver function tests, RMSF = Rocky Mountain spotted fever, RUQ = right upper quadrant, WBC = white blood cell count.

prominent part of their pathogenesis. In Kawasaki syndrome, this process affects the gallbladder wall and results in cystic duct obstruction.

The incidence of gallbladder hydrops complicating Kawasaki syndrome is approximately 15% (76). The typical presentation includes abdominal pain, vomiting, and a right upper quadrant mass. Mild direct hyperbilirubinemia may also be present. The clinical features may mimic intussusception or acute appendicitis. In most cases, gallbladder distention is self-limited, resolving without surgical intervention (77). However, complications of gallbladder necrosis and perforation have been reported (78). The diagnosis of hydrops is made by ultrasonography demonstrating a markedly distended, echo-free gallbladder and a normal-caliber biliary tree. The mainstay of therapy is supportive, with fluid resuscitation, antibiotics, or other therapy aimed at the associated illness. Serial ultrasound examinations can confirm resolution of the condition. Surgery is reserved for the exceedingly rare complication of gallbladder perforation.

Acalculous Cholecystitis

Acalculous cholecystitis is an uncommon entity in infants and children and occurs in an acute and chronic form (Table 23.7). The acute form is most important to recognize because it may present as a surgical emergency. Predisposing factors in pediatric cases of acute acalculous cholecystitis include a previous surgical procedure, burns, multiple transfusions, trauma, and systemic infection. In a recent series of 13 children with acute acalculous cholecystitis, 2 were infected with salmonella; 5 had systemic medical illness including cystic fibrosis, end-stage liver disease, hemolytic-uremic syndrome, and leukemia; and 6 had undergone recent operative procedures, 4 with congenital heart disease and 2 with recent spinal fusions (79). Other infectious conditions associated with acute acalculous cholecystitis include leptospirosis, Rocky Mountain spotted fever, typhoid fever, and, in immunocompromised hosts, infections with cytomegalovirus (CMV), *Candida*, *Aspergillus*, *Giardia*, and *Cryptosporidium* (80). A review of neonates with acute acalculous cholecystitis found that 8 of 10 had systemic infection (81) with bile cultures growing *Escherichia coli*, *Streptococcus viridans*, *Serratia*, and *Pseudomonas*. There are some children with no underlying disease who present with this condition (82).

The pathophysiology is poorly understood but is thought to depend on a number of factors including inflammation of the cystic duct, gallbladder stasis, secondary bacterial invasion, and episodic ischemia. Postsurgical patients who are fasting, and receiving parenteral nutrition and narcotics for pain, are prone to gallbladder stasis. In the severely ill patient in the intensive care unit on inotropic support, or in patients after cardiac surgery, ischemia and hypoperfusion may play a significant role.

Patients with acute acalculous cholecystitis generally present with fever, right upper quadrant pain, and vomiting. Physical examination reveals right sided or generalized abdominal tenderness and a mass may be palpable. Jaundice is present in the minority, but most have leukocytosis and abnormal liver enzymes. Ultrasonography can demonstrate gallbladder distention, with thickening of the gallbladder wall (>3.5 mm), echogenic intraluminal sludge, and a pericholecystic fluid collection. However, it is important to note that a thickened gallbladder wall can also be seen in patients with hypoalbuminemia and ascites without any evidence of cholecystitis (83). Gallbladder wall thickening may represent a local inflammatory process or may be a reflection of a systemic process, and should be interpreted within the clinical context. Radioisotope hepatobiliary scans generally show nonfilling of the gallbladder in the presence of good hepatic uptake and prompt intestinal excretion of the isotope.

Although some cases of acute acalculous cholecystitis can be managed with supportive therapy and antibiotics, most children undergo cholecystectomy or tube cholecystostomy to allow adequate drainage and to prevent complications such as gallbladder necrosis, perforation, and bile peritonitis. Children whose condition is thought to be secondary to infection will often respond to antibiotics and conservative therapy, but most others require surgery. At the time of surgery, the gallbladder is often described as edematous, purpuric, or focally hemorrhagic. Histologically, specimens show polymorphonuclear infiltration, edema, focal hemorrhage, and occasional necrosis, thromboembolisms, and eosinophilic infiltration.

Chronic cholecystitis in children is most often diagnosed in older children (ages 7 to 18 years) without underlying systemic diseases or acute infections. Patients present with chronic symptoms of right upper quadrant pain, nausea, and vomiting (79). Few of these patients have liver enzyme or bilirubin abnormalities and their white blood cell count is normal. Abdominal ultrasonography is not helpful; however, hepatobiliary scanning may show abnormal uptake of the isotope by the gallbladder, and abnormal function measured by delayed gallbladder emptying in response to a fatty meal or intravenous cholecystokinin. In these patients, all symptoms resolve after cholecystectomy; and microscopic examination of gallbladder specimens shows transmural chronic inflammation consisting of lymphocytes, occasional plasma cells, and eosinophils. Rokitansky-Aschoff sinuses are present in some specimens.

Tumors and Other Inflammatory Conditions of the Gallbladder

Neoplastic disorders of the gallbladder are exceedingly rare in children. Embryonal rhabdomyosarcoma is the most frequent malignancy arising from the biliary tree and presenting as obstructive jaundice with dilated bile ducts (Fig. 23.7) (84). The tumor is most often poorly responsive to surgical removal, biliary diversion, and chemotherapy. Carcinoma of the gallbladder has also rarely been reported in children (85). Benign neoplasms, such as adenomas of the gallbladder, have also rarely been reported presenting with symptoms of biliary colic. Resection is recommended because of the malignant potential of these polypoid lesions (86). Adenomyomatosis of the gallbladder, defined as hyperplasia of the mucous membrane, thickening of the muscularis, and Rokitansky-Aschoff sinuses have also been described in children and are often associated with other anomalies (87). Gallbladder polyps have been found in patients with Peutz-Jeghers syndrome (88). Granulomatous lesions in the wall of the gallbladder have been described in patients with Crohn's disease, and vasculitis is seen in patients with polyarteritis nodosa.

Cystic Fibrosis and Biliary Tract Disease

Table 23.8 lists the approximate frequency of the spectrum of hepatobiliary manifestations of cystic fibrosis (CF). As patients live longer, it is becoming clear that an increasing number will manifest significant hepatobiliary disease. In fact, with our current knowledge of the expression of the cystic fibrosis transmembrane regulator (CFTR) gene in intrahepatic and extrahepatic biliary epithelia, and the known involvement of CFTR in chloride and water secretion into bile at the ductal level, it is difficult to understand why all patients with CF do not develop clinical symptoms and signs of liver disease. Autopsy studies have confirmed the presence of focal biliary cirrhosis in the majority of older CF patients, even those who were asymptomatic during life. Other modifying genetic or environmental factors likely play a role in determining the degree of phenotypic expression of the hepatobiliary abnormalities in CF.

The main pathogenesis of the hepatobiliary lesions of CF has been attributed to focal inspissation of biliary secretions, obstruction of small ducts and ductules, the eventual devel-

Table 23.8. Spectrum of hepatobiliary manifestations in children with cystic fibrosis

Feature	Affected (%)[a]
Elevated liver enzymes	9–17
Hepatomegaly	5–30
Cirrhosis	5–10[b]
Neonatal cholestasis	2
Microgallbladder	15–30
Gallstones	8–15
Common bile duct disease (stenosis, strictures, sclerosing cholangitis)	5–10

[a] Wide range reflects differing ages at which patients were studied and whether data was obtained from clinical and radiographic studies or autopsy data.
[b] 5% over 12 years of age; 10% over 25 years of age.

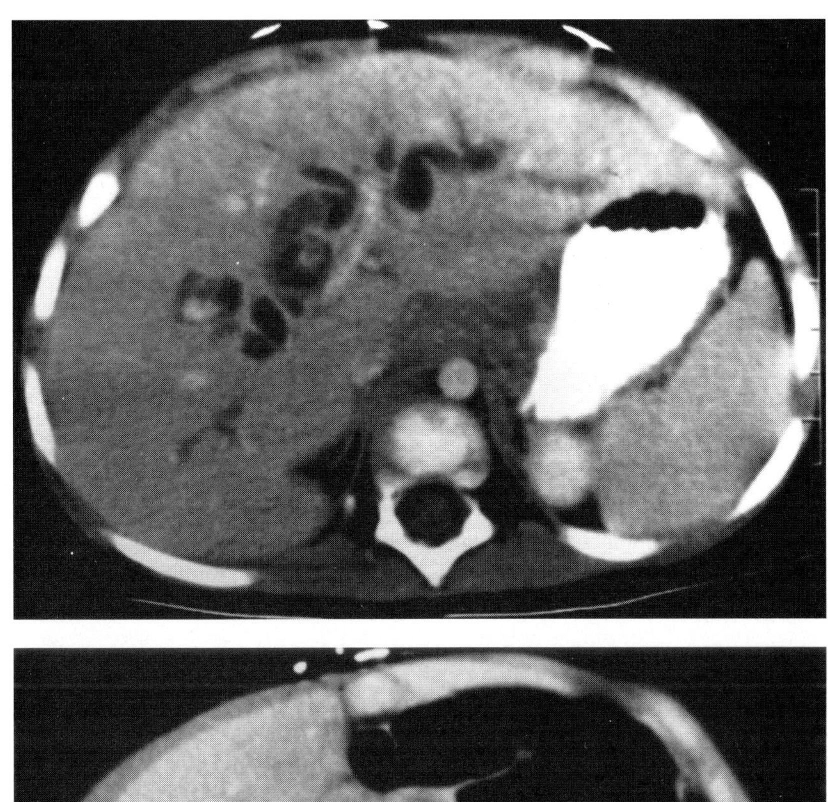

(A)

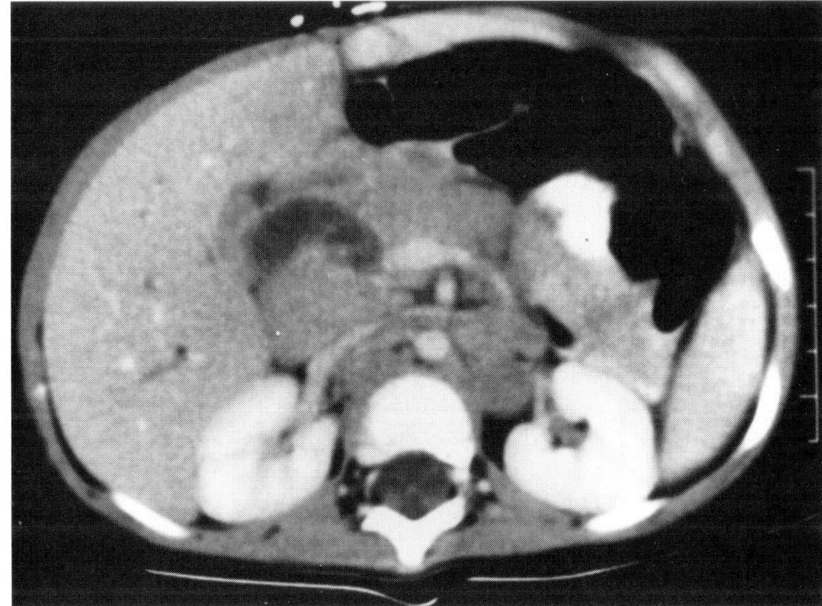

(B)

FIGURE 23.7. *CT scan showing dilatation of the **(A)** intrahepatic and **(B)** extrahepatic biliary tree by a rhabdomyosarcoma in a 2-year-old who presented with obstructive jaundice.*

opment of portal fibrosis, bridging, and eventual cirrhosis. The bile in CF is abnormally viscous, and has an increased concentration of potentially toxic hydrophobic bile acids capable of promoting secondary hepatocyte injury by proinflammatory cytokines, growth factors, or products of lipid peroxidation. Impaired secretion of mucins and other protective proteins from submucosal glands also contributes to the injury pattern. Elaboration of cytokines and growth factors may also directly stimulate collagen synthesis by recruited stellate cells. The progression from cholestasis (decreased bile flow) to focal biliary cirrhosis to multilobular cirrhosis takes years and should be viewed as a continuum. Other intrahepatic lesions seen in CF include steatosis, which may be related to malnutrition, essential fatty acid deficiency, carnitine deficiency, and other dietary factors (89–91); and hepatic congestion resulting from right sided congestive heart failure.

Elevated liver enzymes are found in 9% to 17% of all pediatric patients with CF (92–94), and approximately 5% to 30% have hepatomegaly. Clinically significant liver disease—defined by persistent elevations of liver enzymes, persistent enlargement of a firm liver, and suggested fibrosis and cirrhosis by imaging criteria—is found in 13% to 17% of pediatric patients. Neonatal cholestasis occurs in less than 2% of infants with CF, and is associated with meconium ileus 35% to 50% of the time (95). The incidence of extrahepatic biliary tract disease is much lower with the exception of microgallbladder, which is present in 20% to

30% of patients (96). The remainder of this section deals with the extrahepatic biliary tract abnormalities encountered in children with CF.

Cholelithiasis

Gallstones have been found in 8% to 12% of pediatric patients with CF (97,98) and approximately 25% of adults with CF (99), suggesting that the incidence of cholelithiasis increases with age. Gallstones have not been observed in patients with CF and normal exocrine pancreatic function; thus their occurrence is likely related to malabsorption or to the severity of the underlying biliary secretion abnormality. Initially, the stones in CF patients were thought to be cholesterol gallstones because of presumed increases in fecal bile acid excretion leading to a reduction in the bile acid pool (100). In previous studies, children and adults with CF had been found to have lithogenic bile with high biliary cholesterol concentrations relative to bile acids and phospholipids and bile supersaturated with cholesterol (101). Watkins and associates demonstrated that pancreatic enzyme replacement reduced steatorrhea from 50% to 20% of fat intake, decreased fecal bile acid losses, and produced a doubling of the bile acid pool size (102). More aggressive pancreatic enzyme replacement therapy, and the use of enteric coated preparations and acid blockade to potentiate the efficacy of pancreatic enzymes, may therefore account for the decline in the incidence of gallstones seen in children with CF. However, recent studies have failed to confirm some of these earlier observations, and the radiolucent stones in patients with CF have, in some instances, been found to be pigment stones. This may be related to abnormal motility of the gallbladder in children with CF, resulting in stasis and increased residual gallbladder volumes (103). This finding, coupled with abnormalities of gallbladder mucin secretion, could predispose to nidus and stone formation in the gallbladder.

Cholelithiasis in CF patients is usually asymptomatic but may present with right upper quadrant, back, or right shoulder pain; jaundice, nausea, and vomiting; or pruritus, and elevated levels of alkaline phosphatase, GGT, or bilirubin. Colicky abdominal pain and/or the acute onset of jaundice and acholic stools suggest common bile duct obstruction caused by stones or sludge. Ultrasonography is the first test employed in these circumstances and is most helpful to determine the presence of gallstones, common bile duct stones, and extrahepatic and intrahepatic bile duct dilatation. Hepatobiliary scintigraphy may be useful to suggest biliary obstruction and abnormal gallbladder function. Scintigraphy may be particularly helpful in demonstrating the absence of gallbladder filling that is characteristic of cholecystitis. ERCP is the most sensitive test to reveal strictures, dilatation of bile ducts, stones, and other abnormalities of the biliary tree. Because it is invasive and usually requires general anesthesia and intubation in children with CF, ERCP is reserved for investigating dilated or narrowed bile ducts identified by ultrasonography that may be causing clinical symptoms.

Cholelithiasis in CF patients is not responsive to UCDA therapy (104). If clinical symptoms of gallbladder dysfunction or pain are present or blood tests indicate persistent cholestasis, a laparoscopic or surgical cholecystectomy should be performed unless end-stage liver disease is present and liver transplantation is contemplated. A liver biopsy and intraoperative cholangiogram should always be obtained during any cholecystectomy procedure in a CF patient.

Microgallbladder

In postmortem series, approximately 15% to 30% of patients with CF have atrophy of the gallbladder and atretic cystic ducts (105). Microgallbladders, defined as a gallbladder not exceeding 1.5 cm in length and 0.5 cm in width, are less common in CF patients with liver disease and can occur independently of liver disease. The gallbladder contains translucent, gray mucus, and the assumption is that obstruction to the cystic duct leads to involution and subsequent atrophy of the gallbladder. Although most often asymptomatic, this anomaly is likely responsible for the vast majority of nonvisualized gallbladders in patients undergoing ultrasound, oral cholecystography, or even intravenous cholangiograms. Studies using hepatobiliary scintigraphy have demonstrated that as many as two-thirds of patients with CF without liver disease and one-third of patients with clinical or biochemical liver disease have nonvisualized gallbladders, confirming the high incidence of this anomaly.

Common Bile Duct Disease

Distal common duct strictures have been recognized in infants and children with cystic fibrosis. In these cases, periductal fibrosis appears to compress the common duct as it traverses the head of the pancreas (106,107). Most investigators attribute this condition to external compression due to pancreatic fibrosis, but the radiologic appearance of the common duct at times resembles sclerosing cholangitis, suggesting that intramural fibrosis in the wall of the common duct may also contribute. Patients with distal common duct strictures present with a variety of symptoms, including abdominal pain, steatorrhea, nausea, vomiting, and jaundice (108). Physical examination usually reveals hepatomegaly and occasionally right upper quadrant tenderness. The abdominal pain due to common bile duct strictures in CF patients may be nonspecific and could be mistaken for pain due to distal intestinal obstruction syndrome. Most patients are anicteric, suggesting that the strictures are of limited significance. However, biliary cirrhosis has occurred in these anicteric patients even though the biliary tract obstruction is incomplete (109). Another prominent symptom of a common bile duct stricture is steatorrhea, which is poorly responsive to increasing administration of pancreatic enzymes. In one study, 55% of patients with CF and biliary strictures had malabsorption of over 20% of their fat intake compared with only 18% of controls on similar adequate enzyme therapy. Overall, the above data suggest that recurrent abdominal pain and the persistence of steatorrhea despite compliance with adequate pancreatic enzyme therapy should raise the suspicion of a biliary tract lesion.

Ultrasonography, hepatobiliary scintigraphy, and cholangiography all have a potential role in the assessment of biliary tract strictures. Ultrasonography may or may not demonstrate a dilated common bile duct or gallbladder above the stricture. Hepatobiliary scintigraphy can provide semiquantitative information on hepatic extraction fraction as an assessment of hepatocyte function, and half-clearance times as a measure of biliary obstruction (110). Precise imaging is best achieved with cholangiography, but because of its invasive nature this procedure is only recommended as a prerequisite for surgery.

Sclerosing Cholangitis

Primary sclerosing cholangitis (PSC) is rare in childhood and generally occurs associated with other underlying diseases or unassociated with any underlying disease; and presents either in childhood or in the neonatal period. Table 23.9 shows clinical conditions associated with reported cases of sclerosing cholangitis in children. Sclerosing cholangitis in children may be secondary to repeated bouts of infectious cholangitis after hepatic portoenterostomy surgery for biliary atresia or due to stones, neoplasia, congenitally anomalous ducts, polycystic disease, or trauma. Children infected with human immunodeficiency virus (HIV) or children who have had a bone marrow transplant can develop a cholangiopathy due to CMV or cryptosporidium infection. Some of these conditions are covered elsewhere in this book; this section concentrates on idiopathic PSC in childhood.

Etiology and Pathogenesis

The majority of children with PSC develop the signs and symptoms during childhood and adolescence in association with another underlying disease. These diseases include ulcerative colitis, Crohn's disease, histiocytosis X (Langerhans' cell histiocytosis), other immunodeficiency diseases (including both humoral and T-cell deficiencies), autoimmune chronic active hepatitis (CAH), inflammatory pseudotumor, celiac disease, cystic fibrosis, and sickle cell disease. In adults, 50% to 75% of patients with PSC have concomitant inflammatory bowel disease (IBD), but in children this relationship is seen in only approximately 25% of patients. The complex relationship between PSC and IBD offers several clues about etiopathogenesis, but it does not seem likely that one clinical condition causes the other; nor does this association address the causation of sclerosing cholangitis in the absence of IBD.

A universal model for idiopathic progressive cholangitis in patients with IBD would need to account for immune-mediated destruction of the hepatobiliary tract, perhaps initiated by transient infection, in genetically predisposed individuals who often have concomitant colonic disease. The findings of hypergammaglobulinemia, elevated circulating immune complexes, and circulating autoantibodies provide support for the concept that PSC may be an immunologically mediated disease (111). The presence of circulating antibodies against an epitope shared by colon and bile duct epithelial cells suggests the presence of a common antigenic target for immune attack (112,113). Antibodies to the nuclei of neutrophils and perinuclear immunofluorescent staining of neutrophils have been found in the serum of a large number of patients with PSC, and the presence of these IgG perinuclear anti-neutrophil cytoplasmic antibodies (pANCA) has been found to be 65% sensitive and 100% specific for PSC in adults (114). An analysis of the immunologic features in children with both PSC and autoimmune CAH suggests a different underlying basis for autoimmunity; defective T-cell immunoregulation in CAH and abnormal B-cell activation bypassing T-cells in PSC (115). In addition, the high frequency of HLA-B8 and HLA-DR3/Drwa52 reported in adult patients with PSC and chronic IBD, also encountered in other autoimmune diseases, suggests the possibility of a genetic basis for this disease (116). The relative risk of developing PSC in a patient with ulcerative colitis possessing the HLA-B8, DR3 haplotypes is increased 10-fold over that of normal individuals (117).

The initiating trigger in the immune-mediated destruction of biliary epithelium may be various proinflammatory, bacteria-derived products (lipopolysaccharides, peptidoglycans, or tertiary bile acids) generated in the lumen of an inflamed segment of intestine. This theory has been bolstered by the development of an animal model of PSC occurring in genetically susceptible rats with experimental small bowel bacterial overgrowth (118,119). Methods for blocking the production of these bacterial byproducts and inhibiting their first-pass clearance via the portal vein have prevented the hepatobiliary injury in these rats. However, PSC may develop in children long before symptoms of colonic disease or even after colectomy, seemingly negating a role for the gut as the site of the hepatotoxic factor (120).

Table 23.9. Clinical conditions associated with primary sclerosing cholangitis in childhood

Inflammatory bowel disease
Crohn's disease
Ulcerative colitis
Langerhans' cell histiocytosis
Inherited and acquired immunodeficiencies
Common variable immunodeficiency
T-cell immunodeficiencies
AIDS-associated cholangiopathy
Idiopathic primary sclerosing cholangitis
Neonatal
Non-neonatal
Cystic fibrosis
Celiac disease
Inflammatory pseudotumor

In children with Langerhans' cell histiocytosis (LCH), primary involvement of the bile duct walls with specific histiocytic infiltration or progressive scarring of portal areas leads to distortion of the bile ducts. Ductular necrosis is more prominent in these patients compared to those with IBD and PSC, and this necro-inflammatory process produces a rapid progression to biliary cirrhosis (121). Major biliary strictures, often at the hepatic duct confluence, and the presence of sludge or lithiasis in the intrahepatic bile ducts is more common in PSC associated with LCH.

Chronic viral or opportunistic infections of the biliary tract may play a role in children with congenital immunodeficiency syndromes, those with HIV, and those with acquired immunodeficiency after bone marrow transplantation. CMV DNA has been detected in the liver of small series of patients with PSC; but the typical histologic features of hepatic CMV infection do not resemble those seen in PSC. PSC has developed in children with immunodeficiency syndromes and systemic CMV infection, and in children with immunodeficiency, chronic diarrhea, and cryptosporidial organisms in their stool. However, bile cultures did not grow *Cryptosporidium* or CMV. Reovirus 3, which causes an obliterative cholangitis in a weanling mouse model, has not been found by investigating cultures, immunohistochemical staining, or serologies in patients with PSC.

Clinical Manifestations and Diagnosis

In most series of children with PSC, there seems to be a mild male predominance. Neonatal cholestatic jaundice is present in a minority of patients, but the mean age of initial presentation is 10 years of age in patients with IBD and approximately 3 to 5 years in patients with LCH or immunodeficiency syndromes. Initial signs in the children presenting out of the neonatal period included hepatomegaly in almost all children, splenomegaly and cholestatic jaundice in about 50%, and gastrointestinal bleeding and ascites in approximately 25% (122). Symptoms include abdominal pain in 40%, fever and weight loss in 20%, and pruritus in only 10%. Consanguinity is common in the parents of infants presenting with neonatal PSC. Cholestatic jaundice is universal in infantile PSC but subsides spontaneously in almost all infants by the age of 1 to 12 months. All infants present with elevated GGT and alkaline phosphatase levels but rarely show elevated gamma globulins or the presence of autoantibodies.

Children with PSC and LCH often manifest other lesions including diabetes insipidus, bone lesions, skin lesions, lymphadenopathy, exophthalmos, and pulmonary infiltrates. In most children, cholestasis occurs within 3 years of the onset of LCH, but in a few cholestasis may precede the first signs of histiocytosis by up to 18 months. In children with IBD, the onset of PSC can be insidious, with a significant proportion of them discovered by routine biochemical screening revealing abnormalities of aminotransferases and alkaline phosphatase. In a large retrospective analysis of 555 children with IBD (318 with Crohn's disease, and 237 with ulcerative colitis), only 14 children were identified with persistently elevated alanine aminotransferase levels for greater than 6 months (123). All 14 of these children were found to have chronic liver disease; 10 with PSC, and 4 with autoimmune CAH. Of the 10 with PSC, 8 had ulcerative colitis (3.4% of all patients with ulcerative colitis) and 2 had Crohn's disease (0.6% of all patients with Crohn's disease). All subjects with ulcerative colitis and PSC had disease extending proximal to the rectosigmoid, and both patients with Crohn's disease had colonic involvement. Seven of the 10 patients with PSC had ALT elevations at the time of diagnosis of IBD; and the ALT elevations in the remaining 3 occurred 1.5 to 12.0 years following the diagnosis of IBD. However, there have been several reports of children presenting with clinical features of PSC with no overt gastrointestinal symptoms who were found to have mucosal findings consistent with ulcerative colitis (124,125). This underscores the recommendation that all children diagnosed with PSC should undergo colonoscopy even in the absence of diarrhea, hematochezia, or other symptoms of IBD. The presence of hypergammaglobulinemia or positive autoantibodies (ANA, anti-smooth muscle antibodies, pANCA) is variable in this population.

Ultrasound of the liver and biliary system may not show any clear dilatation of either the extrahepatic or intrahepatic biliary tree. Cholangiography, either via intraoperative techniques, transhepatic cholecystography or cholangiography, or ERCP, remains the technique of choice to diagnose PSC in children. In studies in adults, MRCP has proven as accurate as ERCP in diagnosing PSC but does not provide the therapeutic option of sphincterotomy or stenting primary biliary strictures at the time of the procedure. Changes in the intrahepatic bile ducts are universally seen consisting of irregularities of the duct wall, filling defects, irregular dilatations, rarefaction of secondary branches, complete absence of opacification in some areas, annular strictures alternating with focal dilatation, and long confluent strictures. A major stricture amenable to stenting is seen in a minority of children. Abnormalities of the extrahepatic bile ducts are present in only about 60% of children (Fig. 23.8). In a small number of children with immunodeficiency states, papillary stenosis has been identified (Fig. 23.9). A few patients will have abnormalities seen in the pancreatic duct as well.

Characteristic periductal fibrosis (onion-skin fibrosis) around interlobular bile ducts is visible in percutaneous needle biopsies of the liver in only a minority of children with PSC (Fig. 23.10). More often, histologic findings are limited to portal fibrosis, neoductular proliferation, portal inflammatory cell infiltration and edema, and bile duct inflammation and degeneration. A few patients will present with already established biliary cirrhosis. The presence of piecemeal necrosis may invite confusion and misdiagnosis of autoimmune CAH. At surgery or autopsy the extrahepatic bile ducts may appear as thickened cords. Cross-sectional

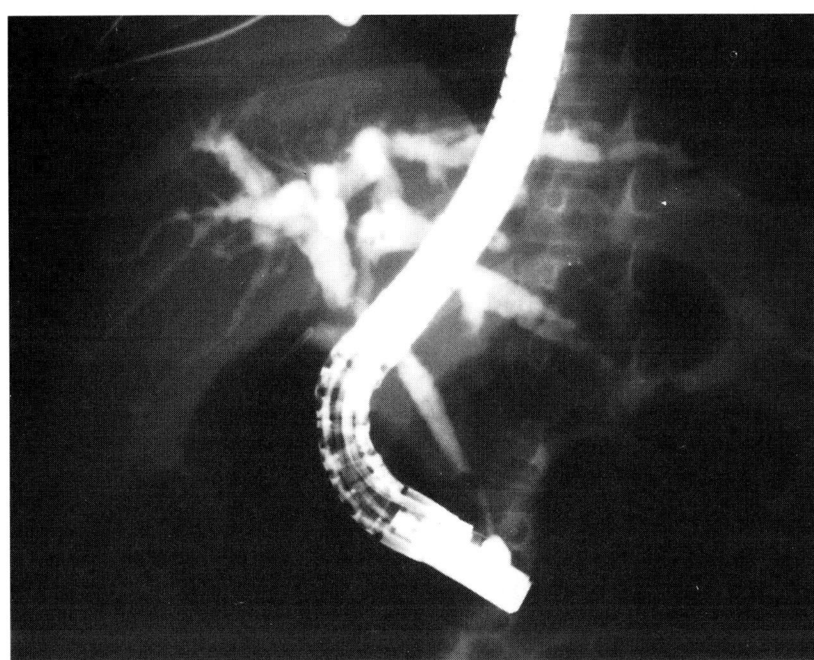

FIGURE 23.8. *Extrahepatic and intrahepatic biliary strictures and saccular dilatations in a 5-year-old child after a bone marrow transplant for severe combined immune deficiency.*

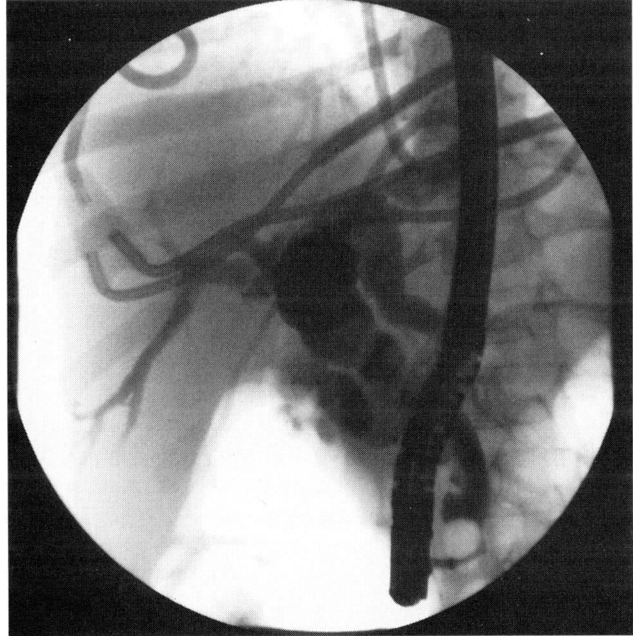

FIGURE 23.9. *Diffuse massive dilatation of the extrahepatic biliary tree seen with ERCP in a 5-year-old child after a bone marrow transplantation with CMV-induced papillitis and papillary stenosis.*

examination will reveal the lumen to be narrowed as a result of concentric fibrous thickening of the wall, with the mucosa unaffected (126).

Treatment and Prognosis

PSC is a severe disease in childhood with up to one-third of patients dying or requiring liver transplantation, and the majority developing signs of portal hypertension with significant gastrointestinal bleeding. The prognosis is worse in children with neonatal PSC and PSC associated with LCH or immunodeficiency syndromes, compared to those with IBD. In one series, the estimated 10-year survival rate on a Kaplan-Meier plot was 35% for children with PSC and LCH as compared to 86% for those with PSC and IBD (122). Most children with IBD examined up to 14 years have remained well, although some develop compensated cirrhosis (123). Whereas PSC accounts for nearly 10% of all liver transplants in North America, it is an uncommon cause of liver transplantation in the pediatric population (127). A recurrence rate of 8.6% has been reported in adult patients undergoing liver transplantation for PSC but does not seem to affect 5-year survival; however, liver transplantation appears to be curative in the few children who have undergone this treatment with no evidence of recurrent PSC after transplant reported to date (122). Hepatocellular carcinoma in the explanted liver has been found in at least one child requiring liver transplantation for PSC, and death from cholangiocarcinoma has likewise been reported in one young adult patient who had initially developed PSC during childhood (128).

In many children with PSC, the goals of therapeutic intervention are to provide symptomatic relief of pruritus and other symptoms; to improve nutrition and growth by ameliorating steatorrhea and preventing fat-soluble vitamin deficiency; and to decrease pain often due to cholangitis or biliary colic. There are anecdotal reports of improvement in biochemical parameters and liver histology in children with PSC treated with prednisone or a combination of prednisone and azathioprine, but no controlled trials have been performed. Studies in adults with PSC have shown that

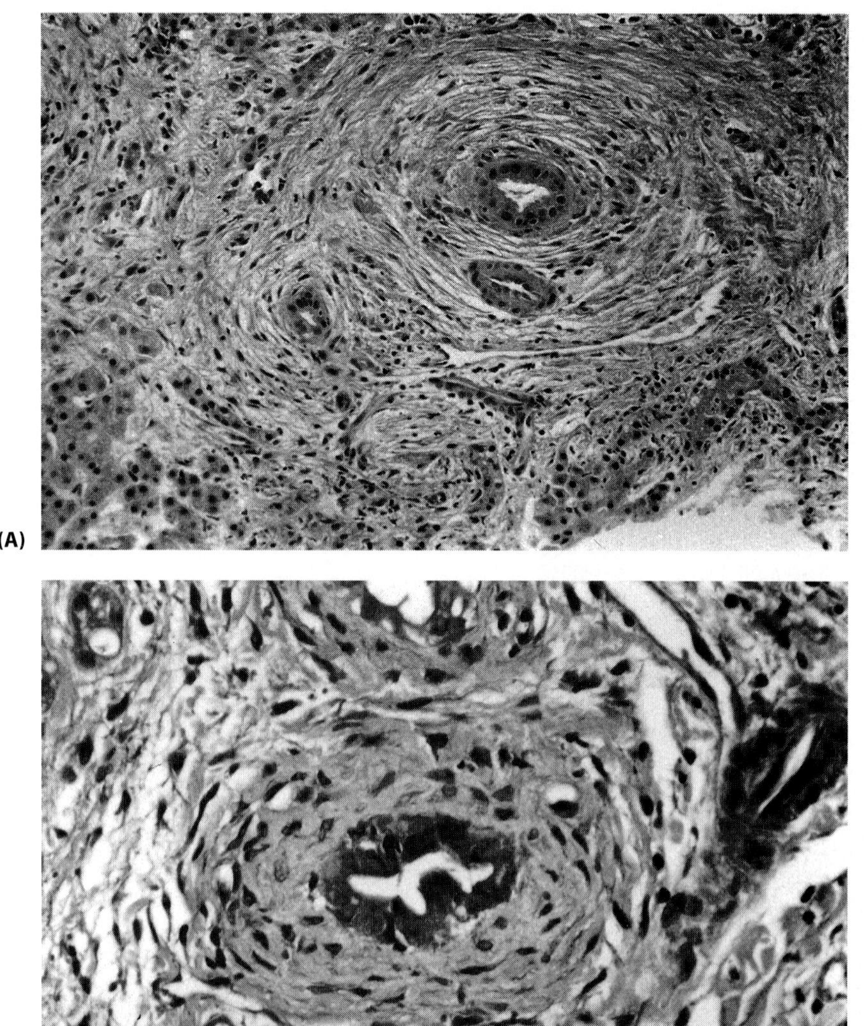

FIGURE 23.10. ***(A)*** *Percutaneous liver biopsy from a 6-year-old child with severe combined immunodeficiency after a bone marrow transplant. The child had developed sclerosing cholangitis. The biopsy shows typical changes of onion-skin fibrosis around interlobular bile ducts (hematoxylin and eosin stain, magnification ×20).* ***(B)*** *Percutaneous liver biopsy of an 18-month-old infant with Langerhans' cell histiocytosis and sclerosing cholangitis (trichrome stain, magnification ×40).*

long-term therapy with UCDA results in a reduction in aminotransferases and alkaline phosphatase and an improvement in clinical symptoms (129,130). A small number of children with PSC have been treated with UCDA. A reduction of over 50% in the ALT level compared to pretreatment levels was observed in five of six children with PSC and IBD within several months of administering UCDA (123). In other cases, a resolution of pruritus and weight gain has been reported (124). Thus UCDA may be beneficial, especially in the early stages of PSC; but whether long-term therapy will alter the natural history is unknown.

Cystic Diseases of the Intrahepatic Bile Ducts

Cystic diseases of the intrahepatic bile ducts represent a wide range of disorders which include both sporadically occurring and inherited conditions. When cysts communicate with the biliary tree, they are more likely to cause clinical disease. Communicating duct cysts are often associated with cholangitis, intrahepatic stone formation, and even rarely neoplasia. Noncommunicating duct cysts are usually asymptomatic, but if sufficiently large can present as an abdominal mass or biliary obstruction. Many of the significant intrahepatic cystic lesions of the bile ducts in children are variations on the theme of ductal plate malformation. Embryologically, the intrahepatic ducts develop by a process of differentiation from the hepatocytes at the margins of the portal tracts. This differentiation results in the formation of the ductal plate, which is then remodeled by duplication and formation into tubular structures that eventually bud off and migrate to the center of the portal tract to become the interlobular bile ducts (131) (Fig. 23.11). The ductal plate cells around the periphery of the portal tract normally involute, but some elements remain to form the ducts of Hering which provide the functional link between the bile canaliculi and the interlobular ducts. This process continues up to 1 month after birth (132). The ductal plate malformation reflects some degree of failure of the normal formation of

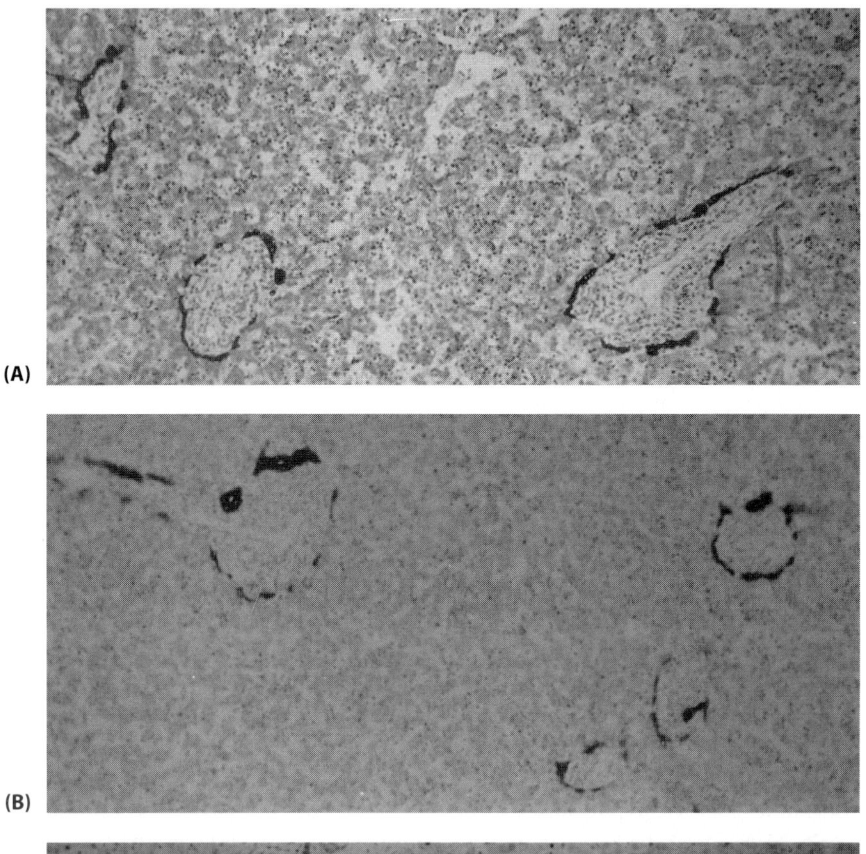

FIGURE 23.11. *Ontogeny of the formation of the interlobular bile ducts. Cytokeratin stains of biliary epithelium.* ***(A)*** *Liver from premature infant (gestational age 22 weeks) showing prominent ductal plate immunoreactivity.* ***(B)*** *Liver from premature infant (age 26 weeks) showing persistent ductal plate immunoreactivity with peripheral ductal formation.* ***(C)*** *Two-month-old full-term infant showing loss of ductal plate immunoreactivity with mature interlobular bile ducts within portal areas. (From Treem WR, et al. Cytokeratin immunohistochemical examination of liver biopsies in infants with Alagille syndrome and biliary atresia. J Pediatr Gastroenterol Nutr 1992;15:73–80.)*

the interlobular bile ducts, and results in a characteristic portal tract lesion consisting of persistence of some remnant of the ductal plate resulting in misshapen, often enlarged ductular structures, an increase in duct elements, and an increase in portal fibrous tissue (133). The ductal plate malformation is found most often in a variety of polycystic diseases seen in childhood, with the prime example being congenital hepatic fibrosis.

Congenital Hepatic Fibrosis

Congenital hepatic fibrosis (CHF) is a prime example of the polycystic diseases affecting the liver in childhood that are inherited, have communicating intrahepatic bile ductular cysts, and are associated with renal polycystic disease. The term congenital hepatic fibrosis was proposed by Kerr et al. (134) in 1961 to describe a disease with characteristic hepatic pathology (ductal plate malformation), portal hypertension, an increased risk of ascending cholangitis, and polycystic disease of the kidneys inherited in an autosomal recessive fashion. Many authors consider CHF to be the same disease as autosomal recessive polycystic kidney disease (ARPKD), although in the latter the renal disease predominates in infancy and early childhood; in CHF the renal disease may be relatively silent until later in life. The genetic defect responsible for ARPKD has been mapped to a 3.8 cM interval on chromosome 6, 6p21.1-p12 (135).

The most common presenting feature of CHF is hematemesis or melena due to variceal bleeding in a child between 3 and 10 years of age (136). However, infants presenting with hepatomegaly alone and older teenage children with ascites, splenomegaly, and encephalopathy have been reported (137). The pathogenesis of the portal hypertension is not fully understood but is thought to be related to the hepatic fibrosis and portal vein abnormalities encountered in these patients. Firm hepatomegaly is present in almost all patients with an especially prominent left lobe. Splenomegaly is commonly present with accompanying thrombocytopenia and hypersplenism. In most patients, the biochemical parameters of hepatic synthetic function are normal and the bilirubin and aminotransferases are likewise normal or only mildly elevated. The sedimentation rate, white blood cell count, and globulin levels can be increased due to chronic cholangitis. Ultrasonography with Doppler assessment of the portal vasculature is helpful and will show evidence of portal hypertension, splenomegaly, intense hepatic echogenicity, and large echogenic kidneys. Portal vein abnormalities including duplication of the intrahepatic branches are common (138). Other vascular abnormalities including cerebral, hepatic, splenic, and renal aneurysms are present in some cases (139).

The pathognomonic intrahepatic features of CHF are characterized by marked dilatation of the intralobular bile ducts, broad bands of portal to portal fibrosis containing abnormal bile ducts, and otherwise preserved basic lobular architecture of the liver parenchyma (no cirrhosis) (Fig. 23.12). Initially, this lesion may be patchy in distribution. These patients are at an increased risk for cholangitis, which at times may be indolent or chronic in nature. All liver biopsy specimens in these patients must be cultured for bacterial pathogens in addition to evaluating them for histologic evidence of cholangitis. Palpable kidneys are sometimes noted at the initial evaluation and may be associated with arterial hypertension (140). At the time of diagnosis of CHF, renal dysfunction is already present in approximately 20% of patients (141). Intravenous pyelography (IVP) can demonstrate a characteristic lesion of enlarged kidneys with alternating dense and lucent streaks radiating out like the spokes of a wheel from the medulla to the cortex.

Portosystemic shunting has been the treatment of choice, as there appears to be a low incidence of postoperative hyperammonemia or encephalopathy (136). Care must be taken in the choice of the surgical shunt to avoid limiting the options of hepatic or renal transplantation later in life. Some children form spontaneous splenorenal shunts or other portosystemic shunts and can be managed with endoscopic and medical management of esophageal varices until hemodynamically significant shunts form. Repetitive bouts of acute cholangitis or chronic indolent cholangitis are the major causes of progressive hepatic failure and death in most series of patients. Thus, an aggressive response to unexplained fever or even serologic evidence of ongoing inflammation in the absence of overt signs of infection is warranted. A diagnostic liver biopsy and aspirate for culture should be performed and antibiotics promptly instituted. Any manipulation of the extrahepatic biliary tree including ERCP examination should be covered with appropriate antibiotics to prevent infection secondary to intrahepatic biliary tract obstruction and stasis.

Caroli's Disease

Caroli's disease was first described in 1958 and is characterized by congenital segmental saccular dilatation of the larger intrahepatic bile ducts (142). There is much confusion over the use of this term because it is often used to describe cases of extrahepatic choledochal cysts associated with intrahepatic dilatation (type IVa choledochal cyst) (Fig. 23.13); cases of isolated biliary cystic dilatation without any evidence of the ductal plate malformation; or any radiographically evident communicating dilatation of the biliary tree. The term Caroli's *syndrome* is often used to describe cases of CHF with prominent intrahepatic ductal dilatation, a high incidence of renal disease, and the characteristic portal fibrosis and ductular abnormalities. Some studies reserve the

(A) 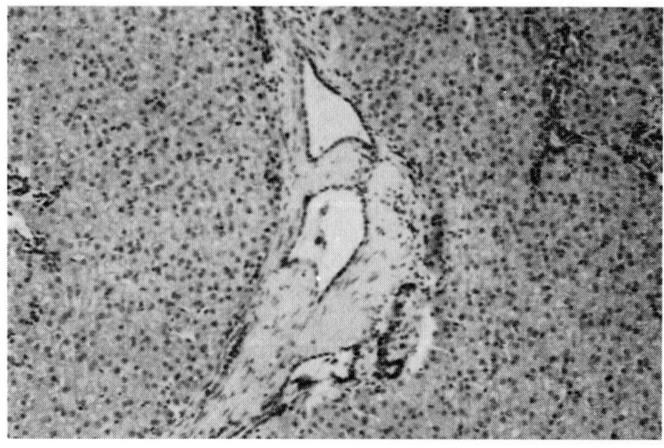

 **(B)**

FIGURE 23.12. *(A) Low-power view of percutaneous liver biopsy in a child with CHF showing the broad bands of fibrous tissue containing enlarged, dilated biliary ducts. (B) High-power view of a portal triad in a patient with CHF showing the enlarged bizarre remnant of the ductal plate encased in marked portal fibrous tissue.*

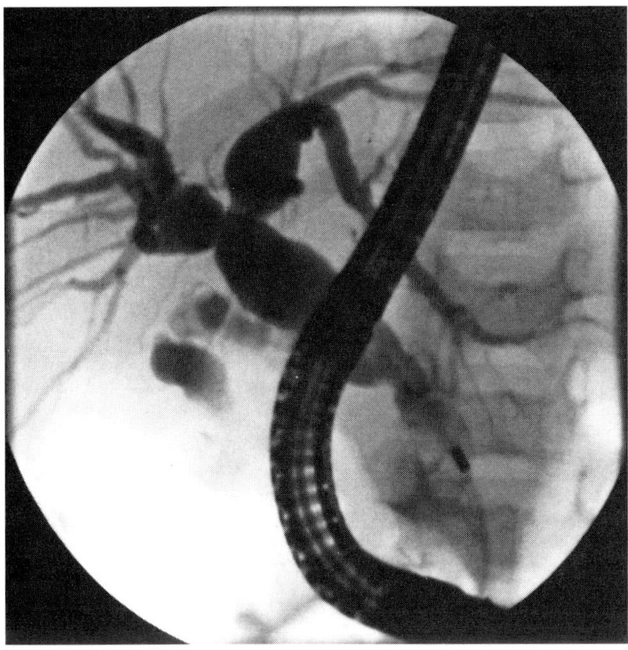

FIGURE 23.13. *ERCP of a 2-year-old child with both extrahepatic and intrahepatic saccular dilatations of the large bile ducts consistent with a type IVa choledochal cyst.*

term Caroli's disease for those patients with prominent saccular dilatation of larger ducts of the *intrahepatic* biliary tree without evidence of intrahepatic fibrosis, or any extrahepatic ductal dilatation (Fig. 23.14). It is considered to be the result of a ductal plate remodeling defect that only affects the large segmental or subsegmental ducts.

Caroli's disease may be universally spread throughout the liver or unilobular (143). In the largest series published to date, which included 12 patients with Caroli's syndrome and 8 with Caroli's disease, polycystic renal disease was present in 42% of those with Caroli's syndrome and 25% of those with Caroli's disease (144). If one includes radiographic or histologic features of medullary sponge kidney or tubular ectasia, a higher percentage of patients have renal lesions. Although it is often associated with ARPKD and autosomal recessive inheritance, there is recent information which suggests an autosomal dominant mode of inheritance with variable penetrance and expressivity (145). Studies of siblings and parents of children with Caroli's disease who themselves are asymptomatic have revealed evidence of intrahepatic biliary cystic lesions.

Caroli's disease is more prevalent in males, and generally presents during late childhood or adolescence with repetitive bouts of abdominal pain, and episodes of cholangitis (64%), clinical evidence of portal hypertension (22%), and radiographic findings of macroscopic bile duct ectasia demonstrated by abdominal computed tomography (CT) scan or ultrasound. There are rare reports of a neonatal presentation associated with neonatal cholestasis, pulmonic

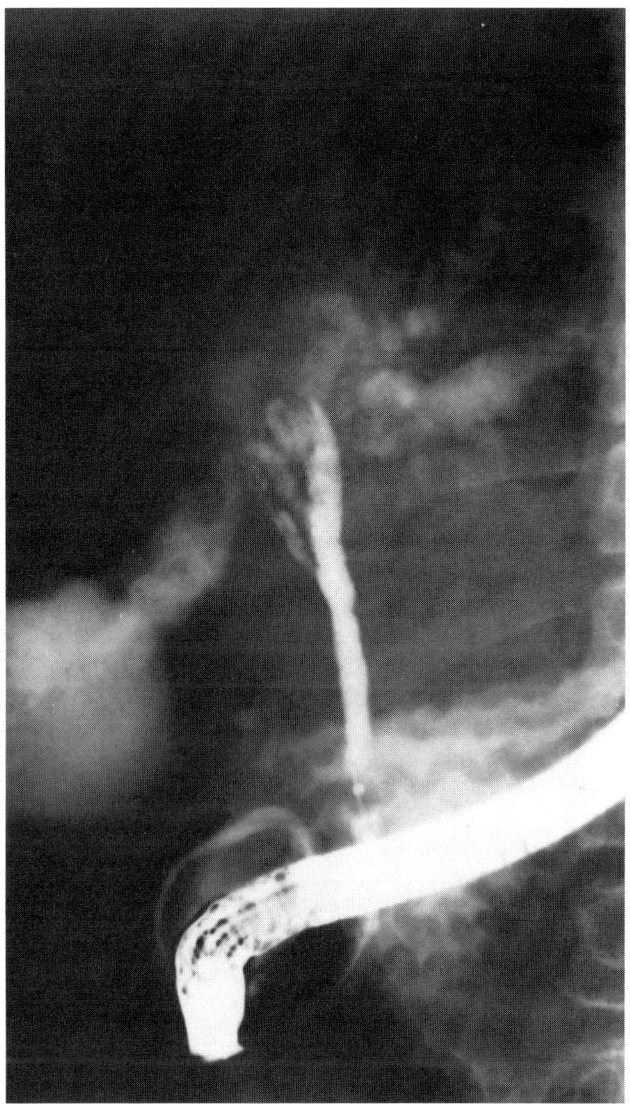

FIGURE 23.14. *ERCP in a 14-year-old child with Caroli's disease, cholangitis, and intrahepatic saccular dilatations of the biliary tree.*

valve stenosis (but no other stigmata of Alagille syndrome), diffuse cystic dilatation of the intrahepatic bile ducts, and enlarged kidneys with rapidly progressive deterioration in renal function (146). Cholangiography confirms the diagnosis and demonstrates continuity of the multiple cystic lesions with the biliary tree. In more advanced cases, biliary sludge formation and intrahepatic stone formation will be present. Black pigmented calcium bilirubinate stones appear as filling defects within the intrahepatic biliary tree. Bile duct strictures and wall irregularities may form as a consequence of repeated episodes of bacterial cholangitis (147). Laboratory studies may demonstrate cytopenias typical of hypersplenism, with elevated alkaline phosphatase, with or without abnormal bilirubin levels. Long-term consequences of repeated bouts of cholangitis, biliary abscesses, and septicemia include cirrhosis, hepatic failure, amyloidosis, and cholangiocarcinoma (148). In those patients with liver failure but without cholangiocarcinoma, the only therapeutic option is liver transplantation. In more focal Caroli's disease, resection of a severely affected lobe may be possible without resorting to total organ replacement.

SUGGESTED READINGS

Balistreri WF, Grand R, Hoofnagle JG, et al. Biliary atresia: current concepts and research directions—summary of a symposium. Hepatology 1996;23:1682–92. A good outline of the current research questions and newer thoughts about biliary atresia.

Desmet VJ. Congenital diseases of the intrahepatic bile ducts: variations on the theme "ductal plate malformation." Hepatology 1992;16:1069–82. Excellent introduction to the pathologic concepts underlying some of the important causes of intrahepatic cholestasis in children.

Krantz ID, Piccoli DA, Spinner NA. Clinical and molecular genetics of Alagille syndrome. Curr Opin Pediatr 1999;11:558–64. Good summary of the newly understood molecular underpinnings of syndromic intrahepatic paucity of the bile ducts.

Trauner M, Meier PJ, Boyer J. Molecular pathogenesis of cholestasis. N Engl J Med 1998;339:1217–27. Excellent explanation of the newly described molecular defects underlying disorders of bile acid, organic anion, and phospholipid transport resulting in profound intrahepatic cholestasis.

REFERENCES

1. Yoon PW, Bresee JS, Olney RS, et al. Epidemiology of biliary atresia: a population-based study. Pediatrics 1997;99:376–82.
2. Balistreri WF, Grand R, Hoofnagle JH, et al. Biliary atresia: current concepts and research directions—summary of a symposium. Hepatology 1996;23: 1682–92.
3. Schweizer P. Treatment of extrahepatic biliary atresia: results and long-term prognosis after hepatic portoenterostomy. Pediatr Surg Int 1986;1:30–6.
4. Carmi R, Magee CA, Neill CA, Karrer FM. Extrahepatic biliary atresia and associated anomalies: etiologic heterogeneity suggested by distinct patterns of associations. Am J Med Genet 1993;45:683–93.
5. Hofmann AF, Popper H. Ursodeoxycholic acid for primary biliary cirrhosis. Lancet 1987;2:398–9.
6. Morecki R, Glaser JH, Johnson AB, Kress Y. Detection of reovirus type 3 in the porta hepatis of an infant with extrahepatic biliary atresia: ultrastructural and immunocytochemical study. Hepatology 1984;4:1137.
7. Brown WR, Sokol RJ, Levin MR. Lack of correlation between infection with reovirus 3 and extrahepatic biliary atresia. J Pediatr 1988;113:670–6.
8. Tarr P, Haas J, Christie D. Biliary atresia, cytomegalovirus, and age at referral. Pediatrics 1996;97:828–31.
9. Riepenhoff-Talty M, Gouvea V, Evans MJ, et al. Detection of group C rotavirus in infants with extrahepatic biliary atresia. J Infec Dis 1996;174: 8–15.
10. Desmet VJ. Congenital diseases of the intrahepatic bile ducts: variations on the theme "ductal plate malformation." Hepatology 1992;16:1069–82.
11. Yokoyama T, Copeland NG, Jenkins NA, et al. Reversal of left-right symmetry: a situs inversus mutation. Science 1993;260:679–82.
12. Silveira TR, Salzano FM, Donaldson PT, et al. Association between HLA and extrahepatic biliary atresia. J Pediatr Gastroenterol Nutr 1993;16:114–17.
13. Bates MD, Bucuvalas JC, Alonso MH, Ryckman FC. Biliary atresia: pathogenesis and treatment. Semin Liver Dis 1998;18:281–93.
14. Ben-Haim S, Seabold JE, Kao SC, et al. Utility of Tc-99m mebrofenin scintigraphy in the assessment of infantile jaundice. Clin Nucl Med 1995;20: 153–63.
15. Zerbini MC, Gallucci SD, Maezono R, et al. Liver biopsy in neonatal cholestasis: a review on statistical grounds. Mod Pathol 1997;10:793–9.
16. Kasai M, Suzuki S. A new operation for "non-correctable" biliary atresia—portoenterostomy. Shijitsu 1959;13:733–9.
17. Altman RP, Lilly JR, Greenfield J, et al. A multivariable risk factor analysis of the portoenterostomy (Kasai) procedure for biliary atresia. Ann Surg 1997;226: 348–55.
18. Ohi R, Ibrahim M. Biliary atresia. Semin Pediatr Surg 1992;1:115–24.
19. Davenport M, Kerker N, Mieli-Vergani G, et al. Biliary atresia: the King's College Hospital experience (1974–1995). J Pediatr Surg 1997;32:479–85.
20. Okazaki T, Kobayashi H, Yamataka A, et al. Long-term postsurgical outcome of biliary atresia. J Pediatr Surg 1999;34:312–15.
21. Goss JA, Shackleton CR, McDiarmid SV, et al. Long-term results of pediatric liver transplantation: an analysis of 569 transplants. Ann Surg 1998;228:411–20.
22. Chardot C, Carton M, Spire-Bendelac N, et al. Prognosis of biliary atresia in the era of liver tranplantation: French national study from 1986 to 1996. Hepatology 1999;30:606–11.
23. Revillon Y, Michel JL, Lacaille F, et al. Living related liver transplantation in children: the "Paresian" strategy. J Pediatr Surg 1999;34:851–3.
24. Holland RM, Lilly JR. Surgical jaundice in infants: other than biliary atresia. Semin Pediatr Surg 1992;1:125–9.
25. Banani SA, Bahador A, Nezakakatgoo N. Idiopathic perforation of the extrahepatic bile duct in infancy: pathogenesis, diagnosis, and management. J Pediatr Surg 1993;28:950–2.
26. Chardot C, Iskandarani F, De Dreuzy O, et al. Spontaneous perforation of the biliary tract in infancy: a series of 11 cases. Eur J Pediatr Surg 1996;6:341–6.
27. Suita S, Shono K, Kinugasa Y, et al. Influence of age on the presentation and outcome of choledochal cyst. J Pediatr Surg 1999;34:1765–8.
28. Ando K, Miyano T, Kohno S, et al. Spontaneous perforation of choledochal cyst: a study of 13 cases. Eur J Pediatr Surg 1998;8:23–5.
29. Shamberger RC, Lund DP, Lillehei CW, Hendren WH. Interposed jejunal segment with nipple valve to prevent reflux in biliary reconstruction. J Am Coll Surg 1995;180:10–15.
30. Saing H, Han H, Chan KL, et al. Early and late results of excision of choledochal cysts. J Pediatr Surg 1997;32:1563–6.
31. Kahn E, Markowitz J, Aiges H, Daum F. Human ontogeny of the bile duct to portal space ratio. Hepatology 1989;10:20–3.
32. Emerick KM, Rand EB, Goldmuntz E, et al. Features of Alagille syndrome in 92 patients: frequency and relation to prognosis. Hepatology 1999;29:822–9.
33. Berard E, Sarles J, Triolo V, et al. Renovascular hypertension and vascular anomalies in Alagille syndrome. Pediatric Nephrology 1998;12:121–4.
34. Krantz ID, Piccoli DA, Spinner NB. Clinical and molecular genetics of Alagille syndrome. Curr Opin Pediatr 1999;11:558–64.
35. Dhorne-Pollet S, Deleuze JF, Hadchouel M, Bonaiti-Pellie C. Segregation analysis of Alagille syndrome. J Med Genet 1994;31:453–7.
36. Oda T, Elkahloun AG, Pike BL, et al. Mutations in the human Jagged1 gene are responsible for Alagille syndrome. Nat Genet 1997;16:235–42.
37. Artavanis-Tsakonas S, Rand MD, Lake RJ. Notch signaling: cell fate control and signal integration in development. Science 1999;284:770–6.
38. Krantz ID, Smith R, Colliton RP, et al. Jagged1 mutations in patients ascertained with isolated congenital heart defects. Am J Med Genet 1999;84: 56–60.
39. Hoffenberg EJ, Narkewicz MR, Sondheimer JM, et al. Outcome of syndromic paucity of interlobular bile ducts (Alagille syndrome) with onset of cholestasis in infancy. J Pediatr 1995;127:220–4.
40. Quiros-Tejeira RE, Ament ME, Heyman MB, et al. Variable morbidity in Alagille syndrome: a review of 43 cases. J Pediatr Gastroenterol Nutr 1999;29: 431–7.
41. Schwarzenberg SJ, Grothe RM, Sharp HL, et al. Long-term complications of arteriohepatic dysplasia. Am J Med 1992;93:171–6.
42. Tzakis AG, Reyes J, Tepetes K, et al. Liver transplantation for Alagille's syndrome. Arch Surg 1993;128:337–9.
43. Cardona J, Houssin D, Gauthier F, et al. Liver transplantation in children with Alagille syndrome—a study of twelve cases. Transplantation 1995;60:339–42.
44. Lee NG V, Ryckman FC, Porta G, et al. Long-term outcome after partial external biliary diversion for intractable pruritus in patients with intrahepatic cholestasis. J Pediatr Gastroenterol Nutr 2000;30:152–6.
45. Emond JC, Whitington PF. Selective surgical management of progressive familial intrahepatic cholestasis (Byler's disease). J Pediatr Surg 1995;30:1635–41.
46. Whitington PF, Whitington GL. Partial external diversion of bile for treatment of intractable pruritus associated with intrahepatic cholestasis. Gastroenterology 1988;95:130–6.
47. Narkewicz MR, Smith D, Gregory C, et al. Effect of ursodeoxycholic acid therapy on hepatic function in children with intrahepatic cholestatic liver disease. J Pediatr Gastroenterol Nutr 1998;26:49–55.
48. Setchell KDR, O'Connell NC. Inborn errors of bile acid biosynthesis: update on biochemical aspects. In: Hofmann AF, Paumgartner G, Stiehl A, eds. Bile acids in gastroenterology: basic and clinical advances. London: Kluwer Academic, 1995:129–36.
49. Balistreri WF. Inborn errors of bile acid metabolism clinical and therapeutic aspects. In: Hofmann AF, Paumgartner G, Stiehl A, eds. Bile acids in

gastroenterology: basic and clinical advances. London: Kluwer Academic, 1995:333–53.
50. Bull LN, Carlton VEH, Stricker NL, et al. Genetic and morphological findings in progressive familial intrahepatic cholestasis (Byler disease [PFIC-1] and Byler syndrome): evidence for heterogeneity. Hepatology 1997;26:155–64.
51. Clayton RJ, Iber FL, Ruebner BH, McKusick VA. Byler disease: fatal familial intrahepatic cholestasis in an Amish kindred. Am J Dis Child 1969;117:112–24.
52. Whitington PF, Freese DK, Alonso EM, et al. Clinical and biochemical findings in progressive familial intrahepatic cholestasis. J Pediatr Gastroenterol Nutr 1994;18:134–41.
53. Bull LN, van Eijk MJT, Pawlikowska L, et al. A gene encoding a P-type ATPase mutated in two forms of hereditary cholestasis. Nature Genet 1998; 18:219–24.
54. Houwen RHJ, Baharloo S, Blankenship K, et al. Genome screening by searching for shared segments: mapping a gene for benign recurrent intrahepatic cholestasis. Nature Genet 1994;8:380–6.
55. Shneider BL. Invited review: genetic cholestasis syndromes. J Pediatr Gastroenterol Nutr 1999;28:124–31.
56. Strautnieks SS, Bull LN, Knisely AS, et al. A gene encoding a liver-specific ABC transporter is mutated in progressive familial intrahepatic cholestasis. Nat Genet 1998;20:233–8.
57. Kagalwalla AF, Al Amir AR, Khalifa A, et al. Progressive familial intrahepatic cholestasis (Byler's disease) in Arab children. Ann Trop Paediatr 1995;15: 321–7.
58. Jansen PLM, Strautnieks SS, Jacquemin E, et al. Hepatocanalicular bile salt export pump deficiency in patients with progressive familial intrahepatic cholestasis. Gastroenterology 1999;117:1370–9.
59. Deleuze JF, Jacquemin E, Dubuisson C, et al. Defect of multidrug-resistance 3 gene expression in a subtype of progressive familial intrahepatic cholestasis. Hepatology 1996;23:904–8.
60. De Vree JML, Jacquemin E, Sturm E, et al. Mutations in the MDR3 gene cause progressive familial intrahepatic cholestasis. Proc Natl Acad Sci U S A 1998;95:282–7.
61. Smit JJM, Schinkel AH, Oude Elferink RPJ, et al. Homozygous disruption of the murine mdr2 P-glycoprotein gene leads to a complete absence of phospholipid from bile and to liver disease. Cell 1993;75:451–62.
62. Trauner M, Meier PJ, Boyer J. Molecular pathogenesis of cholestasis. N Engl J Med. 1998;339:1217–27.
63. Beuers U, Boyer JL, Paumgartner G. Ursodeoxycholic acid in cholestasis: potential mechanisms of action and therapeutic applications. Hepatology 1998; 28:1449–53.
64. Jacquemin E, Hermans D, Myara A, et al. Ursodeoxycholic acid therapy in pediatric patients with progressive familial intrahepatic cholestasis. Hepatology 1997;25:519–23.
65. Waldhausen JHT, Benjamin DR. Cholecystectomy is becoming an increasingly common operation in children. Am J Surg 1999;177:364–7.
66. Debray D, Pariente D, Gauthier F, et al. Cholelithiasis in infancy: a study of 40 cases. J Pediatr 1993;122:385–91.
67. Rescorla FJ. Cholelithiasis, cholecystitis, and common bile duct stones. Curr Opin Pediatr 1997;9:276–82.
68. Al-Salem AH, Qaisruddin S. The significance of biliary sludge in children with sickle cell disease. Pediatr Surg Int 1998;13:14–16.
69. Guelrud M, Mendoza S, Jaen D, et al. ERCP and endoscopic sphincterotomy in infants and children with jaundice due to common bile duct stones. Gastrointest Endosc 1992;38:450–3.
70. Ohnuma N, Takahashi H, Yoshida H, Iwai J. Endoscopic retrograde cholangiopancreatography (ERCP) in biliary tract disease of infants less than one year old. Tohoku J Exp Med 1997;181:67–74.
71. Davidoff AM, Branum GD, Murray EA, et al. The technique of laparoscopic cholecystectomy in children. Ann Surg 1992;215:186–91.
72. Newman KD, Powell DM, Holcomb GWI. The management of choledocholithiasis in children in the era of laparoscopic cholecystectomy. J Pediatr Surg 1997;32:1116–19.
73. Vanderpool D, Klinpensmith W, Oles P. Congenital absence of the gallbladder. Am Surg 1964;30:324.
74. Curtis LE, Sheahan DG. Heterotopic tissues in the gallbladder. Arch Pathol 1969;88:677.
75. Rumley TO, Rodgers BM. Hydrops of the gallbladder in children. J Pediatr Surg 1983;18:138–40.
76. Suddleson EA, Reid B, Woolley MM, et al. Hydrops of the gallbladder associated with Kawasaki syndrome. J Pediatr Surg 1987;22:956–9.
77. Slovis TL, Hight DW, Pilippart AL, et al. Sonography in the diagnosis and management of hydrops of the gallbladder in children with mucocutaneous lymph node syndrome. Pediatrics 1980;65:789–94.
78. Mercer S, Carpenter B. Surgical complications of Kawasaki disease. J Pediatr Surg 1981;16:444–8.
79. Tsakayannis DE, Kozakewich HPW, Lillehei CW. Acalculous cholecystitis in children. J Pediatr Surg 1996;31:127–31.
80. Wong ML, Kaplan S, Dunkle LM, et al. Leptospirosis: a childhood disease. J Pediatr 1977;90:532–7.
81. Traynelis VC, Hrabovsky EE. Acalculous cholecystitis in the neonate. Am J Dis Child 1985;139:893–5.
82. Holcomb GW Jr, O'Neill JA, Holcomb GW III. Cholecystitis, cholelithiasis, and common duct stones in children and adolescents. Am Surg 1980;191:626–35.
83. Patriquin HB, DiPietro M, Barber FE, et al. Sonography of thickened gallbladder wall: causes in children. Am J Roentgenol 1983;141:57–60.
84. Ruyman FB, Raney RB, Crist WM, et al. Rhabdomyosarcoma of the biliary tree in childhood: a report from the Intergroup Rhabdomyosarcoma Study. Cancer 1985;56:575.
85. Iwai N, Goto Y, Taniguchi H, et al. Cancer of the gallbladder in a 9-year-old girl. Kinderchir 1985;40:106.
86. Mogilner JG, Dharan M, Siplovich M. Adenoma of the gallbladder in childhood. J Pediatr Surg 1991;26:223–4.
87. Takiff H, Funkalsrud EW. Gallbladder disease in childhood. Am J Dis Child 1984;138:565–8.
88. Foster DR, Foster DBE. Gallbladder polyps in Peutz-Jeghers syndrome. Postgrad Med J 1980;56:373–6.
89. Wilroy RS, Crawford SE, Johnson WW. Cystic fibrosis with extensive fat replacement of the liver. J Pediatr 1966;68:67–73.
90. Strandvik B, Lultcramtz R. Liver function and morphology during long-term fatty acid supplementation in cystic fibrosis. Liver 1994;14:32–6.
91. Treem WR, Stanley CA. Massive hepatomegaly, steatosis and secondary plasma carnitine deficiency in infant with cystic fibrosis. Pediatrics 1989;83:993–7.
92. Colombo C, Apostolo MG, Ferrari M, et al. Analysis of risk factors for the development of liver disease associated with cystic fibrosis. J Pediatr 1994;124: 393–9.
93. Gaskin KJ, Waters DLM, Howman-Giles R, et al. Liver disease and common-bile-duct stenosis in cystic fibrosis. N Engl J Med 1988;318:340–6.
94. Scott-Jupp R, Lama M, Tanner MS. Prevalence of liver disease in cystic fibrosis. Arch Dis Child 1991;66:698–701.
95. Lykavieris P, Obernard O, Hadchouel M. Neonatal cholestasis as the presenting feature in cystic fibrosis. Arch Dis Childhood 1996;75:67–70.
96. Feigelson J, Mareschal JL, Sauvegrain J. Anomalies of the gallbladder in mucoviscidosis: apropos of 57 cases. Med Chir Dig 1975;4:121–4.
97. Isenberg JN, L'Heureux PR, Warwick WJ, et al. Clinical observations on biliary system in cystic fibrosis. Am J Gastroenterol 1976;65:134–41.
98. Mowat AP. Hepatobiliary lesions in cystic fibrosis. In: Liver disorders in childhood. 2nd ed. London: Butterworths, 1987:277–86.
99. Willi UV, Reddish JM, Teele RL. Cystic fibrosis: its characteristic appearance on abdominal sonography. Am J Radiol 1980;134:1005–10.
100. Weber AM, Roy CC, Morin CL, et al. Malabsorption of bile acids in children with cystic fibrosis. N Engl J Med 1973;289:1001–5.
101. Roy C, Weber A, Morin C, et al. Abnormal biliary lipid composition in cystic fibrosis. N Engl J Med 1977;297:1301–5.
102. Watkins JB, Tercyak AM, Szczepanik P, et al. Bile salt kinetics in cystic fibrosis: influence of pancreatic enzyme replacement. Gastroenterology 1977;73: 1023–8.
103. Santamaria F, Vajro P, Oggero V, et al. Volume and emptying of the gallbladder in patients with cystic fibrosis. J Pediatr Gastroenterol Nutr 1990;10:303–6.
104. Colombo C, Bertolini E, Assaisso ML, et al. Failure of ursodeoxycholic acid to dissolve radiolucent gallstones in patients with cystic fibrosis. Acta Paediatr 1993;82:562–5.
105. Park RW, Grand RJ. Gastrointestinal manifestations of cystic fibrosis: a review. Gastroenterology 1981;81:1143–61.
106. Vitullo BB, Rochan L, Seemayer TA, et al. Intrapancreatic compression of the common bile duct in cystic fibrosis. J Pediatr 1978;93:1060–1.
107. Lambert JR, Cole M, Crozier DN, et al. Intrapancreatic common bile duct compression causing jaundice in an adult with cystic fibrosis. Gastroenterology 1981;80:169–72.
108. Gaskin KJ, Waters DLM, Howman-Giles R, et al. Liver disease and common bile duct stenosis in cystic fibrosis. N Engl J Med 1988;318:340–6.
109. Nagel RA, Westaby D, Javaid A, et al. Liver disease and bile duct abnormalities in adults with cystic fibrosis. Lancet 1989;2:1422–5.
110. Brown PH, Juni JE, Lierberman DA, et al. Hepatocyte versus biliary disease: a distinction by deconvolutional analysis of technetium-99m IDA time-activity

curves. J Nucl Med 1988;29:623–30.
111. El-Shabrawi M, Wilkinson ML, Portmann B, et al. Primary sclerosing cholangitis in childhood. Gastroenterology 1987;92:1226–35.
112. Das KM, Vecchi M, Sakamski S. A shared and unique epitope(s) on human colon, skin and biliary epithelium detected by a monoclonal antibody. Gastroenterology 1990;98:464–9.
113. Takahashi F, Das KM. Isolation and characterization of a colonic autoantigen specifically recognized by colon tissuebound immunoglobulin G from idiopathic ulcerative colitis. J Clin Invest 1985;76:311–18.
114. Duerr RH, Targan SR, Landers CJ, et al. Neutrophil cytoplasmic antibodies: a link between primary sclerosing cholangitis and ulcerative colitis. Gastroenterology 1991;100:1385–91.
115. Mieli-Vergani G, Lobo-Yeo A, MCFarlane BM, et al. Different immune mechanisms leading to autoimmunity in primary sclerosing cholangitis and autoimmune chronic active hepatitis of childhood. Hepatology 1989;9:198–203.
116. Prochazka EJ, Terasaki PI, Park MS, et al. Association of primary sclerosing cholangitis in childhood. Gastroenterology 1987;92:1226–35.
117. Chapman RW. Role of immune factors in the pathogenesis of primary sclerosing cholangitis. Semin Liver Dis 1991;11:1–4.
118. Lichtman SN, Sartor RB, Keku J, et al. Hepatic inflammation in rats with experimental small bowel bacterial overgrowth. Gastroenterology 1990;98:414–23.
119. Lichtman SN, Keku J, Clark SL, et al. Biliary tract disease in rats with experimental bacterial overgrowth. Hepatology 1991;13:766–72.
120. Schrumpf E, Fausa O, Elgjo K, et al. Hepatobiliary complications of inflammatory bowel disease. Semin Liver Dis 1988;8:201–9.
121. Rand EB, Whitington PF. Successful orthotopic liver transplantation in two patients with liver failure due to sclerosing cholangitis with Langerhans cell histiocytosis. J Pediatr Gastroenterol Nutr 1992;15:202–7.
122. Debray D, Pariente D, Urvoas E, et al. Sclerosing cholangitis in children. J Pediatr 1994;124:49–56.
123. Hyams J, Markowitz J, Treem W, et al. Characterization of hepatic abnormalities in children with inflammatory bowel disease. Inflammatory Bowel Dis 1995;1:27–33.
124. Kagalwalla AF, Altraif I, Shamsan L, et al. Primary sclerosing cholangitis in Arab children: report of four cases and literature review. J Pediatr Gastroenterol Nutr 1997;24:146–52.
125. Werlin LS, Glicklich M, Jona J, Starshack RJ. Sclerosing cholangitis in childhood. J Pediatr 1980;96:433–5.
126. Ludwig J. Surgical pathology of the syndrome of primary sclerosing cholangitis. Am J Surg Pathol 1989;13:43–9.
127. Goss JA, Shackleton CR, Farmer DG, et al. Orthotopic liver transplantation for primary sclerosing cholangitis: a 12-year single center experience. Ann Surg 1997;225:472–83.
128. Quigley EMM, LaRusso NF, Ludwig J, et al. Familial occurrence of primary sclerosing cholangitis and ulcerative colitis. Gastroenterology 1983;85:1160–5.
129. Stiehl A, Raedsch R, Rudolph G, et al. Treatment of PSC with ursodeoxycholic acid: first results of a controlled study. Hepatology 1989;10: 602.
130. Hayashi H, Higuchi T, Ichimiya H, et al. Asymptomatic primary sclerosing cholangitis treated with ursodeoxycholic acid. Gastroenterology 1990;99:533–5.
131. Treem WR, Krzymowski GA, Cartun RW, et al. Cytokeratin immunohistochemical examination of liver biopsies in infants with Alagille syndrome and biliary atresia. J Pediatr Gastroenterol Nutr 1992;15:73–80.
132. Van Eyken PV, Sciot R, Callea F, et al. The development of the intrahepatic bile ducts in man: a keratin-immunohistochemical study. Hepatology 1988;8: 1586–95.
133. Desmet VJ. Congenital diseases of intrahepatic bile ducts: variations on the theme "ductal plate malformation." Hepatology 1992;16:1069–83.
134. Kerr DNS, Harrison CV, Sherlock S, et al. Congenital hepatic fibrosis. Quart J Med NS 1961;30:91–117.
135. Mucher G, Wirth B, Zerres K. Refining the map and defining flanking markers of the gene for autosomal recessive polycystic kidney disease on chromosome 6p21.1-p12. Am J Hum Genet 1994;55:1281–4.
136. Alvarez F, Bernard O, Brunelle F, et al. Congenital hepatic fibrosis in children. J Pediatr 1981;99:370–5.
137. Perisic VN. Long-term studies on congenital hepatic fibrosis in children. Acta Paediatr 1995;84:695–6.
138. Odievre M, Chaumont P, Montagne JP, et al. Anomalies of the intrahepatic portal venous system in congenital hepatic fibrosis. Radiology 1977;122: 427–30.
139. King K, Genta RM, Giannella RA, et al. Congenital hepatic fibrosis and cerebral aneurysm in a 32-year-old woman. J Pediatr Gastroenterol Nutr 1986;5:481–4.
140. Kerr DN, Okonkwo S, Choa RG. Congenital hepatic fibrosis: the long term prognosis. Gut 1978;19:514–20.
141. Anand SK, Chan JC, Lieberman E. Polycystic disease and hepatic fibrosis in children. Renal function studies. Am J Dis Child 1975;129:810–13.
142. Caroli J, Soupault R, Kossakowski J, et al. La dilatation polycystique congenitale des voies biliares intrahepatiques. Semin Hôp Paris 1958;34:488–95.
143. Boyle MJ, Doyle GD, Path FRC, MCNulty JG. Monolobar Caroli's disease. Am J Gastroenterol 1989;84:1437–44.
144. Summerfield JA, Nagafuchi Y, Sherlock S, et al. Hepatobiliary fibropolycystic diseases: a clinical and histological review of 51 patients. J Hepatol 1986;2: 141–56.
145. Tsuchida Y, Sato T, Sanjo K, et al. Evaluation of long-term results of Caroli's disease: 21 years' observation of a family with autosomal "dominant" inheritance, and review of literature. Hepatogastroenterology 1995;42:175–81.
146. Keane F, Hadzic, Wilkinson ML, Qureshi S, Reid C, et al. Neonatal presentation of Caroli's disease. Arch Dis Child 1997;77:F145–6.
147. Miller WJ, Sechtin AG, Campbell WL, Pieters PC. Imaging findings in Caroli's disease. Am J Radiol 1995;165:333–7.
148. Hozard JB, Wyatt JI, Hall RI. Epithelial dysplasia in Caroli's disease. Gut 1989; 30:1150–3.

Index

Note: Page numbers followed by f indicate figures; those followed by t indicate tables.

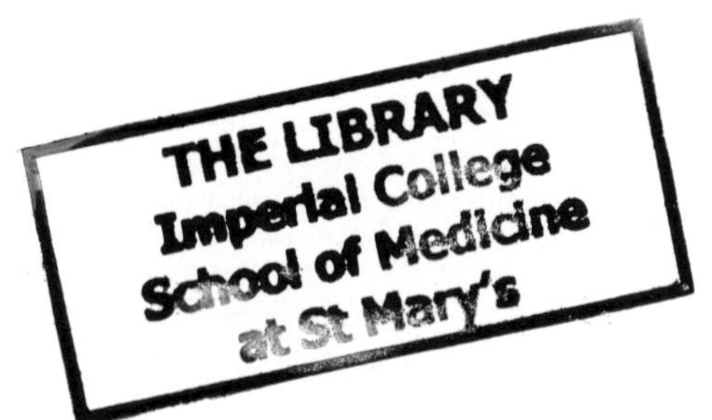